Leading an Academic Medical Practice

Lee B. Lu • Robert J. Fortuna
Craig F. Noronha • Halle G. Sobel
Daniel G. Tobin
Editors

Leading an Academic Medical Practice

Second Edition

Springer

Editors
Lee B. Lu
Baylor College of Medicine
Houston, TX, USA

Craig F. Noronha
Boston University Chobanian & Avedisian School of Medicine
Boston, MA, USA

Daniel G. Tobin
Yale University School of Medicine
New Haven, CT, USA

Robert J. Fortuna
School of Medicine and Dentistry
University of Rochester
Rochester, NY, USA

Halle G. Sobel
Larner College of Medicine
University of Vermont
Burlington, VT, USA

ISBN 978-3-031-40272-2 ISBN 978-3-031-40273-9 (eBook)
https://doi.org/10.1007/978-3-031-40273-9

This Springer imprint is published by the registered company Springer Nature Switzerland AG
The registered company address is: Gewerbestrasse 11, 6330 Cham, Switzerland

Paper in this product is recyclable.

Foreword

The Society of General Internal Medicine (SGIM) is delighted to endorse the second edition of *Leading an Academic Medical Practice*. The inspiration for this important book began in 2002 as a grassroots effort among members of the SGIM Medical Resident Clinic Directors' Interest Group for a formal "orientation handbook." The handbook was shared internally among members and was so well received that many pushed for its growth and expansion. With the collaborative effort of our members, the first edition of this book was published by Springer in 2018. The first edition of *Leading an Academic Medical Practice* was highly popular among the academic medicine community, in part for its pragmatic focus and evidence-based approach. Its success stems from how it addresses the increasing complexity of the academic, regulatory, clinical, and administrative aspects of care delivery in outpatient academic medicine that many academic internists face. Beginning in 2021, SGIM members Lee B. Lu, Robert J. Fortuna, Craig F. Noronha, Halle G. Sobel, and Daniel G. Tobin once again led the effort to produce the second edition of this valuable book. Over 70 SGIM members, all practicing academic general internists, contributed to the authorship of this edition. New chapters in this second edition of *Leading an Academic Medical Practice* include telemedicine, crisis management, social justice, diversity, bias, and healthcare advocacy. The second edition provides valuable clinical and educational guidance to any individual academic faculty who lead and teach in outpatient general internal medicine clinics alongside peers, learners, and patients.

This book is not an "official" statement of practice standards from the SGIM. However, the writing and editorial process involved extensive peer review and represents the culmination of years of work from the authors and editors in collaboration with Springer and members of the SGIM.

About SGIM: SGIM is an international medical society of over 3000 physicians who represent the general internal medicine faculty of medical schools and teaching hospitals in the United States as well as Canada, Europe, South America, and Asia. SGIM members teach medical students, residents, and fellows. They also conduct research intended to foster comprehensive coordinated care of patients across ambulatory and hospital settings, including preventive measures and treatment services. Please learn more about SGIM's mission and activities by visiting us online at http://www.sgim.org/.

Preface

Academic medical practices play a vital role in resident education, patient care, and medical scholarship. In addition, they are uniquely positioned to serve as a beacon for clinical excellence and educational innovation.

Leading an academic medical practice is also uniquely demanding and has become increasingly complex over time. Medical directors for academic medical practices must simultaneously become expert clinicians, administrators, and educators, and they need to use these skills to mobilize resources and engage a wide array of stakeholders. Meeting the needs of graduate medical education programs while caring for patients, engaging in academic scholarship, overseeing clinical operations, spearheading population health initiatives, and safeguarding the financial health of a practice is no easy task.

Recognizing this challenge, in 2015, a small group of physician leaders and academic medical directors from the Society of General Internal Medicine joined together to create a "how-to" guide for medical directors and academic clinicians across the country. After recruiting a remarkable collection of academic physician experts as authors, this group compiled their collective experiences, best practices, and clinical workflows into the first book of its kind to address this need. The first edition of *Leading an Academic Medical Practice* was published in 2018.

Since that time, much has changed. COVID-19 forced academic medical practices to rapidly adapt to the realities of the pandemic, which impacted patients, physicians, and trainees in profound ways. Relatedly, the rise of telehealth, a shifting regulatory landscape, new billing rules, and evolved best practices in care delivery all required a new and updated exploration of the unique needs of academic medical practices. In this milieu, the second edition of *Leading an Academic Medical Practice* was born. More than just an update, this new edition of our book dramatically expands on the first edition and adds new content that is especially relevant to the academic medical practice of today.

As editors for this project, we also want to acknowledge the impact that the COVID-19 pandemic had on our authors and contributors. Several of our authors overcame profound personal and family health crises while writing for the book, and we are immensely grateful for their resilience and dedication. Sadly, while this book was in production, we also lost one of our co-authors, Dr. Laura Whitman, after a long illness. Laura was a tremendously talented, kind, and beloved clinician-educator and medical director at Yale University, and we are privileged and grateful for her contributions to our book.

Finally, this book would not have been possible without the support from our families, and we want to acknowledge the love and support they have given us. Bich Nguyen, Christopher Nguyen, Jonathan Nguyen, Janice Fortuna, Katelyn Fortuna, Allison Fortuna, Ansu Noronha, Elizabeth Noronha, Maria Noronha, Cecilia Noronha, Mark Kautzman, Francis Kautzman, Melissa Held-Tobin, Rebecca Tobin, and Jack Tobin—thank you for putting up with our many long nights of work!

It is our hope that this book will serve as a foundation for medical directors and leaders of academic practices across the United States. This was a labor of love, and we hope that it helps you to take the next step in your journey.

Houston, TX, USA — Lee B. Lu
Rochester, NY, USA — Robert J. Fortuna
Boston, MA, USA — Craig F. Noronha
Burlington, VT, USA — Halle G. Sobel
New Haven, CT, USA — Daniel G. Tobin

Contents

Part I
Clinic Director and Faculty

Chapter 1
Clinic Director Roles and Expectations

Halle G. Sobel and Mark E. Pasanen

Introduction

The clinic director plays an instrumental role in a successful clinic experience for trainees, faculty, staff, and patients. This chapter provides an overview of the general expectations and qualifications of an academic medical clinic director. The responsibilities of a clinic director will be reviewed including the clinical, academic, quality improvement, and administrative missions. Lastly, the relationship between the clinic director and health care administration will be discussed as this can present both challenges and opportunities for the clinic director as well as the overall clinical environment.

Outline

- Background
- Overview of clinic director role
  - General expectations
  - Qualifications
- Principal responsibilities
  - Clinical mission (clinical operations)
  - Academic mission (residency program, resident/medical student education)
  - Quality mission
  - Administrative mission

H. G. Sobel (✉) · M. E. Pasanen
Division of General Internal Medicine, Department of Medicine, University of Vermont Medical Center/Larner College of Medicine at the University of Vermont, Burlington, VT, USA
e-mail: Halle.sobel@uvmhealth.org; Mark.pasanen@uvmhealth.org

L. B. Lu et al. (eds.), *Leading an Academic Medical Practice*,
https://doi.org/10.1007/978-3-031-40273-9_1

- Working with health care administration
- Conclusion

Background

The ambulatory clinic is a critical learning venue for internal medicine residents to master the skills necessary to provide outstanding care in the outpatient clinic. The resident clinic director plays an important role, with responsibility for oversight of the clinical and educational missions for residents while assuring a supportive learning environment. In addition, the clinic director must work closely with faculty and staff, helping navigate the inherent challenges of care delivery in a teaching clinic. Every ambulatory clinic director should strive to foster a resident training experience that will help residents gain the knowledge and skills necessary to practice independently in an outpatient setting and within an inter-professional team. This includes making sure that residents have sufficiently broad exposure to allow for skill development in varied areas of medicine, including acute care, chronic disease management, preventative care, mental health care, substance use disorder care, population management, and practice improvement. The clinic director must keep up with the changing and challenging landscape of medicine and be a champion of quality improvement and patient safety. This typically involves understanding the patient-centered medical home (PCMH) and National Committee of Quality Assurance (NCQA) standards that apply to primary care settings [1]. The clinic director works closely with the entire clinic staff to create a positive experience for residents that balances the education and service needs [2]. He/she serves as a liaison to the residency program director and the residency administrative team [3].

Overview of the Clinic Director Role

General Expectations

In addition to the responsibility of overseeing the resident experience and caring for patients, the resident clinic director may have a variety of other roles. These may include serving as the clinic's medical director, academic roles in residency leadership (such as associate program director, primary care program director, or core faculty), or other clinic and/or educational leadership positions. Because this role is not consistently defined, the salary support and protected time vary from institution to institution.

Qualifications

Clinic directors are expected to be certified by either the American Board of Internal Medicine (ABIM) or the American Osteopathic Board of Internal Medicine (AOBIM) [3]. It is good practice for the resident clinic director to have significant experience in outpatient resident precepting, previous participation in resident educational conferences, and strong leadership skills. In addition, it is important that this individual has excellent communication and problem-solving skills to handle daily issues. Experience in curricula development, resident assessment, quality improvement, panel management, and primary care research are also desirable traits. However, recruiting additional faculty members for these tasks is often necessary, making strong organizational skills essential [4]. The ability to engage with residents, staff, and patients effectively and productively in response to concerns about the resident clinic is another important attribute. Patient and resident physician continuity [5] (see Chap. 6) is important for the resident experience, and team-based care can enhance the resident experience [6].

From an administrative standpoint, he/she will frequently meet with program administration to ensure that patient care and educational goals are aligned and that all Accreditation Council for Graduate Medical Education (ACGME) requirements are being met (see Chap. 8) [7]. This will often involve active engagement in the residency infrastructure, including potential participation in Program Evaluation and Clinical Competency committees. He/she will also collaborate with faculty and the section chief to make sure that the expected work relative value units (wRVUs) and educational value units (EVUs) are well understood and appropriate (see Chap. 3).

Principal Responsibilities

Clinical Mission

During the academic year, the clinic director or delegate begins each year by orienting the new first-year residents to the clinic. Residents meet the staff and become familiar with both the structure and the day-to-day operations of the clinic. Although residents learn the majority of the clinic processes once they start seeing patients in the clinic, they clearly benefit from a well-organized orientation. This often includes arranging for additional electronic health record training that may not be part of the overall graduate medical education (GME) orientation and focuses on outpatient workflows (in-basket management, result notifications, ordering durable medical equipment, etc.). Some programs choose to have ambulatory intern "boot camps" to orient residents to the clinic [8]. Graduating resident panels are often assigned to the new intern or resident (PGY2) panels during the Spring, as this ambulatory handoff process is necessary to ensure that continuity of care for patients is maintained through this time of transition, a key component of high-quality care [8–10].

As the academic year progresses, the clinic director may serve as the point person when clinic protocols develop or change to make sure that all the residents can function well within an ever-evolving system. The clinic director often supervises resident activities that require an attending attestation such as anticoagulation encounters, prior authorization paperwork, and durable medical equipment forms. Given their role as a preceptor in the clinic, the director can also serve as a resource for residents, patients, faculty, and staff on feedback for issues that arise. It is common for resident clinic directors to oversee panel management activities and to provide oversight to result follow-up, chart documentation, consultations, and other tasks that may fall through the cracks when the resident is out of clinic. Some clinic directors may set up a resident coverage system to manage results and messages by residents in the clinic for residents who are out of the clinic. The clinic director should recruit and orient faculty preceptors to ensure that residents work with faculty who are dedicated to the educational and clinical mission of the clinic [3]. Throughout, team-based care should be modeled and taught with a patient-centered approach [2].

Academic Mission

Although patient care is often the focus of the resident continuity clinic experience, making sure that there is a strong educational program is critical. He/she often directs the resident conferences, which require curriculum development, faculty recruitment, and faculty development to ensure a robust curriculum [11]. This may include didactic experiences, small group workshops, resident-led presentations, self-study with electronic resources, quality improvement activities (discussed in Chap. 29), and panel management (discussed in Chaps. 25 and 27). The academic offerings of the clinic must undergo consistent assessment, based on input from evaluations and feedback by the learners.

For programs that offer a primary care track, the clinic director may coordinate the offerings of this track and should help support these residents with particular interest in primary care [12, 13]. Some institutions have a primary care program director who would then work with the clinic director to coordinate electives and academic conferences for the primary care residents.

Many residency programs have formal expectations for resident scholarship, and the clinic director may be requested to assist residents in performing research that is focused on the outpatient setting. As clinic directors may have limited experience or training in research mentorship, working with program leadership is critical to be confident that residents are receiving adequate support to successfully complete these projects.

In addition to the other academic roles, the clinic director is frequently involved in ensuring compliance with program requirements from the Accreditation Council for ACGME and ABIM. This requires close coordination with program leadership, including delivery of effective feedback and evaluation of residents as part of the assessment and support of their progress toward independent practice (see Chap. 10).

Quality Mission

The clinic director must be engaged in the quality improvement initiatives that are ongoing in the outpatient clinic and ensure that residents are aware and involved in this work. For practices that are designated as a PCMH, the clinic director should follow the NCQA guidelines to make sure that accreditation requirements are being met and familiarize residents with these credentialing standards. In addition, features of ongoing primary care transformation, a key aspect of the PCMH, must be openly discussed with residents, with the clinic director ensuring compliance within this system of care [1]. These efforts will guide curriculum development and learner assessment in medical homes. Competencies and entrustable professional activities (EPAs) are tied to many of the clinical tasks, which can be observed and integrated into feedback [14, 15].

With the increasing presence of Accountable Care Organizations (ACOs) and additional available metrics, the clinic director or faculty may review clinical data such as Healthcare Effectiveness Data and Information Set (HEDIS) indicators, patient volume, no-show rate, and patient satisfaction surveys. Additionally, it is important to participate in implementation plans to meet clinic goals based on these metrics, such as diabetes and hypertension management. It is essential for the clinic director to foster a safe environment for quality initiatives and be prepared to innovate and adjust clinic experiences for their trainees in the changing landscape of medicine.

The resident clinic director is also likely to be involved in efforts to review and improve the health of the population the clinic serves. This can include formal training in population health assessment and can blend in nicely with quality improvement projects.

Administrative Mission

In addition to the clinical, academic, and quality missions, it is important to recognize the administrative expectations of the position. For instance, the residency clinic director must negotiate with clinic administration to assure that the clinic has adequate workspace, exam rooms, equipment, and supplies. He/she must also advocate for acceptable clinic staffing, including nursing and assistants along with appropriate access to social work, case management, and pharmacy. He/she must effectively interface with the program director to assure timely clinic schedule availability and advocate for minimizing disruptions to the continuity experience.

As noted above, it is also critical to negotiate adequate support for the clinic director position and to assure that productivity expectations are achievable and sustainable. Clinic directors must provide support to the other preceptors, including assistance in delivering feedback and remediation as well as offering mentoring for junior faculty.

Working with Health Care Administration

Given the broad roles and responsibilities of the clinic director, successful navigation of complex administrative structures is crucial. It is not unusual for the clinic director to have multiple reporting relationships, including program leadership, clinic leadership, and division/department leadership. The competing priorities within the leadership structure can create tension, as issues around clinical productivity and patient access can impact support for teaching time and other non-patient care activities. However, these challenges can also identify opportunities to improve clinical care and learning environment. Throughout these interactions, it is important for the clinic director to appreciate the complexities of health care delivery and medical education, all while making sure to advocate for themselves, their learners, and their patients. In dealing with challenges, they should make sure that all stakeholders understand the role of the teaching clinic and are able to fairly advocate for both patients and learners.

Conclusion

For a successful ambulatory clinic experience, the medical resident clinic director should be an individual with a mastery of patient care, residency education, and office practice management [3]. With approximately one-third of residency time spent in the outpatient setting, a positive clinical and educational experience is a key component of residency training. Clinic directors should be flexible and able to pivot when both small and large emergencies interface with the system such as the COVID-19 pandemic or natural disasters, as effective leadership is critically important. In addition, an excellent training environment can improve patient care and physician satisfaction and promote increased interest in primary care.

References

1. Chang A, Bowen JL, Buranosky RA, Frankel RM, Ghosh N, Rosenblum MJ, et al. Transforming primary care training—patient-centered medical home entrustable professional activities for internal medicine residents. J Gen Intern Med. 2013;28(6):801–9.

2. Wong JG, Fagan M, Pinsker J. Expectations of and for the medical director of the resident's ambulatory clinic. Am J Med 2001;111(1):84-87.
3. Hern T, Talen M, Babiuch C, Durazo-Arvizu R. Patient care management teams: improving continuity, office efficiency, and teamwork in a residency clinic. J Grad Med Educ. 2009;1(1):67–72.
4. Fazio SB, Chheda S, Hingle S, Lo MC, Meade L, Blanchard M, et al. The challenges of teaching ambulatory internal medicine: faculty recruitment, retention, and development: an AAIM/SGIM position paper. Am J Med. 2017;130(1):105–10.
5. Holt SR, Tobin DG, Whitman L, Ellman M, Moriarty JP, Doolittle B. Creating a satisfying continuity clinic experience for primary care trainees. Am J Med. 2021;134(4):547–53. https://doi.org/10.1016/j.amjmed.2020.12.005.
6. Accreditation Council for Graduate Medical Education; American Board of Internal Medicine. The Internal Medicine Milestone Project. http://www.acgme-nas.org/assetts/pdf/Milestones/InternalMedicineMilestones.pdf
7. Esch LM, Bird AN, Oyler JL, Lee WW, Shah SD, Pincavage AT. Preparing for the primary care clinic: an ambulatory boot camp for internal medicine interns. Med Educ Online. 2015;20:29,702.
8. Bennett K, Baxley E, Carter C, Stanek M. Organized continuity panel reassignment. J Grad Med Educ. 2011;3(3):404–7.
9. Donnelly MJ, Clauser JM, Weissman NJ. An intervention to improve ambulatory care handoffs at the end of residency. J Grad Med Educ. 2012;4(3):381–4.
10. Coyle A, Helenius I, Cruz CM, Lyons EA, May N, Andrilli J, Bannet MM, Pinotti R, Thomas DC. A decade of teaching and learning in internal medicine ambulatory education: a scoping review. J Grad Med Educ. 2019;11(2):132–42. https://doi.org/10.4300/JGME-D-18-00596.1.
11. Aagaard E, Kane GC, Conforti L, Hood S, Caverzagie KJ, Smith C, et al. Early feedback on the use of the internal medicine reporting milestones in assessment of resident performance. J Grad Med Educ. 2013;5(3):433–8.
12. O'Rourke P, Tseng E, Chacko K, Shalaby M, Cioletti A, Wright S. A national survey of internal medicine primary care residency program directors. J Gen Intern Med. 2019;34(7):1207–12.
13. Klein R, Alonso S, Anderson C, Vaidya A, Chams N, Kurl A, Lim K, Taylor C, Higgins SM. Delivering on the promise: exploring training characteristics and graduate career pursuits of primary care internal medicine residency programs and tracks. J Grad Med Educ. 2019;11(4):447–53.
14. Quick B, Alexander E, Ramm B, Rachford W, Quinlan J, Broxterman J. Multidisciplinary approach to maximize continuity in an academic internal medicine resident clinic. BMJ Open Qual. 2020;9(2)
15. Doolittle BR, Lim J, Edgar L. Milestones 2.0—a growth mindset for internal medicine residency programs. Am J Med. 2020;133(12):1492–9. https://doi.org/10.1016/j.amjmed.2020.09.003.

Chapter 2
Supervising and Supporting Faculty

Alaka Ray, Priya Radhakrishnan, and Joyce Wipf

Introduction

The academic clinic medical director has complex responsibilities to align patient care, clinic operations, and the clinic's education mission. Successful academic clinics require leadership and collaborative management with academic affiliates and multiple team professions. In this chapter, we describe the role of the medical director in providing oversight of the teaching faculty, including faculty responsibilities for precepting and teaching trainees, supervising patient care, and mentoring and training their learners to achieve graduated autonomy. The clinic director provides resources for faculty, residents, and staff to utilize data tools and work together to improve health metrics, outcomes, access, and equitable care. Academic primary care clinics may serve as a training site for other health professionals in addition to medicine, which expands the medical director roles to support and facilitate education and collaboration to enhance patient care. Partnership with academic program leaders creates an alliance to optimize scheduling, continuity clinic experience, and teaching the next generation of physicians and other health professionals.

A. Ray
Internal Medicine Residency Program, Massachusetts General Hospital, Boston, MA, USA
e-mail: aray2@mgh.harvard.edu

P. Radhakrishnan (✉)
HonorHealth, Scottsdale, AZ, USA
e-mail: Priya.Radhakrishnan@honorhealth.com

J. Wipf
Center of Education for Interprofessional Collaboration, VA Puget Sound, Seattle, WA, USA

Department of Medicine, University of Washington, Seattle, WA, USA
e-mail: joyce.wipf@va.gov; jwipf@uw.edu

L. B. Lu et al. (eds.), *Leading an Academic Medical Practice*,
https://doi.org/10.1007/978-3-031-40273-9_2

Outline

- Overview
- Management of academic clinic faculty
  - Outlining expectations
  - Part-time vs. full-time
  - Compensation and productivity goals
  - Scheduling
  - Clinic call coverage
- Oversight of teaching activities
  - Responsibilities
  - Clinical supervision
  - Clinic operations
  - Clinical coverage
  - Qualification and teaching skills development
  - Supervision and support of scholarly activities
- Conclusion

Overview

Academic faculty are integral to the clinical and medical education in an academic medical practice. A well-structured general internal medicine clinic requires the active engagement of faculty under strong leadership of the clinic director. Academic clinics are complex with faculty and resident physicians only present in clinic part-time due to other responsibilities and commitment to many training sites in partnership with academic affiliates. Yet, the teaching clinic has positive outcomes for patients, faculty, and staff, based on the data from Veterans Affairs (VA) team-based care in interprofessional academic clinics [1–3]. Residents may become "change agents" with participation in quality improvement projects of innovations in care delivery. Academic clinics vary in size, scope, and academic affiliations. There are over 500 internal medicine residency programs, with over 30,000 internal medicine residents in the United States [4]. The clinics that support the primary care and categorical internal medicine programs have various academic affiliations, with the majority being hospital based. The sponsoring institutions include universities, academic medical centers, community-based hospitals, VA, federally qualified health centers, and community health centers. Geographical locations may be urban, suburban, or rural and include underserved populations. According to the Society of General Internal Medicine Medical Resident Clinic Director Interest Group (MRCDIG) 2022 survey, directors reported their resident clinic or practice affiliation as hospital based (63% of respondents), medical school (31%), community (20%), VA (17%), or private practice (3%) [5].

The clinic director has many responsibilities, ranging from overseeing patient care and resident education to many administrative and financial elements of the clinic. Many academic clinics are teaching clinics with residents supervised by precepting faculty and are also the site where these faculty see their own patients. Faculty members can range in clinical effort from part-time to full-time. Some "part-time" faculty may have limited clinical responsibilities with significant administrative, educational, and/or research commitments. Some academic General Internal Medicine (GIM) faculty also attend on the inpatient medical wards for several weeks per year. It is the clinic director's role to support all of these diverse physicians. As primary care is increasingly team based in medical home-type settings, some clinic directors are also responsible for their interprofessional team of advanced practice providers (APPs), clinical pharmacists, and other healthcare professionals who work closely with the residents and faculty in co-managing patients.

Management of Academic Clinic Faculty

Outlining Expectations

In many institutions, the clinic director is directly responsible for the faculty who work in the clinic. In some university-based institutions, this responsibility may lie with the section chief of the division or the chair of the department. Regardless, the clinic director plays an important role in interacting with the faculty and academic leaders on a regular basis and is directly responsible for overseeing the faculty preceptor schedule and faculty development with regard to precepting and teaching conferences. To ensure excellent clinical supervision, teaching skills, and academic progress of faculty, it is essential that residents formally evaluate the precepting faculty. Additionally, the 360 evaluations with peer faculty and clinic staff assessments of the teaching faculty are invaluable. The clinic director must work closely with the resident program leaders to discuss any issues that arise with faculty preceptors.

The clinic director and each faculty member need to be aware of metric tools to monitor clinical care in chronic disease and preventive health, patient satisfaction, and access to care. The clinic structure should have methods for reviewing these data with the faculty member on a periodic basis. Ideally, electronic health records (EHRs) should provide available tools for faculty to independently assess their data, termed population health panel management. Primary care clinics should have built-in protected time for faculty to work with their healthcare team to improve clinical care and outcome measures, with time proportionate to panel size. Additionally, faculty can self-assess their individual productivity metrics, so they can adjust their clinic schedules to meet expectations based on clinical time mapping. This allows the practice to plan for adequate staffing. Goals for faculty members are dependent on many factors and organizational priorities. They often include accountable care objectives, education, research priorities, and quality initiatives. Staying well informed and having input in the organizational and departmental initiatives and priorities are important tasks for the clinic director and enable them to advocate for faculty in a methodical and equitable manner.

During the onboarding process for new faculty, the clinic director and the program director provide input to the section chief, service chief, and department leaders regarding roles and responsibilities as to the expected number of clinical sessions and educational sessions in the teaching clinic. For full-time and regularly scheduled clinic faculty, it is helpful to include quality improvement responsibilities and potential projects with residents, given the need for clinical champions for quality initiatives. The clinic director should provide a formal document outlining expectations for faculty preceptors and can enlist the support of residency program leadership for this task.

Clinical Time: Part-Time vs. Full-Time

Internal medicine residency clinics have variable models of staffing: all full-time employed faculty, combined part- and full-time faculty, or a combination of employed and community-based preceptors. According to the MRCDIG 2022 survey [5], out of 36 respondents, 68% stated that their faculty precepted 1–2 half-days per week; 13% responded that faculty precepted 3–5 half-days per week, and only 6.5% reported that their faculty precepted more than 5 sessions a week on average. In the authors' experience, academic clinics vary in the structure and faculty expectations in their clinical and educational roles. To provide teaching opportunities for all the faculty and enhance broad engagement in the teaching mission, a common design is for each faculty member to have 1–3 half-days per week of dedicated precepting, with the remainder of clinical time for their own direct patient care. The clinic director and support staff should develop a system to manage the preceptor schedules and ensure sufficient clinical coverage when faculty are teaching or in other education, research, or nonclinical activities. It is important for the clinic director to build a culture of wellness and collaboration so that faculty members are encouraged to cover each other [6–8]. Diversity of practice is an essential component for physician longitudinal career satisfaction and joy of practice. Although less common in the past two decades, academic GIM faculty may in some settings choose to maintain inpatient skills and continue to have ward attending rotations for several weeks per year. This requires special efforts for clinic panel size adjustment and panel patient care coverage, although there are potential advantages. Dual career may be a recruitment incentive for recent graduates who wish to maintain skills, broaden internal medicine knowledge base, and expand teaching time. GIM primary care physicians bring disease management skills to wards and expertise in transitions of care.

Compensation and Productivity Goals

Faculty productivity is essential for academic medical centers striving to achieve excellence and national recognition. Most academic departments measure relative value units (RVUs), and some may measure educational value units (EVUs) [9–12].

The Medical Group Management Association (MGMA) and the American Medical Group Association (AMGA) survey reports productivity median RVUs at 4,847 and 4,861 respectively [10, 13]. The clinic director is an integral part of the financial success of the institution and should oversee correct billing and coding practices by faculty preceptors. In our experience, academic internal medicine clinics are often represented as "loss centers" for hospitals and sponsoring institutions. This is a combination of undervaluing of primary care reimbursement and overvaluing specialty care [14]. To overcome institutional bias against primary care, the clinic director must have an understanding of the operating dashboards, expenses, revenue and productivity metrics, downstream revenue generated from testing, and referrals to specialists. Most clinics have administrative leaders such as clinic managers or operational managers who are responsible for day-to-day management. However, understanding the finances of the clinical operations is particularly important for the clinic director. Several professional organizations such as MGMA, AMGA, and Alliance for Academic Internal Medicine (AAIM) have resources for understanding dashboards and in-depth financial education [10, 15, 16].

Most academic institutions use RVUs, billing charges, patients per session, or other encounter standards as a measure of clinical productivity. The academic and administrative work may be compensated based on an hourly rate or a percentage of salary. Some institutions use educational relative value units (eRVUs) to measure and quantify the educational work that academic faculty perform [17]. A simple measure may be the number of visits per day for the entire clinic or the specific preceptor. In VA clinics, the preceptor is assigned in the encounter as the direct primary provider when supervising resident clinic visits. If a preceptor supervises 2–3 residents per half-day in a typical clinic, the volume of patients seen and supervised would meet or exceed the numbers of patients seen if the preceptor had their own clinic session.

Since numbers of patients may fluctuate on a seasonal basis based on resident schedules, academic meetings, and other local factors including the availability of physicians, the clinic director is able to plan on staffing as well as outreach based on projected volumes. Faculty should have the expectation to be flexible in order to meet financial outcomes. For example, to ensure that productivity targets are met and quality measures are addressed, some clinics develop their wellness visits during the summer or holiday months when visit volumes can be lower, leading to sustained numbers of patients. There is an increasing number of organizations that include quality and patient satisfaction measures in the physician compensation structure (i.e., "pay for performance"), either as part of their compensation plans or as part of their arrangements with Accountable Care Organizations or other shared savings programs [18, 19]. The clinic director often also plays the role of the quality director in smaller clinics and serves as the liaison between faculty and administration on the quality targets. Specific metric targets for pay for performance may change over time to include organization "stretch goals" (going beyond the primary aim to expand the target outcome in a defined time; for example, if the usual diabetes type 2 metric is having 80% of patients in a panel with HBA1c <7, it could aim for 90% in target in 1 year). Pay-for-performance metrics must be reviewed in advance with faculty.

Preceptor payment occurs via a number of different models across the country. Many programs compensate preceptors based on the productivity-based revenue from resident clinic sessions they supervise. In other cases, preceptors are paid a stipend based on sessions of precepting or number of residents precepted. Funds for stipends may be set aside from clinical revenue at the practice site or from the division or department budget. Clinics may have agreements with academic affiliate for compensation of teaching, based on indirect funding established for resident training via Medicare and the Accreditation Council for Graduate Medical Education (ACGME) payment system. This includes direct funding for salary support and indirect funding for the cost of training. Less frequently, the clinic site such as the federally funded healthcare centers may have their own federal payment for residents.

Review of clinical productivity for allotted clinical time during regularly scheduled staff meetings is essential to engage the physicians and the staff in the financial success of the clinic and the organization at large. Since financial education is often not a priority in residency education, it is not unusual for faculty to have gaps in their knowledge. Having sessions devoted towards improving the faculty understanding of the finances of the clinics may improve engagement and ownership of the process. Training in high-value care will also impact clinic and healthcare organization costs. Although not regularly accounted by financial review, training the next generation of physicians has financial benefits to the organization when/if potential recruitment of resident clinic graduates to the practice. Research estimates that the cost of recruiting and establishing fully in practice a primary care physician nears twice an annual physician salary [20–22]. Recruiting resident graduates who already are familiar to the culture and system of care will lead to greater initial efficiency and faster up-titration of panel size than external candidates.

The clinic director or a delegate should work with the departmental leadership to understand dashboards such that the faculty can monitor their own performance. It is not unusual for clinic directors to inherit senior faculty who have traditionally been allotted time for research and administrative or educational duties that have changed. Faculty careers evolve over time, and accurate time mapping of active nonclinical responsibilities should be done annually with monitoring of academic progress and productivity of protected time. For example, if an established research-based physician no longer has research funding or ongoing publications, then additional clinical time would be allotted. In such cases, having a dashboard that takes into account educational and research metrics is important.

Scheduling

In the authors' experience, the creation and maintenance of schedules are a complex entity in a resident practice. The term "scheduling" encompasses appointment capacity, maximizing continuity, maintaining physician productivity, and optimizing workflows [23]. It is advisable to meet regularly with key stakeholders including clinic staff and clinic faculty to review the schedules. Regularly reviewing appointment data with the number of arrived patients, no-show rates, and late visits at faculty meetings in a transparent way ensures that all the members of the clinic are engaged. A team-based approach with data-driven quality improvement should be used [24].

There should be an established policy for how to handle patients who arrive late or miss appointments that is transparent to the faculty preceptors, clinic staff, and residents. For example, at the University of Vermont Medical Center, if a patient is 20 minutes late, the faculty preceptor can decide if the patient should be seen or rescheduled. It is advisable to consider how far the patient has traveled and the reason for the visit and to evaluate the psychosocial factors which may impact the ability of the patient to arrive on time. Safety net clinics often have patients who run late due to transportation issues. The Institute of Healthcare Improvement guides on primary care or the Dartmouth Institute Microsystem Academy on the Clinical Microsystem (Improving Health Care by Improving Your Microsystem) provides a good framework for patient-centered management of late arrivals and no-show visits [25–27].

Clinic Call Coverage

Ambulatory clinics vary in the structure of their call coverage, while some may employ residents or other advanced practice providers such as nurse practitioners, and others may not. In our experience, an established workflow for on-call documentation ensuring necessary post-call follow-up should be part of the clinic workflow. It can be helpful to have a telephone medicine curriculum so that residents and new faculty learn this important skill. To maintain high-value care, the clinic director plays an important role in managing utilization of services including emergency room visits and is expected to train faculty, residents, and staff in ensuring that proper care is given at the appropriate time [28]. Clinics need to have a system to immediately address critical lab and imaging results for clinicians who are not available or on leave [29, 30] (see Chap. 5 for details). In authors' experience, a "critical-results" pager may be rotated among clinic faculty, who address and determine if emergency department evaluation or other workup is needed.

Oversight of Teaching Activities

As part of the responsibilities of an academic practice, clinic directors will also have supervision of faculty who precept medical residents or medical students in outpatient clinic. As such, it is useful to have a clear understanding of the resident continuity clinic preceptor role and responsibilities.

Responsibilities

The responsibilities of the clinic preceptor can be summed up in the phrase "the primary supervisor for learners in their outpatient clinical practice" [31, 32]. In most cases, preceptors serve as the "attending of record" for resident patients. Thus, the preceptor is also usually associated with the patients in the resident panel for insurance and medicolegal purposes. Another key responsibility is to serve as a role model in the field of primary care and general medicine. Role modeling is particularly relevant in imparting skills in competencies such as professionalism and communication [33]. Preceptors are also called on to provide mentorship, especially for trainees considering general medicine careers. However, there are several concrete components, as discussed below.

Clinical Supervision

Clinical supervision can take various forms depending on the experience level of the resident and the teaching style of the preceptor. Unlike medical students, residents will obtain the history and physical exam independently. Following this, residents will usually present each patient to the outpatient preceptor. This may be done in a separate office or conference room, but in some cases, preceptors have found it effective to listen to the presentation in the patient's room, allowing the patient to hear the presentation and also facilitating clarifying questions by the preceptor. After reviewing the details of the case together, the preceptor may use various teaching methods to impart teaching points relevant to the case, including the approach to the disease, management, and follow up. Effective teaching requires the preceptor to have multiple content frameworks and teaching strategies. In addition, teaching points must be made in a time-sensitive manner allowing the resident to adhere to the patient schedule [34, 35]. The preceptor may then choose to ask the patient additional questions or examine the patient to clarify the resident's history and physical exam. The resident may then discuss the plan with the patient. At times, the resident may do this in the presence of the preceptor. After the visit has ended and the resident has completed the documentation, preceptors are required to review, addend, and cosign the documentation.

Typically, questions arise outside clinic sessions as well. The clinic preceptor must be available, or the clinic should have a coverage system in place to assist residents outside of continuity clinic sessions with questions regarding patient panel management, patient laboratory testing follow-up, imaging studies, consults, paperwork, or other duties. This includes being available by email, phone, or pager to respond to residents with urgent clinical questions. In most institutions, the clinic preceptor is not the attending of record when a resident patient is admitted to the hospital. However, clinic preceptors should encourage residents to continue monitoring the progress of their hospitalized clinic patients and maintain communication with the inpatient team. This can contribute to strengthening the therapeutic relationship with clinic patients and support the transition of care at discharge. Equally important, residents should discuss any potential medical recommendations with the preceptor and inpatient attending of record for that admission.

There are different clinic supervisory models. Generally, only the supervising preceptors cosign the notes and are responsible for the care of the patients. To ensure continuity between patients, resident physicians, and panel preceptors, the VA Puget Sound Resident Clinic, for example, has the dual supervisory model whereby a resident is paired with a preceptor on a shared panel for 3 years. In addition to the supervising faculty, the panel preceptors are required to cosign every EHR note by their residents, even if they are not directly involved in the care during the specific clinic session. Intervisit care and follow-up of studies post-visit are managed by the resident with the paired panel preceptor, who knows those patients over time. Patient and preceptor continuity is enhanced as the panel preceptor will address issues when the resident is not available, such as prescription renewals, triage of acute needs, or seeing the patient in urgent clinic visits.

There are relevant guidelines from the ACGME regarding the preceptor-to-resident ratio in a clinic, which state that clinics "must maintain a ratio of residents or other learners to faculty preceptor not to exceed four to one." In addition, "Faculty members must not have other patient care responsibilities while supervising more than two residents or other learners" [36]. This ratio is currently utilized as part of the Centers for Medicare & Medicaid Services (CMS) Primary Care Exception Rule that allows preceptors to bill and supervise the entire visit from outside the patient's room if the following requirements are met: the patient is covered by Medicare; the resident has more than 6 months of experience; the 4:1 ratio stated above is maintained; and the preceptor is easily available for any required supervision [37]. As a result, this teaching ratio has been utilized in many continuity clinics, even if the exception rule is not being utilized for billing. In clinics where the resident patients have a broader range of insurers, the exception rule can be challenging to implement equitably since the preceptor's approach to each patient should theoretically be payer blind. Commercial payers usually require that each patient be seen by an attending physician—a rule that can pose difficulties in clinics with fewer teaching faculty. In addition, the literature suggests that the six-month threshold is arbitrary and should be supplemented by an ACGME Milestones-based assessment of each individual resident's readiness to practice under indirect supervision [38, 39]. The University of Washington Internal Medicine Residency Program instituted a requirement across all eight primary care clinic sites that residents be observed and signed off in several specific skills prior to exception rule utilization, including agenda setting; counseling on new medication, behavior change, and screening; history; examination; and advance care planning. Thus, it should be possible to utilize the exception rule while balancing patient safety and resident autonomy.

Clinic Operations

The clinic director oversees clinic operations with a management team that includes nurse manager and administrative manager. We encourage a standing managers' meeting (e.g., weekly) of these individuals with academic leaders such as the section chief to systematically discuss operations such as staffing needs and actions, updates, care metrics, and training program activities. This leadership team also identifies and troubleshoots challenges. Selected meetings have expanded multidisciplinary focus to include clinic supervisors in pharmacy, mental health, social work, and program leaders for women's health, homeless care, telemedicine, and population health. The clinic director also holds standing meetings monthly or bimonthly of the entire clinic staff and preceptors to educate on changes in operations and delivery of care processes, identify clinician challenges, and address questions.

Preceptors must educate residents in effective clinical operations and also assist with patient triage. Preceptors have an important role in orienting and updating residents to clinic structure and workflow, as well as use of the electronic care systems and billing. Preceptors are ideally placed to serve as an outpatient ambassador, as well as by introducing and orienting residents to various clinic supports (i.e., nurse practitioners, nurses, medical assistants, administrative staff, nutritionists, and case managers). When practice-level discussions occur regarding workflow and clinical support, preceptors can serve as a strong advocate for resident physicians to ensure that there is equity in the support that is provided. Often, since residents are usually the most "part-time" providers, workflows need to be adapted to be effective for residents and their patients. Soliciting feedback and input from preceptors and residents on clinic workflows can help improve efficiency and foster team engagement.

Primary care clinics are increasingly team based, such as medical home-type models of care, with evidence of positive outcomes for patients and staff [40, 41]. In training the next generation of physicians and other profession clinicians, academic clinic medical director's scope of supervision is expanding beyond medicine residents, students, and faculty. Clinic faculty of other health professions may have their own trainees and academic affiliates. Training program leaders need to align with the medical clinic director to plan opportunities, including resources such as sufficient exam rooms, computers, and precepting space for training. In 2011, the VA established Centers of Excellence in Primary Care Education (CoEPCE) to transform training from professional "silos" to interprofessional learning and care collaboration [42]. The Centers successfully created and sustained programs with expanded primary care requirements (30% of total clinical training) and innovative curricula. Centers included medical residents and other postgraduate professional trainees, such as advanced practice nursing, pharmacy, psychology, social work, and other professions. Patient outcome measures included study comparison of medical resident clinical care at five VA CoEPCE centers versus VA academic clinics without CoEPCE [1]. Results showed that CoEPCEs had improved diabetes A1c, renal monitoring, mental health referrals, deprescribing polypharmacy, reduced related emergency department visits, and reduced hospitalizations compared to other VA non-CoEPCE academic clinics.

Clinical Coverage

Preceptors are required to assist with resident clinical activities that require attending sign-off, e.g., controlled substance refills, anticoagulation oversight, forms related to outpatient services, and other forms. In some clinics, preceptors also provide coverage for assigned residents' patient panel when a resident is unavailable. In larger programs, this coverage can be offset by any available resident coverage system; however, preceptors should still remain available to provide clinical supervision as needed for the resident who is covering. The literature suggests that residents are less able to attend to "between-visit" work during inpatient rotations rather than electives [43]. Episodic coverage for these "between-visit" tasks can be at least partially provided by preceptors.

Qualifications and Teaching Skill Development

The ACGME states: "Faculty members are a foundational element of graduate medical education—faculty members teach residents how to care for patients." There must be physicians with certification in internal medicine by the American Board of Internal Medicine (ABIM) or the American Osteopathic Board of Internal Medicine (AOBIM) to teach and supervise [36]. Faculty should be primary care physicians in good standing at an approved primary care site affiliated with the residency program.

Precepting faculty should have a deep interest in medical education and mentorship of residents. Programs must have robust faculty development programs, and preceptors should be expected to attend. Attendance to a reasonable number of faculty development events per year should be prioritized and facilitated by the clinic director. Onboarding activities for new preceptors should be available, either through in-person meetings or through asynchronous access to materials. Topics should delineate common outpatient teaching strategies such as One-Minute Preceptor; SNAPPS 6-step learner-centered education model, or Precepting in the Presence of the Patient, as well as guidelines for clinical supervision and billing, evaluations, and well-being [44–46].

360-degree evaluations are a core requirement for medical education. Preceptors should have the opportunity to review their evaluations from residents and discuss their engagement in teaching with a residency program director or associate program director or their section chief on an annual basis. Generally, a successful preceptor will have a demonstrated interest and experience in education, reflected in written evaluations by trainees.

Finally, it should be noted that a genuine alliance between precepting faculty and practice leadership promotes a stronger educational experience for learners. Gupta et al. discussed the concept of "Clinic First" and described six actions that can improve the educational experience of a resident continuity clinic. Four of the six actions—developing a small core of clinic faculty, creating operationally excellent clinics, building stable clinic teams, and engaging residents in practice transformation—are in the bailiwick of the clinic medical director [47]. The goals are for residents to be embedded in the clinic as engaged clinicians with graduated responsibilities, and not viewed as "visitors" to the clinic.

Supervision and Support of Scholarly Activities

Traditionally, academic faculty, particularly core faculty, have an expectation for scholarly work and research. Over the last few decades, there have been dramatic changes in healthcare funding and increasing pressure of clinical productivity. This has resulted in a diminishing relationship between tenure and guaranteed salary for some academic clinics. As a result, there have been significant changes in the scholarly output of GIM faculty if predominantly clinical track with the academic affiliates, which usually have fewer or no requirements for publication and yet provide significant precepting expertise.

All faculty need to make a contribution to the academic culture; defining tracks and identifying core faculty are the first steps towards building and sustaining a culture of scholarship. Faculty with an interest in academic work in the clinic setting usually belong to the clinician-educator or clinician-researcher tracks. The advent of big data and the need for quality improvement due to the shift towards population-based medicine provide a rich opportunity for academic clinicians to pursue academic work with relative ease and in line with the mission of most organizations.

For clinics with faculty in academic tracks requiring scholarship, productivity measures need to consider specific promotion criteria of the academic affiliate, which vary by type of track and institution. For example, physician-scientist track faculty have more limited clinical and teaching, and major requirements for research achievements, publications, and grants contribute to success and reputation. Clinician-educator track faculty in some institutions have required scholarly criteria, curriculum development, and publications, in addition to clinical and teaching excellence and educational leadership.

To retain and recruit outstanding academic track faculty, it is crucially important for the clinic director and section chief to foster an environment of curiosity, discovery, and innovation. This includes setting uniform expectations for proportions of protected time and clinical time based on the type of faculty track and scholarly productivity. The section chief, affiliate division head, and department chair monitor academic progress and encourage mentoring of junior faculty. For clinician-educators who develop curricula and provide a majority of the teaching for the residents and students, developing a rich faculty development program with instructions on how to evaluate curricula provides professional enrichment. In addition, providing support for faculty to present their work at local, regional, or national meetings not only fulfills the ACGME requirements for scholarship, but also helps develop the culture of inquiry. These academic faculty may bring in funding to the healthcare organization via grants, have a percentage of salary paid by the affiliate, or expand educational funding if the clinic site facility receives resident stipends (direct and indirect) as a partner with the affiliate.

While the role of the clinic director is primarily to ensure that the academic clinic runs smoothly, the very nature of the academic enterprise requires commitment to promote scholarship and research. The clinic director needs to partner and work closely with the department chair or division chief to ensure growth of the clinical, research, and scholarly activities; to define academic work distinct from clinical service; and to carve out time for faculty to achieve career goals and promotion in their specific career pathway.

Conclusion

The clinic director has a challenging role. In order to fulfill the responsibilities and expectations, it is important for a clinic director to have leadership and management skills, an understanding of financial and operational metrics, and a passion for mentorship and education in partnership with academic affiliates. A robust organizational structure, in collaboration with other health profession leaders, and clearly delineated expectations for all clinic staff can greatly augment the effectiveness of the clinic director.

References

1. Edwards ST, Hooker ER, Brienza R, et al. Association of a multisite interprofessional education initiative with quality of primary care. JAMA Netw Open. 2019;2(11):e1915943.
2. Tuepker A, Newell S, Nicolaidis C, Reyes ME, González-Prats MC, Skaperdas E, Kansagara D. Veteran patient perspectives and experiences during implementation of a patient-centered medical home model. J Patient Exp. 2018;5(2):107–13. https://doi.org/10.1177/2374373517731602.
3. Newell S, O'Brien B, Brienza R, Dulay M, Strewler A, Manuel JK, Tuepker A. Experiences of patient-centered medical home staff team members working in interprofessional training environments. J Gen Intern Med. 2020;35(10):2976–82. https://doi.org/10.1007/s11606-020-06055-y.
4. Summary of Workforce Trends in Internal Medicine Training—Academic Years 2005/2006 through 2014/2015. http://www.abim.org/about/statistics-data/resident-fellow-workforce-data.aspx
5. MRCDIG SGIM survey 2022. SGIM.
6. American Hospital Association Primary Care Workforce Roundtable. Workforce roles in a redesigned primary care model. http://www.aha.org/content/13/13-0110-wf-primary-care.pdf

7. Shanafelt TD, West CP, Sloan JA, Novotny PJ, Poland GA, Menaker R, Rummans TA, Dyrbye LN. Career fit and burnout among academic faculty. Arch Intern Med. 2009;169(10):990–5.
8. Shanafelt TD, Boone S, Tan L, et al. Burnout and satisfaction with work-life balance among US physicians relative to the general US population. Arch Intern Med. 2012;172(18):1377–85.
9. Hyden M, Wong M. How to measure physician compensation per RVU. August 14, 2013. http://www.mgma.com/practice-resources/mgma-connection-plus/online-only/2013/august/how-to-measure-physician-compensation-per-rvu
10. http://www.mgma.com
11. Stites S, Steffen P, Turner S, Pingleton S. Aligning clinical compensation with clinical productivity: design and implementation of the financial value unit (FVU) system in an academic department of internal medicine. Acad Med. 2013;88(7):946–51.
12. Kairouz VF, Raad D, Fudyma J, Curtis AB, Schünemann HJ, Akl EA. Assessment of faculty productivity in academic departments of medicine in the United States: a national survey. BMC Med Educ. 2014;14:205.
13. Darvis B. Physician compensation still rising in primary care and fast-growing urgent care sector, but flattening is expected. NEJM Career Center; 2021. https://resources.nejmcareercenter.org/article/physician-compensation-still-rising-in-primary-care-and-fast-growing-urgent-care-sector-but-flattening-is-expected/
14. Shi L. The impact of primary care: a focused review. Scientifica. 2012;2012:432892. https://doi.org/10.6064/2012/432892.
15. www.amga.org
16. www.im.org
17. Lessons for Financial Success, MGMA chapter 5 Productivity, capacity and staffing. http://www.mgma.com/about/about-mgma-medical-group-management/about-center-for-research/lessons-chapter-5-productivity-capacity-and-staffing
18. Berkowitz S, Ishii L, Schulz J, Poffenroth M. Academic medical centers forming accountable care organizations and partnering with community providers: the experience of the Johns Hopkins medicine alliance for patients. Acad Med. 2015;91 https://doi.org/10.1097/ACM.0000000000000976.
19. https://www.cms.gov/Medicare/Medicare-Fee-for-Service-Payment/sharedsavingsprogram/Downloads/MSSP-ACO-data.pdf
20. Buchbinder SB, Wilson M, M, Melick CF, Powe NR. Estimates of costs of primary care physician turnover. Am J Managed Care. 1999;5(11):1431–8.
21. Garner BR, Hunter BD, et al. Treatment staff turnover in organizations implementing evidence-based practices: turnover rates and their association with client outcome. J Subst Abus Treat. 2012;42(2):134–42.
22. Salary data by occupation obtained from the Bureau of Labor Statistics, Occupational Employment Statistics: https://www.bls.gov/oes/current/oes_nat.htm#29-0000
23. Stryker C. More effectively schedule patient visits at your practice. Physicians Practice. Practice Your Way. Blog; 2013 Jun 19. http://www.physicianspractice.com/blog/more-effectively-schedule-patient-visits-your-practice
24. Institute of Health care Improvement (www.ihi.org).
25. The Dartmouth Institute, Microsystem Academy (www.clinicalmicrosystem.org).
26. Godfrey M, Nelson E, Batalden P, Wasson, Mohr J, Headrick L. Improving healthcare by improving your microsystem. http://clinicalmicrosystem.org/wp-content/uploads/2014/07/CMAG040104.pdf. Dartmouth Medical School. 2003 Sep 2. Version 2: Rev 4/13/2004.
27. Cassel CK, Guest JA. Choosing wisely: helping physicians and patients make smart decisions about their care. JAMA. 2012;307(17):1801–2.
28. Centers for Medicare & Medicaid Services. Delivery system reform, Medicare payment reform. https://www.cms.gov/Medicare/Quality-Initiatives-Patient-Assessment-Instruments/Value-Based-Programs/MACRA-MIPS-and-APMs/MACRA-MIPS-and-APMs.html.
29. https://www.nationalahec.org/pdfs/vsrt-team-based-care-principles-values.pdf

30. Iglehart JK. Expanding the role of advanced nurse practitioners—risks and rewards. N Engl J Med. 2013;368:1935–41.
31. Kaplan S, Garrett K. The use of logic models by community based initiatives. Eval Program Plann. 2005;28:167–72.
32. McLaughlin J, Jordan G. Logic models: a tool for testing your program's performance story. Eval Program Plann. 1999;22:65–72.
33. Cote L, Laughrea P. Preceptors' understanding and use of role modeling to develop the can MEDS competencies in residents. Acad Med. 2014;89(6):934–9.
34. Cote L, Bordage G. Content and conceptual frameworks of preceptor feedback related to residents' educational needs. Acad Med. 2014;87(9):1275–81.
35. Dugdale DC, Epstein R, Pantilat SZ. Time and the patient-physician relationship. J Gen Intern Med. 1999;14:S34–40.
36. Accreditation Council for Graduate Medical Education. ACGME Program Requirements for Residency Education in Internal Medicine. https://www.acgme.org/globalassets/pfassets/programrequirements/140_internalmedicine_2022v3.pdf
37. Department of Health and Human Services—Centers for Medicare and Medicaid Services. Guidelines for Teaching Physicians, Interns, and Residents. https://www.cms.gov/Outreach-and-Education/Medicare-Learning-Network-MLN/MLNProducts/Downloads/Teaching-Physicians-Fact-Sheet-ICN006437.pdf
38. Tobin DG, Doolittle BR, Ellman MS, Ruser CB, Brienza RS, Genao I. Modifying the primary care exception rule to require competency-based assessment. Acad Med. 2017;92(3):331–4.
39. Accreditation Council for Graduate Medical Education. The Milestones Guidebook. http://www.acgme.org/Portals/0/MilestonesGuidebook.pdf
40. Nelson KM, Helfrich C, Sun H, et al. Implementation of the patient-centered medical home the Veterans Health Administration: associations with patient satisfaction, quality of care, staff burnout, and hospital and emergency department use. JAMA Intern Med. 2014;174(8):1350–8.
41. Reddy A, Wong E, Canamucio C, et al. Association between continuity and team-based care and health care utilization: an observational study of medicare-eligible veterans in VA patient aligned care team. Health Serv Res. 2018;53(Suppl 3):5201–18.
42. Harada ND, Traylor L, Rugen KW, Bowen JL, Scott Smith C, Felker B, Ludke D, Tonnu-Mihara I, Ruberg JL, Adler J, Uhl K, Gardner AL, Gilman SC. Interprofessional transformation of clinical education: the first six years of the veterans affairs centers of excellence in primary care education. J Interprof Care. 2018;2018:1. https://doi.org/10.1080/13561820.2018.1433642.
43. Hom J, Richman I, Chen JH, Singh B, Crump C, Chi J. Fulfilling outpatient medicine responsibilities during internal medicine residency: a quantitative study of housestaff participation with between visit tasks. BMC Med Educ. 2016;16:13941.
44. Neher J, Gordon K, Meyer B, Stevens N. A five-step "microskills" model of clinical teaching. J Am Board Fam Pract. 1992;5:419–24.
45. Wolpaw T, Wolpaw D, Papp K. SNAPPS: a learner-centered model for outpatient education. Acad Med. 2003;78(9):893–8.
46. Power DV, et al. Precepting medical students in the patient's presence: an educational randomized trial in family medicine clinic. Fam Med. 2017;49(2):97–105.
47. Gupta R, Barnes K, Bodenheimer T. Clinic first: 6 actions to transform ambulatory residency training. J Grad Med Educ. 2016;8(4):500–3.

Chapter 3
Faculty Recruitment and Retention

Mohan Nadkarni and Ira Marie Helenius

Introduction

In an ambulatory teaching practice, successful retention and recruitment of high-quality teaching faculty are critical. Shifts in care delivery models that now emphasize efficient patient-centered ambulatory care require a large ambulatory faculty workforce capable of both providing and teaching high-value medical care. This chapter highlights the steps to accomplish successful retention and recruitment identified from the literature. Common barriers and ways to overcome them are discussed. This chapter also provides specific steps of recruitment, contract negotiation, onboarding, and retention. Particular attention is given to retention strategies that help to improve the well-being of faculty in their positions and reduce the incidence of attrition.

Outline

- Background
- Identifying the challenges to recruitment and retention
- Successful recruitment
- Contract negotiation
- Onboarding
- Making retention possible

M. Nadkarni
Division of General, Geriatric, Palliative and Hospital Medicine, University of Virginia Health System, Charlottesville, VA, USA
e-mail: MMN9Y@UVAhealth.org

I. M. Helenius (✉)
University Medical Associates, University of Virginia Health System, Charlottesville, VA, USA
e-mail: IH4B@UVAhealth.org

L. B. Lu et al. (eds.), *Leading an Academic Medical Practice*, https://doi.org/10.1007/978-3-031-40273-9_3

- Creating a culture of connection and flexibility
- Optimize clinical work environments
- Ensuring a mission-based care focus
- Factors to overcome barriers to faculty recruitment and retention

  Value teaching
  Career development
  Faculty development
  Faculty mentoring
  Innovative clinical learning models
  Develop faculty interests
  Nonfinancialincentives
- Conclusion

Background

Recruitment and retention of high-quality clinical educators to internal medicine (IM) residency teaching ambulatory practices have always been an important part of successful leadership. Shifts in care delivery models that now emphasize efficient patient-centered ambulatory care require a large ambulatory faculty workforce capable of both providing and teaching high-value medical care. Even before the pandemic, recruitment and retention of clinical faculty had become increasingly difficult. Data from a 2010 Association of Program Directors in Internal Medicine (APDIM) survey demonstrated that greater than 40% of programs reported difficulty recruiting core ambulatory faculty [1]. In the current environment, the pressures on retaining and recruiting faculty have increased dramatically. Rising rates of physician burnout and effects of "The Great Resignation" of 2021 seen across all sectors of employment, but highly magnified in medicine, have continued to strain the system [2]. Attrition of faculty is costly and time consuming. Specifically, turnover of primary care physicians (PCPs) in the USA has been estimated to add $979 million of excess health care spending in a 2018 study [3]. For an organization, the cost of physician turnover can range from $500,000 to more than $1 million per doctor [4]. This estimate includes recruitment, sign-on bonuses, lost billings, and onboarding costs for replacement physicians. Thus, clinic leadership needs to recognize the critical importance of a strategy to actively recruit and retain a stable core of faculty.

Identifying the Challenges to Recruitment and Retention

Physicians are faced with many stressors that potentially reduce their job satisfaction and lead to increased risk of attrition. Fifty-four percent of physicians leave their practice group within the first 5 years [5]. The Jackson Physician Search and Medical Group Management Association (MGMA) 2021 survey of 181 physicians found that 46% of physicians had considered leaving their current employer for another medical practice and 43% had considered early retirement in the year prior to the survey [6]. In the survey, physicians identified various problems that impacted their job satisfaction: lack of effective two-way communication with management, loss of influence on patient care and scheduling, inadequate support staff and increased administrative burden, loss of meaning and value in their work, fear of instability, being overworked, and lack of recognition.

A 2017 Alliance for Academic Internal Medicine (AAIM)/Society of General Internal Medicine (SGIM) position paper on faculty recruitment, retention, and development identified four problems that are prevalent for faculty in ambulatory teaching clinics [7]: (1) increased workload and stress (driven by increasing clinical volume, lack of time, increasing patient complexity, and workflow modernization), (2) inadequate financial support of teaching, (3) increased demand for ambulatory teaching, and (4) inadequate faculty development.

In the current climate, the effects of the pandemic on the health care workforce cannot be overstated. In a 2020 survey of 20,665 health care workers including 2914 physicians, 1 in 5 physicians reported intention to leave their practice within 2 years [8]. Burnout, fear of exposure, COVID-related anxiety/depression, and workload were found to be the driving factors (see Chap. 38 on burnout). Conversely, physicians who felt highly valued by their organization and who had a strong sense of meaning and purpose in their work were less likely to report intent to leave their jobs.

Successful Recruitment

Recruitment of faculty takes much time, commitment, and attention to detail. The key to success is being able to consistently and effectively communicate the strengths of the program to the right candidates. A program with high levels of retention of faculty will be attractive to potential candidates. Successful recruitment will effectively highlight the program's strengths and the features that make it an attractive place to work.

The first step of recruitment is assessing the needs for the position and then disseminating the information about the job opening out to appropriate venues. Some of the important components of this communication are clear and informative job descriptions, effective use of good advertisement in the right journals/venues including social media, use of professional organizations and meetings (i.e., regional and national SGIM meeting), and use of word of mouth. Taking the step to recruit in areas where minority candidates are reached is imperative and may help minimize any potential recruitment bias.

Once a candidate is identified, ensure clear and quick communication. Consider having a knowledgeable administrative staff member as well as a clinic faculty leader as point persons assigned to always be responsive to the candidate's inquiries. Be transparent about the position and the requirements and explicit about details such as relative value unit (RVU) goals, protected teaching or research time, and any other expectations.

Interview time requires putting the best foot forward. Have the candidate interview with faculty that have similar or complementary interest while emphasizing program diversity. Seeing a variety of faculty members supported by leadership to pursue many different academic endeavors will impress candidates.

The details of the interview day highly influence the candidate's opinion of the position and environment. The applicant's experience should be optimized from beginning to end. Hotel choice, friendly travel assistance, and shared meals with interested, engaged faculty will be critical. Use video technology when necessary, but prioritize in-person meetings.

Assessing and addressing special needs of candidates' family members are vital to success and retention.

Contract Negotiation

Once mutually interested, it is important to negotiate an appealing contract for both parties. Knowing the resources and the salary ranges available to offer and amount of protected time that can be supported is paramount prior to the negotiation. Within that context, be as flexible as possible to meet the needs of the candidate. Items such as remote work, flexible schedules, continuing education, and leadership opportunities are important to discuss. The candidate should leave the negotiation meeting feeling welcomed and understanding the expectations of the position itself.

Onboarding

The first few months of a faculty member's new position are an opportunity to build future success. Clear direction and strong support will help smooth the path for the new faculty member. Commitment, time, and attention to detail are needed in this phase just as they were required during recruitment.

Ensuring that the lines of communication are open will be very important in the first few months. The faculty member should have easy and quick access to the staff who are in charge of administrative tasks of onboarding. Assigning a mentor, such as the clinic medical director or another seasoned clinic faculty member who knows the ropes, will be helpful to ease the transition. A written manual for clinic faculty can be very effective as a way of organizing the information that needs to be relayed to the new member of the team. Such a manual could include items such as the following: lists of websites, phone numbers, and email groups to join; list of teaching/supervising/resident feedback responsibilities; clinical responsibilities when seeing own patients; list of staff/service resources; scheduling rules, processes, and guidelines (i.e., how to make any schedule adjustments); list of resources patients may need outside of clinic; how to use translation services; and how to use the electronic medical record (EMR) most efficiently in the clinic and resources to help, etc.

Other very important steps of the onboarding process are (1) introducing the new faculty member to the whole clinic, including support staff, residents, and faculty; (2) creating a reasonable clinical schedule with a gradual ramp-up to full productivity; (3) making sure that the EMR training is effective and ongoing (general and specific to the clinic); (4) sending an email to the department/division/medical center introducing the new faculty member; (5) introducing candidates to faculty in other clinics/divisions who share interests (work or nonwork related); (6) adding new faculty to critical email lists; and (7) ensuring that the new faculty can physically find their way in the health system.

During the onboarding period, it is the department and clinic leaders' responsibility to create effective and open lines of communication. Frequent and early check-ins will be the building blocks to success. These check-ins will create strong working relationships, will help identify issues that need attention quickly, and will forge a path towards an engaged and confident faculty member who feels empowered and supported by leadership.

Making Retention Possible

Prioritizing the well-being and satisfaction of the faculty in a teaching clinic will be paramount to increase retention and also enable recruitment. The Jackson Physician Search and Medical Management Association group survey identified the top three drivers of physician satisfaction with their employer as [5] (1) effective two-way communication between physician and management, (2) increased/adequate compensation, and (3) decreased administrative burden.

Sinsky C et al. recommended evidence-based approaches to reducing burnout and a focus on ensuring that each faculty feels valued by their organization as potential ways of retaining physicians and other health care workers [8].

Other key areas of focus to maximize retention and ensure adequate recruitment are (1) creating a culture of connection and flexibility, (2) optimizing the clinical environment, and (3) ensuring a mission-based care focus. These three areas are further described below:

Creating a Culture of Connection and Flexibility

It is imperative that leadership maintains strong effective communication strategies with their faculty. Long after onboarding is completed, frequent check-ins remain necessary. Such meetings will help to recognize burnout and to begin meaningful conversations regarding how to improve a struggling faculty member's situation. Showing care for the health and well-being of the faculty's whole family is essential. It is also important to recognize the natural shift in priorities that happens for any employee when their family is challenged by illness or other stressors. Providing flexibility in (1) place of work (practice site home, clinic, hospital); (2) time (part-time, nontraditional work schedules); and (3) job descriptions and career paths will help faculty adjust to challenging situations. If a faculty member does make the difficult decision to step away from work, leadership should try to ensure the stability of their position in the future and make reentry possible once the time arises.

Optimize Clinical Work Environments

Many academic continuity clinics are under-resourced and may not operate efficiently placing significant administrative burden on clinician educator faculty [9]. This can lead to decreased satisfaction and burnout detracting from faculty retention. Focusing specifically on the "quadruple aim" enhancing patient experience, improving population health, and reducing costs, but including work-life balance improvement, can be vital to retention [10]. Advocating for increased administrative and clinical support while involving faculty in quality and efficiency improvement programs may be helpful. Working in a culture which rewards collaborative cooperation amongst faculty (flexible coverage, peer support) creates a positive environment, which can go a long way towards offsetting any financial disincentives that may be inherent in the system. In an analysis of high-functioning primary care practices, the tenets of "Joy in Practice" indicated that optimization of clinical practice can be achieved via focusing on team-based care with distribution of clinical and clerical duties amongst team members, co-location of team members, nonphysician order entry, and enhanced team communication [11].

Ensuring a Mission-Based Care Focus

The sense of participation in a valued mission shared by the faculty as a whole is one of the strongest motivators for many faculty. Whether that be pride in providing the best teaching experience for trainees or, as in many teaching continuity clinics, dedicating the practice to care of vulnerable populations can create an atmosphere of collaboration and support that offsets the challenges of practicing in under-resourced environments. Leaders who identify these core missions and prominently highlight the importance of the mission may often be rewarded by faculty teams who dedicate themselves to providing the highest level of care and education.

Factors to Overcome Barriers to Faculty Recruitment and Retention

The AAIM/SGIM position paper published prior to the pandemic outlined seven factors to consider in order to overcome barriers to faculty recruitment and retention. These seven factors are summarized below [7]:

Value Teaching

One key element in demonstrating institutions placing value on ambulatory teaching is to provide adequate time and compensation for those providing this education. Studies note that teaching during a clinical session adds significant time and complexity to the workday. One study estimated that 30–50 min extra time was spent with learners embedded in an ambulatory clinical session [12]. Additionally, relative value unit (RVU)-based productivity may be compromised during teaching sessions. Clinical educators should not be "penalized" for teaching and should have protected time to teach. Systems which provide "teaching RVUs" to supplement clinical RVUs may be useful in offsetting decreased clinical productivity [13, 14]. Similarly, ramping down the number of patients scheduled per session can enhance teaching performance and highlight the value placed on such educational activity while decompressing clinical pressures. Another mechanism utilized is "mission-based funding," with specific salary support provided for those faculty regularly precepting learners, thus recognizing the inherent clinical productivity losses necessitated by time spent actively teaching and mentoring trainees. Indeed, paying faculty to teach is positively correlated with better teaching evaluations [15]. Freeing up faculty time by the use of scribes or advanced practice providers are other mechanisms to protect faculty time while demonstrating institutional commitment to support clinical teaching.

Career Development: Promotion and Tenure

Academic faculty with large clinical demands may still face traditional pressures to obtain research grants and publish formal peer-reviewed articles, which may not be feasible for clinicians focused on clinical care of patients and direct teaching of trainees.

Promotion criteria must be updated and upgraded to reflect the work of the teaching faculty, which includes recognizing a faculty member's support of the educational mission, curriculum development, mentoring, presentations, and completion of learner evaluations. Faculty members who exhibit excellence in teaching should be recognized and rewarded [16].

Faculty Development

Formal faculty development has been widely recognized as vital to the success of clinician educators and requires sufficient protected time for meaningful engagement. For clinical educators, faculty development should focus on teaching as educational skills, as they are often more comfortable with their clinical skills than with the skills required to teach effectively. Furthermore, implementation of measurement of Milestones, Entrusted Professional Activities, and other recent educational competency requirements may require faculty to learn new skills to function successfully in educational settings [17].

Faculty Mentoring

In addition to faculty development workshops, faculty mentorship must be highly developed in order to successfully retain talented faculty. A position paper published by the Association of Program Directors in Internal Medicine in 2010 on the redesign of residency education in internal medicine highlighted the importance of well-qualified clinician educators to mentor and help develop the skills of junior teaching faculty [18]. Components of peer observation and "learning communities" with an emphasis on faculty collaboration appear to be most successful in supporting clinician educators in their work. A systematic review on mentoring programs found that successful programs included mentor engagement, presence of a steering committee, mentor-mentee relationships, formal curricula, regularly scheduled mentoring activities, and dedicated program funding [19].

Innovative Clinical Learning Models

Recruiting and retaining faculty into sites with innovative clinical learning models which can enhance clinical care and education are an appealing mechanism for attracting faculty committed to clinical education. Innovative educational models which add variety to the teaching environment include use of nontraditional venues such as homeless clinics or prison clinics, incorporating medical students into a clinic, and incorporating specialty clinics or other primary care specialties into a clinic. Changing the resident schedules in clinic can also improve the learning environment; for example, clinics utilizing long block curriculum or increasingly popular X + Y block system can enhance continuity and resident satisfaction while decreasing the stress of simultaneous clinic and inpatient duties [20, 21].

Develop Faculty Interests

Faculty members may have specific niche interests that lend themselves well to the development of a specialized sub-clinic within the regular continuity clinic setting. Examples such as women's health, sports medicine, integrated behavioral care, and high-risk patient or procedure clinics have been reported. Faculty members with a passion in such areas can often spur educational interest amongst trainees and may lead to enhanced faculty satisfaction and retention.

Nonfinancial Incentives

Direct funding for clinician educators as mentioned is important in demonstrating institutional commitment to education. However, other mechanisms of incentivization of the faculty can be employed. Simple interventions such as providing an academic title can assist with career advancement. Providing teaching faculty with extra exam rooms or dedicated parking if possible and other simple recognitions can go a long way to demonstrate appreciation for the work provided. Ambulatory teaching awards, letters of recognition provided to departmental leadership, and certificates of appreciation are all inexpensive but effective interventions, which may enhance faculty satisfaction.

Conclusion

Ambulatory education in the continuity clinic setting is a vital part of medical training. Recruitment and retention of excellent clinician educators can be increasingly difficult. However, focusing on valuing clinician educators as demonstrated by protected teaching time, warding off clinical burnout, educational parity with other academic endeavors, rigorous faculty development, and promotion and tenure advancement, as well as nonfinancial incentives and mission-focused goals can enhance leaders' ability to recruit and retain the highest quality clinician educators. Excellent communication with faculty and flexibility focused on work-life balance are highly important factors in retaining happy productive faculty.

References

1. Willett LL, Carlos A, Estrada CA, Adams M, Arora V, Call S, Chacko K, Chaudhry S, Halvorsen AJ, Hopkins R, McDonald FS. Challenges with continuity clinic and core faculty accreditation requirements. Am J Med. 2013;126(6):550–6.
2. Klotz A. The Covid vaccine means a return to work. And a wave of resignations; 2021. https://www.nbcnews.com/think/opinion/covid-vaccine-means-return-work-wave-resignations-ncna1269018. Accessed 19 Sep 2022.
3. Sinsky CA, Shanafelt TD, Dyrbye LN, Sabety AH, Carlasare LE, West CP. Health care expenditures attributable to primary care physician overall and burnout-related turnover: a cross-sectional analysis, Mayo Clinic Proc, Published online 2/29/2022.
4. https://www.ama-assn.org/practice-management/physician-health/how-much-physician-burnout-costing-your-organization. Accessed 2022.
5. Misra-Hebert AD, Kay R, Stoller JK. A review of physician turnover: rates, causes, and consequence. Am J Med Qual. 2004;19(2):56–66.
6. Jackson Physician Search. Getting Ahead of Physician Turnover in Medical Practices Physician recruitment, engagement, retention and succession planning survey results. Jackson Physician Search in partnership with Medical Group Management Association (MGMA) Oct 19, 2021. https://www.jacksonphysiciansearch.com/white-paper-getting-ahead-of-physician-turnover-in-medical-practices-survey-results/. Accessed 2022.
7. Fazio S, Chheda S, Hingle S, Lo M, Meade L, Blanchard M, Hoellein A, Brandenburg S, Denton GD. The challenges of teaching ambulatory internal medicine: faculty recruitment, retention and development. An AAIM/SGIM position paper. AAIM perspectives. Am J Med. 2017;130(1):105–10.
8. Sinsky C, Brown R, Stillman M, Linzer M. COVID-related stress and work intentions in a sample of US health care workers. Mayo Clinic Proc. 2021;5(6):1165–73.
9. Nadkarni M, Reddy S, Bates CK, et al. Ambulatory-based education in internal medicine: current organization and implications for transformation. Results of a National Survey of Resident Continuity Clinic Directors. J Gen Intern Med. 2011;26(1):16–20.
10. Bodenheimer T, Sinsky C. From triple to quadruple aim: care of the patient requires care of the provider. Ann Fam Med. 2014;12(6):573–6.
11. Sinsky CA, Willard-Grace R, Schutzbank A, Sinsky TA, Margolius D, Bodenheimer T. In search of joy in practice: a report of 23 high-functioning primary care practices. Ann Fam Med. 2013;11:272–8.
12. Bowen JL, Irby DM. Assessing quality and costs of education in the ambulatory setting: a review of the literature. Acad Med. 2002;77:621–80.
13. Yeh MM, Cahill DF. Quantifying physician teaching productivity using clinical relative value units. J Gen Intern Med. 1999;14:617–21.
14. Osborn LM, Sostok M, Castellano PZ, et al. Recruiting and retaining clinician-educators. Lessons learned from three programs. J Gen Intern Med. 1997;12(Suppl 2):S83–9.
15. Ashar B, Levine R, Magaziner J, Shochet R, Wright S. An association between paying physician-teachers for their teaching efforts and an improved educational experience for learners. J Gen Intern Med. 2007;22(10):1393–7.
16. Bowen JL, Salerno SM, Chamberlain JK, et al. Changing habits of practice. Transforming internal medicine residency education in ambulatory settings. J Gen Intern Med. 2005;20(12):1181–7.
17. Holmboe ES, Ward DS, Reznick RK, et al. Faculty development in assessment: the missing link in competency-based medical education. Acad Med. 2011;86(4):460–7.
18. Fitzgibbons JP, Bordley DR, Berkowitz LR, Berkowitz LR, Miller BW, Henderson MC. Redesigning residency education in internal medicine: a position paper from the Association of Program Directors in Internal Medicine. Ann Intern Med. 2006;144:920–6.
19. Sambunjak D, Straus SE, Marušić A. Mentoring in academic medicine: a systematic review. JAMA. 2006;296(9):1103–15.

20. Chaudhry SI, Balwan S, Friedman KA, Sunday S, Chaudhry B, Dimisa D, Fornari A. Moving forward in GME reform: a 4+1 model of resident ambulatory training. J Gen Intern Med. 2013;28(8):1100–4.
21. Harrison J, Ramaiya A, Cronkright P. Restoring emphasis on ambulatory internal medicine training—the 3:1 model. J Grad Med Edu. 2014;6(4):742–5.

Part II
Operational Management

Chapter 4
Academic Scheduling Models: Challenges and Solutions

Craig F. Noronha, Mamta K. Singh, and William G. Weppner

Introduction

Scheduling models for continuity clinics have expanded over the past few decades, ranging from the traditional one half-day per week model to versions of more intense clinic immersion experiences or "X + Y" block models. These seek to balance consistency and access for patients with the increasingly important goals of decreasing simultaneous inpatient and outpatient duties, as well as supporting team and patient continuity and resident wellness. While no one cookie-cutter approach is likely to solve all the challenges a program faces, this chapter reviews different models and the available evidence (or lack thereof) of impacts on important patient and resident outcomes.This chapter reviews ACGME requirements for resident scheduling with a focus on the ambulatory experience. The authors describe the most common scheduling models and illustrate the benefits and challenges with each model. The chapter also highlights a few curricular opportunities that align with ambulatory schedules. A review of recent literature will highlight the impact of scheduling models.

C. F. Noronha (✉)
Department of Medicine, Internal Medicine Residency Program, Boston Medical Center, Boston University Chobanian & Avedisian School of Medicine, Boston, MA, USA
e-mail: craig.noronha@bmc.org

M. K. Singh
Department of Medicine /Primary Care, VA Northeast Ohio Health Care System, Case Western Reserve University School of Medicine, Cleveland, OH, USA
e-mail: Mamta.singh@case.edu

W. G. Weppner
Education, Academic Hospitalist & Geriatrics/Palliative Care Sections, Boise VAMC, Department of Medicine, University of Washington School of Medicine, Boise, ID, USA
e-mail: William.Weppner@va.gov

L. B. Lu et al. (eds.), *Leading an Academic Medical Practice*,
https://doi.org/10.1007/978-3-031-40273-9_4

Outline

- The Accreditation Council for Graduate Medical Education (ACGME) common program requirements
- Current scheduling models
  - Traditional
  - Hybrid
  - X + Y
  - Ambulatory long block
- Evidence of impact:
  - Satisfaction
  - Educational outcomes

    Duty hours and resident wellness
    Systems-based practice and practice-based learning and improvement
    Primary care or ambulatory specialty interest of graduate

  - Clinical outcomes

    Access
    Continuity
    Quality of care
    Diabetic care

- Opportunities provided by scheduling models
  - Non-traditional clinic experiences
  - Specialty clinics
- Conclusion

Common Program Requirements

The Accreditation Council for Graduate Medical Education (ACGME) is a private not-for-profit organization that "sets the standards for US graduate medical education programs and renders accreditation decisions based on compliance with these standards" [1]. The ACGME creates a set of common program requirements that all residency programs must comply with in order to maintain certification. The July 2022 program requirements include several substantial changes including scheduling models and continuity clinic requirements (Box 4.1) [2]. Among the ACGME suggestions for scheduling include encouraging programs to reduce conflicts between inpatient and outpatient responsibilities. They provide specific options including creating schedules that "provide more continuity clinic experiences or an exclusive continuity clinic experience when residents are not on inpatient rotations" [2].

The ACGME has made a concerted effort to create opportunities for residents to engage in individualized training that may prepare them for their intended future career paths. The ACGME requires programs to provide "at least six months of individualized educational experiences to participate in opportunities relevant to their future practice or to further skill/competency development in the foundational areas." Furthermore, the ACGME changed the requirements for a continuity clinic experience to a more generic outpatient setting requirement as opposed to the more prescribed requirement of 130 total clinic sessions in a primary care setting that was required in previous iterations. The ACGME provides several examples of what satisfies outpatient experiences including internal medicine subspecialty clinic, home visits, or even non-medicine clinics [2].

These relaxed regulations potentially provide programs more flexibility with scheduling while also tailoring residency training to trainee-specific interests. The new ACGME requirements indicate that programs provide at least 10 months of outpatient clinical experiences. The requirements highlight that if continuity clinic experiences in a primary care clinic can count towards the required 10 months, then each month is equal to 40 half-day continuity clinic experiences. Residents must have a longitudinal, continuity experience for the duration of their residency training. Thus, if the resident experience is solely located in a continuity clinic setting without other outpatient experiences, they would be required to fulfill 400 total clinics. The author suspects that most programs will aim for a mixture of ambulatory experiences to meet the requirements of 10 total months. To this end, the ACGME specifically notes that 1 month in a subspecialty clinic counts as 1 month of outpatient clinical experience. The individualized educational experiences can count as part of the outpatient requirements if the experiences occur in the ambulatory setting. The ACGME allows for flexibility with outpatient training schedules if they meet the program requirements. This allows programs to utilize systems such as ambulatory long blocks, X + Y scheduling models, or hybrid models to meet these requirements [3–7].

Box 4.1 ACGME Internal Medicine 2022 Requirements

ACGME Internal Medicine Scheduling Requirements—effective July first, 2022 [2].

Total clinical experiences	At least 30 months
Clinical experiences in the outpatient setting	At least 10 months
Longitudinal team-based continuity experience	Duration of the residency training
Continuity clinic experience	1 month = 40 clinics
Individualized educational experiences	At least 6 months

Current Scheduling Models

The flexibility of the new ACGME requirements and the need to reduce the inpatient and outpatient rotation tension have led to different models for ambulatory scheduling. Clinical sites are moving away from the traditional half-day rotations (described below) and adopting a "X plus Y" model, immersive or block or hybrid model [4, 5]. The traditional scheduling model, often dubbed "visitor in clinic," has been shown to contribute to the perception of chaotic ambulatory experiences and can lead to trainee dissatisfaction. This further prompted innovative schedules to reduce the tension between inpatient and outpatient clinical duties [8]. Transitioning to these models within a residency program is a complex process that involves faculty and staff in both the inpatient and outpatient arenas. Thus, programs must carefully weigh the pros and cons for each of the scheduling models to determine what is best for each institution. The authors recommend spending at least a year planning any major schedule changes prior to initiation of a new model, based on our experience with schedule transitions.

Traditional Scheduling

In a traditional scheduling model, residents are scheduled for one half-day of continuity clinic per week throughout their residency. Residents are expected to hand off their inpatient duties to a covering resident or nonresident provider on the particular half-day of their continuity clinic each week. Certain rotations and call schedules may dictate that the resident returns to their inpatient duties after the clinic session. As we could imagine doing the "flip," where a resident spends their time in outpatient and returns to the wards once a week to admit patients, we can see how dysfunctional this approach seems. Invariably, there will be scheduling issues that cannot be reconciled leading to clinic cancelations. The most common issues include cancelations of clinic if the resident is post-call, in an intensive care unit rotation, or possibly on call where they are expected to be admitting patients in the hospital in the afternoon. Other examples include rotations such as night float or away rotations. Inherent in this model is a conflict between the inpatient and outpatient settings [9].

A resident may be caring for a sick inpatient and feel pressure to leave for clinic to see his or her scheduled patients. Similarly, the resident may feel pressure to leave clinic quickly if they are expected to go back to their inpatient rotation after clinic. This typically includes travel between sites, which adds to stress and time and may lead to issues with work-hour restrictions. Covering team members may have an increase in workload with the additional patient care duties, and this may increase stress on the inpatient team. Within this traditional model, some programs may call on residents to cover the inpatient duties of the clinic resident, leading to some discontinuity for the inpatient service. However, in the traditional model, the clinic may pair preceptors with residents on specific half-days, which may be beneficial for continuity between the teaching pairs. The traditional model also provides some predictability, knowing that the resident usually will be there each week.

Hybrid Models

There are multiple programs that use hybrid models integrating combinations of the traditional scheduling model, the ambulatory long block, and the X + Y model. The hybrid model is often a safe transition for programs that cannot abruptly change their schedule to a different structure, especially with a specific cohort of residents. Some programs utilize a traditional scheduling model for the PGY-1 and then transition the PGY-2 and PGY-3 residents into an X + Y model. A hybrid model might be employed by a residency program to allow some flexibility in scheduling, with a more intensive period of clinic exposure. This can be part of efforts to orient residents to clinic at the beginning of residency or to provide them with greater exposure at other times. Some programs follow a traditional model and integrate month-long ambulatory blocks throughout the residency, for example, one long block per postgraduate year so that there would be at least three ambulatory long blocks during the course of residency. Another option is to include multiple ambulatory long blocks in the third year of residency. Yet another alternative is the 1 + 1 model where residents alternate nonambulatory months with ambulatory months. Continuity clinic is only scheduled during ambulatory blocks in this 1 + 1 model. In any hybrid model, consideration should be given to variations in the number of preceptors required and clinic space availability based upon when the long blocks fall.

X + Y Model

This model has become the most popular over the years with about greater than 44% of programs using this scheduling model [4]. In an X + Y scheduling model, the X represents the number of continuous weeks of the nonambulatory portion of the schedule including inpatient wards, ICU rotations, night float rotations, and inpatient electives. The Y represents the number of continuous weeks in the continuity clinic and possibly other ambulatory experiences before returning to the inpatient setting. There are different versions of X + Y models such as 3 + 1, 4 + 2, 5 + 1, and 6 + 2 models. In each case, the Y portion entails a concentrated block of ambulatory clinics and ambulatory experiences. The Y can be scheduled in various ways depending on the resources available. Based on surveys and discussion at the Society of General Internal Medicine Clinic Directors Interest Group, there are typically at least four half-days of continuity clinic per week, and some programs may schedule up to eight sessions per week. Unlike the traditional model, the timing of continuity clinics can be more flexible, allowing for morning clinics and evening clinics without adversely impacting inpatient schedules or work-hour restrictions. Aside from continuity clinics, other unique or specialty clinic opportunities can be built into the ambulatory Y week. Examples include rotations through specialty clinics (e.g., rheumatology clinic), outside community and underserved clinic rotations, and even a second continuity clinic, thus improving residents' exposure to multiple ambulatory settings. Some programs have designed the subspecialty rotations such that the residents rotate through multiple specialty clinics during their residency, doing specific ambulatory blocks in each specialty. For instance, an intern may rotate through three to four different specialties and then rotate through other specialty clinics during their second and third years of residency. Each clinic must also decide on how to schedule preceptors within this model. Some programs have utilized the traditional model where the attendings precept one to two sessions per week and attend clinic every week. This allows preceptors to meet most residents in the program from different Y weeks but also reduces the responsibility they have for any specific group of residents. A more complex scheduling model is to have the preceptors rotate on the same schedule as the residents. For example, in a 3 + 1 system (see Box 4.2), the attendings would have their usual continuity and/or inpatient schedule for the 3 weeks or X part of the model. Then during the Y week, they would ideally precept four or more sessions with the same group of residents. This model improves the continuity between the preceptor and resident given that at least 10% of the trainees' residency will be with the same preceptor or preceptor group. Given these alignment needs, this type of scheduling may be more complicated for the preceptors as it may impact access for their own patients. There are several other advantages and disadvantages to the X + Y scheduling model (Table 4.1).

Table 4.1 Advantages/disadvantages of X + Y scheduling models

Advantages	Disadvantages
Regularly interspersed periods of clinic with weekend (and holidays) off during ambulatory block	Perception of more limited elective time (if ambulatory clinic elective time not counted)
More easily allows for morning, afternoon, and/or evening clinics	Weekend night float/medicine/call transition from wards can limit Monday clinics and electives
Most permutations may work with commonly used 13-block system to allow for scheduling compatibility with other residency programs	May not exactly match ward rotations for collaborating residency programs that are not using a similar X + Y base
Allows for integrated resident cohorts; they may cover for each other when away from clinic and offer more exposure to a smaller group of co-residents for cohesion in a larger program	Interaction of residents in different cohorts may be more limited, if they are not rearranged periodically in the schedule or geographic locations
Fixed clinic scheduling makes identifying follow-up appointments easier in most cases (e.g., within 1 week for close follow-up or in 4/8/12/16/etc. week intervals for a 3 + 1 system, or 5/10/15/20/etc. for a 4 + 1 system)	Limited patient access for acute visits, follow-up calls, completion of forms for the X week period between Y clinic weeks

Table 4.1 (continued)

Advantages	Disadvantages
Better use of resident clinic room space by making it easier to schedule a consistent number of residents each week	Decreases the ability of residents to swap rotations with other residents outside of their cohort
Allows for scheduling of related ambulatory "elective" half-days in specialty settings	Requires programs to find high-quality half-day experiences for residents for non-continuity clinic half-days
Permits flexibility for recurring didactic, quality improvement, panel management lessons; this includes having a set academic half-day to collaborate with faculty or other programs	Requires programs to have staff and support supervision of half-day didactics, quality improvement, and panel management sessions
Increased appreciation for clinic by residents, with decreased perceived conflict with inpatient duties	Increased stress on clinic staff in the management of patients between ambulatory (Y) weeks
Allows for scheduled time off for resident wellness, or personal half-days for appointments, testing, interviews	May convey perception that continuity clinic is "optional" compared to other duties, unless criteria to balance out cancellations are used
Increased appreciation for clinic by residents, decreased stress from transitions between inpatient and ambulatory settings	Increased stress on clinic staff in the management of patients between ambulatory blocks (Y weeks)

Box 4.2 Description of a 3 + 1 Schedule

For each level of resident (R1, R2, R3), we instituted a "3 + 1" schedule which consisted of 3 weeks of more intensive call months (wards/ICU/night medicine) or 3 weeks of electives, which were split by 1 week of ambulatory clinic. During this "+1" ambulatory week, residents typically have 5 half-days of continuity clinic, 1 half-day of dedicated didactics, and 3 half-days of ambulatory electives. Depending on the level of the trainee, dedicated time for required half-day "selectives" (women's health, telehealth, addictions clinic, quality improvement) is assigned. Senior residents also participate in an evening continuity clinic, which permits a half-day off during another part of the week, allowing a longer weekend or daytime off for residents to schedule activities outside of work.

During the 1-week clinic block, approximately half the time is spent in the continuity clinic. There are 3–4 half-days of continuity clinic with two to seven patient visits, depending on the resident level. The "virtual clinic" has one or two face-to-face clinic appointments, and then dedicated time for telemedicine visits, telephone calls, secure messaging, and administrative time. The other half of the ambulatory block time can be used for a flexible schedule of ambulatory electives, didactics, group visits, or panel management time. For example, during a 1-week block, the resident might rotate through four or more affiliated clinics, including more traditional specialties such as gastroenterology, cardiology, nephrology, and dermatology; affiliated services may include insulin titration clinic with a clinical pharmacist, hyperlipidemia clinic, behavioral health clinics such as smoking cessation, endoscopy, physical therapy, women's health clinic, pacemaker clinic, and podiatry, to give some examples. While this does not give trainees an "in-depth" understanding of each discipline, it offers residents exposure to the available services and resources and may improve appropriate use of referrals. It can also serve as a way to "sample" electives that residents may not be exposed to with traditional clinic scheduling systems. Residents may have more choice during the ambulatory block to tailor their clinic sessions to see other clinics, and this may help with career choices. For example, morning clinics are possible because of lack of conflict with morning rounds seen in traditional systems. Evening clinics for patients are also possible, allowing for flexibility in administrative time during the workweek. It is also possible to schedule recurring half-day conferences during ambulatory block for didactics, quality improvement, and panel management. Often, X + Y schedules create "cohorts" of R1/R2/R3s that tend to be together during clinic rotations and possibly the ward as well as educational sessions. This allows members from different cohorts to cross cover in the clinic while the others are away from clinic. For example, in a 3 + 1 schedule, four cohorts of resident groups are created; the residents that are in clinic can be assigned to cover three other residents that are out of clinic on wards, elective or vacation. This can be to cover their colleagues' paperwork, follow up on results, and attend to electronic health record notifications, and even for face-to-face visits for patients with urgent issues.

Ambulatory Long Block

The "ambulatory long block" was created as part of the ACGME's Educational Innovations Projects (EIP) in 2006 [6]. Several residency programs initially trialed the model, and other programs have adopted variations since then. In an ambulatory long block model, residents follow the traditional model of primary care clinics, with one afternoon clinic per week, and then intermittently have weeklong blocks of ambulatory experiences. Another example is the yearlong ambulatory long block where residents follow a traditional residency model with once-weekly afternoon clinics until midway through the second year of residency (Box 4.3). At the midpoint of the second year of residency, they start a 12-month continuous ambulatory clinic schedule until the midpoint of the third year. Given that the long block spans the last 6 months of the PGY-2 and the first 6 months of the PGY-3, there will always be either second-year or third-year residents on the ambulatory long block throughout the academic year. The long block consists of three or more half-day clinics per week for 12 months. During the times when the residents are not in clinic, they rotate on electives and research blocks. In these ambulatory long block periods, due to an increase of the time that the resident is present in the clinic, there is often increased access for their continuity patients. The non-continuity clinic portions of the long block can be designed according to available opportunities (and programmatic needs) in both the outpatient and inpatient setting. There is typically an equal number of residents on the ambulatory long block throughout the academic year, and there is ideally little or no fluctuation in preceptor needs.

Box 4.3 Description of a 12 + 12 Schedule
The Cleveland VA medical Center's of Education in primary care implemented a block immersion model at the program's onset in 2012. Each 12-week block of outpatient experience alternates with a 12-week inpatient experience. Internal medicine residents have one block in postgraduate year 1 (PGY-1), two blocks in PGY-2, and one block in PGY-3. The residents do not have continuity clinic when assigned to inpatient experiences. Cleveland was granted an Accreditation Council for Graduate Medical Education (ACGME) waiver to allow for 12-week absences from continuity clinic. Residents in this practice partnership model are assigned a panel of patients together over 3 years. Each resident pair shares an assigned IM faculty member who provides oversight and supervision. While on the 12-week ambulatory rotation, residents do three half-days of primary care, one half-day of geriatrics or women's health, two half-days of urgent care, one half-day of elective rotation in a subspecialty clinic, one half-day of self-directed learning, one half-day of panel management, and one half-day of didactic lectures in an interprofessional setting.

Evidence of Impact

There are several examples of programs transitioning from traditional to newer models of scheduling in the literature. Many share pre/post-outcomes, which are context specific, but still provide important insights when choosing a model that works for a given program.

Satisfaction

Clinic block scheduling is associated with improved team development and improved learning opportunities [6, 10]. Patient satisfaction evidence is mixed; in one study, it was similar between block and traditional models, but not as good as in a combined system [11]. In another pilot, there was a suggestion of improved patient satisfaction [6].

Clinic block scheduling models are associated with improved resident satisfaction compared to traditional scheduling models [12]. Additionally, there is improved faculty perception of the educational value of clinic [13, 14]. Much of this is likely related to decreased stress of abruptly leaving inpatient duties, decreased distraction by conflicting needs of both inpatient and outpatient care, and improved comfort and empowerment based on time spent in a designated clinical setting. These improvements support a reported increased interest in primary care by residents participating in a block system. Residents reported improved perception that ambulatory medicine is enjoyable to practice [13]. There is also evidence that a dedicated primary care pathway emphasizing clinic block scheduling is associated with an increase in interest in primary care as a career choice [15]. However, there are no published data related to X + Y scheduling and the ambulatory long block data that supports an increased interest in primary care careers. The Association of Program Directors in Internal Medicine 2015 annual survey did not reveal any program director perception of increased interest in primary care careers in programs utilizing X + Y scheduling models [4].

Educational Outcomes

Duty Hours and Resident Wellness

It stands to reason that block ambulatory rotations without night float duties or on-call responsibilities will have a positive impact on resident sleep cycles and well-being. Block rotations have been shown to reduce sleep disturbances, regain diurnal sleep cycle, and improve well-being [12].

Systems-Based Practice and Practice-Based Learning and Improvement

Another advantage of dedicated ambulatory rotations is the opportunity for residents to work with interprofessional team members and develop a continuity panel. This "empanelment" process creates opportunities to engage in population health discussions, practice-based learning improvements at the panel level, or clinic-wide quality improvement (QI) initiatives [16, 17]. As residents have more immersive time in clinic, it allows them to identify system barriers, which they may have been impervious to during half-day clinics. This creates a natural environment to learn QI. As competencies such as practice-based learning improvement and systems-based practice remain challenging to assess in learners, block rotations may have an added benefit of providing an ideal venue to teach QI and help meet these core ACGME competencies [2].

Primary Care Interest or Ambulatory Specialty Interest of Graduate

All these improvements potentially support increased interest in primary care by residents participating in a block system. Residents reported improved perception that ambulatory medicine is enjoyable to practice [15]. There is also evidence that a dedicated primary care pathway emphasizing clinic block scheduling is associated with an increase in interest in primary care as a career choice [18]. However, there is no published data related to X + Y scheduling and the ambulatory long block data that supports an increased interest in primary care careers. There is evidence that continuity of relationships with patients is a strong predictor of likelihood to enter primary care [19].

Clinical Outcomes

Access

Patient's access to care appears to increase in the block system; there are reports of decreased no-show rates [6] and more opportunities for clinical encounters by residents [20]. Residents reported improved patient access to care and improved empanelment, or a more consistent cohort of patients that is assigned to them [13, 14]. Developing a means to schedule acute visits via a practice partner system, in which the attending or other linked provider is prioritized to see the patient, can help to maximize within-team continuity with providers and team members more closely linked to the resident provider. Either way, maintaining access for acute care needs is necessary and may require extra effort to include the primary care provider via sharing of clinic notes to maintain educational understanding of the patient's course.

Continuity

The evidence related to continuity between residents and patients is mixed but overall supports an improvement in continuity, either perceived or measured. One report of a 1-year ambulatory care block pilot program improved visit continuity as defined by increased number of visits with the patient's primary provider, as well as a higher percentage of all visits with that primary provider [6]. However, some changes to X + Y scheduling models have decreased continuity from the patient perspective while simultaneously improving continuity from resident perspective [11, 18, 20, 21]. This means that although a resident in an X + Y system may have more of their clinic slots taken up by their panel, from the patients' perspective, they see that resident less frequently, because they see other providers instead during the X period while the resident is away. A conclusion is that residents in a block system are more likely to have continuity for routine follow-up visits but less likely for acute care visits occurring during the "X" part of the clinic block. Other types of continuity may benefit as well; there is better follow-up on diagnostic tests by residents, better perceived educational continuity, and reduced fragmentation of care in both the inpatient and outpatient settings [13, 14, 20].

Quality of Care

The ultimate goal of internal medicine residency training is to train physicians who will improve patient-related outcomes through high-quality care. Ideally, clinical performance measures and outcomes would be utilized to assess individual trainees and at a larger level potentially evaluate the quality of training for an entire residency program [22, 23]. However, the "challenges of defining, extracting, and measuring clinical performance" are barriers to their use in educational assessment [24]. Despite these limitations, there have been a handful of studies that have attempted to measure the impact of residency scheduling models on clinical outcomes.

Comparison of Scheduling Models in Care of Patients with Diabetes

A 2016 study by Francis et al. compared three diabetic outcomes based on scheduling on 4 models in 12 internal medicine programs [25]. The scheduling models compared were traditional weekly experience; the ambulatory long block, hybrid schedules with a combination of weekly experiences plus additional ambulatory block rotations; and a block or X + Y structure with discrete inpatient and ambulatory rotations. They demonstrated no major differences in overall glycemic control. The block or X + Y scheduling model demonstrated significantly higher performance in several measures including percentage of patients with an LDL <100, percentage of diabetic patients with blood pressure < 130/80, and percentage of patients who had A1c measured in the last year [25].

Ambulatory Long Block

The ambulatory long block was assessed extensively by Warm et al. [6] for both educational and clinical outcomes. They demonstrated an improvement in a variety of process measures and clinical measures including improved diabetes control, increased number of patients with blood pressures within goal, and completion of age-appropriate cancer screening rates. It should be noted that while most reported measures improved after the implementation of the ambulatory long block, a few process measures such as semiannual HbA1cs in 1 year and influenza vaccination rates actually worsened [6].

50:50 Outpatient-Inpatient Model

Wieland et al. studied and evaluated several educational and clinical measures in relation to the implementation of a 50:50 outpatient-inpatient model [18]. They demonstrated no significant improvement in multiple clinical outcomes including blood pressure control and cancer screening.

Opportunities Provided by Scheduling Models

The most recent ACGME updates to internal medicine program requirements are less prescriptive allowing residency programs and clinics to be more flexible and innovative in designing resident schedules [2]. It is important for leadership from both the resident clinic and residency program to work together to take full advantage of opportunities within scheduling models. We will highlight some specific examples of nontraditional opportunities that can be considered within residency training.

Nontraditional Clinic Experiences

The ACGME does not specify when clinics should be scheduled in terms of time of day or days of the week. Resident clinics could potentially be scheduled for evening sessions. At first glance, this may not appear to be appealing to both faculty and residents, but in fact clinicians may favor swapping a morning session for an evening session. An evening clinic is not possible in a traditional schedule where residents have both inpatient and outpatient requirements on the same day. However, in ambulatory long block, hybrid, and X + Y scheduling models, this may be a valuable option. Another option, while less favorable, may be weekend clinic sessions. Any consideration of weekend clinics should be discussed with all stakeholders to ensure that all factors including resident well-being and overall schedule requirements are considered. A weekend clinic in the first weekend of a two-week ambulatory block would be more accepting compared to a weekend clinic on the last weekend before a resident starts an inpatient rotation. A weekend session will most likely be less desirable than a weekday clinic, so trade-offs such as converting two weekday clinics to one weekend session may be acceptable to a resident.

Other options to consider include ambulatory time focused on panel management and population health within the context of the primary clinic experience. For example, residents can spend time focused on managing patients with diabetes via telephone or electronic messaging. Other options include residents working hand in hand with clinic-based population health managers to develop interventions to improve cancer screening rates in their patient panel [26]. Ambulatory time may be reserved for huddles with primary care team members to plan population health interventions or identify specific patient needs in advance of a clinic session [27, 28].

Specialty Clinics

The ACGME requirements have placed a heavy emphasis on individualized training and experiences in specialty care. In fact, the specification that each ambulatory month equates to 40 primary care clinics makes it almost impossible to exclusively utilize a standard primary care clinic to meet all the ambulatory requirements. Resident clinic directors and residency leadership should consider alternative options for ambulatory experiences both within the primary care setting and in other ambulatory settings. Within a primary care clinic, there could be specialized clinics such as office-based substance use disorder treatment clinics, women's health, procedure clinics, or refugee clinics that could all potentially provide unique ambulatory-based training opportunities.

Outside of the primary care clinic setting, rotations in internal medicine subspecialties and non-internal medicine specialties are potential options to enhance resident ambulatory experiences. The ACGME requirements allow residents to develop individualized training matching their future career goals. For instance, a resident interested in cardiology may have a longitudinal cardiology clinic-based rotation throughout their residency. A resident interested in rheumatology may spend time in an orthopedic clinic or physical therapy clinic to provide supplemental opportunities outside of internal medicine training.

Conclusion

There are various scheduling models that can be used in internal medicine residency programs, each with their own benefits and challenges. More recent scheduling models, such as X + Y block models, are designed to increase the amount of time in ambulatory settings while simultaneously reducing the tensions between inpatient and outpatient care responsibilities. Residency programs must work hand in hand with clinic directors to optimize each scheduling model to meet multiple goals including providing excellent patient care, supporting training in ambulatory settings, and maintaining trainee wellness.

References

1. Accreditation Council for Graduate Medical Education. https://www.acgme.org/about-us/overview/#:~:text=The Accreditation Council for Graduate, medical care to all Americans. Accessed 8 May 2022.
2. ACGME Program Requirements for Graduate Medical Education in Internal Medicine. https://www.acgme.org/Portals/0/PFAssets/ProgramRequirements/140_InternalMedicine_2022.pdf?ver=2021-02-19-152614-193.
3. Ray A, Jones D, Palamara K, Overland M, Steinberg KP (2016) Improving Ambulatory Training in Internal Medicine: X + Y (or Why Not?) Despite the Accreditation Council for Graduate Medical. J Gen Intern Med 31:1519–1541.
4. Noronha C, Chaudhry S, Chacko K, McGarry K, Agrawal A, Yadavalli G, Shalaby M. X + Y scheduling models in internal medicine residency programs: a National Survey of program directors' perspectives. Am J Med. 2018;131:107–14.

5. Shalaby M, Yaich S, Donnelly J, Chippendale R, DeOliveira MC, Noronha C. X+Y scheduling models for internal medicine residency programs-a look Back and a look forward. J Grad Med Educ. 2014;6:639–42.
6. Warm EJ, Schauer DP, Diers T, Mathis BR, Neirouz Y, Boex JR, Rouan GW. The ambulatory long-block: an accreditation council for Graduate Medical Education (ACGME) Educational Innovations Project (EIP). J Gen Intern Med. 2008;23:921–6.
7. Thomas KG, West CP, Popkave C, Bellini LM, Weinberger SE, Kolars JC, Kogan JR. Alternative approaches to ambulatory training: internal medicine residents' and program directors' perspectives. J Gen Intern Med. 2009;24:904–10.
8. Keirns CC, Bosk CL. The unintended consequences of training residents in dysfunctional outpatient settings. Acad Med. 2008;83:498–502.
9. Keirns CC, Bosk CL. Perspective: the unintended consequences of training residents in dysfunctional outpatient settings. Acad Med. 2008;83:498–502.
10. Mariotti JL, Shalaby M, Fitzgibbons JP. The 4:1 schedule: a novel template for internal medicine residencies. J Grad Med Educ. 2010;2:541.
11. Francis MD, Thomas K, Langan M, et al. Clinic design, key practice metrics, and resident satisfaction in internal medicine continuity clinics: findings of the educational innovations project ambulatory collaborative. J Grad Med Educ. 2014;6:249–55.
12. Bordley J, Agustin AG, Ahmed MA, Khalid R, Paluso AM, Kobza BS, Spaugy AW, Emens J, Desai SS, Khan A. Restoration of resident sleep and wellness with block scheduling. Med Educ. 2017;51:1241–9.
13. Mariotti JL, Shalaby M, Fitzgibbons JP. The 4:1 schedule: a novel template for internal medicine residencies. J Gr Med Educ. 2010;2:541–7.
14. Chaudhry SI, Balwan S, Friedman KA, Sunday S, Chaudhry B, Dimisa D, Fornari A. Moving forward in GME reform: a 4 + 1 model of resident ambulatory training. J Gen Intern Med. 2013;28:1100–4.
15. Brislen H, Dunn A, Parada A, Rendon P. Addressing the primary care shortage on a shoestring: a successful track in an internal medicine residency. Acad Med. 2016;91:224–8.
16. Kaminetzky CP, Beste LA, Poppe AP, Doan DB, Mun HK, Woods NF, Wipf JE. Implementation of a novel population panel management curriculum among interprofessional health care trainees. BMC Med Educ. 2017;17:264. https://doi.org/10.1186/S12909-017-1093-Y.
17. Watts B, Lawrence RH, Singh S, Wagner C, Augustine S, Singh MK. Implementation of quality improvement skills by primary care teams: case study of a large academic practice. J Prim Care Community Heal. 2014;5:101–6.
18. Wieland ML, Halvorsen AJ, Chaudhry R, Reed DA, Mcdonald FS, Thomas KG. An evaluation of internal medicine residency continuity clinic redesign to a 50/50 outpatient–inpatient model. Springer. 2009;28:1014. https://doi.org/10.1007/s11606-012-2312-1.
19. Peccoralo LA, Tackett S, Ward L, Federman A, Helenius I, Christmas C, Thomas DC. Resident satisfaction with continuity clinic and career choice in general internal medicine. J Gen Intern Med. 2013;28:1020–7.
20. Heist K, Guese M, Nikels M, Swigris R, Chacko K. Impact of 4+1 block scheduling on patient care continuity in resident clinic. J Gen Intern Med. 2014;29:1195–9.
21. Wieland M, Jaeger T, Bundrick J. Resident physician perspectives on outpatient continuity of care. J Grad Med Educ. 2013;4:668–73.
22. Warm EJ, Mathis BR. Ambulatory education: time to move from process to outcome. J Grad Med Educ. 2019;11:143–5.
23. Simpson D, Sullivan GM, Artino AR, Deiorio NM, Yarris LM. Envisioning graduate medical education in 2030. J Grad Med Educ. 2020;12:235–40.
24. Smirnova A, Sebok-Syer SS, Chahine S, et al. Defining and adopting clinical performance measures in graduate medical education: where are we now and where are we going? Acad Med. 2019;94:671–7.

25. Francis MD, Julian KA, Wininger DA, et al. Continuity clinic model and diabetic outcomes in internal medicine residencies: findings of the educational innovations project ambulatory collaborative. J Grad Med Educ. 2016;8:27.
26. Strout EKH, Landrey AR, MacLean CD, Sobel HG. Internal medicine resident experiences with a 5-month ambulatory panel management curriculum. J Grad Med Educ. 2018;10:559–65.
27. Gupta R, Laponis R, Ratanawongsa N, Davis E, Horton C. Teaching teamwork: enhancing resident continuity training in an urban academic clinic. J Gen Intern Med. 2012;27:S567.
28. Goldberg DG, Beeson T, Kuzel AJ, Love LE, Carver MC. Team-based care: a critical element of primary care practice. Transformation. https://home.liebertpub.com/pop. 2013;16:150–6.

Chapter 5
Management of Refills and Electronic Medical Record in-Basket Messages

Chad Henson Martins, Elizabeth Bowles, and M. Danielle King

Introduction

The intervisit interval is underrepresented in formal ambulatory care curricula. This is the time during which the negotiated plan of care will be implemented, monitored, and titrated. It is human nature to focus on matters directly before us, relegating intervisit patient care to the status of afterthought both in professional practice where providers are expected to complete intervisit task in the moments between face-to-face care and in ambulatory care curricula where formal teaching on the intervisit period is uncommon. Both these situations are unfortunate and inappropriate. The intervisit period is a time to strengthen patient-provider relationships, encourage patient engagement in healthcare, and achieve the connectedness with patients that drew providers to outpatient continuity practice. In graduate medical education, the intervisit period is rife with opportunities to learn the skills, knowledge, and attitude to prepare trainees for outpatient practice. It is crucial that the management of patients *between* visits be given dedicated time and similar amounts of support as face-to-face encounters. It is also important that these tasks be framed accurately as representative of the practice of outpatient medicine. The tasks are not scut work or some other demeaningly labeled activity. Refilling medications, reporting results of testing, and responding to patient communications are opportunities for trainees to practice clinical reasoning, grow communication skills, build rapport,

C. H. Martins · E. Bowles (✉)
Primary Care, Alexandria Louisiana Veterans Health Care System, Adjunct Clinical Assistant Professor of Medicine, Tulane University School of Medicine, New Orleans, LA, USA
e-mail: chad.miller@health.slu.edu; Elizabeth.Bowles@va.gov

M. D. King
Department of Medicine, Southeast Louisiana Veterans Health Care System, Tulane University School of Medicine, New Orleans, LA, USA
e-mail: Melissa.King3@va.gov

L. B. Lu et al. (eds.), *Leading an Academic Medical Practice*,
https://doi.org/10.1007/978-3-031-40273-9_5

connect with patients, demonstrate accountability, and prepare for independent practice.

Outline

- Management of medication refills
- In-basket management
- Result notification
- Triaging patient phone calls
- Patient portal messages
- Conclusion

Medication Refills

A key role in resident management is the oversight of medication prescriptions. Each year, between 7000 and 9000 patients die in the United States due to reported medication errors, and the cost of errors related to medication prescriptions exceeds $40 billion [1]. The reported errors and injuries may represent a much smaller proportion of actual harm. Resident education in medication management and reconciliation is represented in several ACGME milestones, yet there is little guidance on the management of medication between visits. This section will emphasize the importance of proper documentation to avoid medication errors between visits as well as the suggested process for managing medication refill requests in between visits (Table 5.1).

Trainees frequently make medication changes during clinical encounters. Blood pressure and diabetes medication titration are among the most common clinical decisions at the point of care. Residents often will start new medications in a visit, either for chronic disease management or for acute care concerns. Moreover, medication therapy is frequently de-escalated or discontinued at clinical encounters due to nonadherence, tolerability concerns, or changes in clinical condition. In order to improve the medication refill process, it is imperative to properly

Table 5.1 ACGME Milestones related to medication management in ambulatory setting [2]

Patient care	1: History 3: Clinical reasoning 5: Patient management—outpatient 6: Digital care (EHR)
Medical knowledge	2: Therapeutic knowledge 3: Knowledge of diagnostic testing
Professionalism	3: Accountability/conscientiousness
Practice-based learning and improvement	1: Evidence-based and informed practice

document this medication changes at the point of care and to reconcile changes to the medication list. Recommendations for in-office medication management include the following:

- Clinical support staff should take inventory of the medication list during the rooming or pre-visit encounter. This includes reconciling the medication list and seeing if refills are needed.
- When managing any medications whose frequency and dosage do not need adjustment, residents should be trained to provide their patients with enough refills to last 12 months. Most insurance providers allow for and encourage 90-day refills, and clinic attendings can work with the EMR builders to make this the default order for commonly prescribed medications. Such a strategy would not be applicable to controlled substances.
- When making dose changes to medications, residents should be encouraged to not only document this in the progress note, but also adjust the medication list accordingly.
- Sometimes, it may be necessary for significant medication adjustments or those for patients who have low health literacy to be communicated directly to the pharmacy. If refills have already been authorized, automated pharmacy refills could continue without this communication.
- For self-limited prescriptions, residents should be encouraged to enter not only a "start" date, but also an "end date" so that these medications can be removed from the medication list upon completion.

We suggest reviewing medication reconciliation expectations with residents formally on an annual basis, as part of both clinic orientation and reorientation for senior-level residents. Additionally, faculty should be aware of these recommendations in order to best oversee the implementation at the office visit and while precepting.

Refill requests can be generated in several ways. Pharmacies can automatically request refills through the EMR. Patients can request refills through patient portal systems, and they can call to request any medication (new or old). We suggest that the initial requests be triaged through clinical support staff, who can be trained to address refill requests systematically to avoid overutilization of physician resources. Some policy examples for refill requests include the following:

- Set a timeline for patient visits in order to obtain refills. For example, most chronic medications require assessment on an annual basis, so the refilling of medications could be denied by support staff until a visit is scheduled. Alternatively, the staff could process the refill request but also call the patient to schedule.

- Flag medications that require laboratory monitoring. While there are no well-validated guidelines on laboratory monitoring for all medications, many classes of medications require intermittent lab testing, for example, monitoring potassium and serum creatinine for patients on ACE inhibitors or diuretics and hemoglobin A1c for those on diabetes medications. Clinical support staff can review the chart for the relevant lab tests prior to forwarding medication refill requests in order to identify patients who will need a clinical visit or lab testing. Some examples are listed in Table 5.2.

Each resident-based clinic will have its own policy for medication refill requests at the provider level. While some larger institutions might have advanced practice practitioners to assist, residents or clinic faculty might take on the responsibility of managing refills of medications prescribed by their peers. Education around therapeutic monitoring, laboratory monitoring, and chart review should occur on an annual basis in order to make sure that medications are correctly renewed. Residents should be instructed to review the chart of each medication requested to verify that:

- The medication is still actively being prescribed at the correct dose and frequency.
- The patient is not overdue for an appointment or laboratory testing.

Table 5.2 Therapeutic drug monitoring of common outpatient medications [3]

Drug	Test	Frequency
ACE inhibitor/angiotensin receptor blocker (ARB)	BMP (hyperkalemia, serum creatinine)	Annually or within 2 weeks of medication change
Allopurinol	BMP (serum creatinine)	Annually
Amiodarone	CBC, LFT, TSH	Annually
Carbamazepine	CBC, CMP (hepatotoxicity, bone marrow suppression)	Annually
Digoxin	BMP (potassium, creatinine), digoxin level	Annually
Diuretics (loops, thiazides, potassium-sparing)	BMP (potassium, serum creatinine)	Annually
Insulin	A1c	Every 3 months (uncontrolled), every 6 months (controlled)
Metformin	BMP (serum creatinine), A1c	Annually, every 3 months (uncontrolled), every 6 months (controlled)
SGLT-2 inhibitors	BMP (serum creatinine), A1c	Annually, every 3 months (uncontrolled), every 6 months (controlled)
Statins	Lipid panel	Annually
Valproic acid	CBC, CMP (hepatotoxicity, bone marrow suppression), valproic acid level	Annually
Thyroid replacement therapy	TSH	Annually or 6 weeks following dose change

- There are no obvious medication interactions or new medical conditions precluding refill of the medication.

Controlled substances are a special consideration. At some training sites, medications listed as Drug Enforcement Agency Controlled Substances will be managed by the attending physician. Other training sites may include trainees in the prescribing and monitoring of controlled substances. If trainees are involved in the prescribing of controlled substances, they should be educated on appropriate prescribing practices. These include use of prescription drug monitoring sites, urine toxicology testing, and overdose risk mitigation strategies. Similarly, trainees must learn to complete all required regulatory documentation and to maintain any certifications and educational requirements at the local, state, or federal level that apply to the clinic. As trainees will immediately be expected to prescribe controlled substance upon achieving independent practice, they are well served in learning the complexities and risks of this particular prescribing practice.

In-Basket Messages

Attending physicians and residents have the unique opportunity to co-manage a panel of patients. Residents have a primary duty to these patients, and the supervising attending shares duty as well as liability. It is imperative that attendings play an active role in the management of residents not only in the clinical encounter, but also in the follow-up and intervisit management that ensues. This is also represented in several ACGME Milestones (Table 5.3).

Result Notification

In the primary care setting, laboratory testing, imaging, and procedures are ordered to assist in the clinical decision-making process. These tests usually result during the intervisit period. The individual who ordered the tests may be on another rotation outside of the clinic or may be on leave. The manager of the clinical practice and medical director need protocols in place for safe handling of these alerts. The vast majority of healthcare systems utilize electronic medical record systems

Table 5.3 ACGME Milestones related to in-basket message management in ambulatory setting [2]

Patient care	5: Patient management—outpatient 6: Digital care (EHR)
Medical knowledge	2: Therapeutic knowledge 3: Knowledge of diagnostic testing
Professionalism	3: Accountability/conscientiousness
Interpersonal and communications skills	3: Communication within healthcare systems

(EMRs) in which test results will be directed to the ordering provider through a process known as "order entry results reporting." The implication of this is that the ordering provider (trainee) will receive the alert about the test results in their personal account in the EMR, but that person may be working at another academic site for several weeks. Some EMRs are structured such that results are reported to both the ordering resident and supervising attending. This may not be possible in all EMR systems. In collaborating with local informatics professionals, the following options could be discussed:

- Configuration of panels where patients are assigned to a trainee provider/attending provider (team), thus enabling alerts to be routed to that team. EMRs capable of this type of configuration often allow tailored selection of the alert types that will result to the "team."
- Use of surrogacy settings: These are settings found in virtually all EMRs that are intended to facilitate coverage when a healthcare team member is on leave. The function directs the EMR to direct all alerts to the surrogate until the setting is turned off or until a preset date.
- Prompt to select additional desingees to be alerted to results at the time of order entry. This is a less optimal option because it increases the number of clicks to complete an action.
- Manual selection of designees at this time of order placement. This is a cumbersome and error-prone option, and it increases cognitive burden because providers must remember to add additional alerte alert designees without a prompt.

Some systems do not use an electronic medical record or do not have remote access options to allow trainees to log into their accounts when rotating at another site. When there is not an option to access the EMR remotely, it might be difficult or impossible for trainees to safely and effectively manage patients in the intervisit interval. A more attending-reliant process will be necessary.

Once strategies are developed to prevent results from languishing in unreviewed inboxes, the academic practice director will need to consider how trainees will be supported in their development and use of intervisit care competencies. The clinic director, in collaboration with the leadership of the training program and trainee leaders, should delineate formal expectations about intervisit patient management to include roles and responsibilities for the stakeholders (trainees, outpatient attending providers, academic clinic director, nursing and support personnel, and training program). The following is a list, not exhaustive, of considerations for inclusion:

- Trainee responsibility for maintaining remote access to EMR
- Frequency of trainee remote log-in to EMR
- Timeframe for results notification (trainee and attending, see below)
- Protected time for outpatient intervisit care management
- Documentation of intervisit care
- Oversight of intervisit care
- Availability of attendings to trainees who are off-site

As noted above, trainees have primary duties to their patients in the intervisit interval. They are also early in their professional development, being pulled in a number of different directions, working long hours, and at risk for fatigue and burnout. In setting expectations, it is helpful to list those times when the trainee will not be expected to attend to issues in their primary care patients. These include vacation, sick leave, and demanding clinical rotations (ICU, etc.). It is not reasonable, fair, or safe to expect trainees to function without downtime or to divert their attention from critically ill patients or large inpatient rosters when an outpatient attending or a trainee rotating on an ambulatory elective can act as a surrogate for outpatients. Clear communication about the start and stop of these times of coverage is crucial to avoid dangerous lapses in the coverage of clinical notifications.

The intervisit period presents a unique challenge in that clinical management conundrums arise when the trainee is not collocated with their partnered attending physician. Residents should be frequently reminded to ask questions if they struggle to determine an assessment and plan based on results so as to ensure a culture of safety and decrease the delay in result notification. The academic site director must ensure that all attendings have shared their contact information with the trainees, that they are responsive to trainee questions, and that they understand that their trainees may need to confer with them outside of standard clinic operating hours. Demonstrating availability and empathy for the trainees' experience will make contact in times of clinical uncertainty more likely and will decrease the likelihood that a trainee opts for unsupervised clinical action instead of trying to contact an attending who is perceived as unavailable.

Resident clinic directors should determine policies of timeliness of result communication and ensure that faculty and trainees are aware of these expectations. A suggested timeframe is as follows:

- Critical results: all healthcare facilities should have a policy for handling critical results
- Urgent abnormal results: 1 business day
- Abnormal results: 1 week (synchronous or asynchronous communication as deemed clinically appropriate). This timeline may seem long until it is recalled that there are many mild abnormalities that require neither action nor urgent discussion (e.g., stably elevated creatinine)
- Normal results: 1–2 weeks (asynchronous communication recommended for the sake of efficiency)

Attendings should screen the results for any urgent abnormalities and, if identified, address these results in collaboration with or independent of the resident physician, dependent upon the resident's schedule. If results are to be addressed in collaboration with the resident, communication to the resident can be through the EMR, but we also recommend direct contact with the resident through HIPAA-compliant methods. Residents should be instructed to communicate these results and document the communication in the patient's chart. Failed attempts at communication with a patient should also be documented. Multiple failed attempts to contact a patient may require escalation of communication method, up to and including registered mail, and in extreme situations, police welfare check, based on the criticality of the issue being communicated.

We suggest that all results requiring action or resulting in an alteration of the management plan are communicated synchronously. Additionally, anticipatory management should be considered when ordering tests (i.e., if a lab is abnormal, the follow-up plan will be ...). If this is properly documented, covering providers can more easily communicate results if the resident is unavailable.

Triaging Patient Phone Calls

In addition to the patient care that occurs in the clinic, a primary responsibility of primary care physicians is managing their patient panel between visits. As discussed above, result communication is one form of intervisit management, but patients can also initiate communication with their providers through phone calls or portal messages. Patients may call the office to discuss medication refills (discussed above), questions related to their last visit, or new concerns. Each resident clinic should determine a workflow for triage of these patient calls in order to facilitate timely communication with their providers. Some challenges to this communication with residents include:

- Rotations spent outside of clinic (wards, ICU, electives, etc.) with limited access to EMR or telephone
- Changes in attending oversight in clinic
- Clinical uncertainty in patient management
- EMR inability to send messages to multiple recipients (for instance, sending a call notification to the resident but not the attending)

While every resident clinic will have a different policy for the management of patient calls, all clinics should ensure that patient calls are returned as quickly as possible, with 24-h callback being the goal. Support staff and call centers can be trained to triage messages in order to limit the number of calls the provider needs to return. For example, a list of critical complaints can be established wherein the staff should immediately recommend emergency evaluation. Support staff can also offer same-day visits for new complaints and close follow-up appointments for patients requesting to be seen.

Patient Portal Messages

As with results reporting in the electronic medical record system, the patient portal system should be explored for configuration options that allow notification of a group of persons to patient communications in the portal. This is an extremely common feature, and it allows multi-professional teams to receive and triage patient requests to the most appropriate person to respond (clerk, LPN, RN, pharmacist, provider). Trainees should be included in these systems along with their attending provider. As recommended with other forms of patient communication, a set of guidelines for timely response should be developed and shared with all team members. When trainees are on leave or on rotations where they are not expected to remotely review alerts, they would be similarly relieved of duty to address patient portal messages.

Management of intervisit patient care is often an unconsidered dimension of the academic clinical practice and medical education. Lack of formal curriculum, competing priorities, and absence of protocols can lead to patient safety vulnerabilities and threats to maintaining positive patient relationships. Strategies to mitigate these risks should include vulnerability analysis, written expectations and protocols, and creation of formal curricula in collaboration with training program leadership.

Conclusion

Management of inter-visit patient care is often an unconsidered dimension of the academic clinical practice and medical education. Lack of formal curriculum, competing priorities, and the absence of protocols can lead to patient safety vulnerabilities and threats to maintaining positive patient relationships. Strategies to mitigate these risks should include vulnerability analysis, written expectations and protocols, and creation of formal curricula in collaboration with training program leadership.

References

1. Wittich CM, Burkle CM, Lanier WL. Medication errors: an overview for clinicians. Mayo Clin Proc. 2014;89(8):1116–25. https://doi.org/10.1016/j.mayocp.2014.05.007. Epub 2014 Jun 27.
2. Accreditation Council for Graduate Medical Education (ACGME) Milestones Guidebook for Residents and Fellows; 2020 https://www.acgme.org/globalassets/pdfs/milestones/internal-medicinemilestones.pdf
3. Raebel MA, Lyons EE, Andrade SE, et al. Laboratory monitoring of drugs at initiation of therapy in ambulatory care. J Gen Intern Med. 2005;20(12):1120–6. https://doi.org/10.1111/j.1525-1497.2005.0257.x

Chapter 6
Maximizing Continuity in Resident Clinic

William G. Weppner, Reena Gupta, and Robert J. Fortuna

Introduction

Continuity of care between a physician and patient is associated with improved quality and efficiency of care, improved patient and provider experience, and better overall clinical outcomes for patients [1–7]. Studies specific to resident training clinics support the assertion that higher continuity is associated with better chronic disease management, improved preventive care, lower administrative burden, and better patient and resident satisfaction [8, 9]. Maximizing continuity of care in residency practice is particularly important to provide quality care to patients and support residency education. Achieving high levels of continuity, however, is challenging in residency practices. This chapter discusses both the importance of continuity and different methods of measuring it. In addition, we will explore means to maximize continuity in teaching clinics using different schedules and models.

W. G. Weppner
Department of Medicine, University of Washington, Seattle, WA, USA

University of Washington-Boise Internal Medicine Residency, Boise, ID, USA

Primary Care Provider, Boise VA Medical Center, Boise, ID, USA
e-mail: William.Weppner@va.gov

R. Gupta
Division of General Internal Medicine, Department of Medicine, San Francisco General Hospital, University of California, San Francisco, CA, USA
e-mail: reena.gupta@ucsf.edu

R. J. Fortuna (✉)
Departments of Internal Medicine, Pediatrics, and Community Health, University of Rochester, Rochester, NY, USA
e-mail: Robert_Fortuna@urmc.rochester.edu

L. B. Lu et al. (eds.), *Leading an Academic Medical Practice*,
https://doi.org/10.1007/978-3-031-40273-9_6

Outline

- The case for continuity
- Types of continuity
- Measuring continuity
- Maximizing continuity
- Conclusion

The Case for Continuity

Studies have demonstrated that continuity of care is associated with improved chronic disease management, including quality of hypertension and diabetes care [1, 4, 10, 11]. Increased continuity is also associated with better delivery of preventative care, including colorectal screening, breast cancer screening, and immunizations [1, 4].

In addition to improved clinical outcomes, continuity is associated with improved satisfaction for both physicians and patients [12, 13]. Longitudinal relationships and continuity of care form the foundation of primary care. Supporting continuity improves provider satisfaction and helps to prevent physician burnout [7, 14, 15]. Enhanced continuity also imparts increased trust of physicians by patients [12]. These influential relationships are also incredibly important to the professional development of trainees. Experiences with continuity of care throughout training can influence career choice. In fact, developing a strong relationship with patients during training is a powerful predictor for entering a primary care specialty [16].

Beyond improvements in clinical outcomes and patient-provider satisfaction, there is evidence that improved continuity is associated with reduced hospital utilization and lower costs of care [3, 17, 18]. As value-based payment structures continue to evolve, patient satisfaction and financial accountability will become increasingly important.

Types of Continuity

Continuity can be defined from both the patient and trainee perspectives [19]. From a patient perspective, the most basic continuity measure indicates the proportion of visits in which a patient is seen by their primary care physician (PCP). From a resident physician perspective, continuity indicates the proportion of a resident's visits that occur with patients from their assigned panel. Both forms of continuity are crucial to consider when developing office scheduling processes and protocols to optimize quality, patient satisfaction, and physician satisfaction in a teaching practice.

The concept of continuity can be further extended to include other members of the clinical team. Some programs include the frequency of the attending–resident precepting dyad to define continuity between a patient and the supervising physician and trainee dyad. Some institutions follow the continuity of the resident team (i.e., supervising physician and team of residents that share a panel of patients). The Veteran Affairs (VA) includes the assigned supervising physician in measures of continuity when considering continuity among resident physicians. With the expansion of team-based care models, continuity between patients and other multidisciplinary team members who help to coordinate care is becoming increasingly important.

Continuity of care is also an important consideration with the expansion of telehealth services. Telehealth may provide valuable opportunities to increase patient-PCP continuity [20].

Measuring Continuity

Residency teaching practices should prioritize measuring and tracking continuity. As one would expect, there are a myriad of different metrics for measuring continuity of care [19]. Continuity indices that are commonly used in training clinic settings include the "Usual Provider of Care" (UPC), "Modified Continuity Index" (MCI), "Modified, Modified Continuity Index" (MMCI), and "Continuity of Care" (COC) (Fig. 6.1). There are strengths and weaknesses for each. The UPC is defined as the proportion of all visits that are with the patient's PCP. The UPC, while easier to interpret, does not take into account dispersion of care among other clinicians [21]. The UPC metric is also less reliable when there are fewer visits. The corresponding metric from the physician's perspective is the PHY ("Continuity for Physician"), which measures the proportion of visits that an individual physician sees his or her own patients in a given timeframe [22].

- Usual Provider of Care (UPC) = n/N
- Continuity of Care Index (COC) = $\Sigma_{i=1}^{k} n^2 - N \ (N \ N - 1)$
- Modified Continuity Index (MCI) = 1-(P/N+0.1)
- Modified Modified Continuity Index = MCI/(1-1/N+0.1)

n = number of visits to a single provider (typically assigned PCP)
N = total number of visits for a single patient to other providers
P = total number of providers seen by a single patient
i = provider rank (index), from 1 to P

Fig. 6.1 Formula for calculating commonly used continuity metrics

Measuring continuity requires sufficient data on the number of visits with health care professionals. Some continuity indices require empanelment of patients to a specific primary care provider (such as UPC), while some do not (COC, MCI, MMCI) [19]. These indices range between 0 and 1; they approach 0 if all visits are with different clinicians, and equal 1 if all visits are with the same clinician. One of the easiest continuity measures to understand is the UPC metric. This is simply the percentage of primary care visits that are with the primary care provider, defined as seen from the patient's point of view. This is commonly used for its ease of calculation and its ready interpretability. For example, a UPC of 0.78 indicates that the patient saw their designated PCP at 78% of all measured primary care (or equivalent) visits. The UPC measure is most commonly measured in the context of all primary care visits, but alternative applications have also been developed. An innovative modification of the UPC continuity measure, used by the Veterans Administration health system, may include emergency department visits inside or outside the VA in the denominator. Continuity is lower if patients visit the emergency department more often, thereby placing responsibility on the primary care team to prevent unnecessary emergency department visits. In the VA system, a stated goal is that 75% of the time, a patient will see their own clinician when they are seen the primary care office or come to the emergency department [23]. The goal is to maximize the number of appropriate visits with the PCP (numerator) while minimizing unnecessary ED utilization and visits with non-continuity providers (denominator).

The MCI and MMCI provides a sense of continuity with a single provider, but also corrects for dispersion among other clinicians [24]. There is some suggestion that the MMCI is more appropriate than UPC, COC, or MCI for resident providers, to adjust for dispersion among other clinicians [24].

How these metrics are interpreted in settings where a resident physician has a panel of patients shared with an attending or "supervising" PCP may vary. In most cases, these metrics focus on visits that occur in the primary care office. However, the type of visits that are counted may be defined in different ways. For example, in VA clinics, continuity is assessed with UPC: the numerator is the encountered visits with the associate PCP (resident) + preceptor PCP (supervising physician), and the denominator is all visits to primary care clinics, urgent care clinics, or emergency department visits. Thus, if a resident sees their own patient in continuity or episodic care clinics, this counts for continuity. If a resident sees a patient that is not their patient but precepts with the panel attending for that patient (and the attending is on the encounter form as a primary or secondary physician), then this counts for continuity.

In order to evaluate resident physician continuity, these metrics can be altered from the patient perspective to the physician perspective. While not as strongly associated with health outcomes, this can be important for the resident's experience in continuity clinic and may be associated with improved physician satisfaction. This metric is commonly evaluated in residency continuity clinic settings when scheduling changes are enacted to make sure that continuity has improved for both patients and providers.

Finally, most of these metrics are based on traditional face-to-face visits in primary care, but the measures can be extended to include telehealth visits. Historically, continuity measures have not accounted for encounters via telephone, video, secure messaging, group visits, or affiliated members of the team, although these interactions certainly contribute to the overall relationship between a provider and patient. As telehealth expands, practices should explicitly measure continuity for both face-to-face and virtual encounters.

Maximizing Continuity

Maximizing continuity is important to support patient and physician satisfaction, as well as to improve quality of care. There are several factors associated with increased continuity of care, including the consistent use of scheduling protocols, increased faculty clinical time, and increased number of resident clinical sessions per week [4]. Several examples are presented in Table 6.1. Having clearly defined scheduling

Table 6.1 Specific approaches to improve continuity in resident teaching clinics

Processes to maximize continuity	Examples
Clinic scheduling protocols	• Make sure that patients are clearly assigned to residents ("empaneled" or clearly designated in the electronic health record banner) • Establish protocols to prioritize continuity for nonurgent follow-up and preventive care visits with the primary resident [4] • Develop processes to assess whether urgent appointments can wait for primary residents. Otherwise, prioritize visit with primary team attending or team of advanced practice providers (APPs) [4] • Advanced access (or "open access") scheduling protocols may improve continuity, but protocols to increase access may decrease UPC [26]
Rescheduling residents pulled from clinic	• Adopt policies that prioritize stable and consistent resident clinic scheduling and prevent residents being pulled from clinic to cover other clinical duties [4] • If cancelling clinics is necessary, it is required that residents are rescheduled in clinic within several days to accommodate patients. Policies should emphasize the importance of clinic time, but not penalize residents [4]
Increased resident ambulatory clinical time and/or panel size	• Examine ways to increase the amount of time spent in clinic by residents • Increasing the number of sessions will improve availability (this increases UPC, but can decrease PHY) [29] • Increasing the number of empaneled patients to a resident increases PHY, but decreases UPC [29]
Thoughtful use of practice partners or advanced practice providers	• If PCP is not available and patients need urgent appointments, schedule with a full-time team anchor clinician or practice partner so that patients see one of the two clinicians for nearly all visits • Identifying a single "anchor" attending, advanced practice provider, or practice partner may increase continuity [4], likely by decreasing dispersion through MMCI or COCI; may not affect UPC or PHY

protocols that prioritize continuity for acute, chronic, and preventive care visits is an essential component of maintaining continuity in resident practices. These scheduling protocols will be unique to each practice and must balance the need for continuity with the need for maintaining access for patients. The balance between continuity and access will be partially contingent upon the amount of time that residents are available in clinic.

Maximizing the time that residents are in clinic is also a critical component to support continuity. The Accreditation Council for Graduate Medical Education (ACGME) has established core requirements outlining requirements for longitudinal continuity experience in the outpatient setting [25]. Although this establishes the minimal requirements, the absolute number of sessions required per week is not prescribed, and the optimal number of sessions to maximize continuity is not known. However, programs with increased number of resident clinical sessions per week are typically able to provide greater availability and continuity to patients and residents.

Resident panel size also influences continuity. Panel size should be determined based on residents' availability to care for those patients. The number of sessions residents are in clinic and the number of patients seen per session should guide overall panel size. In addition to the amount of time spent in clinic and the size of resident panels, practices should consider the structure of the schedule. There is mixed evidence regarding continuity in block schedules compared with continuity in traditional schedules [26]. In the largest study of block vs. traditional vs. hybrid scheduling, UPC was highest in the block model and lowest in traditional weekly; PHY was the lowest in block model, but subject resident-perceived continuity was the highest hybrid model [27, 28].

Rescheduling clinics for residents who are pulled to support inpatient needs is another important measure to consider when developing processes to maintain resident and patient continuity [4]. This requires programmatic and institutional recognition of the importance of outpatient training and patient access to their resident physician. Rescheduling policies also discourage residents from being pulled unnecessarily from ambulatory rotations.

Thoughtful integration of advanced practice providers (APPs), who may be nurse practitioners or physician assistants, can also support patient continuity with resident physicians. APPs are important members of ambulatory teams who can help improve access to care for patients. At the same time, APP visits may also hinder direct patient continuity with their resident physician. This can be reduced by having clear scheduling protocols that prioritize scheduling with resident PCP unless the patient has a need for an urgent appointment and the PCP is not available. Individual clinics must balance the competing needs for maintaining access for patients while prioritizing continuity with residents. This balance will be different for each program. In many teaching practices, patients are seen by numerous providers when their resident or faculty PCP is not available. Having a designated full-time team anchor clinician and clear scheduling protocols that require scheduling appointments with this single alternate team provider when the PCP is not available can greatly improve the continuity experience for patients.

Conclusion

Based on a review of the available evidence, continuity of care appears closely associated with all aspects of the "quadruple aim" including improving care outcomes, enhancing patient and provider experience, and lowering costs [30]. Residency teaching practices should place a high priority on measuring and tracking continuity and implementing strategies to maximize continuity of care for their patients and trainees.

References

1. Atlas SJ, et al. Patient-physician connectedness and quality of primary care. Ann Intern Med. 2009;150(5):325–35.
2. Cabana MD, Jee SH. Does continuity of care improve patient outcomes? J Fam Pract. 2004;53(12):974–80.
3. De Maeseneer JM, et al. Provider continuity in family medicine: does it make a difference for total health care costs? Ann Fam Med. 2003;1(3):144–8.
4. Fortuna RJ, et al. Factors associated with resident continuity in ambulatory training practices. J Grad Med Educ. 2016;8(4):532–40.
5. Gupta R, Bodenheimer T. How primary care practices can improve continuity of care. JAMA Intern Med. 2013;173(20):1885–6.
6. Saultz JW, Lochner J. Interpersonal continuity of care and care outcomes: a critical review. Ann Fam Med. 2005;3(2):159–66.
7. Schultz K, Delva D, Kerr J. Emotional effects of continuity of care on family physicians and the therapeutic relationship. Can Fam Physician. 2012;58(2):178–85.
8. Connolly MJ, et al. Continuity and health outcomes in resident clinics: a scoping review of the literature. Cureus. 2022;14(5):e25167.
9. Stepczynski J, et al. Factors affecting resident satisfaction in continuity clinic-a systematic review. J Gen Intern Med. 2018;33(8):1386–93.
10. Dearinger AT, et al. The effect of physician continuity on diabetic outcomes in a resident continuity clinic. J Gen Intern Med. 2008;23(7):937–41.
11. Fisher M, et al. Continuity of care and hypertension control in a university-based practice. Ethn Dis. 2007;17(4):693–8.
12. Mainous AG 3rd, et al. Continuity of care and trust in one's physician: evidence from primary care in the United States and the United Kingdom. Fam Med. 2001;33(1):22–7.
13. Reddy A, et al. The effect of primary care provider turnover on patient experience of care and ambulatory quality of care. JAMA Intern Med. 2015;175(7):1157–62.
14. Ellman MS, et al. Continuity of care as an educational goal but failed reality in resident training: time to innovate. J Grad Med Educ. 2016;8(2):150–3.
15. Hirsh DA, et al. "continuity" as an organizing principle for clinical education reform. N Engl J Med. 2007;356(8):858–66.
16. Peccoralo LA, et al. Resident satisfaction with continuity clinic and career choice in general internal medicine. J Gen Intern Med. 2013;28(8):1020–7.
17. Nyweide DJ, et al. Continuity of care and the risk of preventable hospitalization in older adults. JAMA Intern Med. 2013;173(20):1879–85.
18. Weiss LJ, Blustein J. Faithful patients: the effect of long-term physician-patient relationships on the costs and use of health care by older Americans. Am J Public Health. 1996;86(12):1742–7.

19. Saultz JW. Defining and measuring interpersonal continuity of care. Ann Fam Med. 2003;1(3):134–43.
20. Imlach F, et al. Telehealth consultations in general practice during a pandemic lockdown: survey and interviews on patient experiences and preferences. BMC Fam Pract. 2020;21(1):269.
21. Phan K, Brown SR. Decreased continuity in a residency clinic: a consequence of open access scheduling. Fam Med. 2009;41(1):46–50.
22. Darden PM, et al. Comparison of continuity in a resident versus private practice. Pediatrics. 2001;108(6):1263–8.
23. Office of Quality Safety and Value. VHA facility quality and safety report, veterans health Administration Office of Information and Analytics, 2012. Department of Veterans Affairs; 2012.
24. Magill MK, Senf J. A new method for measuring continuity of care in family practice residencies. J Fam Pract. 1987;24(2):165–8.
25. Accreditation Council for Graduate Medical Education (ACGME). ACGME program requirements for graduate medical education in internal medicine. Effective July 1, 2022.
26. Walker J, et al. Continuity of Care in Resident Outpatient Clinics: a scoping review of the literature. J Grad Med Educ. 2018;10(1):16–25.
27. Francis MD, et al. Clinic design, key practice metrics, and resident satisfaction in internal medicine continuity clinics: findings of the educational innovations project ambulatory collaborative. J Grad Med Educ. 2014;6(2):249–55.
28. Francis MD, et al. Clinic design and continuity in internal medicine resident clinics: findings of the educational innovations project ambulatory collaborative. J Grad Med Educ. 2015;7(1):36–41.
29. Francis MD, et al. Effect of number of clinics and panel size on patient continuity for medical residents. J Grad Med Educ. 2009;1(2):310–5.
30. Bodenheimer T, Sinsky C. From triple to quadruple aim: care of the patient requires care of the provider. Ann Fam Med. 2014;12(6):573–6.

Part III
Resident Clinic Requirements and Expectations

Chapter 7
Outpatient Billing and Coding and Center for Medicare & Medicaid Services Billing Rules

Lee B. Lu, Scott V. Joy, and Jeannine Z. Engel

Introduction

Knowing the complexities of outpatient billing is critical to optimizing financial success in a general internal medicine clinic. With a current focus in academic medical centers on visit volume and clinical productivity as measured in work relative value units (wRVUs), faculty and clinic directors must understand the visit types and preventive services that are provided by the general internist, the documentation requirements for each of these services, and how to appropriately code and bill for the services provided. This chapter highlights the history of physician reimbursement including the impact of the Public Health Emergency (PHE) on physician billing, basics of outpatient billing and coding for evaluation and management visits with emphasis on the 2021 documentation changes, telemedicine visits, care management services, and preventive visits and services. Clinical examples will illustrate how to maximize wRVUs and revenue in a general internal medicine practice.

L. B. Lu (✉)
Department of Medicine, Baylor College of Medicine, Houston, TX, USA
e-mail: lblu@bcm.edu

S. V. Joy
HealthONE Physician Services Group, HCA Graduate Medical Education, Continental Division, Englewood, CO, USA
e-mail: scott.joy@healthonecares.com

J. Z. Engel
Department of Medicine, University of Virginia, School of Medicine, Charlottesville, VA, USA
e-mail: zdw5zv@hscmail.mcc.virginia.edu

L. B. Lu et al. (eds.), *Leading an Academic Medical Practice*,
https://doi.org/10.1007/978-3-031-40273-9_7

Outline

- History of physician reimbursement for medical services
- The COVID pandemic PHE
- The basics of billing and coding, emphasis on 2021 documentation changes
- New/established patient billing
- Telemedicine billing and coding
- Preventive visits
- Screening visits
- Medicare services
  - Annual wellness visits
  - Care management services
  - Home healthcare oversight
  - Coding and billing for counseling services.
- Modifiers
- Relative value units
- Maximizing revenue
- Conclusion

History of Physician Reimbursement for Medical Services

The United States (US) Congress created Medicare in 1965. At that time, Congress did not want physicians to have a disincentive to treat Medicare patients; thus, Medicare allowed for locally determined "reasonable" charges. In an attempt to standardize medical services, the American Medical Association (AMA) created Current Procedural Terminology (CPT) in 1965 to codify medical services and procedures but did not assign a financial value to each CPT code. Without any financial checks in the system, fees rose. In 1976, the Congress implemented the Medicare Economic Index, which limited fee increases by tying them to inflation rates, and in 1986, the Congress froze fee increases, due to budgetary constraints. This led to physicians, physician advocacy groups, and government to engage in endless sparring to address stakeholders' concerns that continue today. Some highlights of the historical timeline and interventions relevant to general internal medicine billing and coding are as follows [1]:

1986: Physician Payment Review Commission provided independent advice regarding Medicare spending, which continues today as the Medicare Payment Advisory Commission (MedPAC) [1997].

1989–1992: Resource-based relative value scale (RBRVS) was created as a result of the Omnibus Budget Reconciliation Act with the intent to streamline physician fee scales and reduce disparities in reimbursements. RBRVS assigns relative value units (RVUs) to various aspects of physician activities and forms the basis for determining Medicare reimbursements.

1991–1992: The Relative Value Scale Update Committee (RUC) was created by the AMA to advise the Center for Medicare & Medicaid Services (CMS) and Congress on "refining" RBRVS. This group remains controversial as the majority of voting members represent subspecialty services and not primary care.

1997: Sustainable Growth Rate (SGR) was a method that CMS used to calculate Medicare reimbursement. It was tied to the gross domestic product (GDP) and maintained budget neutrality. When expenditures exceeded targets, CMS enacted payment cuts, which could only be altered by an act of the Congress. This led to an ongoing series of temporary financial patches, commonly referred to as the "doc fix."

2010: The Patient Protection and Affordable Care Act (PPACA, ACA, or Obamacare) was signed by President Obama. It established the Annual Wellness Visit and Center for Medicare & Medicaid Innovation (CMMI) to evaluate new payment models for physicians, including Accountable Care Organizations (ACOs) and Comprehensive Primary Care (CPC), providing coverage for services and testing meeting the U.S. Preventive Services Task Force (USPSTF) grades A and B recommendations.

2015: Medicare Access and Children's Health Insurance Program (CHIP) Reauthorization Act (MACRA) of 2015 ended the SGR formula, which threatened clinicians participating in Medicare with potential payment cliffs for 13 years [2]. MACRA created the Quality Payment Program to provide new tools and resources to give patients with Medicare the best possible care. Physicians and practices can choose how to participate in the Quality Payment Program, based on practice size, specialty, location, or patient population.

There are two tracks a physician can choose to participate in, which are advanced alternative payment models (APMs) or the merit-based incentive payment system (MIPS).

For practices deciding to participate in an advanced APM, through Medicare Part B, they may earn an incentive payment for participating in an innovative payment model. Practices deciding to participate in traditional Medicare Part B will participate in MIPS earning a performance-based payment adjustment.

Each calendar year, data for various patient-driven quality performance metrics can be submitted under MIPS. Based on the submitted metrics, a practice or practice group may be eligible for an incentive payment or a penalty 2 calendar years later. This is a budget-neutral program, so the incentives and penalties must balance out. For 2022, the maximum bonus is 9% and the maximum penalty is −9%. The MIPS program is updated yearly as part of the Physician Fee Schedule (PFS) final rule.

2019–2020: In the 2019 Medicare Physician Fee Schedule (MPFS) final rule, CMS finalized radical changes in the Outpatient Evaluation and Management (E/M) documentation and coding framework [3]. However, they deferred the implementation of these changes until 2021. The proposals included eliminating low-level new patient visit code (99201) and offering two payments, one for office levels 2–4 and a second higher payment for level 5 visits. They continued to differentiate payments for new and established visits. The intent was to simplify documentation requirements and reduce clinician burden. Essentially, CMS proposed that the clinician could choose how to document. Choices included using the long-standing framework, using medical decision-making only, or using time. For the combined level 2–4 visits, the minimum documentation would follow the 1995/97 E/M level 2 framework. Based on this proposal, CPT convened a workgroup and revised the E/M documentation requirements. Ultimately, CMS accepted the CPT-proposed changes in the MPFS 2021 Final Rule. The 2021 outpatient E/M documentation requirements will be outlined in detail later in the chapter.

Over the same period, CMS proposed and finalized a supplemental add-on code for visit complexity, GPC1X, later assigned G2211. This code was valued at 0.33 RVUs and could be added to any level of service for "**Visit complexity inherent to evaluation and management** associated with primary medical care services that serve as the continuing focal point for all needed health care services." On December 22, 2020, Congress passed a massive stimulus bill (over 5,000 pages), which included a 3-year delay on the implementation of this code or any similar code [4].

Other new billing opportunities during this time frame include virtual check-ins (**G2012** and **G2252**) as well as remote evaluation of recorder video or images (**G2010**). In 2020, CPT added codes **99421**: Online digital evaluation and management service, for an established patient, for up to 7 days' cumulative time, during the 7 days, 5–10 minutes. Code **99422** allows 11–20 minutes, and **99423** accounts for 21 or more minutes [5].

The COVID Pandemic and Public Health Emergency

The coronavirus pandemic and Public Health Emergency (PHE) opened new reimbursement opportunities for non-face-to-face services as well. In March 2020, CMS published many blanket waivers in an effort to decrease burden on physicians and facilities, as well as increase access to care for Medicare beneficiaries during the COVID-19 pandemic [6]. Particularly important to primary care, telemedicine including audiovisual and telephone-only visits were generally reimbursable regardless of the location of the patient or the physician. Payment for these visits has evolved significantly over the course of the pandemic and is currently variable from state to state. In addition, CMS added RVU value for telephone-only visits, which in the past were not reimbursed. Ultimately, CMS increased the value of a telephone encounter to be equivalent to face-to-face or telemedicine visit based on time. This PHE implementation emphasized the importance of any visit during the pandemic and encouraged providers and facilities to advance their telemedicine platforms. The downside was that many of these reimbursement opportunities might disappear depending on the evolution of the COVID PHE. The chapter was prepared prior to the ending of PHE on May 11, 2023. Though PHE has ended, telephone visits are still reimbursable by Medicare. Eventually, telephone-only visits may go back to zero value, and the vast majority of primary care practices may not qualify as originating sites for telemedicine reimbursement from Medicare. The Society of General Internal Medicine (SGIM) Health Policy Committee is an excellent way to keep apprised of the changing reimbursement landscape [7].

**Due to the evolving changes in CMS regulations, please see the statement at the end of the chapter for the updates.*

The Basics of Billing and Coding: Big Changes in 2021

As noted previously, in January 2021, CPT and CMS finalized major changes in the outpatient evaluation and management documentation requirements. The impetus for these changes was the proposed MPFS 2019 and final rule from CMS, which included leveling of payment and documentation requirements for level 2–4 visits, along with complexity add-on codes for continuity-type practices and clinicians. There was a whirlwind of feedback from the healthcare community, and ultimately, the CPT editorial panel took on the task of revising the 25-year-old guidelines using an appointed workgroup with open meetings, allowing for broad feedback. The new guidelines were accepted by the editorial panel and ultimately by CMS as codified in the MPFS 2021 final rule.

For many years, there were two CMS documentation guidelines, the E/M 1995 and 1997 versions. In the 1995/1997 E/M guidelines, history and physical examination required multiple system documentation in addition to medical decision-making to meet certain levels of services (LOS). The complexity and cumbersome requirements added burden to physicians' work-life. In January 2021, the new outpatient E/M guideline went into effect with the goal of reducing irrelevant documentation. It allows time-based billing and eliminates the billing code of 99201 for new patients. In this section, we will review the definition of new and established patients, describe the new 2021 E/M guidelines, compare the old and new E/M guidelines, and provide clinical case examples for determination of LOS.

New/Established Patient Billing and Coding

New patient definition [8]—by Current Procedural Terminology (CPT) definition—a patient who has not received any care and professional services from the physician, or another physician of the same specialty who belongs to the same group practice within the past 3 years. New patient outpatient CPT codes are 99202-99205.
Established patient definition [8]—a patient who has received care from the physician or another physician of the same specialty who belongs to the same group practice within the past 3 years. Established patient outpatient CPT codes are 99212-99215.

One nuance for the clinic medical director to consider is how a new patient is defined within the context of the broader health system, especially if the outpatient clinician previously cared for the patient in the inpatient setting. Although this nuance is beyond the scope of this chapter, the medical director is encouraged to reach out to their administrative and financial support offices for further guidance.
2021 Outpatient E/M Guidelines—same documentation for both established and new patients.

History—only relevant history

Review of systems—relevant positives and negatives

Physical examination—relevant physical examination
Reviewed laboratory and imaging studies—specify which studies and analysis of studies
Assessment and plan—level of services depends on medical decision-making (MDM) or is **time based**

Comparison of 1995/1997 with 2021 E/M Guideline Documentation

1995/1997 E/M guidelines **must meet many requirements and documentation in the components of history and physical exam** to bill the levels of services [9, 10]. 2021 E/M guidelines allow limited documentation in history and physical examination [11].

2021 E/M guidelines for new and established patients

CPT code	History and exam	MDM	Time (min)
99202	Only relevant history and physical exam	Straightforward	15–29
99203		Low	30–44
99204		Moderate	45–59
99205		High	60–74
99212	Only relevant history and physical exam	Straightforward	10–19
99213		Low	20–29
99214		Moderate	30–39
99215		High	40–54

Medical Decision-Making

Number of diagnoses, amount and complexity of data to be reviewed and analyzed, and risk of complications and/or morbidity or mortality of patient management

Level of service based on MDM [12]
Only requires two or three elements

CPT	Number of diagnoses	Complexity of data	Risk
99202 99212	1 self-limited	Minimal	Minimal

CPT	Number of diagnoses	Complexity of data	Risk
99203 99213	≥2 self-limited or minor problems Or 1 stable chronic condition Or 1 acute uncomplicated	Meet 1 out of 2 I. any 2 of the following—Review external notes, review results of each unique tests, order each unique test II. Independent historian	Low (e.g., allergic rhinitis, simple sprain, controlled hypertension)
99204 99214	≥1 chronic condition with exacerbation Or ≥2 stable chronic conditions Or 1 new problem with uncertain prognosis Or 1 acute problem with systemic manifestation	Meeting 1 out of 3 I. any combination of 3—Review external notes, review results, order tests, independent historian II. Independent interpretation of tests III. Discussion with external physicians about management and test results	Moderate – Prescription of medications – Minor surgery – **Social determinants of health (new 2021 E/M)** (e.g., uncontrolled diabetes mellitus [DM], pyelonephritis, food insecurity)
99205 99215	≥1 chronic condition with severe exacerbation Or ≥1 acute or chronic condition with threat to life	Meeting 2 out of 3 I. any combination of 3—Review external notes, review results, order tests, independent historian II. Independent interpretation of tests III. Discussion with external physicians about management and test results	High – Referral to emergency department – Hospitalization – Emergent major surgery – Decision does not resuscitate code status or de-escalate care due to poor prognosis (e.g., stroke, acute coronary syndrome, lung mass)

Time

When choosing a billing level based on time for outpatient E/M codes, the rules around what time can count changed in January 2021. While not perfect, the changes are an improvement over the previous restrictions. Beginning in January 2021, all time spent by the billing physician or qualified healthcare professional (QHP) on the date of service can be counted. Both face-to-face and non-face-to-face time can be included. Examples of activities that can count in this time include:

- Preparing to see the patient
- Obtaining and/or reviewing separately obtained history
- Performing a medically appropriate examination and/or evaluation

- Counseling and educating the patient/family/caregiver
- Ordering medications, tests, or procedures
- Referring and communicating with other healthcare professionals (when not separately reported)
- Documenting clinical information in the electronic or other health record
- Independently interpreting results (not separately reported) and communicating results to the patient/family/caregiver
- Coordinating care (not separately reported) [13]

Activities that cannot be counted toward total time:

- Time spent on a calendar day other than the date of service
- Time spent on services that are separately reportable/reimbursed
- Clinical staff time
- Time spent teaching residents or students (please see sections of GC/GE modifiers for details)

CPT	Time (min)	CPT	Time (min)
99202	15–29	99212	10–19
99203	30–44	99213	20–29
99204	45–59	99214	30–39
99205	60–74	99215	40–54

Physicians should document their total time spent and the activities that they performed as part of the time-based service. One example of a possible documentation "smart phrase" is given below:

My total time on this date was *** minutes, which included the following activities {drop down}. This time is independent and nonoverlapping.

An example of drop-down list of activities (adapted from the University of Virginia Health Epic System):

Preparing before the patient visit
Collecting and/or reviewing history
Performing physical examination and/or evaluation
Counseling and educating patients and caretakers
Ordering medications, tests, and studies
Referring and discussing management with others
Documenting clinical information in the electronic or other health record
Interpreting results independently (not separately reported)
Coordinating care (not separately reported)
*** (free text)

For visits that go beyond the upper time threshold, there is a prolonged service code:

99417—Prolonged office or other outpatient E/M services (beyond the total time of the primary procedure which has been selected using total time), requiring total time with or without direct patient contact beyond the usual service, on the date of the primary service, each 15 min (list separately in addition to codes 99205 and 99215 for office or other outpatient evaluation and management services).

This code should be added only if **billing is based on time**, and only to the code 99215 or 99205. CPT directions for this code outline its use as follows:

"Code 99417 is only used when the office or other outpatient service has been selected using time alone as the basis and only after the minimum time required to report the highest-level service (i.e., *99205 or 99215) has been exceeded by 15 min. To report a unit of 99417, 15 min of additional time must have been attained. Do not report 99417 for any additional time increment of less than 15 min"* [13].

CMS did not agree with the minimum time requirement and added their own prolonged service code, G2212, stating that it should be added to the maximum time interval for the service, not the minimum. Physicians and other health professionals need to be aware of this discrepancy in the expectations for the use of the prolonged service codes based on time.

Codes	Time range (min)	CPT: times to add 99417 (min)	CMS: times to add G2212 (min)
99205	60–74	75–89	89–103
99215	40–54	55–69	69–83

Split-Shared Visits in the Clinic

When the physician and QHP perform an E/M as a split-shared visit, the time spent by each can be summed for the total time. The time spent by each professional must be medically necessary, and any time spent together (reviewing the patient's data, discussing a plan, seeing the patient) can only be counted once—either by the physician or by the QHP. On January 2022, CMS changed the split-shared rules for facility-based outpatient clinics [14]. The rules now state that payment will be made to the practitioner who performs the substantive portion of the visit. Beginning in January 2023, CMS defines the substantive portion as more than half of the time spent. During a transition year in 2022, CMS allowed the substantive portion to be one of the three key E/M components (history, exam, or MDM) OR more than half of the time. Each clinician should document their contribution to the split-shared service, whether time or a key component. Time can be summed. If billing based on time and QHP spends more than half of the total time, the claim will be submitted under their name and (generally) paid at 85% of the physician rate.

E/M Visits with Residents or Students

When seeing patients with medical students, **only time spent by the billing physician can be counted if billing is based on time**. When precepting residents and billing with the GC modifier, the same caveat applies. Only the time spent by the billing physician should be counted. In both of these scenarios, if the billing physician spends time observing the student or resident taking the history and/or performing an exam as part of the patient's visit, this time can be counted. For primary care resident clinics who operate under the primary care exception (GE modifier), CMS clarified in the 2022 PFS final rule that time CANNOT be used to select a visit level. Only MDM may be used in GE encounters, "to guard against the possibility of inappropriate coding that reflects residents' inefficiencies rather than a measure of the total medically necessary time required to furnish the E/M services" [15].

More details about the GE/GC modifiers and specifics of the primary care exception are outlined later in the chapter.

When would a physician use time for billing over medical decision-making? It really depends on the individual practice style and the patient characteristics. Consider the following scenarios:

- Did you spend a considerable amount of time preparing for the visit **on the date of service**, collecting a history, or performing an exam? You can only count time on the date of service only. If you pre-chart the day prior, or complete your notes on the days after clinic, you cannot count this time.
- Did the patient's care require that you personally engage with other physicians or review complex data?
- Is this a patient who does not meet level 5 MDM criteria, but takes level 5 time?
- Are you seeing a partner's patient (established for you) who is taking more time because you do not know them like your own patients?
- Do you routinely complete your notes on the date of service? If so, you can count this time toward total visit time.

Clinical Examples

Example #1
A 60-year-old male with well-controlled hypertension and hyperlipidemia returns to the resident clinic for routine follow-up. Also, he reports 3 days of left knee pain after hiking with grandkids 5 days prior.

HTN: doing well on meds; blood pressure is controlled. Denies dizziness.

For cholesterol: on atorvastatin; no muscle ache.

Medications and allergies are reviewed.

Physical exam: vital signs: normal including blood pressure—120/72

Heart: RRR, S1 and S2

Lungs: clear

Left knee: full range of motion, no erythema, no warmth
A/P:

1. HTN, well controlled on lisinopril 20 mg and HCTZ 25 mg daily. Order BMP today. Continue current medications. Refills done.
2. Hyperlipidemia on atorvastatin 20 mg daily. Last lipids 9 months ago, reviewed. No side effects. Continue treatment. Counseling provided: diet and exercise.
3. Left knee pain. Acute. Consistent with overuse. Exam reassuring. Over-the-counter diclofenac gel recommended. Acetaminophen PRN. Call in 2 weeks if not resolving, for physical therapy referral.

Attending went in to examine the patient with the resident.

Level of service based on MDM-99214

CPT	Number of diagnoses	Complexity of data	Risk
99214	≥1 condition with exacerbation or ✓**≥2 chronic conditions** or ✓**1 new problem with uncertain prognosis** or 1 acute problem with systemic manifestation	Meeting 1 out of 3 I. Any combination of 3—review external notes, ✓**review results**, ✓ **order tests**, independent historian II. Independent interpretation of tests III. Discussion with external physicians about management and test results	✓**Moderate** ✓Prescription of medications – Minor surgery – Social determinants of health (new 2021 E/M)

Level of service based on time:
Attending personally spends 25 min on the date of service involved in the care of this patient. This time includes reviewing the medical record for details of medication history and most recent refills, listening to the presentation from the resident, personally performing an exam, and discussing plans for the patient's knee pain with the patient. Finally, there is additional time reviewing and editing the resident's documentation and placing the attending attestation. **Based on time, 25 minutes would allow for billing 99213**. Therefore, the attending does not document time and submits 99214-GC (a higher level) for LOS based on MDM.

Diagnoses managed	Complexity of data	Risk	Overall code for MDM	Overall code for time
2 stable chronic plus 1 new with uncertain prognosis	BMP ordered, prior lipid panel reviewed	Prescription drug management	Need 2/3, drop data	25 min
Meets 99214	Meets 99213	Meets 99214	**99214**	99213

Example #2:
A 55-year-old established female with hypertension and diabetes presents with crying spells and insomnia.
She reports that her symptoms started gradually in the past 2 months. She would have crying spells for "no reason" in addition to having a difficult time falling asleep. She would wake up in the middle of the night sobbing. Due to disrupted sleep, she would fall asleep at work. She is worried about these episodes and is afraid that things will get worse.
As for her blood pressure, she takes lisinopril, and her blood pressure is 130/78 at home.
She is on metformin 500 mg bid for her DM.
On further questioning, she stated that 6 months ago, her husband passed away unexpectedly from a heart attack due to COVID while they were vacationing in Idaho celebrating their anniversary. He was previously healthy. During the trip, they both felt tired and did not think much of it. While in the hotel room, he suddenly became unresponsive and breathless. She tried to use her phone to call 911, but the phone did not work. She ran out in the hallway, but no one could hear her. Finally, she used her husband's cell phone and got connected to 911. The 911 respondent walked her through on how to perform CPR on him until EMS arrived. They continued CPR, and his pulse returned. In the emergency department, they told her that he had suffered a massive heart attack. He was then transferred to intensive care. At that time, she found out that he had contracted COVID. She went back to her hotel and shortly after received a call from the hospital that he coded again and they could not revive him. In shock and desperation, she felt the world had crashed onto her. She was all alone away from home. With the help of the hotel manager, she got tested and was confirmed to have COVID. Subsequently, her oxygen level dropped and was admitted to the hospital. Finally, she was discharged, had her husband cremated, and flew home. She thought she was doing OK for 6 months that had passed, but is now with all these symptoms. She does not have suicidal or homicidal thoughts. She does not have children.
PE: vital signs normal with BP 128/70
She appears tired
Mood—tearful at times
The patient's response to the PHQ-9 depression screening questionnaire is positive
At the last visit about 1 month ago, laboratory studies were done.
Her basic metabolic panel was normal, hgba1c 6.4, and TSH was normal.
A/P:
Depression and insomnia—patient does not want to be on medication; I contacted the psychologist to schedule an urgent appointment
DM: at goal; continue metformin
HTN: continue lisinopril

Level of service based on MDM 99214

CPT	Number of diagnoses	Complexity of data	Risk
99214	≥1 chronic condition with exacerbation or ✓**≥2 stable chronic conditions** or ✓**1 new problem with uncertain prognosis** or 1 acute problem with systemic manifestation	Meeting 1 out of 3 I. Any combination of 3—review external notes, ✓**review results**, order tests, independent historian II. Independent interpretation of tests ✓**III. Discussion with external physicians about management and test results**	✓**Moderate** –✓Prescription of medications – Minor surgery – Social determinants of health (new 2021 E/M)

Level of service based on time:
The total time on this date and for this encounter was 71 minutes, which included the following activities:

Preparing to see the patient, performing a medically appropriate examination and/or evaluation, counseling and educating the patient, ordering medications, referring and communicating with other healthcare professionals, and documenting clinical information in the electronic health record.

This time is independent and nonoverlapping and qualifies **level 599215 (40–54 min) + 99417**

Diagnoses managed	Complexity of data	Risk	Overall code for MDM	Overall code for time
2 stable chronic plus 1 new but self-limited	Discuss with external physician about management	Prescription drug management	Need 2/3	71 min
Meets 99214	Meets 99214	Meets 99214	99214	**99215+ 99417**

In this scenario, billing by time allows a higher level of service from level 4 to level 5 plus prolonged service code to truly reflect the work done by the physician.

Telemedicine Billing and Coding

Since the beginning of the COVID pandemic on March 6, 2020, with PHE, CMS started to allow telemedicine visits to be performed by physicians and advanced practice providers, regardless of location. Telemedicine visits permit physicians and healthcare professionals to continue chronic medical disease management and address certain acute conditions. In this section, the focus will be mainly on telemedicine outpatient billing and coding. The section of telemedicine in this book will cover the history of telemedicine, special telemedicine considerations, and clinic workflow in an academic medical practice with learners (Chaps. 12–14).

Telephone (Audio) Only [16]

During PHE, telephone (audio) only was used by clinicians to care for patients who did not have access or did not feel comfortable using technological devices to perform video-audio visits. Though PHE has ended, telephone (audio) only is still allowed, but this may vary state by state. CMS will determine when the reimbursement for audio-only CPT codes will end.

The service cannot be originated from the related E/M service within the last 7 days and will not lead to E/M service within the next 24 hours.

CPT code	Time (min)
99441	5–10
99442	11–20
99443	21–30

For telephone audio-only visit documentation, few elements are required:

- Patient has consented for telemedicine visits
- Place of service
- People who are on the call with the patient
- Chief complaint or reason for call
- Relevant history and laboratory results
- Assessment and plan
- Time spent on medical discussion

Level of services—add 93 modifier to the appropriate CPT code

Audio and Video Telemedicine Visits [5, 17]

During PHE under the 1135 waiver with expansion of telehealth, many video chat modalities were allowed. For example, products such as Apple FaceTime, Facebook Messenger video chat, Google Hangouts video, WhatsApp video chat, Zoom, Skype, Doximity, and Doxy.me, or electronic health record with video-audio capability, enabled clinicians and their patients to conduct a video chat visit privately.

Please note that the list of products is incomplete and not intended to promote a specific product. Though PHE has ended, audio and video telemedicine are still permitted.

Documentation—same as in person visits except with limitation of certain systems of physical exam.

CPT codes for new patients (99202-99205)

CPT codes for established patients (99212-99215)

Add modifier 95

Virtual Check In (for Established Patients Only)

G2012—initiated by patient to communicate with their physician through telephone or any telecommunication device to discuss whether an in-person visit is needed

G2010—a virtual evaluation of a video recording or images sent by patients

E-visits (Initiated by Established Patients Through Online Patient Portal)

For physicians:

99421—online digital management, cumulative time for up to 7 days, 5–10 min

99422—online digital management, cumulative time for up to 7 days, 11–20 min

99423—online digital management, cumulative time for up to 7 days, 21 or more minutes

For qualified nonphysician healthcare professionals (e.g., physical therapist, behavioral therapist):

G2061—online digital management, cumulative time for up to 7 days, 5–10 min

G2062—online digital management, cumulative time for up to 7 days, 11–20 min

G2063—online digital management, cumulative time for up to 7 days, 21 or more minutes

Preventive Visits [18]

The value of routine physical exams in general internal medicine practice continues to be debated [19].

These services can be billed using preventive visit codes for non-Medicare patients. Preventive exams for Medicare patients fall under the Welcome to Medicare exam and initial/subsequent Annual Wellness Visits.

CPT codes for preventive visits are as follows:

New patient:

99385 (18–39 years of age)

99386 (40–64 years of age)

Established patient:

99395 (18–39 years of age)

99396 (40–64 years of age)

Preventive services are bundled services, and thus documenting preventive visits is more straightforward than E/M coding. The following documentation is required:

- Include a comprehensive history of past, family, and social history as well as assessment/history of pertinent risk factors, and physical exam (components based on age and risk factors)
- Describe the status of chronic, stable problems that are not "significant enough to require additional work"
- Describe the management of minor problems that do not require additional work
- Document that a conversation occurred about age-appropriate counseling, screening labs, and tests, and order these labs/tests as appropriate
- Document that shared decision-making occurred in regard to recommended vaccines that are relevant to patients' age and risk factors and that vaccines were appropriately ordered

Screening Visits [20]

Prostate Cancer Screening

Screening for prostate cancer remains controversial. It is a shared decision between physicians and patients.

CPT code: G0103—prostate-specific antigen test (PSA)

Annually, for all male Medicare beneficiaries aged 50 and older, co-payment/coinsurance and deductible are applied

Screening Pelvic Examinations

CPT: G0101—cervical or vaginal cancer screening and pelvic and clinical breast exam
All female Medicare beneficiaries, annually if at high risk or childbearing age with abnormal Pap test within the past 3 years
Every 2 years for women at normal risk for Medicare patients (please note that the screening frequency may be different for non-Medicare patients based on the U.S. Preventive Services Task Force)
Co-payment/coinsurance and deductible waived

Depression Screening

CPT code: G0444—annual depression screening, 15 min.
All Medicare beneficiaries covered; co-payment/coinsurance/deductible waived
Must be furnished in a primary care setting that has staff-assisted depression care supports in place
Tip: Have your staff administer a Patient Health Questionnaire (PHQ) 2 to all patients once a year during the check-in process.

Medicare Services

The Annual Wellness Visit

Created as part of the Affordable Care Act, the Annual Wellness Visit (AWV) has high potential to increase revenue for a general internal medicine practice [20].

Who can deliver the AWV?

1. Any primary care (PC) practitioner (MD, DO, NP, PA)
2. Any health professional "under direct supervision in the suite and immediately available to the PC provider"
3. Someone other than the provider billing for the service, which can include health educators, nutritional professionals, and others; no credentialing requirements

When is a patient eligible?

1. Medicare patients after the completion of their first year of Medicare participation can receive their initial AWV (G0438) and can receive this only once
2. After the initial AWV, each year, patients are eligible for subsequent AWVs (G0439).

What are the requirements of an AWV?

Tip: For the first year a patient participates in Medicare, they are eligible for the Welcome to Medicare Visit, or Initial Preventive Physical Examination, described later in this chapter.

1. Medical history (tip: updated problem list can address this requirement)
2. Medications, prescription, and nonprescription (over-the-counter medications, herbal products)
3. Family history
4. List of "current providers and suppliers" regularly involved in the patient's care
5. Basic vital signs (height, weight, blood pressure, body mass index)
6. Detection of cognitive impairment based on provider's best judgment (no specific test recommended)
7. Review of individual's "potential" risk factors for depression (no instrument specified)

Tip: A PHQ-2 works well here.

8. An assessment of functional ability based on direct observation or the use of appropriate screening questions or screening questionnaire focused on the following:

   (a) Hearing
   (b) Activities of daily living (ADL)
   (c) Fall risk
   (d) Home safety

Tip: A standard health risk assessment (HRA) form can help greatly here and is worth the effort to create one for the office practice. At a minimum, the HRA should include demographic data, self-assessment of health status, psychosocial risks, behavioral risks, and activities of daily living. Also, the forced whisper test and the get up and go test can be quickly performed in a general internal medicine setting to assess hearing and gait instability/fall risk.

9. A written schedule for the USPSTF recommendations and Advisory Committee on Immunizations
10. A list of risk factors and conditions for which primary, secondary, or tertiary interventions are recommended (highly discretionary)
11. Written advice or referral to appropriate health education or prevention services or programs

Tip: Giving a patient a senior guide to resources will meet these criteria, along with specific referrals if needed such as physical therapy if fall risk is identified.

With proper planning and teamwork, these visits can be performed in less than 30 min and generate significant revenue to the practice: Creating smart phrases in electronic health record (EHR) can reduce the keystrokes required to document these elements.

AWVs can be combined with other general internal medicine NEW and ESTABLISHED E/M codes such as 99202–99205 and 99212–99215 using the 25 modifier. Documentation must clearly reflect that more than a wellness visit has occurred.

Tip: This can be done in the assessment by using ICD-10 for health maintenance for the AWV, and then using ICD-10 s for the acute or chronic medical conditions also discussed, with a specific plan for each of these conditions clearly documented.

The Initial Preventive Physical Examination (IPPE), also known as the "Welcome to Medicare Preventive Visit":

The goals of the IPPE are health promotion and disease prevention and detection.

Medicare pays for one IPPE per beneficiary per lifetime for beneficiaries within the first 12 months of the effective date of the beneficiary's first Medicare Part B coverage period [21, 22].

Components of the IPPE and required elements with smart phrases or templated checklists within the EHR can be very helpful at documenting and meeting these requirements.

1. Review the beneficiary's medical and social history, including:
   (a) Past medical/surgical history (experiences with illnesses, hospital stays, operations, allergies, injuries, and treatments)
   (b) Current medications and supplements (including calcium and vitamins)
   (c) Family history (review of medical events in the beneficiary's family, including diseases that may be hereditary or place the beneficiary at risk)
   (d) History of alcohol, tobacco, and illicit drug use
   (e) Diet and physical activity
2. Review the beneficiary's potential risk factors for depression and other mood disorders. Use any appropriate screening instrument for beneficiaries without a current diagnosis of depression from various available screening tests recognized by national professional medical organizations to obtain current or past experiences with depression or other mood disorders.
3. Review the beneficiary's functional ability and level of safety. Use any appropriate screening questions or standardized questionnaires recognized by national professional medical organizations to review, at a minimum, the following areas:
   (a) Hearing impairment
   (b) Activities of daily living
   (c) Fall risk
   (d) Home safety
4. Exam requires the following:
   (a) Height, weight, body mass index, and blood pressure
   (b) Visual acuity screen
   (c) Other factors deemed appropriate based on the beneficiary's medical and social history and current clinical standards

5. End-of-life planning, which is verbal or written information provided to the beneficiary about the beneficiary's ability to prepare an advance directive in case an injury or illness causes the beneficiary to be unable to make healthcare decisions and whether or not you are willing to follow the beneficiary's wishes as expressed in the advance directive.
6. Educate, counsel, and refer based on the previous five components. Based on the results of the review and evaluation services in the previous five components, provide education, counseling, and referral as appropriate.
7. Educate, counsel, and refer for other preventive services which include a brief written plan, such as a checklist, for the beneficiary to obtain:

A once-in-a-lifetime screening electrocardiogram (EKG/ECG), as appropriate
Appropriate screenings and other preventive services covered by Medicare
The CPT codes for the IPPE are:

G0402—Initial preventive physical examination: face-to-face visit, services limited to new beneficiary during the first 12 months of Medicare enrollment (wRVU = 2.60).

G0403—Electrocardiogram, routine ECG with 12 leads: performed as a screening for the initial preventive physical examination with interpretation and report.

G0404—Electrocardiogram, routine ECG with 12 leads: tracing only, without interpretation and report, performed as a screening for the initial preventive physical examination.

G0405—Electrocardiogram, routine ECG with 12 leads: interpretation and report only, performed as a screening for the initial preventive physical examination.

Care Management Codes

Transition Codes: 99495–99496 [23].

In 2013, CMS allows Transition Care Management (TCM) codes 99495 and 99496 to be used by physicians (any specialty) and the following nonphysician practitioners (NPPs) who are legally authorized and qualified to provide the services in the state in which they are furnished:

Certified nurse-midwives (CNMs)
Clinical nurse specialists (CNSs)
Nurse practitioners (NPs)
Physician assistants (PAs)

The services must be provided within the first 30 days post-inpatient discharge.

Documentation must have the date of initial discharge, date of post-discharge communication with patient or caretaker, date of the first face-to-face visit, medication reconciliation, and complexity of medical decision-making (moderate or high).

CPT code 99495

1. Communication (direct contact, phone, or electronic) with the patient and/or caregiver within 2 business days of discharge—this can be done by licensed clinical staff (non-physician practitioners).

   A member of the care team must make an interactive contact with the beneficiary and/or caregiver, as appropriate, within 2 business days following the beneficiary's discharge to the community setting. The contact may be via telephone, email, or face-to-face (video chat was not included as a modality in this code). For Medicare purposes, attempts to communicate should continue after the first two attempts in the required 2 business days until they are successful. If the two or more separate attempts are made in a timely manner and are documented in the medical record but are unsuccessful, and if all other TCM criteria are met, the service may be reported. Physicians or qualified health professionals may furnish the following non-face-to-face services: Obtain and review discharge information (e.g., discharge summary or continuity of care documents); review need for or follow-up on pending diagnostic tests and treatments; interact with other healthcare professionals who will assume or reassume care of the beneficiary's system-specific problems; provide education to the beneficiary, family, guardian, and/or caregiver; establish or reestablish referrals and arrange for needed community resources; and assist in scheduling required follow-up with community providers and services.
2. A face-to-face visit within 7 calendar days of discharge.
3. At a minimum, the following information must be documented in the beneficiary's medical record:

   Date of discharge
   Date of an interactive contact with the beneficiary and/or caregiver
   Date of the furnished face-to-face visit

   The complexity of medical decision-making (moderate or high)

CPT code 99496

1. Communication (direct contact, phone, or electronic) with the patient and/or caregiver within 2 business days of discharge
2. A face-to-face visit within 14 calendar days of discharge
3. Documentation requirements as noted in 99495
4. The complexity of medical decision-making (moderate or high)

Chronic Care Management Services

In 2015, CMS began paying for chronic care management services furnished to Medicare beneficiaries with multiple chronic conditions [24]. These services are generally non-face-to-face services provided over a calendar month by clinical staff and/or the physician or QHP. Additional codes have been added including physician/QHP-specific codes and principal care management codes to allow for the longitudinal management of a single chronic disease.

There are a number of required criteria for these codes; some of them are listed below:

- Multiple (two or more) chronic conditions expected to last at least 12 months, or until the death of the patient, **OR** one complex chronic condition expected to last at least 3 months
- Chronic conditions place the patient at significant risk of death, acute exacerbation/decompensation, or functional decline
- Comprehensive care plan is established, implemented, revised, or monitored
- Patient consent for the service

There are three general categories of care management: chronic care management (CCM, 99437, 99439, 99490, 99491), complex chronic care management (CCCM 99487, 99489), and principal care management (PCM 99424, 99425, 99425, 99427). The codes are further defined and valued by whether the service is primarily delivered by clinical staff or by the physician/QHP. For many academic primary care practices that are facility based, there has been concern that the services which are provided primarily by clinical staff cannot be billed at these clinics as the staff are generally employed by the facility. CMS has advised that these codes CAN be billed at facility-based clinics [25]. In addition to the MPFS claim for the physician/QHP time, there is an allowable "facility fee" billed under the Outpatient Prospective Payment System (OPPS) to compensate for the use of staff time. To implement CCM in a medical practice, one must review all of the requirements for these service codes.

Home Health Care (HHC) Oversight

The Affordable Care Act included provisions that increased physician responsibility for overseeing the utilization of ongoing home health care services [26].

The Home Health Care Oversight CPT codes are:

G0180, physician certification

G0179, physician recertification

These codes are meant to reimburse physicians for their time spent establishing HHC plans, communicating with HHC agencies, and reviewing form 485s (the Home Health Certification and Plan of Care Form).

The following documentation is required (EHR smart phrases and templates are very helpful):

- A physician must certify that a patient is eligible for Medicare home health services, and physician who establishes the plan of care must sign and date the certification.

- The patient needs intermittent skilled nursing care, physical therapist, and/or speech-language pathologist services.
- Reason the patient is confined to the home (i.e., homebound).
- A plan of care has been established and will be periodically reviewed by a physician.
- Services will be furnished while the individual was or is under the care of a physician.
- A face-to-face encounter—occurred no more than 90 days prior to the home health start of care date or within 30 days of the start of the home health care—was related to the primary reason the patient requires home health services and was performed by a physician or allowed nonphysician practitioner.
- The certifying physician must also document the date of the face-to-face encounter.

Coding and Billing for Counseling Services

Coding and billing for common counseling services offered in a general internal medicine practice are underutilized. Understanding these codes and documentation requirements can improve and generate revenue to medical practices. Below are CPT codes that are covered by Medicare. Medicaid and commercial insurance coverage for these CPT codes vary. These CPT codes can be billed as add-on services for an E/M visit with a 25 modifier.

Advanced Directive Counseling [27, 28]

CPT Codes:

99497—Advance care planning including the explanation and discussion of advance directives such as standard forms (with completion of such forms, when performed), by the physician or other qualified healthcare professionals: first 30 min, face-to-face with the patient, family member(s), and/or surrogate.

99498—Each additional 30 min (list separately in addition to code for primary procedure).

Examples of appropriate documentation would include an account of the discussion with the beneficiary (or family members and/or surrogate) regarding the voluntary nature of the encounter, documentation indicating the explanation of advance directives (along with completion of those forms, when performed), who was present, and the time spent in the face-to-face encounter. Must spend a full 30 minutes to bill for this service.

Counseling to Prevent Tobacco Use [29]

CPT Codes:

99406—Smoking and tobacco-use cessation counseling visit, 3–10 min

99407—Smoking and tobacco-use cessation counseling visit, greater than 10 min

Medicare outpatient and hospitalized beneficiaries are covered (co-payment/coinsurance and deductible waived) and those who meet the following:

1. Use tobacco, regardless of whether they exhibit signs/symptoms of tobacco-related disease
2. Competent and alert at the time of counseling
3. Counseling furnished by a qualified physician or other Medicare-recognized practitioner
4. Two cessation attempts are covered per 12-month period. Each attempt may include a maximum of four intermediate or intensive counseling sessions.

Therefore, the total annual benefit covers up to eight smoking cessation counseling sessions in a 12-month period.

Tip: For counseling, use the 5 As as a template for documentation.

Assess: Ask about/assess behavioral health risk(s) and factors affecting the choice of behavior change goals/methods.

Advise: Give clear, specific, and personalized behavior change advice, including information about personal health harms and benefits

Agree: Collaboratively select appropriate treatment goals and methods based on the patient's interest and willingness to change the behavior

Assist: Using behavior change techniques (self-help and/or counseling), aid the patient in achieving agreed-upon goals by acquiring the skills, confidence, and social/environmental supports for behavior change, supplemented with adjunctive medical treatments when appropriate.

Arrange: Schedule follow-up contacts (in person or by telephone) to provide ongoing assistance/support and to adjust the treatment plan as needed, including referral to a more intensive or specialized treatment.

Alcohol Misuse Screening and Counseling [30]

CPT Codes:

G0442—Annual alcohol misuse screening, 15 min

To bill for this, the clinicians must spend a minimum of 8 minutes performing the screening. This can include both the screening and the documentation. The time spent should be documented. Screening must be performed, documented, and billed before counseling sessions are billed.

G0443—Brief face-to-face behavioral counseling for alcohol misuse, 15 min.

According to the USPSTF (2004), alcohol misuse includes risky/hazardous and harmful drinking, which places individuals at risk for future problems, and, in the general adult population, risky or hazardous drinking is defined as >7 drinks per week or >3 drinks per occasion for women and > 14 drinks per week or > 4 drinks per occasion for men.

All Medicare beneficiaries are eligible for alcohol screening (G0442) once a year, and co-payment/coinsurance and deductible are waived

Medicare beneficiaries who screen positive are eligible for counseling under the following conditions:

They are competent and alert at the time of counseling.

Counseling may be furnished by qualified primary care physician and can be done up to 4 times a year. The primary care clinicians should document the time spent counseling as part of their documentation.

The behavioral counseling intervention should be consistent with the five As approach that has been adopted by the USPSTF.

Intensive Behavioral Therapy for Cardiovascular Disease [31]

CPT code G0446—Annual, face-to-face intensive behavioral therapy (IBT) for cardiovascular disease (CVD), individual, 15 min.

Coverage of IBT for CVD, referred to as a CVD risk reduction visit, consists of the following three components:

1. Encouraging aspirin use for the primary prevention of CVD when the benefits outweigh the risks for men age 45–79 years and women 55–79 years
   *In October 2021, the USPSTF posted a draft statement that primary prevention for CVD with aspirin for ages 40–59 with 10% and greater cardiovascular risk is grade C and should be individualized. They recommend against the use of aspirin in adults aged 60 and older.
2. Screening for high blood pressure in adults aged 18 years and older.
3. Intensive behavioral counseling to promote a healthy diet for adults with hyperlipidemia, hypertension, advancing age, and other known risk factors for cardiovascular and diet-related chronic disease

The behavioral counseling intervention for aspirin use and healthy diet should be consistent with the five As approach that has been adopted by the USPSTF.

Intensive Behavioral Therapy (Obesity) [32]

CPT Codes:

G0447—Face-to-face behavioral counseling for obesity, 15 min

G0473—Face-to-face behavioral counseling for obesity, group (2–10), 30 min

Medicare pays for intensive behavioral therapy (IBT) for beneficiaries with a body mass index of 30 or greater. This service may be performed by a primary care physician, OB/GYN physician, nurse practitioner, physician assistant, or certified clinical nurse specialist. In CMS's decision memo to support covering the service, they said that the service may be performed incident to a physician service by ancillary personnel.

"In the primary care office setting, Medicare may cover these services when billed by the primary care physician or practitioner and furnished by auxiliary personnel under the conditions specified under our regulation at 42 CFR Section 410.26(b) (conditions for services and supplies *incident to a physician's professional service*)." The benefit includes:

- One face-to-face visit every week for the first month
- One face-to-face visit every other week for months 2–6
- One face-to-face visit every month for months 7–12, if the beneficiary meets the 3 kg weight loss requirement during the first 6 months

The Medicare co-pay and deductible are waived for this service.

These services may be provided on the same day as an E/M service or a wellness visit (for Medicare patients), but the time of the counseling must be distinct from the other E/M services.

Be sure to document the time and nature of the counseling in the note.

Modifiers

Coding Nuances to be Aware of in a General Internal Medicine Practice

Modifier 25 [18, 33]

When providing a problem-oriented E/M service or procedure with a preventive visit, the modifier 25 should be added to be paid for both services. Modifier 25 is appropriate when there is a "significant, separately identifiable evaluation and management service by the same physician on the same day." If the second service requires enough additional work that it could stand on its own as an office visit, use modifier 25. Preventive codes include both classic annual exams for commercial insurance and Medicare Annual Wellness Visits. When submitting both services, make sure that the documentation clearly supports both a preventive ICD-10 code and a problem-based code, with linkage of the appropriate diagnosis codes to the CPT codes to facilitate billing:

G0438 (Medicare AWV) diagnosis (dx) code Z00.00 (encounter for general adult medical examination)

99214-25 dx codes I12.9 (hypertensive chronic kidney disease) and E11.9 (T2DM, no complications)

Attach modifier 25 to the problem-oriented E/M code instead of the preventive service code.

If a procedure was done in addition to the preventive service, attach the 25 modifier to the preventive visit code.

Modifiers to Use When Supervising Resident Physicians [34, 35]

Modifier GC

When an E/M service is provided by interns or residents under a teaching physician in an approved Graduate Medical Education program, GC modifier must be used.

For documentation, these are examples given by CMS:

- "I performed a history and physical examination of the patient and discussed his management with the resident. I reviewed the resident's note and agree with the documented findings and plan of care."
- "I was present with resident during the history and exam. I discussed the case with the resident and agree with the findings and plan as documented in the resident's note."
- "I saw and evaluated the patient. I reviewed the resident's note and agree, except that the picture is more consistent with pericarditis than myocardial ischemia. Will begin NSAIDs."

Modifier GE for Primary Care Exception

The Primary Care Exception (PCE) is allowed for Graduate Medical Education programs if they qualify and meet certain specific requirements. This exception allows teaching physicians to bill for indirectly supervised care. Teaching physicians must see all interns' patients during the first 6 months of training and use the GC modifier.

To use the primary care exception, a primary care center must attest the following requirements:

1. The center is located in an outpatient department of a hospital or another ambulatory center, which patient care provided by residents is tied to a teaching hospital.
2. The residents must have completed more than 6 months of residency training.
3. The ratio of teaching faculty to residents does not exceed 1:4.
4. The teaching faculty must be in proximity to provide immediate availability.
5. The teaching faculty must not have other responsibilities such as the direct supervision of other nonresident or medical student learners.
6. The teaching faculty must review medical records and document the participation.
7. The primary care center is the site for patients to receive continuity of care provided by the residents during their residency training.

The modifier **GE** should be used for Primary Care Exception instead of GC, which is used when patients are physically seen and examined by attending physician.

The levels of services for PCE are 99202, 99203, 99212, and 99213 (level three is the highest level that can be billed for Medicare-only patients if not seen by an attending physician).

During the COVID-19 PHE, this restriction was waived, and **all levels of E/M services could be billed using the GE modifier.** In addition, supervision for both GE and GC clinics were done via real-time audiovisual communication, allowing for both flexibility and decreased risk of exposure to COVID [36]. When PHE ended, the billing of higher than level 3 when using GE is no longer allowed; remote supervision is extended until December 2024. * *Please see an updated statement of PHE at the end of the chapter.*

The Healthcare Common Procedure Coding System (HCPCS) codes are included in the primary care exception.

G0402—Initial preventive physical examination, face-to-face encounter for new beneficiary during the first 12 months of Medicare enrollment

G0438—First Annual Wellness Visit

G0439—Subsequent Annual Wellness Visit

Note: **The Transition of Care codes are not eligible for the primary care exception**.

If Transition of Care visits are performed in a teaching setting, the attending physician must see the patient to use the Transition of Care codes.

An example for documenting the Primary Care Exception is as follows: "I have reviewed with the resident Dr. _____'s medical history, physical examination, diagnosis, and results of tests and treatments and agree with the patient's care as documented in the resident's note."

Relative Value Units for E/M Visits, Preventive Visits, and Services

RVUs are composed of three components: physician work RVU, practice expense RVU, and malpractice RVU [37].

Medicare mandates' updating of RVUs every 5 years, and CMS, has delegated the task to the RUC, a committee of the AMA. Also charged to review RVUs is the MedPAC, an independent federal body that the Congress established in 1997 to analyze access, quality of care, and other issues affecting Medicare.

The Medicare conversion factor (CF) is a scaling factor that converts the geographically adjusted number of RVUs for each service in the Medicare physician payment schedule into a dollar payment amount. Adjustments in the CF have been based on three factors [38]:

- The Medicare Economic Index
- An expenditure target "performance adjustment"
- Miscellaneous adjustments including those for "budget neutrality"

The calendar year 2022 conversion factor is $34.6062 [39].

To calculate wRVU for each CPT code, use https://www.aapc.com/practicemanagement/rvu-calculator.aspx [40].

New patient office visit CPT code	wRVU (2022)	Established patient office CPT code	wRVU (2022)
99202	0.93	99212	0.70
99203	1.60	99213	1.30
99204	2.60	99214	1.92
99205	3.50	99215	2.80
99417	0.61	99417	0.61

CPT code (audio only)	wRVU (2022 PHE valuation)
99441 (5–10 min)	0.70
99442 (11–20 min)	1.30
99443 (20–30 min)	1.92

CPT code	Description	wRVU (2022)
G0444	Depression screening	0.18
G0402	IPPE (Welcome to Medicare exam)	2.60
G0438	Initial Medicare Annual Wellness Visit	2.60
G0439	Subsequent AWV	1.92
99496	Transitional care management (TCM), high complexity. FTF visit within 7 days of DC	3.79
99495	TCM moderate complexity (14 days post-DC)	2.78
G0180	Home health oversight, original certification	0.67
G0179	Home health oversight, recertification	0.45
99497	Advanced care planning, first 30 min	1.50
+99498	Advanced care planning, each additional 30 min	1.40
99406	Smoking and tobacco-use cessation 3–10 min	0.24
99407	Smoking and tobacco-use cessation >10 min	0.50
G0442	Annual alcohol screening 15 min	0.18
G0443	Brief alcohol misuse counseling	0.45

Maximizing Revenue

How to Optimize Practice Revenue in a General Internal Medicine Practice: Putting it All Together

1. Schedule face-to-face appointments that have the highest value

2. Take full advantage of billing/coding for counseling and preventive services using the 25 modifier
3. Develop systems to bill for non-face-to-face work
4. Avoid the GE modifier for complex patients
5. Bill for Home Health Care Certifications

1. Schedule face to face appointments that have the highest value

The table below is a ranking of Medicare visit types and relative value units, from highest value to lowest value.

Visit type	CPT code	wRVU
Transition of care 7 days + high MDM	99496	3.79
Transition of care 14 days + moderate MDM	99495	2.78
Medicare annual wellness visit (initial)	G0438	2.60
New patient	99204	2.60
Medicare AWV subsequent	G0439	1.92
Established patient	99214	1.92
New patient	99203	1.60
Established patient	99213	1.30

Most General Internal Medicine patient schedules are filled with established patient visits, E/M codes 99213 and 99214.

Evaluating the opportunity costs of how a general internist's time can best be spent to result in optimal practice financial success, the wRVUs favor schedules that prioritize Transition Care Management visits. Annual Wellness Visit's wRVUs are similar to new patient office visits at level 4 (99204). Note that the wRVU for a 7-day TCM visit (3.79 wRVU) is 2x higher than that of an established patient presenting for follow-up of three chronic conditions, which most likely represents a 99214 visit (1.92 wRVU).

Be sure to monitor inpatient census, and always be open to scheduling a 7-day TCM visit type.

Leave some slots in the clinic schedule for Annual Wellness Visits. This is a good way to talk to patients about their health and wellness and also a way to improve the financial health of the practice.

2. Take full advantage of billing/coding for counseling and preventive services with the 25-modifier

Build a process that systematically screens patients once a year for depression (a PHQ-2 works well), tobacco use, and alcohol use (an Audit-C works well). Medical assistants can ask these questions and/or give the patient a handout of the questionnaires.

For example, a 68-year-old male patient who presents for follow-up of hypertension, diabetes, and hyperlipidemia.

- If the patient is qualified for the Initial Annual Wellness Visit, it can be completed in addition to using the 25 modifier if the three chronic conditions are addressed and the treatment plans are documented.
- This would generate wRVUs of 2.60 for the AWV and 1.92 for the 99214 follow-up visit = 4.52 wRVU.

For the same patient, even without AWV, screening and counseling services can help generate more wRVU to this 99214 follow-up visit.

- Screening for depression (G0444, wRVU 0.18) and alcohol use (G0442, wRVU 0.18) can generate an additional 0.36 wRVU.
- If the screening test is positive for tobacco use and/or alcohol use, counseling using a 5 As template for tobacco counseling (99406, 0.24 wRVU) and alcohol misuse (G0443, 0.45 wRVU) will generate an additional 0.69 wRVU.
- The patient with hypertension, hyperlipidemia, and diabetes is a candidate for Intensive Behavioral Therapy for Cardiovascular Disease. Using the 5 As approach, an additional 0.45 wRVU can be added.
- By creating a workflow that systematically screens for and delivers counseling services, a simple 99214 visit with wRVU of 1.92 can be increased to a 99214 visit (1.92 wRVU) plus 0.36 + 0.69 + 0.45 = 3.42 wRVU.

Advanced Directive Counseling code can also add 1.50 wRVU.

A ranking of Medicare preventive services and relative value units is shown in the table below.

Preventive service	CPT	wRVU
Advanced Directive Counseling	99497	1.50
Alcohol Misuse Counseling	G0443	0.45
Intensive Behavioral Therapy for Cardiovascular Disease	G0446	0.45
Counseling to prevent tobacco use 3–10 min	99406	0.24
Alcohol Misuse Screening	G0442	0.18
Depression Screening	G0444	0.18

3. Develop systems to bill for non-face-to-face work

As more care is delivered outside of the periodic clinic visit, academic practices must embrace and develop systems to deliver and bill for non-face-to-face care. Care management services or digital e-visits and virtual check-ins are services that physicians and practices are already providing. Each of these categories requires patient consent and has potential co-payment for the services. Each would undoubtedly require process development within the institution's EHR. But there would be great potential for revenue as well as RVU-based accounting of the work being done by practices as health systems move toward population health models.

CPT code	Description	Staff type	wRVU
99490	Chronic care management first 20 min	Clinical staff	1.0
99439	CCM, each additional 20 min (may use ×2)	Clinical staff	1.0
99491	CCM, first 30 min	Physician/ QHP	1.50
99437	CCM, each additional 30 min	Physician/ QHP	0.71
99487	Complex chronic care management (CCCM), first 60 min	Clinical staff	1.81
99489	CCCM, each additional 30 min	Clinical staff	1.0
99426	Principal care management, first 30 min	Clinical staff	1.0
99427	Each additional 30 min	Clinical staff	0.71
99424	Principal care management, first 30 min	Physician/QHP	1.45
99425	Each additional 30 min	Physician/QHP	1.0
99421	Online digital E/M 5–10 min	Physician/QHP	0.25
99422	Online digital E/M 11–20 min	Physician/QHP	0.50
99423	Online digital E/M 21+ min	Physician/QHP	0.80
G2010	Remote evaluation of recorded image or video	Physician/QHP	0.18
G2012	Virtual check-in	Physician/QHP	0.25
G2252	Virtual check-in 11–20 min	Physician/QHP	0.50

4. <u>Avoid the GE modifier for complex patients</u>

Did a resident just sign out a complicated established patient with three chronic medical conditions, and/or a new problem with further workup required? Take the opportunity to bill at a higher level by going in to see that patient and avoid the use of the GE Primary Care Exception for complex patients.

5. <u>Bill for Home Health Care Certifications.</u>

Physicians express frustration at completing paperwork with no reimbursement. There is an excellent opportunity to get paid for reviewing Home Health Care Certification and care plans.

Take advantage of creating a template/smart phrase in EHR for documenting the requirements. A suggested checklist is as follows:

The patient is homebound because (list reason).

Physical findings supporting homebound status include (describe why homebound).

The patient is under my care, and I have authorized home health services and certify that they are necessary (describe what home care is offering).

The patient last seen in the office to address Home Health Care was (must occur no more than 90 days prior to the home health start of care date or within 30 days of the start of the home health care).

Not only will this checklist allow the billing for Home Health Certification, but it also provides an excellent tool to teach interns/residents what elements of documentation are required for Home Health Care.

A Cautionary Statement

Both undercoding and overcoding can carry risk. While it is rare to have external audits of professional services, they do happen. Knowledge of the coding guidelines as well as good documentation are the best defense. Most academic centers have compliance personnel who can be excellent resources when questions come up around specific codes and their documentation requirements. Professional societies such as the SGIM, the American College of Physicians, and the American Academy of Family Physicians also have online resources.

Conclusion

The success of an academic medicine clinic is determined not only by having an outstanding ambulatory curriculum but also by generating maximum revenue to provide more ancillary resources and support faculty and clinic personnel. Understanding the billing and coding requirements will allow teaching physicians to apply all the possible billable services to achieve maximum wRVUs. This knowledge can further be passed on to house staff to prepare them for their future clinical practice.

*This chapter was prepared prior to the ending of PHE on May 11, 2023. As of September 2023, audio-visual and telephone-only telemedicine visits are reimbursed by Medicare through December 2024. Reimbursement of these services by Medicaid and commercial insurance may vary based on location. The ability to bill all levels of outpatient E/M under Primary Care Exception (GE modifier) expired at the end of PHE. However, teaching physicians can continue to supervise remotely in all settings except high risk or surgical procedures through December 2024 [41].

References

1. Well PH. How did we get here? A brief history of government involvement in physician reimbursement. http://www.sgim.org/File%20Library/SGIM/Resource%20Library/Forum/2009/SGIM-November-2009-WEB.pdf
2. https://qpp.cms.gov/
3. https://www.ama-assn.org/system/files/2018-11/pfs-qpp-final-rule-sum11-8.pdf
4. https://www.cms.gov/files/document/2021-01-07-mlnc-se.pdf
5. https://www.cms.gov/newsroom/fact-sheets/medicare-telemedicine-health-care-provider-fact-sheet

6. COVID-19 Emergency Declaration Blanket Waivers for Health Care Providers (cms.gov).
7. Health Policy Committee I sgim.org
8. https://www.cms.gov/outreach-and-education/medicare-learning-network-mln/mlnproducts/downloads/eval-mgmt-serv-guide-icn006764.pdf
9. https://www.cms.gov/outreach-and-education/medicare-learning-network-mln/mlnedweb-guide/downloads/95docguidelines.pdf
10. https://www.cms.gov/outreach-and-education/medicare-learning-network-mln/mlnedweb-guide/downloads/97docguidelines.pdf
11. https://www.aapc.com/evaluation-management/em-codes-changes-2021.aspx
12. https://www.ama-assn.org/system/files/2019-06/cpt-revised-mdm-grid.pdf
13. Current procedural terminology: CPT 2021. American Medical Association; 2020.
14. Medicare Claims Processing Manual. Chapter 12. Section 30.6.18: Split (or Shared Visits). (Rev. 11288; Issued: 03-04-22; Effective: 01-01-22; Implementation: 02-15-22).
15. https://www.cms.gov/newsroom/fact-sheets/calendar-year-cy-2022-medicare-physician-fee-schedule-final-rule
16. https://www.aafp.org/family-physician/patient-care/current-hot-topics/recent-outbreaks/covid-19/covid-19-telehealth/coding-scenarios-during-covid-19/audio.html
17. https://www.hhs.gov/sites/default/files/telehealth-faqs-508.pdf
18. Owolabi T, Simpson I. Documenting and coding preventive visits: a physician's perspective. Fam Pract Manag. 2012;19(4):12–6.
19. https://www.choosingwisely.org/clinician-lists/society-general-internal-medicine-general-health-checks-for-asymptomatic-adults/
20. https://www.cms.gov/medicare/prevention/prevntiongeninfo/medicare-preventive-services/mps-quickreferencechart-1.html
21. https://www.cms.gov/Outreach-and-Education/Medicare-Learning-Network-MLN/MLNProducts/preventive-services/medicare-wellness-visits.html
22. Cuenca AE. Making Medicare wellness visits work in practice. Fam Pract Manag. 2012;19(5):11–6.
23. https://www.cms.gov/Outreach-and-Education/Medicare-Learning-Network-MLN/MLNProducts/Downloads/Transitional-Care-Management-Services-Fact-Sheet-ICN908628.pdf
24. https://www.cms.gov/Outreach-and-Education/Medicare-Learning-Network-MLN/MLNProducts/Downloads/ChronicCareManagement.pdf
25. https://www.cms.gov/medicare/medicare-fee-for-service-payment/hospitaloutpatientpps/downloads/payment-chronic-care-management-services-faqs.pdf
26. https://www.cms.gov/Outreach-and-Education/Outreach/NPC/Downloads/2014-12-16-HHBenefit-HL.pdf
27. https://www.cms.gov/Medicare/Medicare-Fee-for-Service-Payment/PhysicianFeeSched/Downloads/FAQ-Advance-Care-Planning.pdf
28. https://www.cms.gov/outreach-and-education/medicare-learning-network-mln/mlnproducts/downloads/advancecareplanning.pdf
29. https://www.cms.gov/Medicare/Prevention/PrevntionGenInfo/medicare-preventive-services/MPS-QuickReferenceChart-1.html#TOBACCO
30. https://www.cms.gov/medicare/prevention/prevntiongeninfo/medicare-preventive-services/mps-quickreferencechart-1.html#ALC_MISUSE
31. https://www.cms.gov/medicare/prevention/prevntiongeninfo/medicare-preventive-services/mps-quickreferencechart-1.html#CARDIO_IBT
32. https://www.cms.gov/medicare/prevention/prevntiongeninfo/medicare-preventive-services/mps-quickreferencechart-1.html#OBESITY_IBT
33. Felger TA, Felger M. Understanding when to use Modifier-25. Fam Pract Manag. 2004;11(9):21–2.

34. https://www.cms.gov/outreach-and-education/medicare-learning-network-mln/mlnproducts/downloads/teaching-physicians-fact-sheet-icn006437.pdf
35. https://www.cms.gov/Regulations-and-Guidance/Guidance/Transmittals/2019Downloads/R4283CP.pdf
36. https://www.cms.gov/files/document/se20011.pdf
37. https://www.cms.gov/Outreach-and-Education/Medicare-Learning-Network-MLN/MLNProducts/Downloads/How_to_MPFS_Booklet_ICN901344.pdf
38. https://www.ama-assn.org/practice-management/medicare-physician-payment-schedules
39. https://www.aafp.org/journals/fpm/blogs/gettingpaid/entry/updated_fee_schedule.html
40. https://www.aapc.com/practicemanagement/rvu-calculator.aspx
41. https://www.cms.gov/files/document/teaching-hospitals-physicians-medical-residents-cms-flexibilities-fight-covid-19.pdf

Chapter 8
ACGME Requirements and Accreditation Issues

Craig F. Noronha and Mark E. Pasanen

Introduction

This chapter reviews the role of the Accreditation Council for Graduate Medical Education (ACGME) in residency education with a specific focus on the ambulatory experience for internal medicine residents. There will be specific descriptions of requirements that clinic directors need to be aware of in the realms of scheduling, assessment, and site obligations. Common program challenges and opportunities in residency clinics are highlighted.

Outline

- Background
- Residency program requirements
- Primary care clinic site requirements
- Faculty requirements
- Resident requirements
- Scheduling requirements
- Assessment and feedback
- Working and learning environment
- Common opportunities and challenges
- Conclusion

C. F. Noronha (✉)
Department of Medicine, Internal Medicine Residency Program, Boston Medical Center, Boston University Chobanian and Avedisian School of Medicine, Boston, MA, USA
e-mail: craig.noronha@bmc.org

M. E. Pasanen
Department of Medicine, University of Vermont Medical Center/Larner College of Medicine at the University of Vermont, Burlington, VT, USA
e-mail: Mark.pasanen@uvmhealth.org

L. B. Lu et al. (eds.), *Leading an Academic Medical Practice*,
https://doi.org/10.1007/978-3-031-40273-9_8

Background

The ACGME is a private nonprofit organization that accredits residency programs based on a set of standards. Accreditation is conferred through ongoing evaluation by the ACGME with the goal of ensuring that residency programs provide a high-quality educational environment [1]. The ACGME standards are delineated in the Common Program Requirements, which apply to all residency and fellowship programs [2]. The ACGME also sets specialty-specific requirements that are designed to encompass the core elements expected for training in the specified field. A portion of the Internal Medicine Program Requirements outlines requirements for continuity clinic experiences including expectations for faculty, required continuity clinics for each resident, and frequency of assessments [1]. It is important for academic clinic directors to understand these requirements in order to maintain certification for the residency program. Failure to meet these requirements can result in residency programs being placed under increased scrutiny from the ACGME and, in the worst-case scenario, the program being placed on probation or terminated. Clinic directors should work with residency program leadership to ensure that the resident clinic experience is meeting ACGME requirements while also balancing the needs and resources of the clinic.

In 1999, the ACGME established six overarching clinical competency domains to form a foundation for education and assessment of graduate trainees. Ten years later, the ACGME began to transform its accreditation system to focus on competency-based outcomes. The Next Accreditation System (NAS), born from this work, had three main goals: "to enhance the ability of the peer-review system to prepare physicians for practice in the twenty-first century, to accelerate the ACGME's movement toward accreditation on the basis of educational outcomes, and to reduce the burden associated with the current structure and process-based approach" [3]. The NAS introduced educational milestones, described as "developmentally based, specialty-specific achievements that residents are expected to demonstrate at established intervals as they progress through training" [3]. The six core competencies were further subdivided into these milestones to highlight educational outcomes expected for each resident to achieve during residency. A residency's Clinical Competency Committee (CCC) is responsible for reviewing all resident evaluations, makes recommendations to promote trainees to their next level of training, and identifies when they are ready for independent practice. The CCC is also responsible for providing summative assessments of each trainee's progression in each milestone, which are submitted to the ACGME twice per year. Further information regarding milestone-based feedback and assessment can be found in Chap. 10. In July 2021, the ACGME updated the internal medicine milestones, introducing Milestones 2.0. These updated milestones addressed several issues with the first iteration of milestones including integrating "growth mindset concepts" and removing negative phrases such as "critical deficiencies" [4].

Another component of the NAS was the introduction of the Clinical Leaning Environment Review (CLER), which was designed to provide assessments and feedback to academic institutions in six areas: "patient safety, health care quality, care transitions, supervision, duty hours and fatigue management/mitigation, and professionalism" [5]. The CLER program includes periodic ACGME-sponsored site visits to institutions with graduate medical education programs. The CLER representatives meet with organizational leaders such as chief medical officers and graduate medical education leaders along with residents and faculty representatives from multiple residencies/fellowships. At the end of the visit, the CLER representatives meet with organizational leadership to review their assessment and feedback. Continuity clinics and clinic faculty may be included in the CLER visit, so it is important for clinic leadership to be aware of CLER-related discussions from hospital and residency leadership.

In July 2022, the ACGME Program Requirements for Internal Medicine underwent significant changes, and one of the goals is to encourage increased flexibility for both programs and residents to individualize training to better support resident career goals [6]. As part of those changes, the ACGME Internal Medicine Residency Review Committee (RRC) made substantial changes, including the elimination of many of the detailed requirements for the longitudinal clinic experience. This gives programs the opportunity to re-examine their structure and schedule but retains many of the core tenets for the continuity clinic experience.

Residency Program Requirements

The ACGME requires residents to have supervised training over a broad range of experiences for a total of 36 months, with a minimum of 30 months of "clinical experience." Over the 3 years, at least 10 months must be in the inpatient setting and at least 10 months in the outpatient setting (which includes time in longitudinal continuity clinic). Residency rotations must be structured to minimize conflicts between inpatient and outpatient responsibilities. In addition, there must be "a longitudinal, team-based continuity experience for the duration of the program." The program requirements provide further specifics, stating that the longitudinal experience would preferentially be in a general internal medicine continuity clinic but that an internal medicine sub-specialty clinic could qualify if all learning environment criteria are met.

Primary Care Clinic Site Requirements

The primary longitudinal clinic site for each individual resident should ideally remain constant over the 3 years of training to assure the development of long-term therapeutic relationships with a panel of patients. This clinic experience will often be in a site at the sponsoring institution but can be located in a variety of other settings, including a physician group practice or federally qualified health center. For any clinic site that is not directly under the sponsoring institution, a program letter of agreement (PLA) is required, which must be renewed every 10 years and be approved by the Designated Institutional Official (the individual in the organization who oversees all graduate medical education). For all clinics, there needs to be a clearly defined site director who is accountable for resident education. In addition, it is recommended that teaching faculty be identified and that there are specific policies and procedures that govern resident education, including specifics around teaching, supervision, and evaluation. The patient population should be representative of a broad spectrum of clinical disorders and conditions typically managed by internists. For patients in whom there is limited or no physical contact, opportunities for telemedicine services should be made available. As residents need to have opportunities to perform procedures relevant to career planning, longitudinal sites may be asked to provide such opportunities for common outpatient procedures (arthrocentesis, skin biopsy, etc.) for those residents interested in outpatient or procedural careers.

Faculty Requirements

As noted above, it is important for residency longitudinal clinics to identify the teaching faculty. Supervising faculty do not have to have an academic appointment, but they must be board certified either by the American Board of Medicine or the American Osteopathic Board of Internal Medicine. It is acceptable for a non-internist with appropriate qualifications to teach and supervise residents, such as a family medicine physician who has been approved by the site director and program director. Faculty must demonstrate a commitment to the education of residents and pursue faculty development to enhance their skills annually. Examples of faculty development include efforts to improve skills related to teaching quality improvement and/or patient safety. Additional faculty development can include engagement in training to improve personal or resident well-being and efforts to improve patient care. These faculty development experiences should be reported to residency program leadership annually.

Resident Requirements

One of the primary motivations behind the requirement for a longitudinal outpatient experience is the recognition of the importance of long-term relationships with patients. Therefore, it is critical that residents serve as the primary physician for their panel of patients, with responsibility for preventive health, acute health issues, and chronic disease management. In addition, residents must be involved in care coordination across health care settings and between clinic visits. Residents must demonstrate competence in respect and responsiveness to diverse patient populations, including but not limited to diversity in gender, age, culture, race, religion, disabilities, national origin, socioeconomic status, and sexual orientation. Additionally, they must develop skills in counseling, diagnosis, and treatment of adult diseases and conditions. Residents must also have the opportunity to develop longitudinal relations with supervising faculty members.

Scheduling Requirements

In the past, the ACGME Program requirements have provided specific guidelines for the required number of clinic sessions and the maximum time allowed away from their continuity clinic. As of the 2022 update, there is no longer this degree of specificity. Instead, the language of the requirements simply requires a longitudinal experience over the entire 3 years of residency. It will be crucial for outpatient faculty and leaders to continue to advocate for the critical importance of the continuity experience. If there are major changes implemented by programs to decrease or weaken the experience, it will potentially be to the detriment of their development as an independent physician and may impact faculty by decreasing their opportunities for teaching.

Assessment and Feedback

Residents in longitudinal experiences, such as continuity clinic, must be assessed at least every 3 months usually with a standardized evaluation form. This evaluation must be submitted to the residency program and should be available for the resident to review. Clinic faculty should work with program leadership to assure that these evaluations are not too onerous to complete and provide constructive feedback to the residents. In addition, program leadership will be responsible for linking these evaluations to the ongoing milestone-based competency assessments. Longitudinal clinic often provides an opportunity for highly effective feedback, given the consistency of supervisor relationships, and therefore the clinic evaluations are critical. While assessment is a description of a trainee's performance over a period of time, feedback is timely and specific descriptions of a behavior coupled with actionable suggestions for improvement. This is particularly notable for the milestones focusing on outpatient management and commitment to personal growth, which is assessed by a resident seeking and incorporating performance data. Residents should regularly provide rotational evaluations on the longitudinal clinic experience and the faculty they work with. In addition to residents receiving regular feedback, faculty must receive assessment on their teaching performance at least annually.

Working and Learning Environment

At each site, there must be regular monitoring of the clinical learning and working environment to assure excellent resident experience and education. This includes assurances that resident education is not being adversely affected by the presence of other providers or learners. However, longitudinal clinic can often provide an opportunity to participate in inter-professional teams, a priority noted in the program requirements. During clinic sessions, an individual faculty member in clinic must not be responsible for more than four residents or other learners. Additionally, if supervising >2 residents/learners, they must not have any other patient care responsibilities. In general, residents must be able to attend medical, dental, and/or mental health visits during working hours, so it is important for clinic directors to familiarize themselves with their local program approaches to meeting that requirement. Clinic sites should be expected to provide accommodations for resident disabilities, working closely with human resources and program leadership. Given the high frequency of burnout during residency and beyond, clinic faculty and leadership should notify program leadership for any recognized concerns around resident well-being.

Common Opportunities and Challenges

The ACGME Program Requirements define standards and obligations for residency programs and academic institutions to maintain certification. Meeting the standards set by the ACGME can be challenging requiring cooperation between multiple stakeholders, investment of resources, and advanced planning. However, the ACGME guidelines can also be considered as an opportunity to reinvent and reinvigorate clinic efforts. Clinic directors can use the requirements as a basis for advocating for support for residency-related efforts. Within the context of the 2022 ACGME Program Requirements, we will highlight a handful of specific areas in the program requirements that present unique opportunities and challenges.

Population Health

The ACGME 2022 Program Requirements specify that residents "demonstrate the ability to manage the care of patients using population-based data" [6]. The ACGME also emphasizes that residents "need experience using, understanding, and analyzing population health data" to improve the health outcomes of their patients [6]. The ACGME purposely leaves the details of population health integration vague to allow for academic institutions and clinics develop programs that match their current resources and data availability.

The most cited barrier to integration of population health into clinical care is the lack of access to population data. While electronic medical systems can collect numerous data points, most were originally designed as electronic medical records and ordering systems as opposed to being designed as tools for population health. Clinicians and population health managers often struggle to obtain actionable population health data [7–9]. Residency programs and clinics can advocate for designs of electronic medical system-integrated dashboards to support and enhance population health endeavors [10]. Clinic leadership should work with their local health informatics staff to understand the barriers and potential options for population health data access. Initially, it may be important to focus on 1–2 common disease processes, such as diabetes mellitus or hypertension, and identify a handful of quality or population health-related goals to focus on.

While it is essential to develop and design population health data access for clinicians and clinic staff, it is also equally important to consider curricula or tools to guide both trainees and faculty in the use of population health data. A clinic- or residency-level quality improvement project can help focus efforts while also providing skills and experiences with population health [11, 12]. For further information, please refer to Chap. 25 on population health and quality.

Continuity

The ACGME requires that residents have a "a longitudinal team-based continuity experience for the duration of the program through which they develop a long-term therapeutic relationship with a panel of patients" [6]. The ACGME does not specifically define what continuity means aside from identifying that there must be a long-term relationship between the resident and their panel of patients. The American Academy of Family Physicians defines continuity of care as "the process by which the patient and his/her physician-led care team are cooperatively involved in ongoing health care management toward the shared goal of high-quality, cost-effective medical care" [13]. The ACGME emphasizes that the care of patients in the primary care setting should be team based but should allow "patients to understand that the resident is "their" primary care doctor, and residents to see the continuity clinic patients as "their" patients" [6]. Above all else, the primary care clinic experience should foster the development of long-lasting relationships between patients and residents. These efforts should be done in conjunction with the development of a robust team-based care model that will provide high-quality care for patients even when residents are working in nonambulatory settings. If possible, clinics may consider setting continuity goals for example X number of visits per session that a resident has with patients on their panel [14, 15]. Based on this data, clinics may consider interventions to increase continuity such as resident clinic-specific training for front-desk staff to ensure that residents' patients are scheduling with their primary care provider.

Outside of the patient-primary care relationship, primary care clinics may want to consider approaches to encourage continuity between residents and attending preceptors. Depending on the scheduling model utilized for resident clinics, preceptors may be a vital safety net for resident patients between clinic sessions. Preceptor schedules can be modified to enhance patient and resident-preceptor continuity. For example, in an X + Y model, preceptors could potentially precept on a specific afternoon every week, and thereby end up working with a different group of residents every week. Alternatively, preceptors may be scheduled to match the resident schedule such that a preceptor only precepts during the +Y week. This approach will mean that preceptors will have intense weeks where they work closely with a smaller group of residents. If the preceptor works with the same grouping of residents over a period, they can become acquainted with patients and can act as a form of continuity when graduating residents transfer their patients to incoming interns.

Conclusion

One of the many roles for the residency clinic site director is to offer a rewarding experience for residents and faculty, all while ensuring compliance with ACGME requirements summarized in the table. This includes collaborating closely with the residency program leadership to be certain that all relevant requirements are addressed and to identify priorities for the outpatient setting. In addition, the longitudinal clinic provides an excellent opportunity for constructive resident feedback and evaluation as they work toward achievement of developmental milestones. The requirement that residents care for their patients over the 3-year span leads to excellent opportunities for work on population health and quality improvement, which are the key elements of program requirements. Numerous complexities arise in developing a well-balanced clinical experience for residents, given the challenges in balancing between the inpatient and outpatient needs. To provide the best ambulatory training, resident longitudinal clinics must instill efficient, patient-centered care while giving appropriate attention to the resident experience and the learning environment.

ACGME Ambulatory Specific Requirements as of July 1st, 2022	
Required ambulatory experience	At least 10 months in the outpatient setting
Calculation of time devoted to longitudinal experience as portion of outpatient setting	One month = 4 weeks, 20 days, or 40 half-days of clinic
Specific primary care clinic requirements	No specific number of clinics required
Max interval between primary care clinics	No requirements

ACGME Ambulatory Specific Requirements as of July 1st, 2022	
Primary care/continuity clinic requirement	Must have a longitudinal team-based continuity experience for the duration of residency
Clinic settings that can be considered outpatient experiences	Primary care clinic, internal medicine sub-specialty clinics, non-medicine clinics, walk-in clinics, and home care visits
Definition of continuity clinic experience	A longitudinal, team-based, continuity experience through which they develop a long-term therapeutic relationship with a panel of patients
Resident continuity clinic experience in same clinic throughout residency	ACGME **suggests** that residents will remain in the same clinic throughout the 36 months to maintain continuity of care for their patient panel. ***staying in the same clinic throughout residency is not required by the ACGME***
Days off	Residents must be scheduled for a minimum of 1 day in seven free of clinical work and required education (when averaged over 4 weeks)
Primary care physician definition for residents	Residents must serve serving as the primary physician for a panel of patients, with responsibility for chronic disease management, management of acute health problems, and preventive health care for their patients
Faculty-to-trainee ratio	Faculty cannot supervise >4 trainees (residents and other learners)
Faculty responsibilities when supervising residents	If >2 trainees (residents and other learners), faculty cannot have other patient care responsibilities
Electronic medical system (EMS) access	Must have access to an electronic health record, but not required at every clinical site

References

1. Overview of ACGME." https://www.acgme.org/about-us/overview/. Accessed 4 Nov 2021.
2. ACGME Common Program Requirements July 2022. https://www.acgme.org/what-we-do/accreditation/common-program-requirements/. Accessed 15 Nov 2021.
3. Nasca TJ, Philibert I, Brigham T, Flynn TC. The next GME accreditation system—rationale and benefits. New Engl J Med. 2012;366(11):1051–6. https://doi.org/10.1056/NEJMsr1200117.
4. Doolittle BR, Lim J, Edgar L. Milestones 2.0—a growth mindset for internal medicine residency programs. Am J Med. 2020;133(12):1492–9. https://doi.org/10.1016/J.AMJMED.2020.09.003.
5. Clinical Learning Environment Review (CLER). https://www.acgme.org/what-we-do/initiatives/clinical-learning-environment-review-cler/. Accessed 16 Nov 2021.
6. ACGME. ACGME 2022 Program Requirements for Graduate Medical Education in Internal Medicine. https://www.acgme.org/Portals/0/PFAssets/ProgramRequirements/140_InternalMedicine_2022.pdf?ver=2021-02-19-152614-193. Accessed 22 Dec 2021 [Online].
7. A. Dagliati et al., "A dashboard-based system for supporting diabetes care," JAMIA, vol. 25, no. 5, pp. 538–547, May 2018, doi: https://doi.org/10.1093/jamia/ocx159.
8. Few S. Dashboard confusion: a clear understanding of dashboards requires delving beneath the marketing hype. Intell Enterp. 2004;

9. Roberts DH, et al. Design and measurement of quality improvement indicators in ambulatory pulmonary care: creating a 'culture of quality' in an academic pulmonary division. Chest. 2009;136(4):1134–40. https://doi.org/10.1378/chest.09-0619.
10. Epstein JA, Noronha C, Berkenblit G. Smarter screen time: integrating clinical dashboards into graduate medical education. J Grad Med Educ. 2020;12(1):19–24. https://doi.org/10.4300/JGME-D-19-00584.1.
11. J. Oyler, L. Vinci, J. K. Johnson, and V. M. Arora, "Teaching internal medicine residents to sustain their improvement through the quality assessment and improvement curriculum.," J Gen Intern Med, vol. 26, no. 2, pp. 221–225, Feb. 2011, doi: https://doi.org/10.1007/s11606-010-1547-y.
12. Tentler A, Feurdean M, Keller S, Kothari N. Integrating a resident-driven longitudinal quality improvement curriculum within an ambulatory block schedule. J Grad Med Educ. 2016;8(3):405–9. https://doi.org/10.4300/JGME-D-15-00371.1.
13. Continuity of Care, Definition of. https://www.aafp.org/about/policies/all/continuity-of-care-definition.html. Accessed 17 Feb 2022.
14. Milano SJ. Resident continuity clinic: an oxymoron? J Gen Intern Med. 2010;25(4):572–3.
15. Dubé K, Gupta R, Kong M, Knox M, Bodenheimer T. Continuity of care in residency teaching practices: lessons from 'bright spots'. Perm J. 2018;22:18. https://doi.org/10.7812/TPP/18-028.

Chapter 9
Resident Clinic Orientation and Expectations

Emily Fondahn and Daniel S. Kim

Introduction

Every July, approximately 1/3 of the medicine residents will change during the transition to a new academic year with graduating residents departing and new interns starting. This transition requires a comprehensive and effective orientation and onboarding for the new interns in the outpatient clinic(s). Orientation should not be viewed as a single lecture but rather as a series of activities and resources designed to develop proficient and efficient interns and residents. The clinic structure and guidelines should be reassessed each year to ensure the most efficient workflow and a smooth transition for the new interns. While not exhaustive, this chapter serves as a broad overview and basic guideline to organize the clinic orientation.

Outline

- Overview of key elements of clinic orientation
- Clinical topics to cover during orientation
- Orientation methods
- Clinic processes and practices
- Attending orientation
- Conclusion

E. Fondahn (✉)
Department of Medicine, University of Missouri, Columbia, MO, USA
e-mail: efhfr@health.missouri.edu

D. S. Kim
Utilization Management, Providence St Jude Medical Center, Fullerton, CA, USA
e-mail: Daniel.kim3@stjoe.org

L. B. Lu et al. (eds.), *Leading an Academic Medical Practice*,
https://doi.org/10.1007/978-3-031-40273-9_9

Overview of Key Elements of Clinic Orientation

The transition from medical student to resident is a steep learning curve. Trainees have to not only learn the medicine but also quickly adapt and acclimatize to different clinical learning environments, which can be abrupt, stressful, and exhausting [1]. New trainees will often rely on talking to other residents for advice and learning about attending preferences for preparation [2]. Multiple different options exist for orientation and onboarding activities, which should be linked to important components of the clinical learning environment (Table 9.1).

Table 9.1 Elements of the clinical learning environment

Trainee perspective	Theme description	Orientation approach
Why am I here?	Educational goals	Elicit learner goals for clinic/rotation
	Learning opportunities	Describe patient population
Who is the team?	Team members, roles, and relationships	Introduce team members and roles
		Post pictures of team members
What do I do?	Resident role, expectations, tools, and resources	Describe resident's patient care and educational responsibilities
		Discuss clinical cases to highlight situations that require asking for help and how to obtain assistance
		Review evaluation and assessments
Where are things?	Location of patients and resources in physical workspace	Create a clinic map Provide an electronic or paper copy of clinic information
	Location of data and information in virtual space	Review patients' charts
When do things happen?	Clinical and educational schedules	Create a schedule or calendar
		Share workflow diagrams for common patient care processes
How do I navigate patient care and learning?	Navigating the healthcare systems	Share tips of how to get things done
	Patient safety and continuous improvement	Deliver tutorials for specific clinical skills

Adapted from Resources for clinical learning environment orientation by Gifford et al. [2]

Clinic Topics to Cover During Orientation

The curriculum to cover during orientation may seem endless. Each clinic will have specific processes and policies that should be personalized and incorporated into orientation. Below is a basic list of topics to serve as a framework for clinic orientation.

- **Key clinic components**
  - Hours of operation
  - Address
  - Clinic leadership contact information
  - Daily clinic schedule
  - Clinic layout
- **Team members and roles**
  - Attending physicians
    - Contact information
    - Role in clinic
    - Policies regarding staffing and when attending sees the patient
  - Nurses
  - Medical assistants
  - Advanced practice providers
  - Clinic administrators (practice manager, clinical nurse manager, etc.)
  - Support staff
  - Ancillary providers (pharmacists, social workers, nutritionists, and diabetes educators)
  - Interpreter services
- **Clinic workflow**
  - Type of patient visits (new, return, physical, urgent)
  - Check-in process
    - Patient registration
    - Rooming patient, including if flag system used
    - Required questions and documentation such as smoking status and advanced directives
    - Location of nursing documentation
  - Checkout process
    - Laboratory location and services
    - Medication prescribing
    - Referral appointments
    - Test scheduling
    - Ancillary staff appointments
  - Task system: how residents receive notifications about patient phone calls, results, and refill requests

- **Residents' workflow**
  - Staffing patients with attendings

    Where and when to present patients to faculty preceptors
    Which patients need to be seen by the attending
    General guidelines for information to include in oral presentation
    Documentation guidelines

  - How to write a note

    Types of notes

    - Office visit note
    - Telephone call documentation
    - Patient letter

    Documentation components and policies

    - Attending attestation
    - Health maintenance
    - Cut and paste policy
    - Timeline for note completion

  - Order entry

    Medication prescriptions and refills
    Medication list creation, input into electronic medical record (EMR) and reconciliation
    Lab order entry
    Imaging and procedure order entry
    Prior authorization information

  - Referrals

    How to refer to a specialist
    Where referral notes are located in the EMR
    How to make nonphysician referrals (dentist, physical therapy, home health, etc.)

  - Clinic treatments

    Vaccinations available in clinic
    Medications available in clinic
    Procedures performed in clinic
    Emergency department/direct admission process

Orientation Methods

- **Didactic lecture:** These sessions are typically included in orientation activities at the start of the year or can be done during the first clinic rotation and cover a broad overview of the clinic. These sessions are often done as a didactic lecture but can be recorded and made available online. Research prior to the COVID pandemic found that trainees perceived the quality and utility of orientation presentations to be similar whether in-person or recorded [3]. Other clinics are exploring the use of virtual tours and videos as a way to familiarize trainees with clinics prior to starting in a clinic [4].

- Strengths

  Live sessions offer opportunity for questions
  Can include many residents in one session

- Limitations

  Poor retention of material presented
  May seem overwhelming or out of context

• **Electronic medical record training**: Residents will likely have EMR training completed as part of their general orientation. If the clinic site has a different EMR, residents will need additional training for that system. A refresher EMR session can be useful in the fall, to reinforce how to use the EMR once the residents have been practicing in clinic for a few months. These sessions should also cover in-basket management for common tasks that the residents will encounter.

- Strengths

  Hands-on training in a computer lab
  Sessions led by EMR support staff
  Usually high yield
  Short clips can be recorded and placed on website
  Can have residents demonstrate how to do certain tasks

- Limitations

  May seem out of context or overwhelming to someone that has not worked in that system
  May be temporally separated from clinic rotations
  Difficult to assess resident's retention and application of knowledge
  No one may be available from EMR support staff for help while in clinic

• **Intern shadowing of a senior resident or attending:** The Primary Care Medicine Clinic at Washington University started to assign interns to senior residents for their first clinic session a few years ago. This first session allows the intern to see the flow of the clinic firsthand from a senior resident or attending. Interns can use a checklist to ensure that they observe important elements of the clinic visit (Table 9.2).

- Strengths

  Allows interns to observe workflow in the clinical context before they start seeing their own patients
  Provides opportunity to practice common tasks, like prescription writing or order entry

Table 9.2 Intern shadowing resident checklist

These should be observed by the intern while shadowing a resident:
Clinic layout
• Exam rooms
• Printer stations
• Clinic mailboxes
• Physician work rooms
• Conference room
• Break room
• Offices for clinic staff (social work, diabetic educator, anticoagulation nurse, pharmacists)
Electronic medical record
• Verify that log-in and password work for EMR
• Lookup schedule
• Lookup patient
• See appointment tab (previous appointments, upcoming appointments)
• Start a new note
• Write a new prescription and send to pharmacy
• Order a lab/study
• Make a referral
• Review tasks/in-basket
Clinic flow
• Observe residents evaluating a patient
• Observe residents staffing with attending
• Observe residents checking out a patient
• Learn where to find hallway/exam room assignments and charge nurse

– Limitations

Decreases the number of patients seen in clinic and delays the first clinic session for interns

Dependent on interaction between the intern and resident/attending

Requires administrative work to arrange shadowing schedule

Depending on the size of the program, may need residents and attending willing to have interns shadow

- **Resident/attending shadowing of an intern:** A senior resident or attending shadows an intern for a clinic session. These sessions allow interns to obtain formative feedback about clinic performance and have questions answered about the clinic in a real-time setting by a senior resident/attending. The resident/attending can use a checklist to ensure that they observe important elements of the clinic visit (Table 9.3).

Table 9.3 Resident shadowing intern checklist

Verify that the intern knows how to:
• Start a note
• Place a referral
• Write a prescription
• Order a lab or study
Patient evaluation
• Assess the intern's ability to take a thorough and focused history.
• Does the intern:
• Evaluate too few/too many problems in a visit?
• Spend too much time going through the entire problem list?
• Have difficulty prioritizing problems?
• Interrupt the patient frequently?
• Perform a focused physical exam?
• Evaluate the patient's medication list?
• Take a focused review of systems?
• Update key information?
Evaluate the intern's use of the EMR during the patient encounter
• Make poor eye contact with the patient due to looking at computer?
• Spend too much time/too little time looking up patient info before the visit?
• Have difficulty writing prescriptions, ordering labs, making referrals, etc.?
Attending presentation
• Is the intern able to give an accurate and organized presentation to the attending?
• Is any information left out during the presentation?
• Does the intern have a clear problem list and plan?
Organization
• Does the intern come to clinic prepared?
• Does the intern spend too much/too little time looking up patients prior to seeing them?
• Is the intern able to handle late patients or patients moved onto their list?
• How many patients does the intern see? Does the intern stay on time?
Notes
• Are the notes written in a timely manner based on clinic guidelines?.
• Is there any information missing in the notes?
• Are the problem list, allergies, and medication list updated?
• Does the plan accurately reflect what is discussed at the visit?

- Strengths

  Empowers interns to have an active role of seeing patients and using EMR with supervision
  Provides opportunity for the senior resident/attending to answer questions about the EMR, clinic resources, and workflow
  Allows the senior resident/attending to provide immediate feedback regarding efficiency, patient interactions, presentations, and notes
  Incorporates the feedback into an evaluation to verify that the intern is achieving specific milestones
  Can have this session later in academic year to address gaps in knowledge
  Can be incorporated into direct observation evaluations

- Limitations

  Decreases the number of patients seen in the clinic if senior resident taken off the schedule
  Dependent on the interaction between the intern and resident
  Requires administrative work to arrange shadowing schedule
  Depending on the size of the program, may need many residents and attending willing to shadow the interns

- **Ambulatory boot camps:** Given that interns will start residency with a wide range of ambulatory training, an intern ambulatory boot camp can be created for the beginning of the year. One program developed case-based didactic sessions of common ambulatory topics and orientation to the clinic and electronic medical record. The knowledge scores improved from 43.6% pretest to 76.1% posttest [5].

  - Strengths

    Assesses baseline knowledge of the interns
    Level-sets the knowledge for common ambulatory topics
    Increases confidence of interns in ambulatory topics

  - Limitations

    Requires significant work coordinating didactic sessions with faculty
    Can add additional delays to orientation training
    Unclear if boot camp will have impact on clinical skills or performance

Clinic Processes and Practices

- **Patient safety and quality:** Patient safety and quality improvement (QI) initiatives are becoming ubiquitous in clinics. At a minimum, residents should have a clear understanding of adverse event reporting regarding what to report and how to report this information. Additionally, residents should know what the clinical quality metrics and quality improvement projects are, how they are measured, and what the residents are required to do for these QI projects.

- **Telehealth:**
  - Patient phone calls: Most interns will have little to no experience with an answering service or responding to patient telephone calls. Typical signals used in patient care, such as a physical exam, lab results, and visual cues, are not available on the phone. Other limitations may include residents covering for each other or lack of time/outside distractions when taking phone calls. Furthermore, they will need explicit instruction on policies and expectations regarding patient portals. Residents should know what the expectations are for answering patient phone calls, especially after hours and weekends. Next, they should receive instructions outlining the type of patient information to be received, the triaging service, and the appropriate time frame and method for returning a call (personal or clinic phone, patient portals, hospital operator, etc.). In addition, residents should be given information about any telephone medicine policies such as narcotic refills over the phone, who covers patient calls at night and for vacation, and documentation of telephone conversations. Finally, contact information for a supervising physician should be provided if they are uncertain on how to handle a patient phone call. Residents may want to practice these phone calls using clinical vignettes or role-playing [6].
  - Virtual visits: With the expansion of telehealth visits in primary care due to the COVID pandemic, learning how to conduct virtual visits with patients has become an important component of orientation [7]. The American Association of Medical Colleges (AAMC) has developed telehealth skills needed for healthcare professionals [8]. At a minimum, residents should be aware of when and how to use telehealth visits and how to remotely evaluate and care for a patient. They must also be cognizant of privacy, legal, patient safety, and ethical issues pertinent to telehealth. Chapters 13 and 14 cover telemedicine clinical workflow and education, respectively.

- **Lab and test management:** One anxiety-provoking moment for most new residents is what to do with an abnormal test result. Often, new interns do not have enough clinical experience to know how to manage an abnormal result. Throughout the year, this knowledge deficit decreases as residents gain more experience and didactic education. Residents should be given contact information for supervising physicians in case they need assistance interpreting a lab or radiology study. Expectation on timely result management should be included in the orientation. Chapter 5 discusses EMR in basket management.
- **Clinical skills and procedures:** Incoming residents will have a wide variety of experiences with common outpatient procedures. For example, some residents may feel comfortable performing a pelvic exam, Papanicolaou (PAP) smear, and wet prep, whereas other residents may have limited experience. These procedures will need to be supervised, at least initially, in the resident's training. The residents should be encouraged to log all procedures that they perform with the attending.
- **Precepting patients:** The patient presentation to the attending is a critical component to the patient encounter. These presentations need to be simultaneously efficient and cover all important information. Reisman et al. described the eight tips for presenting patients in an academic primary care clinic (Table 9.4) [9]. These tips, adapted to the local environment, will likely be helpful for residents.

Table 9.4 Tips for presenting patients

Provide a preamble	Brief overview to orient attending to patient case. For example: "This is a patient who may need hospital admission"
Appreciate the difference between the case presentation and the written note	The note should contain the subjective, objective, assessment and plan (SOAP) structure. The presentation may be more conversation.
Preceptors will have different styles	Attendings may prefer a more structured presentation, some may interrupt frequently, or some may listen to the whole presentation, and then ask questions.
Ask for bedside precepting	Presenting directly in front of the patient adds to patient-centered care, can save time, and ensures that the patient's story is correct.
Do not look at notes while presenting	The history of present illness (HPI) should be told from memory, while medications and lab results can be referred to paper notes and/or on EMR.
Ask for feedback	If there is a particular area where feedback is needed, preface this need to the attending prior to the presentation.
Ask for explanation	Request guidelines or articles from the attending, especially if it is a new topic to enhance understanding of the clinical decision-making.
Communicate with other team members	Ask others about significant issues and request being alerted to information about shared patients.

- **Resident and attending assessment.**
  - Resident assessment by an attending: At orientation, residents should learn when and how they will be assessed by an attending. These assessments can be either summative or formative evaluations. Residents should be provided information about the milestones that will be assessed during their clinic rotations. Other assessments that will be done on a clinic rotation, such as a 360 evaluation performed by other team members or patient feedback, should also be communicated during orientation.
  - Attending assessment by residents: Residents should have the opportunity to assess the clinic attendings throughout the year. Clinic orientation should include the process of how clinic attendings are assessed, when the assessments are completed, and which attendings the resident will assess. Information about how to address concerns regarding an attending should be provided.
- **Teaching expectations for residents**
  - Ambulatory clinics use a variety of teaching methods, including morning report, lecture series, or online modules. Examples of resident teaching can include case presentation for ambulatory report, 30-minute didactic session, or creation of a brief evidence-based medicine handout. If residents are required to teach as part of the ambulatory curriculum, they should be provided a schedule in advance and clear expectations for the sessions. Information should include:

Learning objectives for presentation
What needs to be prepared by the resident (if applicable)

- PowerPoint slides
- Handouts

Example of an "ideal" presentation
Date of presentation
Required readings
If and how residents will be evaluated

- **Resources for residents**
  - Having reference materials available to residents and faculty through the year is crucial.
  - Clinic handbooks or manuals: Provide a written description of the clinic with all important information and resources

    Strengths

    - Depending on the needs of residents, can be very in-depth or more high-yield
    - Can be accessible from a residency website
    - Can include pictures and descriptions to create standard work
    - Can include clinic policies and procedures

    Limitations

    - Must be updated on an yearly basis
    - Often not read by residents
  - Website: A clinic website can provide updated information throughout the year.

    Strengths

    - Place to store PowerPoints, schedules, and manuals

    Limitations

    - Need administrator to update
    - May want some of the information on a password-protected part of the website
    - Need internet
  - Shared secure storage.

    Strengths:

    - Place to store PowerPoints, schedules, and manuals
    - Can be updated more frequently than printed materials
    - Secure

Limitations

- All members of clinic may have trouble accessing depending on how access is granted
- Need internet
- No notification of when new material is posted

– Plan for updates: The orientation materials should be updated at least yearly. This process should include a multidisciplinary team including clinic leadership, nursing, current residents, and support staff. An "Important Updates" can be added to the orientation materials annually to highlight changes from previous years for current residents and attendings.

Attending Orientation

New clinic attendings will similarly need a comprehensive orientation to clinic. Some of the orientation requirements will depend on if the attending is a recent graduate who may need detailed information about medical billing, or if they are new to the healthcare system, then they will need information about the EMR and workflow. Some of the information may be covered for attendings through other orientations they are required to attend by the health system or department. Clinic-specific topics worthwhile to include for attendings are:

- General information
  - When to arrive and where to go
  - Typical number of patients staffed per session
  - Guidelines for using primary care exception versus when patients must be seen by attending
  - Expectations for following up on laboratory, imaging, and referral information
  - Resident assignments for attendings
- Assessments
  - Which residents will need to be assessed
  - How assessments are completed
  - How residents assess attendings
- Billing and coding
  - Use of primary care exception
  - Process for coding
  - Key drivers for coding specificity

Conclusion

Given the new influx of residents each year, maintaining an organized system and outlining a thorough orientation process are keys to an efficient clinic system and aiding resident transition. A structured orientation program can improve resident self-confidence and ensure baseline competencies while the residents transition into a new clinic [10]. While each academic clinic will have different requirements and needs, this chapter provides a basic checklist and starting point for the clinic orientation process.

References

1. Sturman N, Tan Z, Turner J. "a steep learning curve": junior doctor perspectives on the transition from medical student to the health-care workplace. BMC Med Educ. 2017;17(1):92.
2. Gifford KA, Choi E, Kieffer KA. Resources for clinical learning environment orientation. Med Educ Online. 2022;27(1):2013404.
3. Andolsek KM, Murphy G, Pinheiro S, Petrusa E, Tuck T, Weinerth J. Efficacy and efficiency of webcast orientations versus live resident orientations: results of a 2-year survey. J Grad Med Educ. 2010;2(1):136–40.
4. Feltz K, Skelly N, MacFadden L, Wetering J. 360-degree perspective: improving hospital orientation with interactive virtual tour. AAOS Now [Internet]; 2022. https://www.aaos.org/aaosnow/2022/jan/residency/residency02/. Accessed 17 Mar 22.
5. Esch LM, Bird AN, Oyler JL, Lee WW, Shah SD, Pincavage AT. Preparing for the primary care clinic: an ambulatory boot camp for internal medicine interns. Med Educ Online. 2015;20:29702.
6. Reisman AB, Brown KE. Preventing communication errors in telephone medicine. J Gen Intern Med. 2005;20(10):959–63.
7. Alexander GC, Tajanlangit M, Heyward J, Mansour O, Qato DM, Stafford RS. Use and content of primary care office-based vs telemedicine care visits during the COVID-19 pandemic in the US. JAMA Netw Open. 2020;3(10):e2021476-e.
8. Consensus E. Telehealth skills for health care professionals. Telemedicine and e-Health. 2021;27(7):820–4.
9. Reisman AHF, Brienza R. Eight tips for presentation patient in an academic primary care clinic. SGIM Forum. 2016;39(2):1–2.
10. Hiraoka M, Kamikawa G, McCartin R, Kaneshiro B. A pilot structured resident orientation curriculum improves the confidence of incoming first-year obstetrics and gynecology residents. Hawaii J Med Public Health. 2013;72(11):387–90.

Chapter 10
Resident Milestones, Assessments, and Feedback

Craig F. Noronha, Jillian Catalanotti, and Mia Marcus

Introduction

Feedback and assessment are essential elements of residency training, providing trainees descriptions of their performance with goals of individual growth and development. Feedback is formative and based on concrete observations of a trainee's performance, typically in a time-limited period. Feedback should be concrete and actionable. Assessment is generally summative, providing a more encompassing review of a trainee's performance over a period of time. Clinical faculty are responsible for delivering high-quality feedback and assessment but may be faced with barriers to doing so. This chapter addresses feedback and assessment within the clinic setting and provides sample tools to deliver feedback and assess trainees.

C. F. Noronha (✉)
Department of Medicine, Internal Medicine Residency Program, Boston Medical Center, Boston University Chobanian & Avedisian School of Medicine, Boston, MA, USA
e-mail: craig.noronha@bmc.org

J. Catalanotti · M. Marcus
Department of Medicine, Division of General Internal Medicine, The George Washington University, Washington, DC, USA
e-mail: jcatalanotti@mfa.gwu.edu; mmarcus@mfa.gwu.edu

L. B. Lu et al. (eds.), *Leading an Academic Medical Practice*,
https://doi.org/10.1007/978-3-031-40273-9_10

Outline

- Feedback
  - Barriers to effective feedback
  - Ways to overcome barriers to feedback
  - What makes feedback effective
  - Continuity clinic feedback pearls (styles and methods)
  - Feedback focused faculty development
  - Feedback tools and models
- Assessment
  - Milestones assessment
  - Clinic faculty members' roles in assessment
  - Assessment tools
- Clinic-specific situations
  - Asynchronous care
  - Outpatient procedures
- The struggling learner
- Conclusion

Feedback, Assessment, and Milestones in the Continuity Clinic

At its core, medical education furnishes environment, information, and experiences needed for learners to acquire knowledge, skills, and attitudes that will be requisite to practice as a physician in the future [1, 2]. The Accreditation Council for Graduate Medical Education (ACGME) states that the purpose of graduate medical education is to "prepare physicians to deliver safe, high-quality medical care." Residency programs are tasked with providing clinical experience and education for residents with the ultimate goal of preparing them to provide high-quality patient care without supervision [1].

This chapter reviews best practices in giving formative feedback and performing assessment of resident performance in the continuity clinic setting. We also describe the process of learner assessments by continuity clinic preceptors within the greater context of the work of Clinical Competency Committees and ACGME requirements.

Feedback

Assessment in competency-based medical education (CBME) relies on frequent and regular context-specific feedback [3–5]. Feedback is information given to learners to reinforce appropriate and correct inappropriate clinical behavior. It is a crucial

Table 10.1 Feedback versus assessment

	Feedback	Assessment
Formality	Informal	Formal
Mode	Usually verbal	Written
Frequency	Higher frequency	Lower frequency
Awareness	Usually kept between faculty and learner	Reported to program office via electronic system
Goal	Formative	Summative
Time period	Current performance	Past performance
Examples	Attending gives specific direct feedback regarding knee exam after resident examines a patient	Attending fills out assessment form of a resident describing overall performance in the primary care clinic over the last 3 months

component of any learning environment [6–8]. There are several key differences between feedback and assessment in medical education (Table 10.1). In resident continuity clinic, feedback is most effective when it reflects residents' self-assessment and affects their performance [9–11]. Ongoing feedback in medical education is a set of repeated information and reaction cycles with the goal of enhancement of clinical skills and achievement of the intended goals [12]. The process of feedback involves learner knowledge of the expected competencies, comparing those competencies to the learner's own level of work and taking action to close the gap between the two. Formative feedback on resident performance in core competencies within milestones contributes to summative decisions regarding advancement in training [13]. Most importantly, the ultimate goal of resident feedback is to facilitate the development of competent independent physicians who provide excellent clinical care to patients.

Barriers to Effective Feedback

A recurrent theme in medical education is that learners feel that they do not receive adequate feedback, both in quantity and quality. Barriers to effective feedback fall into four major categories:

Setting/context: These types of barriers include lack of time for direct observation of learner and for feedback giving, conflicting clinical responsibilities, environmental distractions, and onerous nature of form completion. These factors may lead to disengagement of both faculty and residents. In addition, delays in submitting feedback documentation may make it harder to give concrete, specific feedback as details are forgotten over time [14, 15].

Sociopsychological factors: These barriers include perceived threat to resident self-esteem and autonomy, fear of causing tension and harm in the educator-learner relationship, skepticism about the credibility of the source, and apprehension when feedback is incongruent with resident self-assessments [7, 16–18].

Resident factors: Barriers specific to the resident receiving the feedback include emotional responses to constructive feedback, perceiving feedback-seeking as burdensome and anxiety-provoking, and perceiving the feedback process as summative rather than formative, leading to concerns about performance. The latter also leads to selection bias when residents can choose an encounter to be observed. For example, a resident choosing a part of the patient interaction that they already excel in to be observed for feedback protects their sense of self-worth at the expense of a learning opportunity [9, 11, 14, 19].

Preceptor factors: Barriers specific to the faculty member giving the feedback include lacking skill and experience in giving feedback, apprehension around balancing reinforcing with corrective feedback, worry about feeling "mean" or "unkind" when giving constructive feedback [20, 21], and concern that documenting constructive feedback may have larger impacts on resident progress, such as non-promotion.

Institutional learning and feedback culture: Learning environments that lack longitudinal relationships and promote learner autonomy contribute to a culture in which constructive feedback is avoided. It is essential to foster a culture in which feedback is normalized and expected, thus creating an institutional growth mindset of feedback giving and seeking [21, 22].

Ways to Overcome Barriers to Feedback

Continuity clinics should have protected and allocated time for feedback built into the clinic schedule at predetermined points of the year. Regular direct observation of residents must be coupled with timely formative feedback. It is important to incorporate the practice of informal conversations and coaching (as opposed to forms and checklists) with specific actionable feedback, creating teaching moments.

The process of feedback should be focused on the potential *for* learning rather than the assessment *of* learning [23]. The language and tone of feedback ought to be kind and supportive, while the content must be specific and direct. Feedback should be framed in the context of expected milestones and competencies, rather than feedback about a person. Goal-directed feedback with action plans for improvement yields residents motivated to improve.

The longitudinal nature of continuity clinic is the ideal setting in which to promote a strong trusting relationship between faculty and residents, and thus a positive feedback culture [24, 25]. In most programs, clinic faculty members work with the same residents throughout their training. A faculty member's baseline knowledge of a resident's strengths and weaknesses is invaluable in the process of growth that can occur with effective feedback [20].

It is essential to create a positive feedback culture in which both faculty and residents feel comfortable and are expected to participate in feedback conversations. Prioritization should be given to regular feedback, promotion of direct observation of learners, and regular faculty training [26].

What Makes Feedback Effective

Feedback is in essence a conversation between the feedback sender and the feedback recipient. It is a complex interactive two-way interpersonal exchange. Effective feedback is crucial for developing resident professionalism, communication skills, performance, and documentation [4, 27]. When done well, feedback can motivate learners, improve their learning, and enhance their professional growth [28]. According to feedback recipients, there are three major components of effective feedback [13, 29].

Feedback content: Early positive recognition of what the learner is doing right or well is appreciated by the learner. This promotes confidence in the resident to be more receptive to receiving the ensuing constructive or corrective feedback. Constructive feedback that is specific, clear, direct, and honest is also highly valued. Feedback should be tied to explicit common goals and action plans.

Method of delivery: Frequent, both formal and informal (ad hoc, or "off the cuff"), feedback is appreciated. Timing of the feedback should be as close to the observed resident behavior as possible with deliberate time set aside for feedback. It should be given in a private 1:1 setting and should be delivered using a supportive nonjudgmental and empathetic tone.

Interaction with feedback giver: The learner needs to be actively engaged in the process, given opportunities to respond and react to feedback as well as to ask questions.

Giver credibility: Giver credibility is demonstrated through respect, professionalism, likeability, knowledge, and experience level. The longitudinal nature and strength of the relationship between the receiver and sender of feedback are also a critical aspect of effective feedback. Giver credibility enhances effectiveness of feedback.

Continuity Clinic Feedback Pearls (Styles and Methods)

- *Timing:* Give feedback early so there is time to improve [3, 4]. Scheduled versus unscheduled directly observed encounters are both valuable, but unscheduled ones can happen more frequently and can yield a more authentic representation of resident skills on which to focus feedback [30].
- *Setting:* Base feedback on direct observation as much as possible. Set aside quiet, dedicated time to ensure privacy and minimize interruptions [3].
- *Language:* Use specific neutral and objective language that focuses on changeable behaviors rather than personality traits [31].
- *Methods:* Different methods include brief/informal feedback (in the moment, quick teaching point), formal feedback (5–20 minutes, following a presentation or observed patient interaction, occurring once a month), and major feedback (scheduled, 15–30 minutes, occurring 3–4 times per year) [32]. Best practice is to provide a combination of these methods. Methodology may include checklists

Table 10.2 Resident scenarios

Resident type	Feedback approach
High-performing resident	Coaching conversation
Resident with insight gaps	Directive feedback
Overly confident resident	Mediating to encourage shift from being defensive to empathizing with the patient
Emotionally distressed resident	Mentoring/supporting

or open-ended feedback; each has its own advantages and disadvantages. Checklists give structure and discussion points from which to pivot but can be onerous and may not necessarily present an accurate global reflection of intended feedback. Open-ended feedback forms can be vague and insufficient. Using a combination of these is likely wise.

- *Style:* Start with self-feedback by the learner prompted by open-ended questions. Points made by the learner can then be reinforced by the feedback giver. Conclude with an action plan that is collaborative. Set up a time for a follow-up feedback session, even if brief.
- *Know your resident:* Being able to individualize feedback to different residents is an important consideration. Each resident has their own unique contexts and expectations [3]. It can be particularly challenging for faculty to provide residents at extreme ends of the spectrum—those performing at a high level or failing to meet expectations—effective feedback [33]. See some approaches that may match particular resident scenarios in Table 10.2.

Feedback Focused Faculty Development

Given the complexity of the feedback process, formal ongoing periodic faculty training is necessary. Feedback giving is a skill, and often feedback givers are not well prepared for it [34]. Training should involve formal education using multimedia resources (e.g., video vignettes) [35] as well as deliberate practice [36]. One- to two-hour workshops twice a year can go a long way in advancing feedback givers' skill sets. A robust faculty development program is the foundation for a healthy and successful feedback culture. Resources for faculty development are available at MedEdPORTAL, professional societies or organizations, and potentially at the local institutional level.

Feedback Tools and Models

Feedback tools and models should be intuitive, easy to follow, and frequently used [37, 38]. However, there is no perfect feedback tool. Quality of care is an inherently difficult to measure end point.

Medication Initiation Feedback Form

Example from Boston Medical Center/Boston University School of Medicine

Instructions:

Document whether you observe the resident possessing the specific skills. Please be accurate in your assessment of the resident. It is NOT expected that a resident has mastered all these skills but rather that they receive feedback on their observed encounter. Proficiency in these skills is expected over 12-36 months of residency. This does not assume that the resident conducts the entire discussion. Please evaluate the portion the resident conducted; and if the preceptor intervened, please provide specific feedback.

Reviews drug allergies in chart and with patient			
No	Partially	Yes	N/A
o	o	o	o
Understands the relevant pathophysiology, pharmacology and indication for the medication			
No	Partially	Yes	N/A
o	o	o	o
Understands what follow up testing is required for the new medication (follow up chem 7, A1c, etc.)			
No	Partially	Yes	N/A
o	o	o	o
Communicates risks and benefits of the medication and alternatives to the patient			
No	Partially	Yes	N/A
o	o	o	o
Uses language the patient could understand			
No	Partially	Yes	N/A
o	o	o	o
Engages in shared decision making regarding the initiation or change of the medication			
No	Partially	Yes	N/A
o	o	o	o
Gives the patient the opportunity to ask questions			
No	Partially	Yes	N/A
o	o	o	o
Confirms patient understanding of the medication plan; asks the patient to repeat back in their own words			
No	Partially	Yes	N/A
o	o	o	o
Is able to independently manage the encounter (explains the rationale for the medication and answers all questions to the patient and attending's satisfaction)			
No	Partially	Yes	N/A
o	o	o	o
Preceptor needs to take over a portion of the discussion.			
No	Partially	Yes	N/A
o	o	o	o

What are the resident's strengths in this session?

What are the resident's areas for improvement?

Fig. 10.1 Medication initiation feedback form

Direct clinical observation of residents: The mini-clinical evaluation exercise (mini-CEX) is a valuable tool for resident skill development. In continuity clinic, it is an essential method for creating feedback that both reinforces and coaches behavior and skills that are necessary to becoming competent clinicians [30]. Checklists of clinical skill domains (such as professionalism, interpersonal/communication, electronic health system [EHS] use, diagnostic acumen, negotiation of the healthcare system, and medical knowledge) can be used by both faculty preceptors and residents (self-assessment) after the observed encounter and then reviewed and discussed together in a coaching feedback session (Figs. 10.1 and 10.2). Residents can then develop concise goals for their clinical practice over the ensuing weeks. Brief follow-up session can be scheduled to check on the status of implementing and

Structured Clinical Observation Example

Structured Clinical Observation form (SCO)

Please observe the resident in either data gathering and/or information giving. Place a check by each item for behaviors that were observed.

Y	N	N/A	Data Gathering: History of Present Illness, Past Medical History, Medications/allergies, Social History, Family History, Review of Systems
			Allows patient to complete opening statement
			Starts with open ended questions
			Avoids use of leading questions
			Limits questions with multiple parts (question stacking)
			Elicits patient's beliefs about causes of the illness or problem
			Asks about remedies or therapies used to address chief complaint (traditional or non-traditional)
			Asks for clarification if necessary
			Explicitly elicits patient's expectations regarding the visit
			Summarizes and confirms information given by the patient
			Proceeds with logical sequencing of questions
Y	N	N/A	Information Giving: explains diagnosis, medicine, procedures, gives counseling, addresses chronic disease management, follow-up
			Limits use of jargon and/or explains medical terms if used
			Explains diagnosis
			Explains management plan
			Explains need for follow-up
			Explicitly asks for patient input in management plan

Fig. 10.2 Structured Clinical Observation form (SCO)

			Asks patient for their understanding of treatment plan (teach back method)
			Solicits questions
			Asks about patient's ability to follow treatment plan
			Explains when, why, how patient should contact physician

Y	N	N/A	Interpersonal Skills
			Introduces self
			Addresses patient by name after initial introductions
			Avoids interrupting patient
			Actively listens using nonverbal techniques (e.g. eye contact, nodding)
			Expresses empathy (e.g. using tone of voice, "That must be hard for you")
			Explicitly recognizes patient's feelings or concerns (e.g. "you seem upset")
			Deals effectively with language barriers

Key Feedback Points:

1.____

2.____

3.____

Time Spent Observing:___min.
Time Spent in Feedback:_min.

Resident Signature: ______________________

Preceptor Signature: _____________________

Adapted from L Lane, MD and R Gottlieb, MD, Jefferson Medical College

By E Hamburger, MD, S Cuzzi, MD and D Coddington, MD, Children's National Medical Center

Modified by Mia Marcus, MD, George Washington University Hospital

Fig. 10.2 (continued)

achieving these goals [24]. In essence, a coaching session workflow might look something like this: previsit huddle, before directly observed patient encounter reviewing checklist; resident self-assessment using the same checklist; focused coaching/feedback session with faculty observations; setting goals for improvement; and one-month check-in on progress towards goals [24].

R2C2 model: This is an evidence-based facilitated feedback model with four phases: (1) build rapport and ***R***elationship, (2) explore ***R***eactions, (3) explore ***C***ontent, and (4) ***C***oach for performance change [37–39].

This model provides structure and flow to the feedback discussion. The *first* phase of building rapport and relationship sets the stage for trust and openness. The *second* phase of exploring reactions encourages residents through self-assessment to be more accepting of feedback. In the *third* phase, faculty assist residents in understanding the content of the feedback especially as it relates to expected competencies and milestones. The *fourth* phase involves coaching residents to close the performance gap and setting goals and plans to achieve this. This model was designed by Sargeant et al. as a model to help faculty and residents to discuss their assessments, feedbacks, and goals, but we feel that this model could be easily rendered for use in immediate feedback after an observed encounter.

Assessment

Feedback provides information for a trainee related to their performance in a set task, which is used to guide future improvement. In contrast, assessment is a summative combination of feedback and other data points that provides a judgment of competency in a set of domains. Ideally, feedback exchanges with trainees will identify key elements included in an assessment, but in most cases, it is not realistic for trainees to receive feedback related to every domain detailed in a summative assessment.

Medical education has transformed to focus on competency-based medical education (CBME), which establishes the standard level of competence expected for independent practice [2, 3, 40]. In CBME, trainees progress based on the assessment of their competence in several domains as opposed to progression based solely on time in training. To this end, the ACGME and the American Board of Medical Specialties have identified six core competencies necessary for a practicing physician (Fig. 10.3). These six core competencies form the scaffolding from which all resident learning, experiences, and assessments are created.

6 Core Competencies - ACGME and American Board of Medical Specialties
1. Patient care and procedural skills
2. Medical knowledge
3. Practice-based learning and improvement
4. Interpersonal and communication skills
5. Professionalism
6. Systems-based practice

Fig. 10.3 Six core competencies—ACGME and American Board of Medical Specialties

Milestones Assessment

ACGME released its Milestones assessment approach in 2011 and subsequently refined it with Milestones 2.0 in July 2021 [41]. Table 10.3 reviews the key changes between the 1.0 and 2.0 version of the Milestones. Each core competency is divided into 2–6 subcompetencies (Fig. 10.4). Distinct milestones, or observable behaviors demonstrating levels of achievement for each subcompetency, help to anchor assessment and calibrate faculty and trainee expectations for satisfactory progression of achievement.

Milestones delineate five levels to indicate progression "from novice to expert" [41]. Levels do not correspond to postgraduate year of education [41], nor are they meant to be scored relative to others at the same training level, but rather compared to the level expected of a fully competent practicing physician (designated level 4). The target is to achieve level 4, previously designated "ready for unsupervised practice," by the time of graduation from the residency program on each subcompetency, but achieving this level is not a requirement for graduation. New trainees may not be used to nonrelative assessments and may be disheartened to see achievement of only level 2 milestone scores. Similarly, faculty on the Clinical Competency Committee may require training to recalibrate their assessments, recognizing that even a high-achieving intern may be performing at a level 2–3 on Milestones.

ACGME does not intend for Milestones assessments to be copied verbatim to create evaluation tools used by faculty, but rather requires that twice per year the Clinical Competency Committee (CCC) review all residents' evaluation data and use it to generate an assessment of milestone achievement by each resident for each

Table 10.3 Key similarities and differences between Milestones versions 1.0 and 2.0

	Milestones 1.0	Milestones 2.0
Number of competencies	6	6 (unchanged)
Number of subcompetencies	22	20
Subcompetency language	Describes performance of activity (e.g., "develops and achieves comprehensive management plan for each patient")	Names activity in short, discrete phrases (e.g., "history," "physical examination," "clinical reasoning")
Settings for assessment of each subcompetency	Unspecified	Some subcompetencies specify outpatient, inpatient, telemedicine. Others are unspecified.
Levels of assessment	1–5 1 = "critical deficiency" 4 = "ready for unsupervised practice" 5 = "aspirational"	1–5 "Novice to expert" Level 4 specified as graduation *goal* but not graduation *requirement*
New topics assessed in subcompetencies	NA	Clinical reasoning Digital health Physician role in healthcare system Quality improvement Divides professionalism into professional behavior, ethical principles, accountability/ conscientiousness, and Well-being

Patient Care 5: Patient Management – Outpatient				
Level 1	Level 2	Level 3	Level 4	Level 5
Identifies opportunities to maintain and promote health	Develops and implements management plans to maintain and promote health	Develops and implements plans to maintain and promote health, incorporating pertinent psychosocial and other determinants of health	Develops and implements value-based (high-value) comprehensive plans to maintain and promote health	
Formulates management plans for a common chronic condition, with guidance	Develops and implements management plans for common chronic conditions	Develops and implements management plans for multiple chronic conditions	Develops and implements value-based (high value) comprehensive management plans for multiple chronic conditions, incorporating pertinent psychosocial and other determinants of health	Creates and leads a comprehensive patient-centered management plan for the patient with highly complex chronic conditions, integrating recommendations from multiple disciplines
Formulates management plans for acute common conditions, with guidance	Develops and implements management plans for common acute conditions	Develops and implements an initial management plan for patients with urgent or emergent conditions in the setting of chronic comorbidities	Develops and implements value-based (high value) management plans for patients with acute conditions	Develops and implements management plans for patients with subtle presentations, including rare or ambiguous conditions
☐ ☐	☐ ☐	☐ ☐	☐ ☐	☐ ☐

Comments:

Not Yet Completed Level 1 ☐
Not Yet Assessable ☐

Fig. 10.4 Example subcompetency in Milestone 2.0: Patient Care 5. Note that in version 2.0, the subcompetencies are shorter phrases listing discrete activities, rather than the longer descriptive versions used in version 1.0. Level 1 is no longer labeled "Critical Deficiency." Additionally, some subcompetencies, such as Patient Care 5, now include specific clinical settings for assessment

subcompetency. Milestone assessments are reported to ACGME twice per year, to the American Board of Internal Medicine (ABIM) at the conclusion of each academic year, and, upon graduation, a resident's final milestone assessment is shared with future fellowship program directors as applicable to inform the continued trajectory of their training.

Continuity clinic provides several unique opportunities for evaluation, and as such can provide important information needed by the CCC for Milestones assessments of residents. Although most subcompetency assessments should be informed by observable activities in both in- and outpatient settings (e.g., Patient Care 1: History, Patient Care 2: Physical), others may be best observed by continuity clinic preceptors (e.g., Patient Care 5: Patient Management—Outpatient and Patient Care 6: Digital Health).

Additionally, improving via performance audit is a subcompetency of the Practice-Based Learning and Improvement (PBLI) core competency and ensures that our residents are trained to deliver high-quality and efficient health care. Resident continuity clinics can adopt a practice-based improvement curriculum, which incorporates longitudinal practice feedback, educational sessions, self-reflection, and involvement in quality improvement (QI) to improve both process and clinical outcome measures [25]. The universal use of EHS allows for extensive, resident-specific, detailed, and frequent availability of data. An X + Y scheduling model makes such a curriculum feasible with dedicated didactic and preclinic educational time [42].

Clinic Faculty Members' Roles in Assessment

According to ACGME requirements, continuity clinic must be a "longitudinal continuity experience in which residents develop a continuous, long-term therapeutic relationship with a panel of general internal medicine patients" [43]. Competency-based evaluations of performance in continuity clinic must be completed at least once every 3 months. The continuity clinic provides an ideal setting for ongoing assessment of residents' performance in multiple subcompetencies given the variety of skills and knowledge required to care for patients in the primary care clinic setting. The unique longitudinal experience of the continuity clinic, as opposed to the short, multiweek "block rotation" experiences that make up most of a resident's schedule, allows clinic preceptors to monitor the progress of residents over a three-year period. In a 2008 survey, internal medicine program directors reported that 32% of struggling residents were identified in the continuity clinic setting [44].

Assessment Tools

Continuity clinic preceptors may be tasked with assessing and documenting resident performance in a single encounter or synthesizing a trainee's skills over a several month period. Perhaps the most common single-encounter assessment is the mini-CEX [45]. Many programs require completion and documentation of a certain number of mini-CEXs among other program requirements; however, in order for these assessments to be valid and consistent within an organization, faculty development is vital. Faculty development may include case-based discussions, after viewing recorded standardized patient encounters as vignettes, to allow faculty to practice assessment skills and calibrate assessment with each other. Open discussions with input from institutional medical educator leaders can help develop standards for competency assessments among faculty [3].

Resident clinic directors should work in conjunction with residency program leadership to identify goals and tools for assessment and to train faculty in proper use of the tools chosen. As with all evaluation tools, a balance must be struck between the desires to obtain highly detailed information, ease of use, and practical limitations on faculty time. An example of a quick assessment tool is provided, and it can be modified based on institutional specific needs (Fig. 10.5, Mini-CEX).

In addition to single-encounter assessments, summative assessments by primary care clinic faculty are a valuable component of the overall assessment of a resident's performance. For this reason, faculty development opportunities for continuity clinic preceptors should also target summative assessment skills and knowledge. Faculty development sessions can be used to calibrate faculty assessments and to gain familiarity with institutional evaluation tools. Because ACGME requires evaluations of resident performance in continuity clinic at least once every 3 months, programs may utilize different evaluation tools at different times of the year or allow preceptors to focus on a different subset of skills at different times. Institutions can use approaches that are best for their faculty and learners; some may prefer multiple checklist item assessment tools utilizing Likert-type responses, while others may lean towards more free text responses. It is recommended that evaluation tools be selected or developed collaboratively to meet the needs of learners, programs, faculty, and clinical competency committee.

Preceptor Evaluation of PGY 1 Continuity Clinic
****Boston Medical Center/Boston University School of Medicine****

Instructions:

Please complete each question to the best of your ability. Continuity Clinic Evaluations will be completed twice a year by the assigned preceptor and discussed with the resident. Additionally, please take a moment to discuss the resident's clinic performance with co-preceptors; we ask that you provide feedback that reflects the whole precepting team.

Bias in Evaluation Language:

In order to make these evaluations most helpful to the recipient and to mitigate bias that can unknowingly affect assessments, please provide comments on OBSERVABLE BEHAVIORS (rather than personality traits) and use SPECIFIC EXAMPLES to support the observations you include. Biases to be aware of may include, but are not limited to, unconscious biases based on one's race/ethnicity, religion, sexual orientation, gender identity, or disability or other cognitive biases due to anchoring, availability bias, confirmation bias, groupthink, or reliance on gist,

Please provide a brief description of the resident's performance in clinic during the last several months. We ask that you be as specific as possible and if you can highlight both the strengths and areas of improvement for this resident:

Obtains accurate, relevant, hypothesis driven history Patient Care 1: History Milestone					
Not Yet Completed Level 1	Level 1	Level 2	Level 3	Level 4	Level 5
	Elicits and reports a comprehensive history for common patient presentations, with guidance Seeks data from secondary sources, with guidance	Elicits and concisely reports a hypothesis driven patient history for common patient presentations Independently obtains data from secondary sources	Elicits and concisely reports a hypothesis driven patient history for complex patient presentations Reconciles current data with secondary sources	Efficiently elicits and concisely reports a patient history, incorporating pertinent psychosocial and other determinants of health Uses history and secondary data to guide the need for further diagnostic testing	Efficiently and effectively tailors the history taking, including relevant historical subtleties, based on patient, family, and system needs Models effective use of history to guide the need for further diagnostic testing
Develops diagnostic and therapeutic plans, which fit current guidelines Patient Care 3: Clinical Reasoning Milestone					
Not Yet Completed Level 1	Level 1	Level 2	Level 3	Level 4	Level 5
	Identifies opportunities to maintain and promote health Formulates management plans for a common chronic condition, with Guidance Formulates management plans for acute common conditions, with guidance	Develops and implements management plans to maintain and promote Health Develops and implements management plans for common chronic conditions Develops and implements management plans for common acute conditions	Develops and implements plans to maintain and promote health, incorporating pertinent psychosocial and other determinants of health Develops and implements management plans for multiple chronic conditions Develops and implements an initial management plan for patients with urgent or emergent conditions in the setting of chronic comorbidities	Develops and implements value based (high-value) comprehensive plans to maintain and promote health Develops and implements value based (high value) comprehensive management plans for multiple chronic conditions, incorporating pertinent psychosocial and other determinants of health Develops and implements value based (high value) management plans for patients with acute conditions	Creates and leads a comprehensive patient centered management plan for the patient with highly complex chronic conditions, integrating recommendations from multiple disciplines Develops and implements management plans for patients with subtle presentations, including rare or ambiguous conditions
	Applies relevant knowledge to patient care Medical Knowledge 1: Applied Foundational Sciences Milestone				
Not Yet Completed Level 1	Level 1	Level 2	Level 3	Level 4	Level 5

Fig. 10.5 Preceptor evaluation of PGY 1 continuity clinic

	Explains the scientific knowledge (e.g., physiology, social sciences, mechanism of disease) for normal function and common medical conditions	Explains the scientific knowledge for complex medical conditions	Integrates scientific knowledge to address comorbid conditions within the context of multisystem disease	Integrates scientific knowledge to address uncommon, atypical, or complex comorbid conditions within the context of multisystem disease	Demonstrates a nuanced understanding of the scientific knowledge related to uncommon, atypical, or complex conditions
	Seeks and incorporates feedback Practice-Based Learning and Improvement 2: Reflective Practice and Commitment to Personal Growth Milestone				
Not Yet Completed Level 1	Level 1	Level 2	Level 3	Level 4	Level 5
	Accepts responsibility for personal and professional development by establishing goals Identifies the factors that contribute to gap(s) between ideal and actual performance, with guidance	Demonstrates openness to performance data (feedback and other input) to inform goals Analyzes and reflects on the factors which contribute to gap(s) between ideal and actual performance, with guidance Actively seeks opportunities to improve	Seeks performance data episodically, with adaptability, and humility Institutes behavioral change(s) to narrow the gap(s) between ideal and actual performance Designs and implements an individualized learning plan, with prompting	Seeks performance data consistently with adaptability, and humility Challenges one's own assumptions and considers alternatives in narrowing the gap(s) between ideal and actual performance Independently creates and implements an individualized learning plan	Models consistently seeking performance data with adaptability and humility Coaches others on reflective practice Uses performance data to measure the effectiveness of the individualized learning plan and when necessary, improves it
	Maintains accurate, complete and timely electronic medical records Patient Care 6: Digital Health Milestone				
Not Yet Completed Level 1	Level 1	Level 2	Level 3	Level 4	Level 5
	Uses electronic health record (EHR) for routine patient care activities	Expands use of EHR to include and reconcile secondary data sources in patient care activities	Effectively uses EHR capabilities in managing acute and chronic care of patients	Uses EHR to facilitate achievement of quality targets for patient panels	Leads improvements to the EHR
Accountability/Conscientiousness Professionalism 3: Accountability/Conscientiousness Milestone					
Not Yet Completed Level 1	Level 1	Level 2	Level 3	Level 4	Level 5
	Performs administrative tasks and patient care responsibilities, with prompting	Performs administrative tasks and patient care responsibilities in a timely manner in routine situations	Performs administrative tasks and patient care responsibilities in a timely manner in complex or stressful situations	Proactively implements strategies to ensure that the needs of patients, teams, and systems are met	Creates strategies to enhance other's ability to efficiently complete administrative tasks and patient care responsibilities

Fig. 10.5 (continued)

Clinic-Specific Situations

Asynchronous Care

Asynchronous care is defined as health care for patients that is not performed in real time. For example, store-and-forward collection of images, patient portal communications, and interdisciplinary electronic consults are forms of asynchronous care [46]. At the very least, residents, within their role as primary care clinicians, practice asynchronous care by being responsible for the management of laboratory and imaging results that they ordered in continuity clinic. As asynchronous care becomes increasingly ubiquitous with the increasing popularity of portals for electronic patient-physician communication, it is imperative that residency programs develop opportunities for observation and assessment of residents performing these activities. One barrier to faculty observing asynchronous care is that many of these interactions may occur when the trainee is not working in the ambulatory space.

Additionally, peculiarities of particular electronic health records may make it easy for residents to provide asynchronous care with varying degrees of faculty knowledge. As an initial step, programs should set the expectation that preceptors be involved at some level in asynchronous care. This could take the form of including preceptors on electronic messages, having residents discuss plans based on result findings with faculty before executing them, or having preceptors review or cosign phone notes. More formally, dedicated time could be set aside to have residents provide asynchronous intervisit care under the direct supervision of faculty. Such a dedicated intervisit time period approach adds complexity to both resident and faculty scheduling and may result in slower turnaround of patient results but provides potential benefits of improved patient care and opportunities for teaching, assessment, and feedback.

Outpatient Procedures

Multiple procedures may be performed in the primary care setting including pelvic exams, arthrocentesis, and minor surgical procedures. Over time, accrediting organizations have moved away from requiring proficiency in specific procedures for graduation. The most recent edition of the ACGME Internal Medicine Milestones does not include any specific procedure performance requirements [41]. Similarly, ABIM also states that while procedures are essential to the practice of internal medicine, they only require that residents have the opportunity to develop procedure-related competencies, which relate to their intended field of practice after residency [47]. Thus, there are no specific requirements for residents to demonstrate procedure competency in the primary care setting unless they are planning a career in primary care. However, each residency program can define specific requirements for their residents. For example, if a program believes that it is important for all their graduates to be able to perform pelvic exams, they may make it a program-specific requirement for residents to demonstrate competency in this procedure. In this case, programs must decide how to determine competency, which may include a combination of case log volume and specific evaluation of procedural performance ability by continuity clinic preceptors.

The Struggling Learner

Faculty will invariably work with a struggling resident at some point. In response to a 2008 survey of internal medicine program directors, 73.5% reported having residents who were having difficulty [48]. The clinic preceptor's role in these instances is multifaceted including providing performance-based feedback and assessment, while also identifying when deficiencies are not corrected despite specific feedback and guidance. In the case of a struggling resident, it is important that preceptors engage educational leaders in discussions to express their concerns. Depending on the system, concerns may be first brought up to a chief resident, residency clinic director, associate program director, or residency evaluation committees. These educational leaders may work behind the scenes to garner additional information from other sources and may convey information to the CCC. In most cases, the clinic preceptor's main role is to provide support for the resident in the continuity clinic setting and to ensure that all patients receive excellent care. It is the CCC or other program leadership's responsibility to determine higher stakes assessments and potentially the need for specific interventions or remediation. These may involve clinic preceptors if clinic-related interventions or assessments are needed [49].

Conclusion

The resident primary care clinic experience is an integral part of internal medicine training providing skills, knowledge, and experience with the care of patients in the ambulatory setting. The internal medicine milestones "represent a road map for the development of residents as they advance in clinical skills, knowledge, and values" [3, 40].

Feedback provides concrete descriptions of a trainee's performance in a specific activity coupled with actionable suggestions for improvement. Information discussed during feedback exchanges and other data should be synthesized to develop a formal assessment of a trainee's performance. The resident clinic director should work in cooperation with residency program leadership to optimize the competency-based assessment of residents in the primary care clinic setting with a shared goal of training residents to become a highly competent physician.

References

1. Accreditation Council for Graduate Medical Education [Internet]. [cited 2022 May 8]. https://www.acgme.org/about-us/overview/#:~:text=The Accreditation Council for Graduate, medical care to all Americans.
2. Green ML, Aagaard EM, Caverzagie KJ, Chick DA, Holmboe E, Kane G, et al. Charting the road to competence: developmental milestones for internal medicine residency training. J Grad Med Educ. 2009;1(1):5–20.
3. Holmboe ES, Iobst WF. ACGME Assessment Guidebook [Internet]. [cited 2021 Nov 8]. https://www.acgme.org/globalassets/PDFs/Milestones/Guidebooks/AssessmentGuidebook.pdf
4. Celeste Eno P, Ricardo Correa MD E, Nancy H Stewart D, Jonathan Lim M, Mary Elizabeth Westerman M, Eric S, Holmboe M, et al. Milestones guidebook for residents and fellows [Internet]; 2020 [cited 2022 May 8]. https://www.acgme.org/globalassets/pdfs/milestones/milestonesguidebookforresidentsfellows.pdf
5. Norcini J, Anderson B, Bollela V, Burch V, Costa MJ, Duvivier R, et al. Criteria for good assessment: consensus statement and recommendations from the Ottawa 2010 conference. Med Teach. 2011;33(3):206–14.

6. Holmboe E. Realizing the promise of competency-based medical education. Acad Med. 2015;90(4):411–3.
7. Ramani S. Reflections on feedback: closing the loop. Med Teach. 2016;38:206.
8. Van De Ridder JMM, Stokking KM, McGaghie WC, Ten Cate OTJ. What is feedback in clinical education? Med Educ. 2008;42(2):189–97.
9. Tripodi N, Feehan J, Wospil R, Vaughan B. Twelve tips for developing feedback literacy in health professions learners. Med Teach. 2020;43:960.
10. Eva KW, Armson H, Holmboe E, Lockyer J, Loney E, Mann K, et al. Factors influencing responsiveness to feedback: on the interplay between fear, confidence, and reasoning processes. Adv Heal Sci Educ. 2012;17(1):15–26.
11. Ladonna KA, Ginsburg S, Watling C. "Rising to the level of your incompetence": what physicians' self-assessment of their performance reveals about the imposter syndrome in medicine, vol. 93. Academic Medicine. Lippincott Williams and Wilkins; 2018. p. 763–8.
12. Boud D, Molloy E. Rethinking models of feedback for learning: the challenge of design. Assess Eval High Educ. 2013 Sep;38(6):698–712.
13. Branfield Day L, Miles A, Ginsburg S, Melvin L, et al. Resident perceptions of assessment and feedback in competency-based medical education: a focus group study of one internal medicine residency program. Acad Med. 2020;95(11):1712–7.
14. Bing-You RG, Trowbridge RL. Why medical educators may be failing at feedback. JAMA. 2009;302(12):1330.
15. Algiraigri AH. Ten tips for receiving feedback effectively in clinical practice. Med Educ Online. 2014;19(1):25141.
16. Hemmer PA, Karani R. Let's face it: we are biased, and it should not be that way. J Gen Intern Med. 2019;34(5):649–51.
17. Young JQ, Sugarman R, Schwartz J, O'Sullivan PS. Overcoming the challenges of direct observation and feedback programs: a qualitative exploration of resident and faculty experiences. Teach Learn Med. 2020;32(5):541–51.
18. Ramani S, Könings KD, Mann KV, Pisarski EE, Van Der Vleuten CPM. About politeness, face, and feedback: exploring resident and faculty perceptions of how institutional feedback culture influences feedback practices. Acad Med. 2018;93(9):1348–58.
19. Moroz A, Horlick M, Mandalaywala N, Stern T, D. Faculty feedback that begins with resident self-assessment: motivation is the key to success. Med Educ. 2018;52(3):314–23.
20. Kogan JR, Conforti LN, Bernabeo EC, Durning SJ, Hauer KE, Holmboe ES. Faculty staff perceptions of feedback to residents after direct observation of clinical skills. Med Educ. 2012;46(2):201–15.
21. Ramani S, Könings KD, Mann KV, Pisarski EE, van der Vleuten CPM. About politeness, face, and feedback. Acad Med. 2018:1.
22. Ramani S, Könings KD, Ginsburg S, van der Vleuten CPM. Twelve tips to promote a feedback culture with a growth mind-set: swinging the feedback pendulum from recipes to relationships. Med Teach. 2019;41(6):625–31.
23. Lefroy J, Watling C, Teunissen PW, Brand P. Guidelines: the do's, don'ts and don't knows of feedback for clinical education. Perspect Med Educ. 2015;4(6):284–99.
24. Graddy R, Reynolds SS, Wright SM. Coaching residents in the ambulatory setting: faculty direct observation and resident reflection. J Grad Med Educ. 2018;10(4):449.
25. Haynes C, Yamamoto M, Dashiell-Earp C, Gunawardena D, Gupta R, Simon W. Continuity clinic practice feedback curriculum for residents: a model for ambulatory education. J Grad Med Educ. 2019;11(2):189.
26. Natesan SM, Krzyzaniak SM, Stehman C, Shaw R, Story D, Gottlieb M. Curated collections for educators: eight key papers about feedback in medical education. Cureus. 2019;11(3)
27. McCutcheon S, Duchemin AM. Formalizing feedback: introducing a structured approach in an outpatient resident clinic. Acad Psychiatry. 2020;44(4):399–402.
28. Omer AA, Abdularhim M. The criteria of constructive feedback: the feedback that counts. J Heal Spec. 2017;5(1):45.

29. Bing-You RG, Paterson J, Levine MA. Feedback falling on deaf ears: residents' receptivity to feedback tempered by sender credibility. Med Teach. 1997;19(1):40–4.
30. Rea J, Stephenson C, Leasure E, Vaa B, Halvorsen A, Huber J, et al. Perceptions of scheduled vs. unscheduled directly observed visits in an internal medicine residency outpatient clinic. BMC Med Educ. 2020;20(1):1–9.
31. Ramani S, Krackov SK. Twelve tips for giving feedback effectively in the clinical environment. Med Teach. 2012;34(10):787–91.
32. Branch WT Jr, Paranjape A. Feedback and reflection: teaching methods for clinical settings. Acad Med. 2002;77(12):1185–8.
33. Roze des Ordons A, Cheng A, Gaudet J, Downar J, Lockyer J. Adapting feedback to individual residents: an examination of preceptor challenges and approaches. J Grad Med Educ. 2018;10(2):168.
34. MedEdPublish CK, Moroz A, Carmody K, Moroz AA. Thank you for your feedback? An imperative to improve feedback givers' skills. scholar.archive.org. 2018;7:51.
35. Moroz A, King A, Kim B, Fusco H, Carmody K. Constructing a shared mental model for feedback conversations: faculty workshop using video vignettes developed by residents. AAMC. 2019;15(15):10821.
36. Bing-You R, Varaklis K, Hayes V, Trowbridge R, Kemp H, McKelvy D. The feedback tango: an integrative review and analysis of the content of the teacher⇓learner feedback exchange. Acad Med. 2018;93(4):657–62.
37. Sargeant J, Armson H, Driessen E, Holmboe E, Konings K, Lockyer J, et al. Evidence-informed facilitated feedback: the R2C2 feedback model. MedEdPORTAL Publ [Internet]; 2016 [cited 2019 Jul 2];12(12). https://www.mededportal.org/publication/10387
38. Sargeant J, Mann K, Manos S, Epstein I, Warren A, Shearer C, et al. R2C2 in action: testing an evidence-based model to facilitate feedback and coaching in residency. J Grad Med Educ. 2017;9(2):165–70.
39. Sargeant J, Lockyer J, Mann K, Holmboe E, Silver I, Armson H, et al. Facilitated reflective performance feedback: developing an evidence-and theory-based model that builds relationship, explores reactions and content, and coaches for performance change (R2C2). Acad Med. 2015;90(12):1698–706.
40. Doolittle BR, Lim J, Edgar L. Milestones 2.0 – a growth mindset for internal medicine residency programs. Am J Med. 2020;133(12):1492–9.
41. ACGME Internal Medicine Milestones 2.0 [Internet]; 2021 [cited 2022 Jun 14]. https://www.acgme.org/globalassets/PDFs/Milestones/InternalMedicineMilestones.pdf
42. Shalaby M, Yaich S, Donnelly J, Chippendale R, DeOliveira MC, Noronha C. X+Y scheduling models for internal medicine residency programs-a look Back and a look forward. J Grad Med Educ. 2014;6(4):639–42.
43. ACGME Common Program Requirements July 2022 [Internet]. [cited 2021 Nov 15]. https://www.acgme.org/what-we-do/accreditation/common-program-requirements/
44. Gebauer S, Steele E. Questions program directors need to answer before using resident clinical performance data. J Grad Med Educ. 2016;8(4):507.
45. Mini-CEX | ABIM.org [Internet]. [cited 2021 Nov 9]. https://www.abim.org/program-directors-administrators/assessment-tools/mini-cex.aspx
46. Reed T, Tuckson V, Edmunds M, Hodgkins ML. Telehealth. N Engl J Med. 2017;377(16):1585–92.
47. American Board of Internal Medicine Policies for Certification [Internet]. [cited 2022 May 8]. https://www.abim.org/Media/splbmcpe/policies-and-procedures.pdf
48. Dupras DM, Edson RS, Halvorsen AJ, Hopkins RH, McDonald FS. "Problem residents": prevalence, problems and remediation in the era of Core competencies. Am J Med. 2012;125(4):421–5.
49. ACGME Clinical Competency Committee. [cited 2021 Nov 9]. https://www.acgme.org/globalassets/PDFs/Milestones/Guidebooks/Purpose-of-a-CCC.pdf

Chapter 11
Academic Year-End Resident Panel Transfer: Models, Methods, and Best Practices

Lisa Ochoa-Frongia, Lee Bach Lu, and Anne Rosenthal

Introduction

Serving as a primary care provider to a panel of patients for three years is a cornerstone of the internal medicine residency ambulatory experience. Academic practices face the unique challenge of transferring resident patient panels to new providers each year as residents graduate. In this chapter, we examine the literature on end-of-year resident panel transfers, present different models of resident panel transfer, and discuss methods and best practices for the transfer process. We include an evaluation of the benefits and challenges of the models.

Outline

- Overview
- Models of panel transfer
  - Model 1: Panel transfer to new interns
  - Model 2: Panel transfer to rising second-year residents
  - Model 3: Transfer of individual patients based on clinical complexity
- Best practices for end-of-year panel transfer
- Conclusion

L. Ochoa-Frongia · A. Rosenthal (✉)
Department of Medicine, University of California San Francisco, San Francisco, CA, USA
e-mail: Lisa.Ochoa-Frongia@ucsf.edu; Anne.Rosenthal@ucsf.edu

L. B. Lu
Department of Medicine, Baylor College of Medicine, Houston, TX, USA
e-mail: Lblu@bcm.edu

L. B. Lu et al. (eds.), *Leading an Academic Medical Practice*,
https://doi.org/10.1007/978-3-031-40273-9_11

Overview

Each June, as internal medicine residents graduate from their three-year programs, it is estimated that over one million patients of over 9000 resident primary care providers (PCPs) [1] undergo a transfer of care. In the process of this transition, patient-provider relationships that have developed over two to three years are disrupted, and patients are most often transferred from more experienced residents to residents with less experience [2]. The organizational and logistical effort involved in orchestrating the simultaneous transfer of large numbers of patients is substantial. These factors make the academic end-of-year panel transfer process a critical time for patient safety and satisfaction. Although the topic has received far less attention than the risks associated with inpatient handoffs, available analyses suggest that academic year-end transfers of patients include a high risk of lost follow-up and missed care opportunities. For example, in 2008, one residency program found that only 48% of the patients of graduating residents saw a new PCP within the following year, including 43% of those patients who had been identified as highest risk [3]. In addition, their analysis uncovered significant delays in the follow-up of abnormal test results, many missed cancer screenings, and deficiencies in chronic disease management. In 2010, one internal medicine program found that 19% of highest-risk patients had not been seen in the 6 months following resident PCP graduation. They also uncovered high rates of test results that were pending upon resident graduation that did not receive appropriate follow-up [4].

Despite the impact on quality of care and patient experience associated with the departure of third-year residents, the majority of residency programs have not historically had a formal end-of-year panel transfer process. A 2013 survey of Medicine-Pediatrics programs found that only 46% had a defined end-of-residency handoff process [5], and in a 2014 Association of Program Directors in Internal Medicine survey, only 34% of respondent programs reported having a year-end ambulatory handoff system [6]. In recognition of the importance of a structured care transition protocol, the Accreditation Council for Graduate Medicine Education (ACGME) emphasizes the importance of transitions of care in patient safety. The Council does not, however, provide specific guidelines on end-of-year panel transfer. Transitions in care have been a focus for the Clinical Learning Environment Review [7].

When the University of California San Francisco (UCSF) Center for Excellence in Primary Care performed a review of residency programs nationally, they found that one feature of the most effective programs is a clear and defined process for year-end panel transfer. Their High-Functioning Primary Care Residency Clinics: Building Blocks for Providing Excellent Care and Teaching stipulate under Building Block 3: Empanelment—"includes clear processes that exist for reassigning panels when residents graduate, with protocols to ensure that patients do not get lost in transition" [8].

Existing Models for Panel Transfer

Model 1: Panel Transfer to New Interns

When graduating residents complete their residency, their panel is transferred to incoming interns.

When:

- The transfer usually takes place at the start of the academic year, once new interns have started internship.

How:

1. Graduating third-year residents perform handoffs by documenting a transfer summary in the progress note of the last visit. They may not be able to physically sign out to the new interns due to a lack of overlapping clinic time.
2. The clinic administrative team sends letters to patients to inform them of the PCP change.
3. Nursing and administrative teams keep a list of graduating resident patients to be scheduled into interns' templates when available.

Advantages:

1. Patients are cared for by the same resident physician for the duration of the three years of their PCP's residency training.

Disadvantages:

1. Patient panel transfer and reassignments cannot be done until intern clinic templates open shortly before the academic year begins.
2. New interns are inexperienced with the healthcare system and have limited clinical experience to treat complex patients.
3. Intern clinic templates are small with limited availability, further delaying patient care due to lack of access. New interns may not be able to absorb a large panel from graduating third-year residents.
4. Depending on residency program schedules, new interns may not start their continuity clinic until August or September, which can further delay patient care.
5. This model often means that patients do not have an active resident PCP for a short time between third-year resident graduation and the first clinic day for interns. Electronic medical record (EMR) in-basket monitoring for patients of the departed third-year resident may need to be delegated to another resident physician or faculty.
6. New interns face challenges in managing the in-basket at the beginning of the academic year due to lack of clinical and systems training.

Model 2: Panel Transfer to Rising Second-Year Residents

When graduating residents complete their residency, their panel is transferred to rising second-year residents.

When:

- The panel transfer panel can start as early as three to four months prior to third-year resident graduation.

How:

1. Graduating third-year residents can leave detailed transfer notes and schedule patients to see rising second-year residents in a time frame they find clinically appropriate.
2. The graduating resident can physically introduce patients to their new PCP (the rising second-year resident).
3. For complex patients, graduating residents leave detailed notes and can arrange to call or meet with rising second-year residents to sign out though this may be time intensive.
4. The clinic administrative team sends letters to patients to inform them of the PCP change.

Advantages:

1. The rising second-year residents are already active users in the EMR system, so reassignments can be done in a timely manner.
2. Rising second-year residents are familiar with the healthcare system and are more experienced in caring for more complex patients.
3. There are opportunities for patients to be introduced in-person to their newly assigned PCP even before third-year residents graduate and leave their clinic practice.
4. Rising second-year residents are more experienced in addressing patient care items found in their in-basket such as results and patient calls.
5. For handoffs, third-year residents can easily contact the rising second-year residents to discuss complex patients.
6. Depending on the scheduling system, rising second-year resident clinic schedules may be available months before the new academic to make the transition easier. The transfer can take place months before the graduating resident departs.
7. This model requires less supervision from clinic faculty and less administrative work as the schedule overlap between graduating third-year residents and rising second-year residents means no gap in active PCP as long as the rising second-year resident is available to assume the PCP role prior to the third-year resident graduating.

Disadvantages:

1. Rising second-year panels might be too large and unable to absorb all graduating third-year panels, forcing panel fragmentation and a possible delay in PCP transition for some patients.
2. Patients are under the care of resident physicians for only two years, leading to more frequent PCP changes.

Model 3: Transfer of Individual Patients Based on Clinical Complexity

Graduating residents triage patients in their clinic panel to different levels of acuity or complexity. Complex patients are assigned to more experienced clinicians, such as a faculty member, if the practice is a shared resident-faculty practice, or a rising R2. Less complex patients will be assigned to incoming interns. This model requires more labored administrative reassignment of select patients.

When:

- The process for this model begins five to six months prior to third-year resident graduation and concludes in fall of the next academic year.

How:

1. Five to six months prior to third-year resident graduation, the third-year residents are asked to assign the patients in their panel to three tiers based on degrees of complexity and acuity of medical or psychosocial conditions. Patients in the tier of highest complexity are prioritized for transfer to the soonest available experienced clinician, prior to graduating third-year resident completion of residency. Patients in descending tiers of acuity are transferred later in the academic year. Outlines considerations and the approach to triaging panels of patients into three tiers. Prior literature outlining characteristics of high-risk patients in resident panels includes many of the below considerations [4, 9] Table 11.1.

Table 11.1 Approach to triaging patients by complexity and acuity

	Tier 1: Highest complexity/acuity	Tier 2: Moderate complexity/acuity	Tier 3: Lowest complexity/acuity
Target for percentage of panel placed in category	5–10%	30%	60–65%
Medical complexity and acuity	Multiple, active chronic conditions New diagnoses requiring active management or care coordination (e.g., diabetes, malignancy) Recent (especially multiple) ER visits or hospitalizations	A few active chronic conditions requiring regular visits	One or no chronic medical conditions
Anticipated PCP visit frequency	5+ visits per year	2–5 visits per year	One visit per year
Psychosocial considerations	Severe challenges with social determinants of health (e.g., low health literacy, unhoused, lack of resources actively impacting health)	Some challenge with social determinants of health or need for additional resources	No unmet psychosocial needs
Communication considerations	Actively or frequently message/contact clinic team or PCP outside of scheduled visits	Occasionally message/contact clinic team or PCP outside of scheduled visits	Seldom or never message/contact clinic team or PCP outside of scheduled visits

2. A clinic administrative team manages the transfer process, making direct outreach and scheduling patients in the two tiers of highest complexity (~35–40% of all departing third-year residents' patients). The remainder of the patients receive a letter via mail and/or patient portal directing them to call to schedule their transfer appointment.
3. Departing third-year residents are directed to document transfer notes in the EMR as the progress note for that visit during their last scheduled visit with each patient.
4. Departing third-year residents may arrange direct handoffs or discussions with the designated new PCP for complex patients.
5. The clinic administrative team sends letters to patients to inform them of the PCP change.

Advantages:

1. In this model, the most complex patients are shepherded through the panel transfer process, and special needs (e.g., need for reassignment to an attending physician or a particular schedule or language concordance) can be met.
2. Interns (who in many programs have limited time in clinic during intern year) do not receive a partial or full panel of patients and can build their patient panel, allowing for gradual learning and mastery of clinic systems.

Disadvantages:

1. A high degree of administrative oversight and time is required in transferring patients to various providers over the course of a process that takes many months.
2. Fragmentation of panels may contribute to patient confusion and patients being lost to follow-up.
3. Patient safety challenges may arise if patients are currently without a designated PCP, though continuity advanced practice practitioners (APPs) may manage these patients while in the process of transfer. This is feasible only for academic medical practices which have AAPs in their primary care team.
4. Nonresident providers (APPs and attending physicians) may be asked to accept generally high-acuity and complex patients into their own panels.

Multiple models of patient panel transfer for senior residents completing residency exist in academic clinics and are described in the literature. Most of these models assume the patient-centered best practice of empaneling a group (panel) of patients to a single primary care provider. These models include transferring a full panel from a departing resident to (1) incoming intern or (2) second-year resident [3, 4, 6], or (3) dividing a departing resident panel among multiple incoming residents and stratifying patients by complexity and acuity. In this section, we will outline, compare, and contrast these models. The authors of this chapter have direct experience with the main models outlined here. Based on our review of the literature, it appears to be most common for academic medical practices to transfer departing resident patient panels to interns or second-year residents. Table 11.2 provides a summary and comparison of these 3 models.

Table 11.2 Comparison of year-end resident panel transfer models

	Model 1: Transfer full panel to intern	Model 2: Transfer full panel to second-year resident	Model 3: Hybrid model
Model description	Graduating third-year resident panels to new interns	Graduating third-year resident panels to rising second-year residents	Transfer panel to various physicians or advanced practice providers based on patient acuity and complexity
Transfer schedule	At the start of a new academic year	3–4 months prior to the end of the academic year	Most complex patients transferred at the end of the academic year; less complex transferred in new academic year
Frequency of patient transition to new PCP	Every 3 years	Every 2 years	Every 3 years
Sign-out method (between departing and new provider)	– Detailed progress notes – Letters to notify patients	– Detailed progress notes – Letter to notify patients – Physically introduce patients to new PCP when possible – Call and sign out to new PCP on complex patients	– Detailed progress notes – Letter to notify patients – Physically introduce patients to new PCP when possible
Intern/resident workload to manage new patient panel	High workload for interns may not be able to handle complex patients	Moderate workload	Low intern workload
Preceptor workload to oversee panel	High workload to oversee panel and help manage in-basket laboratory results	Minimal workload	Moderate workload
Administrative workload required for model	High workload to keep a list of patients and schedule them	Minimal workload	High workload to oversee complex transfer process
Patient safety considerations	Significant concerns: timely appointments, loss of follow-up	Some patients may experience gap between providers but less risk than model #1	Some patients are lost to follow-up; many have gaps between departed PCP and new PCP
Burden on nonresident providers accepting transfers	Little	Little	Some faculty or APPs with open panels in a shared practice may be asked to accept complex patients for transfer

Best Practices for End-of-Year Panel Transfer

Regardless of the model chosen for transferring patients, there are practices that facilitate a safe and smooth transition of care. Table 11.3 outlines best practices for clinic managers, faculty, and departing trainees in addition to the new PCP during the transfer process.

Table 11.3 Best practices for all clinics in year-end resident panel transfer

Clinic manager and faculty roles	
– Prepare patients	– Orientation to transfer process by clinic and outgoing provider.
	– Letter explaining transfer process. If possible, include the name of new PCP and any upcoming scheduled appointments. – See UCSF's CEPC Transforming Teaching Practices Empanelment Toolkit for a sample patient transfer letter (Appendix 3, p. 14) [10].
	– Consider sending a phone call, text, or patient portal message around the time of transfer.
– Orient residents, preceptors, and staff	– Create a curriculum for residents – Example: Teaching Video and Workshop Exercises: Putting the Patient First: Engineering Patient-Oriented Clinic Handoffs (EPOCH) [11]
	– Orient residents to a standardized process for patient handoff
	– Include attending in sign-out communications for high-risk patients
– Use a structured process	– Provide a risk stratification rubric to prioritize higher risk patients – Expedite appointments for the highest-risk patients – Ensure that a process is in place to confirm successful transfer
	– Provide protected time for residents to review and prepare their panel – For example, one clinic session for panel review and stratification, one session for preparing transfer notes or off-service summaries
	– Create a standard transfer note template – Consider creating an EMR smart phrase or other template to capture active problems and needed follow-up
	– Determine how handoffs will take place (via email, face-to-face, phone, or virtual session between residents or entirely within the EMR)
– Dedicate staffing and resources	– Designate a staff member to oversee the transfer process (empanelment manager or transitions coordinator)
	– Maintain a tracking system to ensure that patients are not lost to follow-up
	– If patients are empaneled with a team, ensure team continuity

Clinic manager and faculty roles	
Departing resident roles	
– Prepare patients	– Orient patients early and often to the panel transfer process
	– Express confidence in the incoming PCP and clinic team
	– Ensure that patients know how to contact the clinic during care transition
– Prepare the medical record	– Write a transfer/off-service summary, at minimum for the highest complexity patients – Include: Brief (2–3 line) summary with patient identifiers, list of active problems with plan, and list of new PCP active items to follow-up (such as important pending labs or studies, specialist referrals)
New PCP roles	
– Orient patients	– Orient patients to your role as new PCP. Express confidence in the care the prior PCP and patient undertook together
– Review the medical record	– Review the transfer/off-service summary left by departing PCP

Conclusion

The graduation of residents and transition of care to a new PCP represent a high-risk time for patient safety in academic medical clinics. The loss of continuity and patient relationships associated with third-year resident departure is associated with delays in follow-up and gaps in care. While having a structured transfer process is critical to successful navigation of patient transition, U.S. academic medical clinics have implemented these processes to a variable degree. This chapter has described three existing models for end-of-year transfer of patients and outlined some best practices for facilitating safe and effective handoffs. All programs should establish a structured process for the safe transition of primary care patients, though the details will vary based on the structure of practices and local operational and programmatic resources and needs.

References

1. Resident & Fellow Workforce Data [Internet]. ABIM. American Board of Internal Medicine; 2021 [cited 2021 Nov 7]. Available from: https://www.abim.org/about/statistics-data/resident-fellow-workforce-data/
2. Young JQ, Niehaus B, Lieu SC, O'Sullivan PS. Improving resident education and patient safety: a method to balance initial caseloads at academic year-end transfer. Acad Med. 2010;85(9):1418–24. https://doi.org/10.1097/ACM.0b013e3181eab8d0.
3. Caines LC, Brockmeyer DM, Tess AV, Kim H, Kriegel G, Bates CK. The revolving door of resident continuity practice: identifying gaps in transitions of care. J Gen Intern Med. 2011;26(9):995–8. https://doi.org/10.1007/s11606-011-1731-8.

4. Pincavage AT, Ratner S, Prochaska ML, Prochaska M, Oyler J, Davis AM, Arora VM. Outcomes for resident-identified high-risk patients and resident perspectives of year-end continuity clinic handoffs. J Gen Intern Med. 2012;27(11):1438–44. https://doi.org/10.1007/s11606-012-2100-y.
5. Donnelly MJ, Clauser JM, Tractenberg RE. Current practice in end-of-residency handoffs: A survey of internal medicine-pediatrics program directors. J Grad Med Educ. 2013;5(1):93–7.
6. Phillips E, Harris C, Lee WW, Pincavage AT, Ouchida K, Miller RK, Chaudhry S, Arora VM. Year-End Clinic Handoffs: A National Survey of Academic Internal Medicine Programs. J Gen Intern Med. 2017;32(6):667–72. https://doi.org/10.1007/s11606-017-4005-2. Epub 2017 Feb 14.
7. ACGME program requirements for graduate medical education in internal medicine. Accreditation Council for Graduate Medical Education; 2020.
8. UCSF center for excellence in primary care high-functioning primary care residency clinics: Building blocks for providing excellent care and teaching. American Association of Medical Colleges; 2016. https://fcm.ucsf.edu/sites/g/files/tkssra541/f/wysiwyg/Bodenheimer%20et%20al%2C%20High-Functioning%20Primary%20Care%20Residency%20Clinics.pdf
9. Pincavage AT, Prochaska M, Dahlstrom M, Lee WW, Beiting KJ, Ratner S, Oyler J, Vinci LM, Arora VM. Patient safety outcomes after two years of an enhanced internal medicine residency clinic handoff. Am J Med. 2014;127(1):96–9. https://doi.org/10.1016/j.amjmed.2013.09.024. Epub 2013 Oct 8.
10. Gupta R, Knox M, Willard-Grace R, Kong M, Bodenheimer T. Transforming teaching practices toolkit for empanelment in teaching practices. [Internet] UCSF Center for Excellence in Primary Care; 2018. https://cepc.ucsf.edu/sites/cepc.ucsf.edu/files/Toolkit%20_Empanelment%2018-0829.pdf
11. Pincavage A, Lee WW, Ratner S, Prochaska M, Davis A, Saathoff M, et al. Teaching video and workshop exercises; "Putting the patient first: Engineering patient-oriented clinic handoffs (epoch)." [Internet] MedEdPORTAL. 2014. https://www.mededportal.org/doi/10.15766/mep_2374-8265.9686

Part IV
Telehealth & Telemedicine

Chapter 12
History and Overview of Telehealth

Syed N. Imam and Anna Rubin

Introduction

Telehealth is an efficient health care delivery method that is expanding the landscape of medical practice and becoming an integral part of the healthcare infrastructure. Telehealth is broadly defined as the use of communications technologies to provide health care from a distance, inclusive of asynchronous telehealth, remote patient monitoring and mobile health devices [1]. Telemedicine is a subset of telehealth that more narrowly refers to the remote delivery of clinical care through HIPAA-compliant technology.

In this chapter, we briefly describe the history of telemedicine, review different types of telemedicine, and outline benefits and limitations. Additionally, we discuss important features of a telemedicine portal and present essential resources related to legislation, regulations, and networking.

Outline
- History
- Types of telehealth and telemedicine
- Telehealth requirements
- Benefits and limitations
- Legislation and regulations

S. N. Imam (✉)
Baylor College of Medicine, Houston, TX, USA

Connected Care Michael E. DeBakey VA Medical Center, Houston, TX, USA
e-mail: syed.imam@bcm.edu

A. Rubin
Department of Medicine, The George Washington University School of Medicine and Health Sciences, Washington, DC, USA
e-mail: arubin@mfa.gwu.edu

L. B. Lu et al. (eds.), *Leading an Academic Medical Practice*,
https://doi.org/10.1007/978-3-031-40273-9_12

- Disparities in telehealth
- Conclusion

History

Innovative applications of technological inventions in medicine have shaped patient care through the years. In 1879, just 3 years after the invention of the telephone, an article in the Lancet described using the telephone to reduce unnecessary physician office visits [2].

In 1925, an influential publisher, Hugo Gernsback, foresaw telemedicine. He published a description of a device that doctors would use in the future and called it Teledactyl. Teledactyl was based on its Greek root words of tele, meaning far, and dactyl, meaning finger. The futuristic device would make it possible to "feel at a distance" and would allow the remote examination of a patient by using robotic fingers and a screen [3] (Fig. 12.1).

One of the earliest and most famous uses of hospital-based telemedicine was in 1959 when a closed-circuit television link was established between the Nebraska Psychiatric Institute and Norfolk State Hospital, marking the first telemedicine psychiatric consultation platform [4].

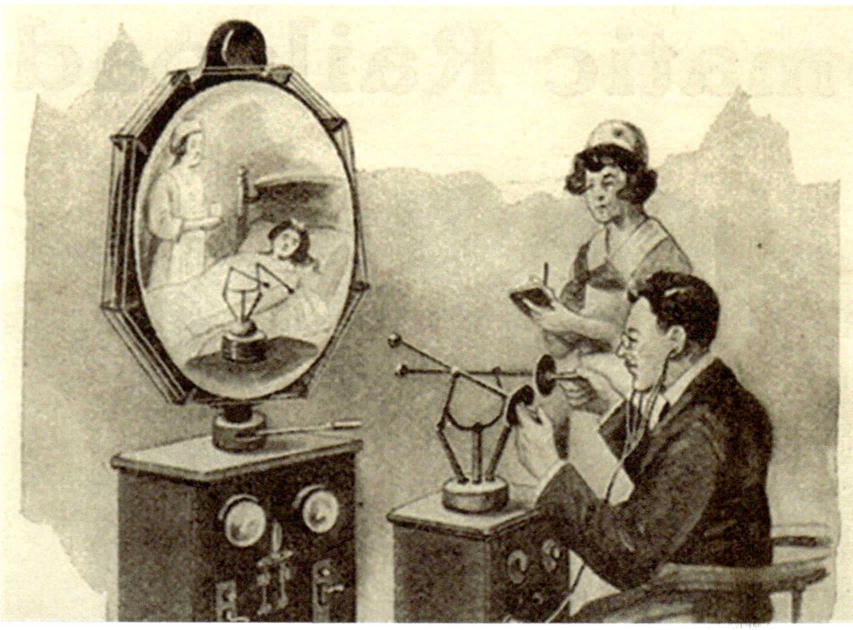

Fig. 12.1 Diagnosis by teledactyl predicted by H. Gernsback in February, 1925 issue of Science and Invention

The growth of telemedicine remained slow prior to the COVID-19 pandemic. Medicare's insurance reimbursement structure was one of the major barriers to the growth of virtual visits, despite available technology and patient interest. In 2019, Medicare began making payments for brief communications or virtual check-ins, which are short patient-initiated communications with a health care practitioner. Medicare Part B separately pays clinicians for E-visits, which are non-face-to-face patient-initiated communications through an online patient portal.

In March 2020, the unprecedented circumstances of the COVID-19 pandemic triggered changes in the reimbursement structure and resulted in exponential growth of telemedicine. Effective March 6, 2020, Centers for Medicare & Medicaid Services (CMS) issued an expansion of telehealth with the 1135 Waiver [5]. The 1135 Waiver allowed CMS to waive certain requirements during the COVID-19 national public health emergency. Prior to this waiver, Medicare could only pay for telehealth on a limited basis. Under this new waiver, Medicare pays for office, hospital, and other visits completed via telehealth across the country, including in the patient's home. During the pandemic, the reimbursement for telehealth visits was paid at the same rate as in-person visits by Medicare and by many private insurances. As circumstances evolve, there will likely be ongoing shifts in the regulation and reimbursement of telemedicine.

Types of Telemedicine and Telehealth

The terms telehealth and telemedicine are often used interchangeably, but there are subtle differences. Telemedicine is a subset of telehealth. Telehealth is a broader term than telemedicine and encompasses additional tools used in the training of physicians, medical education, meetings, and other health care-related activities [1]. Telemedicine more narrowly refers to remote clinical services [6]. They both generally refer to the exchange of medical information from one site to another through electronic communications to improve a patient's health [7, 8].

There are four basic types of telehealth, and some platforms combine two or more types to provide more comprehensive services [9].

Synchronous telehealth: Synchronous telehealth is a live two-way audiovisual link established between a patient and a clinician. It includes any video call or live chat that allows a clinician to communicate with a patient in real time. This interaction is the most well-known type of technology-based health care service referred to as telehealth or telemedicine.

Asynchronous telehealth: Asynchronous telehealth is based on a transmission of a recorded health history to a health practitioner, usually a specialist. Asynchronous telehealth is also known as "store-and-forward" telehealth. It involves specialized technology that allows a patient's data to be collected, stored in a secure cloud-based platform, and later retrieved by another treating professional, often in a different location. Current applications include obtaining and forwarding tele-retina scans and tele-dermatology images.

Remote patient monitoring (RPM): RPM uses connected electronic tools to record personal health data in one location for review by a clinician in another location, usually at a different time. RPM enables providers to record and monitor a patient's health data remotely. RPM is often recommended for patients with chronic diseases like diabetes or heart failure. An important advantage of RPM is that it provides frequent monitoring at a lower cost. For example, daily remote weight monitoring with the use of a connected/smart scale assists in the management of patients with heart failure. Clinicians receive alerts when there is a significant increase in weight suggestive of a heart failure decompensation, allowing for timely therapeutic intervention to decrease the need for hospitalization or emergency visit.

Mobile health (mHealth): Mobile health includes health care augmented through mobile devices. Mobile smart devices have the ability to collect continuous data about a person's behavior or condition that may benefit specific aspects of their health. For example, smartphones and smart wearable devices, like the iWatch, can monitor a variety of factors such as pulse rate, electrocardiography, and falls. Apps are also available to encourage healthier lifestyles and behaviors by providing heart-rate variability scores, sleep cycles, movement tracking, weight changes, dietary intake, and more. In addition to collecting continuous medical data, mobile health offers the potential to amplify important public health information. The information may include targeted texts and notifications about disease outbreaks.

Telehealth Requirements

Synchronous telemedicine visits require specific technological components, including appropriate hardware, peripherals, and software. The provider should have the technical capacity to integrate patient data into the visit, guide the patient through a provider-directed self-examination, and utilize peripherals to augment examination. Peripherals are devices separate from a laptop, tablet, or smartphone that collect and transmit high-definition audio, video, images, and other health data from the patient to a provider.

The hardware required of the patient is a smart device with video call capability. Patients can use a smart phone, tablet, laptop, or desktop. Peripherals at home that the patient may use include thermometers, blood pressure machines, pulse oximeters, and glucometers. If the patient is at a health care facility, a telemedicine cart may be available to use. Telemedicine carts are systems that integrate cameras, displays, and network access to bring remote physicians to the side of the patient. Telemedicine carts offer peripherals not available at home, such as a digital stethoscope, digital otoscope, dermatoscope, or other devices that optimize diagnostic accuracy.

Telehealth platforms must use a HIPAA-compliant secure video conferencing application. The application should be compatible with different operating systems and smart devices to allow access to a larger patient population.

Available software platforms offer various capabilities, such as online scheduling, virtual check-in, and virtual waiting rooms. Other systems facilitate billing and secure payments, perform automated patient insurance eligibility checks, and offer online co-pay collection. Some systems are integrated into the EHR and offer automated appointment reminders, clinical protocols, and secure document sharing.

Benefits and Limitations of Telehealth

Benefits of Telehealth

Telehealth is a valuable tool in modern health care and offers many benefits to both patients and clinicians. Table 12.1 outlines the advantages of telehealth across multiple domains. For instance, telehealth offers greater flexibility, reduced time away from work, and reduced transportation costs for patients. Telehealth also eliminates the potential spread of nosocomial infections in waiting and exam rooms.

Telehealth can also benefit clinicians and practices. Virtual visits are not limited by space constraints and overhead. Clinicians may enjoy greater efficiency and increased availability to patients, as there are fewer no-shows and cancellations. In theory, the number of ancillary staff and time spent by the staff are reduced in virtual visits.

Table 12.1 Benefits of telehealth

Benefit	Description
Improved access to care	• Easier access for patients, including patients with disabilities, mobility constraints, and those living in rural areas • Eliminates distance barrier
Convenience	• Comfort and privacy of own home • Less time off from work or need for childcare
Decreased risk of nosocomial infections	• Minimizes physical contact and infection transmission
Opportunity for preventative care and chronic disease management	• Improves access to preventive care and allows for close follow-up • Remote patient monitoring allows for tighter management of chronic diseases, such as diabetes and heart failure
Reduced costs for patients	• Less time (travel + visit) • Fewer secondary costs (childcare, gas, etc.)
Reduced expenses	• May need less support staff and fewer exam rooms
Potential for additional revenue	• Efficiencies may allow care to be provided to more patients
Patient satisfaction	• Improved access and convenience may result in increased patient satisfaction

Telehealth is useful as a complement to face-to-face care as well as a replacement health care service in some cases. Patients in rural areas often face challenges in receiving comprehensive medical care, particularly in specialty services. Telemedicine offers the option of point-of-care consultation with remotely available specialists.

Additionally, by expanding access to care and improving practice efficiency, telehealth offers the potential to augment chronic disease management and reduce health care costs for a system burdened by chronic health conditions. Ninety percent of the nation's $3.8 trillion in annual health care expenditures are for people with chronic and mental health conditions [10, 11]. In response, the VA developed a telehealth program for the management of chronic diseases. Patients are educated and monitored remotely through the use of technology. This program has resulted in reduced cost of care, decreased hospitalizations, decreased length of stay, and decreased readmissions [12].

The implementation of telehealth has generally yielded high levels of satisfaction among both patients and clinicians. One study of telemedicine by Massachusetts General Hospital demonstrated that "nearly all (patients) perceived the quality of care or communication to be the same or better than traditional and familiar office visits." In fact, 12.6% of patients report that the quality of telehealth care was better than an in-person visit [13]. Physicians who are engaged in telehealth also report high levels of satisfaction with patient care and specialist consultations [14].

Potential Limitations of Telehealth

In addition to the many benefits of telehealth, there are some potential limitations as described in Table 12.2.

Table 12.2 Limitations of telehealth

Limitation	Description
Insurance coverage	• Not all insurers cover telemedicine • Regulations constantly changing
Protecting medical data privacy	• Telemedicine session accessed on a public or unencrypted network may not be secure, putting patient data at risk
Licensing issues	• State laws vary, and clinicians may not be able to practice medicine across state lines
Technological barriers	• Digital platform selection • Patient tech literacy • Weak connection • Security and compliance with privacy laws
Limited physical examination	• Limited ability to perform a complete physical exam despite provider-directed self-examination and peripherals
Disparities in use	• Unequal broadband access • Disparities in tech literacy • Language barriers and difficulty incorporating an interpreter • Limited access may amplify existing health disparities

Legislation and Regulation Resources

Laws and regulations around telehealth are continuously evolving. There are several resources available to ensure that all legalities of telehealth care are met.

- The Health Resources and Services Administration's (HRSA) site Telehealth.HHS.gov provides resources for health care providers and patients about the latest federal efforts to support and promote virtual health care. It includes information on access and equity, as well as on recent research and available funding opportunities in telehealth.
- Clinicians may extend their reach through telehealth by obtaining multiple state licenses. The Interstate Medical Licensure Compact (IMLC) www.imlcc.org facilitates the process for obtaining a medical license in participating US states for physicians who want to practice in multiple states.
- The American Telemedicine Association (ATA) (Americantelemed.org) is a non-profit organization that was established in 1993. The goal of the organization is to bring together medical professionals, government, telecommunication companies, and other groups to advance telehealth and virtual care. The ATA educates about telemedicine and ensures uniform quality in the delivery of telehealth services by developing standards and guidelines.

Disparities in Telehealth

With the increase in utilization of telemedicine, there is a growing body of literature describing disparities in its use, many of which reflect the broader health care disparities that exist in the USA. Approximately 43% of low-income Americans do not have broadband internet service at home, and Black and Latino patients are less likely than whites to have broadband service at home [15]. In a large single-center study evaluating telehealth use in the first month of the public health emergency, patients of non-white race and patients from rural zip codes used telehealth less often. Of those who utilized telemedicine, older patients, Black patients, and patients with Medicaid and Medicare insurance were more likely to have a phone-only visit [16]. Similar findings have been reported in other large studies [17]. In response, the federal Infrastructure Investment and Jobs Act, passed in November 2021, dedicated over $42 billion to investment in broadband infrastructure and made narrowing the digital divide a national priority [18].

Conclusion

Telehealth is an efficient health care delivery method, which will continue to revolutionize and augment traditional health care delivery. Standardization, user-friendliness of platforms, security of data exchange, affordable peripherals, universal availability of high-speed internet, and appropriate reimbursement are all important for widespread adoption and equitable access of telehealth.

While telemedicine is not a substitute for all face-to-face visits, it has proven to be a critical tool in patient care, especially during the COVID-19 pandemic, in which health care experienced an explosion of telehealth services. Telehealth has grown into an effective alternative for patients and providers to complement in-person care in many situations. In addition, it is a proven cost-effective health care delivery method and offers the potential to improve access to care for underserved populations, though barriers to digital health equity must continue to be addressed [19]. With future technological advances, engagement with patients, and policy changes, telehealth will further solidify its role as an invaluable tool in the future of medicine.

References

1. Telehealth medlineplus.gov. Accessed 14 June 2022. https://medlineplus.gov/telehealth.html
2. Institute of Medicine & Board on Health Care Services. National Academies Press; 2012. The role of telehealth in an evolving health care environment: workshop summary. Accessed 22 Feb 2022. https://www.ncbi.nlm.nih.gov/books/NBK207145/
3. Telemedicine Predicted in 1925. With video screens and remote-control arms, any doctor could make a virtual house call. Matt Novak, March 14, 2012. Hugo Gernsback, Science and Invention Magazine, February 1925. Smithsonian Magazine. Accessed 22 Feb 2022. https://www.smithsonianmag.com/history/telemedicine-predicted-in-1925-124140942/
4. Brown FW. Rural telepsychiatry. Psychiatr Serv. 1998;49(7):963–4.
5. Medicare Telemedicine Health Care Provider Fact Sheet | CMS. Accessed 22 Feb 2022. https://www.cms.gov/newsroom/fact-sheets/medicare-telemedicine-health-care-provider-fact-sheet
6. UDS Manual 2021. Published online 2021. Accessed 28 Sep 2022. https://bphc.hrsa.gov/sites/default/files/bphc/datareporting/pdf/2021-uds-manual.pdf
7. What is telehealth? HealthIT.gov. Accessed 22 Feb 2022. https://www.healthit.gov/faq/what-telehealth
8. What is telehealth? - CCHP (cchpca.org). Accessed 22 Feb 2022. https://www.cchpca.org/what-is-telehealth/
9. Telemedicine and Telehealth | HealthIT.gov. Accessed 22 Feb 2022. https://www.healthit.gov/topic/health-it-health-care-settings/telemedicine-and-telehealth
10. Buttorff C, Ruder T, Bauman M. Multiple chronic conditions in the United States. Santa Monica, CA: Rand Corp; 2017. https://www.rand.org/content/dam/rand/pubs/tools/TL200/TL221/RAND_TL221.pdf. Accessed 22 Feb 2022.
11. Martin AB, Hartman M, Lassman D, Catlin A, National Health Expenditure Accounts Team. National Health Care spending in 2019: steady growth for the fourth consecutive year. Health Aff (Millwood). 2021;40(1):14–24.
12. Darkins A, Kendall S, Edmonson E, Young M, Stressel P. Reduced cost and mortality using home telehealth to promote self-management of complex chronic conditions: a retrospective matched cohort study of 4,999 veteran patients. Telemed J E Health. 2015;21(1):70–6.
13. Donelan K, Barreto EA, Sossong S, Michael C, Estrada JJ, Cohen AB, Wozniak J, Schwamm LH. Patient and clinician experiences with telehealth for patient follow-up care. Am J Manag Care. 2019;25(1):40–4.
14. Hoff T, Lee DR. Physician satisfaction with telehealth: a systematic review and agenda for future research. Qual Manag Health Care. 2022;31:160. https://doi.org/10.1097/QMH.0000000000000359. Epub ahead of print.

15. Who has home broadband? Internet/Broadband Fact Sheet. Pew Research Center. https://www.pewresearch.org/internet/fact-sheet/internet-broadband/?menuItem=2ab2b0be-6364-4d3a-8db7-ae134dbc05cd. Accessed 14 June 2022.
16. Pierce RP, Stevermer JJ. Disparities in use of telehealth at the onset of the COVID-19 public health emergency. J Telemed Telecare. 2020;29:1357633X20963893. https://doi.org/10.1177/1357633X20963893. Epub ahead of print.
17. Eberly LA, Kallan MJ, Julien HM, Haynes N, Khatana SAM, Nathan AS, Snider C, Chokshi NP, Eneanya ND, Takvorian SU, Anastos-Wallen R, Chaiyachati K, Ambrose M, O'Quinn R, Seigerman M, Goldberg LR, Leri D, Choi K, Gitelman Y, Kolansky DM, Cappola TP, Ferrari VA, Hanson CW, Deleener ME, Adusumalli S. Patient characteristics associated with telemedicine access for primary and specialty ambulatory care during the COVID-19 pandemic. JAMA Netw Open. 2020;3(12):e2031640. https://doi.org/10.1001/jamanetworkopen.2020.31640. Erratum in: JAMA Netw Open 2021 Feb 1;4(2):e211913.
18. Rodriguez JA, Carmel S, Bates DW. Digital inclusion as health care—supporting health care equity with digital-infrastructure initiatives. N Engl J Med. 2022;386:1101–3. https://doi.org/10.1056/NEJMp2115646.
19. Barbosa W, Zhou K, Waddell E, Taylor Myers E, Dorsey R. Improving access to care: telemedicine across medical domains. Annu Rev Public Health. 2021;42(1):463–81.

Chapter 13
Telemedicine Clinical Workflow

Katherine Otto Chebly and Catherine Anne Varnum

Introduction

Prior to the COVID-19 pandemic, most academic medical practices did not routinely deliver telemedicine-based healthcare. Existing telehealth services were not standardized and faced logistical and technological barriers to routine uptake [1, 2]. The pandemic has since transformed telemedicine into a pillar of healthcare delivery in academic medical centers, and various best practices have been generated for virtual workflows [3–6].

Medical directors and academic leaders need to develop a pragmatic framework for the creation of an effective telemedicine workflow, including delineation of team roles. In this chapter, we discuss these topics as well as areas where telemedicine visits may differ from in-person care, highlighting evidence-based techniques for a virtual physical exam. We also present recommendations for harnessing telemedicine's accessibility to ensure equitable healthcare.

K. O. Chebly (✉)
Division of General Internal Medicine and Clinical Innovation, Department of Medicine, New York University Langone Health, New York, NY, USA
e-mail: katherine.otto@nyulangone.org

C. A. Varnum
Division of General Internal Medicine, Medical Faculty Associates, George Washington University, Washington, DC, USA
e-mail: Cvarnum@mfa.gwu.edu

L. B. Lu et al. (eds.), *Leading an Academic Medical Practice*,
https://doi.org/10.1007/978-3-031-40273-9_13

Outline

- The virtual medical home: workflows and roles
  - Virtual check-in
  - Virtual intake by medical assistant
  - Virtual outtake by medical assistant
- The patient-clinician telemedicine encounter
  - Preparing for the visit
  - Conducting the visit
  - Concluding the visit
- Documentation
- Optimizing the telemedicine workflow for accessibility & equity
- Conclusion

The Virtual Medical Home: Workflow and Roles

The virtual medical home is an approach to the provision of telemedicine services that emphasizes team-based, coordinated, comprehensive, patient-centered care. The virtual medical home strives to reflect a medical practice's existing infrastructure to optimize service delivery and ensure that patients receive efficient and high-quality care (see Fig. 13.1). The structure and staffing needs of a telemedicine clinic workflow differ slightly from that of in-person encounters but reflect similar principles and processes.

Virtual Check-In: Similar to in-person check-in, virtual visit check-in can be done with the support of a clinical associate (clerk or medical assistant). Patients can be checked in through a video or telephone platform, and some portals provide the option for virtual check-in directly by the patient without clinic staff involvement, using the portal itself, email, or text messaging. In advance of a telemedicine visit, patients should be provided with clear check-in instructions and opportunities for real-time technical support to ensure that visits are not missed due to technical challenges.

Redundant backup processes should be in place to ensure that the patient is checked in to—and remains connected to—the appointment. Patients should be asked to provide their location and confirm backup contact information in the case of digital disconnection. If a patient is not checked in within a specific interval from the appointment, clinic staff should have, and be familiar with, a protocol to reach out to the patient and troubleshoot any connectivity issues. Special consideration is required for patients using the telemedicine platform for the first time, patients with limited digital literacy, non-English-speaking patients, and patients with hearing loss.

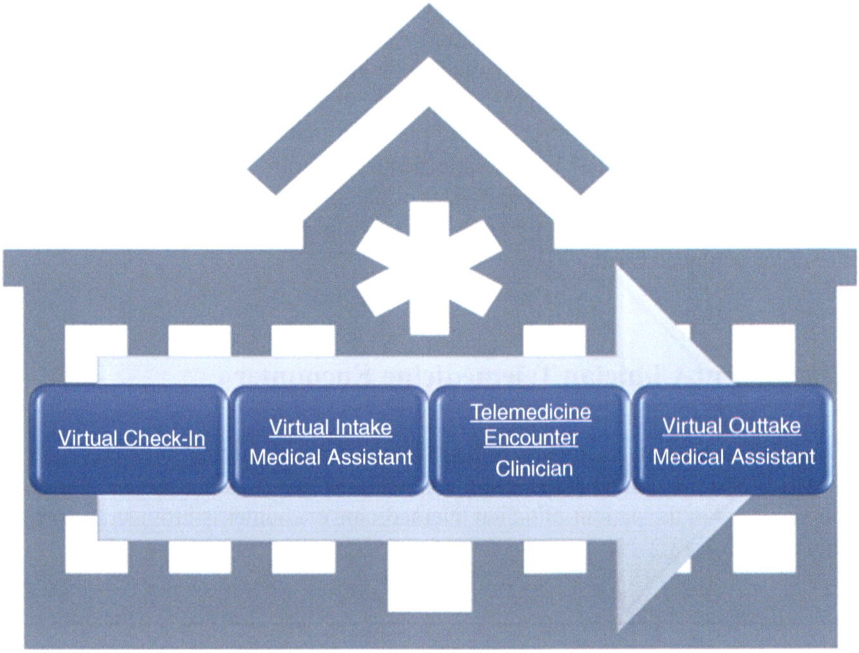

Fig. 13.1 The virtual medical home

If a patient cannot be reached, clinics must have a protocol in place to arrange a follow-up with the patient. It is important to clarify the reason for the no-show; that is, was there a patient scheduling issue, were there technological difficulties, or is the patient acutely ill? Throughout this process, clinical staff can assess a patient's technologic competency and determine if they are appropriate for future virtual visits.

Virtual Intake and Rooming: During the virtual intake, and rooming process, a medical assistant or nurse can connect with the patient to obtain information that will help improve the efficiency of the encounter. In some offices, this process is accomplished within the virtual check-in, and in others, it is a separate process by a different staff member. A medical assistant can ask the patient if there are any updates to their medication list, conduct disease-specific or age-appropriate screenings, and request and document historic or current vital signs obtained with home equipment. Patients with chronic conditions like hypertension and diabetes, in particular, should be asked during the intake to have home blood pressure measurements and blood sugar records available during the visit. In some virtual platforms, a patient can complete a majority of these tasks independently, without initial contact from a medical assistant.

Telemedicine Encounter: Guidelines and considerations for conducting a telemedicine encounter are detailed in Section "The Patient-Clinician Telemedicine Encounter".

Virtual Outtake: Comprehensive virtual outtake of a telemedicine encounter is essential to ensure that a patient understands when and how to follow up on their individual plan. The same medical assistant who facilitated virtual intake can also manage outtake procedures, including sharing a digital summary of the encounter, sent through either patient portal, e-mail, or physical mail. Patients should also be supported to schedule necessary follow-up appointments, labs, imaging, and referrals. Some patient portals provide self-scheduling features, allowing the patient to directly schedule recommended consultations as long as the order is placed for it.

The Patient-Clinician Telemedicine Encounter

The patient-clinician interaction in a synchronous telemedicine encounter includes many of the same principles as an in-person encounter. A framework to summarize the key steps in the patient-clinician telemedicine encounter is provided below as a checklist (Fig. 13.2).

Prepare for Visit

- Determine if appropriate for telemedicine
- Ensure private, quiet space
- Optimize accessibility
- Troubleshoot technology

Conduct Visit

- Set agenda together
- Review available data
- Confirm medications
- Conduct focused physical exam

Conclude Visit

- Confirm follow-up plan with teach back
- Document visit
- Clarify return precautions

Fig. 13.2 The patient-clinician telemedicine checklist

Preparing for the Visit

Prior to starting a virtual visit, pre-charting should be performed with a focus on the appropriateness of the visit for telemedicine. In situations when a patient's condition is appropriate for virtual care, telemedicine visits have been shown to be as effective or more effective than in-person visits. For example, telemedicine visits have been associated with improvements in medicine reconciliation and medication adherence after hospitalization [7], decreased hospital readmissions [8], and control of hypertension equivalent to that achieved through in-person visits [9]. Telemedicine has also been shown to allow clinicians to effectively screen and treat patients with symptoms of COVID-19, with the added benefit of decreasing visits to emergency departments [10].

Once pre-charting is completed and prior to starting the telemedicine visit, clinicians should ensure that they are in a quiet and private environment, free of ambient noise, with a closed door. The room should be well lit with the clinician being clearly visible and not backlit. The backdrop for the telemedicine session should be medically appropriate and without distractions. A sign on the door or other notice should be placed alerting others that the clinician or staff member is in a telemedicine session and therefore unavailable.

Planning for telemedicine encounters also requires careful consideration of potential obstacles to virtual connection. In studies of telemedicine accessibility, common reasons for patients to decline telemedicine services included self-perceptions of lacking necessary skills to use the internet or a computer, and those most likely to decline telemedicine care were patients of older age and lower income levels [11]. Additionally, while telemedicine visits are seen as acceptable when they increase convenience or decrease cost, telemedicine may be inappropriate if privacy cannot be guaranteed, or if there are limitations to conducting an appropriate physical exam [12]. It is thus important to assess if a patient feels confident and comfortable using the technology required for a telemedicine visit, whether they have adequate privacy, and what type of symptoms need to be evaluated.

Considering these preparation factors, it can be helpful to script a standard telemedicine patient welcome and clinician introduction for use once a patient has been virtually "roomed" by clinical staff. After entering the virtual room, we recommend clinicians obtain consent and introduce themselves; an example script is provided below (see Fig. 13.3). A standardized opening allows clinicians to ensure that the patient is prepared for and consenting to a telemedicine visit. As with an in-person visit, all accompanying persons (family, friends, aides) should be identified after the introduction, and the patient should provide permission that they are present during the visit.

Finally, preparation for a telemedicine encounter requires developing fluency with the clinic's telemedicine platform. It is helpful if all clinicians have a baseline of troubleshooting knowledge, as well as readily available contact information to obtain technological support from trained colleagues.

"Hi, I am Doctor/NP/PA/ Resident Physician/ Student Doctor ____, and I work at ____. Before we start, can you please verify your name and date of birth as well as where you are located? This is a billable telemedicine encounter, provided via a secured, confidential, real-time 2-way video connection. It will not be recorded. There are risks associated with any communication technology but we have taken all reasonable precautions to secure and protect this exchange. Do you give your permission and consent to proceed? If our connection is lost, I will attempt to contact you via the number you have provided which I have listed as ______. Do you have any questions before we begin the visit?"

Fig. 13.3 Sample clinician introduction script

Conducting the visit: Conducting an effective telemedicine visit begins with setting a visit agenda in collaboration with the patient. It is important to set expectations regarding the type of care that is possible to deliver during a telemedicine encounter, and best practices suggest that shared decision-making can easily be incorporated into a telemedicine visit workflow [13].

Data collection during a telemedicine encounter may be augmented by access to the patient's home environment. Being virtually in a patient's home ensures access to already recorded data and provides an opportunity for the patient to show how they use diagnostic devices (i.e., blood pressure cuff) and medical treatments that, if misused, could provide explanations for the patient's condition (i.e., improper asthma inhaler technique). Other diagnostic data can be collected as easily during telemedicine visits as during in-person visits. For example, PHQ/GAD surveys, cognitive assessment questionnaires, and symptom scoring systems for COPD or asthma can be conducted during patient intake, and results reviewed by the clinician during the encounter.

To support the telemedicine encounter, additional technologies, such as mobile health platforms, can be incorporated in to improve data collection for chronic disease management. Mobile phone-based applications have been found to assist in both monitoring and management of conditions like atrial fibrillation and heart failure [14]. Self-monitoring of blood pressure with personal devices is associated with lower systolic blood pressure [15–17]. Additionally, patient self-reporting, via mobile phone applications, has been found to improve patient-clinician interactions and to support patients in better understanding their condition (i.e., hypertension) and how their daily behaviors affect health outcomes [18]. Telemedicine visits can be used to review this information and coach patients on how to effectively interpret and act on data collected by these monitoring technologies.

Medication reconciliation is an essential component of high-quality care and avoidance of medical errors. The nature of a telemedicine visit's broadcast into a patient's home uniquely allows the clinician to verify possession of correct medications and identify any discrepancies: finding medications that are unnecessary or not indicated, or medications a patient is meant to be taking but does not possess. Clinicians can also ask patients to demonstrate how they fill a pill box, ask how they set and manage reminder alarms for medication, and ask about medication storage techniques that may affect the likelihood of adherence.

A focused physical exam can be completed during a telemedicine encounter and can generate important clinical information to assist with diagnosis and disease management. While some virtual exam elements translate more effectively to decision-making over a video connection (i.e., visual dermatologic assessments or conversation-based psychiatric evaluations [19]), there are other validated virtual physical examination components that can generate actionable findings [20, 21]. For example, in one study evaluating how to assess acute abdominal pain over telemedicine, patients were able to self-palpate their abdomen with a smartphone (with native accelerometer that calibrated with physician's remote guidance); this showed 95% sensitivity and specificity in matching a physician's abdominal palpation [22]. Another study found high-to-complete concordance between telemedicine (remote auscultation) and in-person pulmonologist consultations regarding pulmonary exam findings and diagnostic suspicions [23]. Additional examples of effective exam maneuvers in telehealth have been studied and are summarized in Table 13.1.

Table 13.1 Virtual exam maneuvers

Organ system	Standard visual-based exam maneuvers	Exam augmented by peripheral devices
Constitutional	• General appearance through observation	• Blood pressure, pulse rate, temperature, pulse oximetry, respiration rate, and weight measured by common home devices, smartphone applications, or wearable technologies
Ophthalmologic [25]	• Assess extraocular movements, pupillary response, conjunctival pallor, scleral icterus	• Digital retinal imaging with remote specialist review and consultation [26]. New technology allows for images to be captured with a smartphone, but images are obtained by a trained healthcare worker in a clinical setting and not at home by the patient [27] • Use of online Snellen chart with assistance in the home to test visual acuity and fields
Ear, nose, mouth, neck [28]	• Assess hearing • Observe auricle, facial motor movements, and thyromegaly/goiter	• A trained healthcare worker can use office-based assistive devices with cameras to accurately inspect the nares, turbinates, and oral cavity, and then transmit images to a specialist for review, but cannot be done at home by a patient

(continued)

Table 13.1 (continued)

Organ system	Standard visual-based exam maneuvers	Exam augmented by peripheral devices
Cardiovascular [29, 30]	• Assess presence and rhythm of distal pulses, with participation from patient • Observe lower extremity edema • Virtual assessment of jugular venous distention is challenging, but sometime possible	• Remote cardiac, respiratory, and abdominal auscultation can be conducted with an electronic stethoscope if the patient is in location with access (i.e., in a care facility with trained personnel)
Respiratory [31, 32]	• Observe respiratory distress, accessory muscle use, chest expansion symmetry, and lower extremity edema • Observe dyspnea on exertion by monitoring patient as they walk briskly • Listen for wheezing or cough (ask patient to inhale and exhale deeply)	
Gastrointestinal	• Assess abdominal pain severity, presence of guarding. Observe abdominal distension, hernia, or masses. • Visual assessment of ascites is challenging, remotely.	
Genitourinary	• Assess costovertebral angle tenderness with assistance from another participant in the home • Before considering a remote visual inspection of the GU area, it is essential to obtain patient consent, involve a virtual clinic chaperone, and ensure patient privacy in their physical location and the clinician's	
Musculoskeletal [33–36]	• Assess passive and active range of motion with joint-specific maneuvers, and inspect swelling or deformities • Assess strength, joint warmth with assistance from a patient or another participant	
Dermatologic [37]	• Inspect skin for discoloration, rashes, and swelling	
Neurological [38]	• Assess mental status, gait, cranial nerves (pupils, eye movement, facial strength, dysarthria, neck flexion, tongue movement), motor exam including involuntary movements (asterixis, tremors), coordination, and gait	

Table 13.1 (continued)

Organ system	Standard visual-based exam maneuvers	Exam augmented by peripheral devices
Psychiatric [39, 40]	• Observe mental status, pace of speech, linearity of thought process, affect, mood lability, patients can complete PHQ-9/GAD-7	
Hematologic, immunologic	• Observe significant lymphadenopathy, ecchymoses, and petechiae • Unreliable concordance has been noted between in-person and telemedicine lymph node exam [41]	

The provision of care can also be equally or more effective in the virtual environment. A systematic review of tele-video versus in-person care for depression found that patients receiving telepsychiatry found relief from depressive symptoms equal to or superior to that of in-person care [24].

Concluding the visit: At the conclusion of the patient's telemedicine visit, patients may receive an electronic summary but will not be provided a physical copy of follow-up instructions. For this reason, it is vital to use teach-back strategies to confirm a patient's understanding of the plan going forward. It is also essential to confirm that the patient has documentation of medication changes, ideally through the electronic medical record (EMR) portal. Utilizing the patient portal in this way is advantageous as it also allows clinicians to share electronic resources and education material.

Documentation

Documentation for telemedicine visits is similar to that for in-person visits; however, it should include several additional components [42–45]:

1. Consent statement (written or verbal).
2. Type of visit (audiovisual vs. audio only).
3. Length of visit.
4. Patient and clinician location.
5. Identification of clinician, patient, and other parties involved in the visit.

The list of documentation requirements has evolved rapidly during the expansion of telemedicine during the COVID-19 pandemic. As a result, regulations may change, and new best practice guidelines are likely to emerge over time. We recommend clinic leadership keep this in mind, monitoring for potential changes and communicating regular updates to clinicians.

"This visit was completed via secure, real time two-way connection [audio-visual/ audio-only] with the patient. The patient provided [oral/ written] consent to engaging in a telemedicine exam and encounter. I have certified the location and identity of the patient to the best extent possible.

Face-to-face time during this encounter:
Non-face-to-face time for this encounter: (time preparing to visit, reviewing separately obtained history, ordering medications, tests or procedures, referring and communicating with other healthcare professionals, documenting clinical information, care coordination, and communication of results with patient)
Total time:

My location (distant site):
Patient location (originating site):

Optional: This encounter was completed [with/without] technical interruptions that could impact my provision of care. [If so, elaborate on impact]"

Fig. 13.4 Sample telemedicine visit documentation

In order to ensure compliance and ease documentation, we recommend a standardized telemedicine note template. Figure 13.4 provides sample documentation to support the telemedicine visit note.

Optimizing the Telemedicine Workflow for Accessibility and Equity

While telemedicine offers an opportunity to strengthen patient access to healthcare, and thus improve equity, the telemedicine workflow must be designed intentionally to consider patient demographic and psychosocial factors in order to avoid diminishing equitable care. Patients who opt into telemedicine care are more likely to have higher formal educational attainment, be employed, and have access to technology devices [46]. Patients with low formal education, lower technology literacy, and lower general health literacy face barriers that impair the adoption of telemedicine [47]. Older adults and low-income adults in the USA are less likely to own a smartphone, and adults with lower educational attainment are less likely to have home broadband [48]. It is thus possible that older patients and those with socioeconomic and educational disadvantages could be unintentionally excluded from the benefits of telemedicine care, leading to widened gaps in existing health inequities.

The Association of American Medical Colleges' recent report on *Competencies in Telehealth and Virtual Care* highlights the need for clinicians to ensure access to and equity of care provided via telemedicine [49]. Specifically, the report establishes the need for recognition and mitigation of biases during telemedicine visits and appropriate accommodation of each patient's specific needs and circumstances. The concept of "digital determinants of health" (i.e., access to digital resources, digital health literacy) and core digital health equity principles (i.e., measuring and seeking to improve digital access and involvement of vulnerable groups in the design of digital services) are both key to ensuring equitable telemedicine workflows [50]. Disparities in technology access can also be addressed through referrals to community health workers who can visit patients' homes, or referrals to community organizations that provide internet access and digital health literacy training [51]. Resources provided by CMS and other national health organizations are also available, with targeted materials for patients with disabilities, non-English-speaking patients, and rural populations.

Webside Manner and Communication Best Practices

Effective communication strategies in telemedicine are essential to provide high-quality care to all patients. The study of clinicians' "webside manner" has produced a set of communications best practices in telemedicine, which mirror interpersonal competencies essential for care in the in-person setting, including rapport-building, active listening, appropriate response to emotional cues, clear information sharing, and shared decision-making [52, 53]. Patient satisfaction with telemedicine care has been shown in a randomized trial to match and even exceed that of in-person visits when physicians are focused and attentive [54]. While this is possible in an ideal setting, patient concerns persist that clinicians offering telemedicine care are less attentive, less capable of establishing a provider-patient relationship, or unaware that a patient needs to ask a question [55]. Studies of the communication style of physicians during in-person and telemedicine visits validate these concerns; some suggest that clinicians can be more prone to dominating conversations and controlling dialogue while providing care virtually [56]. A systematic review further identified the need for improved interpersonal skills during telemedicine visits [57]. Engaging in patient-centered conversation and exploring patient perspectives and concerns about telemedicine visits can optimize the workflow to benefit all patients, especially for vulnerable populations more prone to being affected by potential inequities.

Conclusion

The effective integration of telemedicine into a clinic workflow in an academic medical practice requires a well-trained team of staff and clinicians who understand their specific roles and responsibilities within the patient encounter. The structure of a virtual encounter should mirror that of an in-person encounter and take a strong patient-centered approach. Patient satisfaction with telemedicine care has the potential to match and even exceed that of in-person visits when physicians are focused and attentive, but the real-world application of telemedicine often falls short of this ideal. With a thoughtful and intentional approach—including increased awareness of privacy and accessibility concerns, modifications to the routine physical exam, and attentiveness to patient comfort with the digital medium—telemedicine offers the potential to provide high-quality care comparable to that of in-person care. Finally, clinicians should be trained to provide high-quality care through a lens of health equity, with particular attention to patients from vulnerable populations, to ensure that workflows are inclusive and responsive to patient needs and circumstances.

References

1. Tuckson RV, Edmunds M, Hodgkins ML. Telehealth. N Engl J Med. 2017;377:1585–92. https://doi.org/10.1056/NEJMsr1503323.
2. Cowan KE, McKean AJ, Gentry MT, Hilty DM. Barriers to use of Telepsychiatry: clinicians as gatekeepers. Mayo Clin Proc. 2019;94(12):2510–23. https://doi.org/10.1016/j.mayocp.2019.04.018.
3. Ha E, Zwicky K, Yu G, Schechtman A. Developing a telemedicine curriculum for a family medicine residency. PRiMER. 2020;4:21. https://doi.org/10.22454/PRiMER.2020.126466.
4. AMA Telehealth Implementation Playbook. [Internet] The American Medical Association. [cited 30, March 2022]. https://www.ama-assn.org/system/files/2020-04/ama-telehealth-implementation-playbook.pdf
5. Planning your Telehealth Workflow. [Internet] HHS. [cited 30, March 2022]. https://telehealth.hhs.gov/providers/planning-your-telehealth-workflow/
6. National TRC Webinar—Mapping and Designing Telehealth Clinic Workflows. [Internet] TRC. [cited 30, March 2022]. https://www.youtube.com/watch?v=ZfcEdT5ZRD0
7. Noel K, Messina C, Hou W, Schoenfeld E, Kelly G. Tele-transitions of care (TTOC): a 12-month, randomized controlled trial evaluating the use of Telehealth to achieve triple aim objectives. BMC Fam Pract. 2020;21(1):27. https://doi.org/10.1186/s12875-020-1094-5.
8. O'Connor M, Asdornwised U, Dempsey ML, Huffenberger A, Jost S, Flynn D, Norris A. Using Telehealth to reduce all-cause 30-day hospital readmissions among heart failure patients receiving skilled home health services. Appl Clin Inform. 2016;7(2):238–47. https://doi.org/10.4338/ACI-2015-11-SOA-0157.
9. Levine DM, Dixon RF, Linder JA. Association of structured virtual visits for hypertension follow-up in primary care with blood pressure control and use of clinical services. J Gen Intern Med. 2018;33(11):1862–7. https://doi.org/10.1007/s11606-018-4375-0.
10. Shah M, Patel K, Popa D, et al. Use of telemedicine to expedite and expand care during COVID-19. West J Emerg Med. 2021;22(5):1028–31. Published 2021 Aug 19. https://doi.org/10.5811/westjem.2021.4.51317.
11. Foster A, Horspool KA, Edwards L, Thomas CL, Salisbury C, Montgomery AA, et al. Who does not participate in telehealth trials and why? A cross-sectional survey. Trials. 2015;16:258. https://doi.org/10.1186/s13063-015-0773-3.
12. Powell RE, Henstenburg JM, Cooper G, Hollander JE, Rising KL. Patient perceptions of telehealth primary care video visits. Ann Fam Med. 2017;15(3):225–9. https://doi.org/10.1370/afm.2095.
13. Griffith M, Siminerio L, Payne T, Krall J. A shared decision-making approach to telemedicine: engaging rural patients in glycemic management. JCM. 2016;5:103.
14. MacKinnon GE, Brittain EL. Mobile health technologies in cardiopulmonary disease. Chest. 2020;157:654–64.

15. McManus RJ, Mant J, Haque MS, et al. Effect of self-monitoring and medication self-titration on systolic blood pressure in hypertensive patients at high risk of cardiovascular disease: the TASMIN-SR randomized clinical trial. JAMA. 2014;312:799.
16. McManus RJ, Mant J, Franssen M, et al. Efficacy of self-monitored blood pressure, with or without telemonitoring, for titration of antihypertensive medication (TASMINH4): an unmasked randomized controlled trial. Lancet. 2018;391:949–59.
17. Sheppard JP, Tucker KL, Davison WJ, et al. Self-monitoring of blood pressure in patients with hypertension-related multi-morbidity: systematic review and individual patient data meta-analysis. Am J Hypertens. 2020;33:243–51.
18. Bengtsson U, Kjellgren K, Hallberg I, Lundin M, Mäkitalo Å. Patient contributions during primary care consultations for hypertension after self-reporting via a mobile phone self-management support system. Scand J Prim Health Care. 2018;36:70–9.
19. Hersh W, Helfand M, Wallace J, Kraemer D, Patterson P, Shapiro S, Greenlick M. A systematic review of the efficacy of telemedicine for making diagnostic and management decisions. J Telemed Telecare. 2002;8:197–209.
20. Ansary AM, Martinez JN, Scott JD. The virtual physical exam in the 21st century. J Telemed Telecare. 2021;27:382–92.
21. Benziger CP, Huffman MD, Sweis RN, Stone NJ. The Telehealth ten: a guide for a patient-assisted virtual physical examination. Am J Med. 2021;134:48–51.
22. Myers DR, Weiss A, Rollins MR, Lam WA. Towards remote assessment and screening of acute abdominal pain using only a smartphone with native accelerometers. Sci Rep. 2017;7:12,750.
23. Pacht ER, Turner JW, Gailiun M, Violi LAD, Ralston D, Mekhjian HS, John RCSt (1998) Effectiveness of telemedicine in the outpatient pulmonary clinic. Telemed J 4:287–292.
24. Guaiana G, Mastrangelo J, Hendrikx S, Barbui C. A systematic review of the use of Telepsychiatry in depression. Community Ment Health J. 2021;57:93–100.
25. The Ocular Telehealth SIG. Telehealth resources for eye care during COVID-19 [Internet]. Arlington, VA: American Telemedicine Association; 2020. [cited 2022 Mar 30]. 7 p. https://www.americantelemed.org/resources/telehealth-resources-for-eye-care-during-covid-19/
26. Cavallerano AA, Cavallerano JD, Katalinic P, Blake B, Rynne M, Conlin PR, Hock K, Tolson AM, Aiello LP, Aiello LM. A telemedicine program for diabetic retinopathy in a veterans affairs medical center—the Joslin vision network eye health care model. Am J Ophthalmol. 2005;139:597–604.
27. Tan CH, Kyaw BM, Smith H, Tan CS, Tudor Car L. Use of smartphones to detect diabetic retinopathy: scoping review and meta-analysis of diagnostic test accuracy studies. J Med Internet Res. 2020;22:e16658.
28. Huntley C, Boon M, Ishman S, Capasso R, Crawford J, D'Agostino MA, Hoff P. Virtual otolaryngologic management of sleep apnea patients: lessons learned from COVID -19 pandemic. Laryngosc Investig Otolaryngol. 2021;6:564–9.
29. Oseran AS, Afari ME, Barrett CD, Lewis GD, Thomas SS. Beyond the stethoscope: managing ambulatory heart failure during the COVID-19 pandemic. ESC Heart Failure. 2021;8:999–1006.
30. Mishra K, Edwards B. Cardiac outpatient Care in a Digital age: remote cardiology clinic visits in the era of COVID-19. Curr Cardiol Rep. 2022;24:1–6.
31. Raza T, Joshi M, Schapira R, Agha Z. Pulmonary telemedicine—a model to access the subspecialist services in underserved rural areas. Int J Med Inform. 2009;78:53–9.
32. Heravian A, Fortenko A, Olsen E, Greenwald P, Chang BP, Gutierrez CM, Kessler D. Virtual powers of observation: a telemedicine approach for the suspected COVID-19 patient. J Emerg Manag. 2021;18:45–8.
33. Laskowski ER, Johnson SE, Shelerud RA, Lee JA, Rabatin AE, Driscoll SW, Moore BJ, Wainberg MC, Terzic CM. The telemedicine musculoskeletal examination. Mayo Clin Proc. 2020;95:1715–31.
34. Pinnamaneni S, Lamplot JD, Rodeo SA, Swensen-Buza S, Lawton CD, Dines JS, Young WK, Taylor SA. The virtual shoulder physical exam. HSS J. 2021;17:59–64.

35. Wright-Chisem J, Trehan S. The hand and wrist examination for video Telehealth encounters. HSS J. 2021;17:70–4.
36. Lamplot JD, Pinnamaneni S, Swensen-Buza S, Lawton CD, Dines JS, Nawabi DH, Young W, Rodeo SA, Taylor SA. The virtual shoulder and knee physical examination. Orthop J Sports Med. 2020;8:232596712096286.
37. Bashshur RL, Shannon GW, Tejasvi T, Kvedar JC, Gates M. The empirical foundations of Teledermatology: a review of the research evidence. Telemed e-Health. 2015;21:953–79.
38. Al Hussona M, Maher M, Chan D, Micieli JA, Jain JD, Khosravani H, Izenberg A, Kassardjian CD, Mitchell SB. The virtual neurologic exam: instructional videos and guidance for the COVID-19 era. Can J Neurol Sci. 2020;47:598–603.
39. Chipps J, Brysiewicz P, Mars M. Effectiveness and feasibility of telepsychiatry in resource constrained environments? A systematic review of the evidence. Afr J Psych. 2012; https://doi.org/10.4314/ajpsy.v15i4.30.
40. O'Keefe M, White K, Jennings JC. Asynchronous telepsychiatry: a systematic review. J Telemed Telecare. 2021;27:137–45.
41. Akhtar M, Van Heukelom PG, Ahmed A, Tranter RD, White E, Shekem N, Walz D, Fairfield C, Vakkalanka JP, Mohr NM. Telemedicine physical examination utilizing a consumer device demonstrates poor concordance with in-person physical examination in emergency department patients with sore throat: a prospective blinded study. Telemedicine and e-Health. 2018;24:790–6.
42. Telehealth Department of Health and Human Services (HHS). Best practice guides [Internet]. Rockville, MD: Health Resources and Service Administration [updated 2022 March 25; cited 2022 July 20]. http://telehealth.hhs.gov/providers/best-practice-guides/
43. Bowen R, Warner D. Building new policies and procedure to incorporate telehealth [internet]. J AHIMA; 2021 [cited 2022 Jul 20]. https://journal.ahima.org/page/building-new-policies-and-procedures-to-incorporate-telehealth
44. Smith WR, Atala AJ, Terlecki RP, Kelly EE, Matthews CA. Implementation guide for rapid integration of an outpatient telemedicine program during the COVID-19 pandemic. J Am Coll Surg. 2020;231:216–222e2.
45. Houser SH, Flite CA, Foster SL, Hunt TJ, Morey A, Palmer MN, Peterson J, Pope RD, Sorensen L. Building best practices for Telehealth record documentation in the COVID-19 pandemic. Perspect Health Inf Manag. 2022;19:1e.
46. Liaw WR, Jetty A, Coffman M, Petterson S, Moore MA, Sridhar G, Gordon AS, Stephenson JJ, Adamson W, Bazemore AW. Disconnected: a survey of users and nonusers of telehealth and their use of primary care. J Am Med Inform Assoc. 2019;26:420–8.
47. Alvarado MM, Kum H-C, Gonzalez Coronado K, Foster MJ, Ortega P, Lawley MA. Barriers to remote health interventions for type 2 diabetes: a systematic review and proposed classification scheme. J Med Internet Res. 2017;19:e28.
48. Perrin A. Mobile technology and home broadband 2021. [Internet]. Washington, DC: Pew Research Center; 2022. [cited 2022 Mar 30]. 19 p. https://www.pewresearch.org/internet/2021/06/03/mobile-technology-and-home-broadband-2021/
49. AAMC. New and emerging areas in medicine series: telehealth competencies across the learning continuum [Internet]. Washington, DC: AAMC; 2021 [cited 2022 Mar 30]. 27 p. https://store.aamc.org/downloadable/download/sample/sample_id/412/
50. Crawford A, Serhal E. Digital health equity and COVID-19: the innovation curve cannot reinforce the social gradient of health. J Med Internet Res. 2020;22:e19361.
51. Sheon AR, Bolen SD, Callahan B, Shick S, Perzynski AT. Addressing disparities in diabetes management through novel approaches to encourage technology adoption and use. JMIR Diabetes. 2017;2:e16.
52. Elliott T, Matsui EC, Cahill A, Smith L, Leibner L. Conducting a professional telemedicine visit using high-quality Webside manner. Curr Allergy Asthma Rep. 2022;22:7–12.
53. Chua IS, Jackson V, Kamdar M. Webside manner during the COVID-19 pandemic: maintaining human connection during virtual visits. J Palliat Med. 2020;23:1507–9.

54. Agha Z, Schapira RM, Laud PW, McNutt G, Roter DL. Patient satisfaction with physician–patient communication during telemedicine. Telemed e-Health. 2009;15:830–9.
55. Gordon HS, Solanki P, Bokhour BG, Gopal RK. "I'm not feeling like I'm part of the conversation" patients' perspectives on communicating in clinical video Telehealth visits. J Gen Intern Med. 2020;35:1751–8.
56. Agha Z, Roter DL, Schapira RM. An evaluation of patient-physician communication style during telemedicine consultations. J Med Internet Res. 2009;11:e36.
57. Henry BW, Block DE, Ciesla JR, McGowan BA, Vozenilek JA. Clinician behaviors in telehealth care delivery: a systematic review. Adv in Health Sci Educ. 2017;22:869–88.

Chapter 14
Telemedicine in Medical Education

Dianne L. Goede and Sarai Ambert-Pompey

Introduction

Telemedicine adoption in clinical practice rapidly accelerated through 2020, requiring both faculty and learners to simultaneously navigate a new care delivery modality. In the setting of this rapid expansion, the Association of American Medical Colleges (AAMC) established foundational competencies in telemedicine for recent medical school graduates, residency graduates, and practicing physicians. The academic medical practice provides learners both the clinical experience and faculty supervision to develop the necessary telemedicine skills. We aim to outline the role of the academic medical practice in the support of telemedicine education for medical students and residents.

This chapter addresses important considerations for clinical practices, including competency-based telehealth education, recommendations for tailored experiences at both undergraduate medical education (UME) and graduate medical education (GME) levels, faculty development, and scheduling logistics.

Outline

- Competency-based medical education
  - AAMC telehealth competencies
  - ACGME telehealth competencies

D. L. Goede (✉)
University of Florida, College of Medicine, Gainesville, FL, USA
e-mail: Dianne.roberts@medicine.ufl.edu

S. Ambert-Pompey
University of Washington, Seattle, WA, USA

Boise VA, Boise, ID, USA
e-mail: Sarai.Ambert-Pompey@va.gov

L. B. Lu et al. (eds.), *Leading an Academic Medical Practice*,
https://doi.org/10.1007/978-3-031-40273-9_14

- ACGME supervision requirements
- Teaching of telemedicine
- Scheduling spectrum of telemedicine clinics
- Equitable and inclusive telemedicine
- Special consideration: trauma informed care telehealth strategies
- Conclusion

Competency-Based Medical Education

The explosive use of telemedicine through recent years heightened the need for comprehensive telehealth competencies for all physicians. In response to evolving clinical needs and available technologies, both the AAMC and the ACGME have adopted telehealth competencies to ensure that learners achieve desired training outcomes [1, 2].

AAMC Telehealth Competencies

The Association of American Medical Colleges (AAMC) Telehealth Competencies consist of six domains, each of which includes three tiers directed at different stages in physician development (student, resident, faculty). The six domains include goals around patient safety, access and equity, communication, data management, technology, and ethical practices in telehealth (Table 14.1).

The six domains are each further divided into three tiers directed at different stages in student, resident, and faculty development. Tier one consists of physicians entering residency training or recent medical school graduates. Tier two includes recent residency graduates entering medical practice, and tier three consists of experienced faculty physicians [2]. As an example, Table 14.2 depicts the specific competencies for each tier of domain III.

These competences provide clear targets and a useful framework for learners to set goals toward advancement of their skills in telehealth.

Table 14.1 AAMC telehealth competencies

AAMC telehealth competency six domains
Domain I: Patient safety and appropriate use of telehealth Clinicians will understand when and why to use telehealth and how to assess patient readiness, patient safety, practice readiness, and end-user readiness. **Domain II: Access and equity in telehealth** To promote equitable access to care, clinicians will understand telehealth delivery that addresses and mitigates cultural biases as well as physician bias for or against telehealth and that accounts for physical and mental disabilities and non-health-related individual and community needs and limitations.
Domain III: Communication via telehealth Clinicians will effectively communicate with patients, families, caregivers, and health care team members using telehealth modalities. They will also integrate both the transmission and receipt of information with the goal of effective knowledge transfer, professionalism, and understanding within a therapeutic relationship.
Domain IV: Data collection and assessment via telehealth Clinicians will obtain and manage clinical information via telehealth to ensure appropriate high-quality care. **Domain V: Technology for telehealth** Clinicians will have basic knowledge of technology needed for the delivery of high-quality telehealth services.
Domain VI: Ethical practices and legal requirements for telehealth Clinicians will understand the federal, state, and local facility practice requirements to meet the minimal standards to deliver health care via telehealth. Clinicians will maintain patient privacy while minimizing risk to the clinician and patient during telehealth encounters, putting the patient's interest first, and preserving or enhancing the doctor-patient relationship.

©The Association of American Medical Colleges (AAMC) Adapted from 2021 Telehealth Competencies Across the Learning Continuum [2]

ACGME Telehealth Competencies

Similar to the AAMC, the Accreditation Council for Graduate Medical Education (ACGME) expects residents to achieve competency in six domains spanning patient care and procedural skills [3]. The domains are broken into five levels of competency to help enable the learner and program to determine trajectories of professional development in narrative terms [3]. Digital health is categorized as a sub-competency within the core patient care competency and is detailed in Fig. 14.1 [4].

Reviewing the sub-competency milestones focused on digital health will help identify the resident's trajectory of professional development in this area and focus on areas for improvement.

Table 14.2 Domain III: Communication via telehealth

Entering residency (recent medical school graduate)	Entering practice (recent residency graduate) *All prior competencies +*	Experienced faculty physician (3–5 years post-residency) *All prior competencies +*
1a. Develops an effective rapport with patients via real or simulated video visits, attending to eye contact, tone, body language, and nonverbal cues	1b. Develops an effective rapport with patients via video visits, attending to eye contact, tone, body language, and nonverbal cues	1c. Role models and teaches effective rapport-building with patients via video visits, attending to eye contact, tone, body language, and nonverbal cues
2a. Assesses the environment during real or simulated video visits, such as attending to disruptions related to privacy, lighting, sound, and attire	2b. Establishes therapeutic relationships and environments during video visits, such as attending to disruption related to privacy, lighting, sound, and attire	2c. Role models effective therapeutic relationships and environments during telehealth encounters
3a. Explains how remote patients' social supports and health care providers can be incorporated into telehealth interactions and the care plan (e.g., asynchronous communication and the storage and forwarding of data)	3b. Determines situations in which patients' social supports and health care providers should be incorporated into telehealth interactions, with the patients' consent, to provide optimal care	3c. Role models and teaches how to incorporate patients' social supports into telehealth interactions, with the patients' consent, to provide optimal care

©The Association of American Medical Colleges (AAMC) Adapted from 2021 Telehealth Competencies Across the Learning Continuum [2]

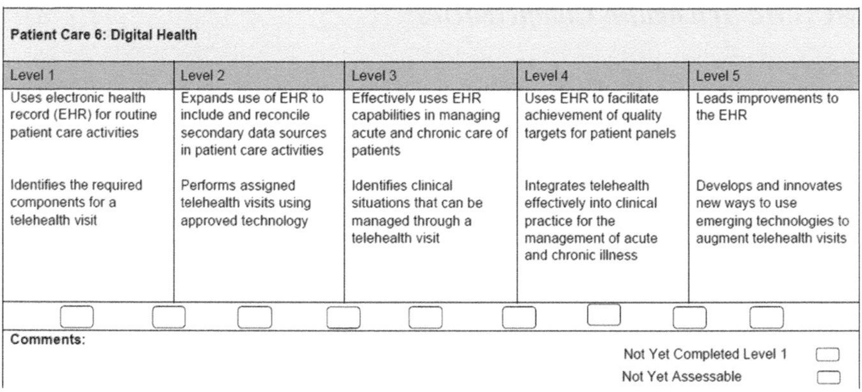

Patient Care 6: Digital Health				
Level 1	Level 2	Level 3	Level 4	Level 5
Uses electronic health record (EHR) for routine patient care activities	Expands use of EHR to include and reconcile secondary data sources in patient care activities	Effectively uses EHR capabilities in managing acute and chronic care of patients	Uses EHR to facilitate achievement of quality targets for patient panels	Leads improvements to the EHR
Identifies the required components for a telehealth visit	Performs assigned telehealth visits using approved technology	Identifies clinical situations that can be managed through a telehealth visit	Integrates telehealth effectively into clinical practice for the management of acute and chronic illness	Develops and innovates new ways to use emerging technologies to augment telehealth visits

Comments:

Not Yet Completed Level 1

Not Yet Assessable

Fig. 14.1 ACGME digital health competency. ©2020 Accreditation Council for Graduate Medical Education (ACGME) [4]

ACGME Supervision Requirements

The ACGME program requirements allow for residents and fellows to participate in the use of telemedicine to care for patients [5]. The provision of telemedicine services still requires faculty supervision - either direct supervision, or in certain circumstances, indirect supervision.

Direct Supervision

Effective July 2021, the ACGME common program requirements allow programs the option of permitting direct supervision through the use of telecommunication technology [6]. Direct supervision allows the supervising physician to either directly supervise the visit in the telehealth room or monitor patient care through appropriate telecommunication technology [6].

Indirect Supervision

The ACGME also allows for indirect supervision of residents and fellows performing telehealth visits in some circumstances. The ACGME states "residents and fellows who are capable of providing this service (telemedicine) with indirect supervision available or immediately available are covered under the indirect supervision requirements" [7]. Residents may be indirectly supervised only after 6 months of training in clinics covered under the primary care exception.

Teaching of Telemedicine

Ensuring Faculty Buy-in

As with any new technology and workflow, ensuring faulty buy-in is critical to successful adoption. The increased reliance on electronic health record (EHR) technology and clinician frustrations associated with EHR use may bias some faculty against emerging telehealth technologies. Acknowledging limitations in the use of telehealth is important when discussing adoption of telehealth into clinical practice with faculty. However, the adoption of telehealth competencies by both the AAMC and the ACGME cements the need for faculty engagement and teaching of telehealth. Ensuring that faculty are comfortable with telemedicine prior to their involvement with learners is a key step to optimizing the learners' clinical experience.

Faculty with significant interest in the field may further seek involvement and contribute to the didactic or simulation portions of these curricula [8]. In addition, faculty need to be prepared to oversee and evaluate the telemedicine experience for UME and GME learners across the developmental competencies and milestones spectrum.

Teaching the Delivery of Telemedicine

Prior to a telemedicine clinic visit, faculty should orient the learner to the telemedicine technology and review the learner's educational goals for the session [9]. During the visit, faculty should ensure that the learner is actively involved in the visit and moving toward independently interviewing and examining the patient as appropriate to their training level. Following the visit, faculty should provide the learner with feedback on their telemedicine clinical skills and the next steps for improvement. Hovaguimian et al. (2021) developed an excellent framework for faculty reference when preparing for telemedicine teaching sessions (Fig. 14.2) [10].

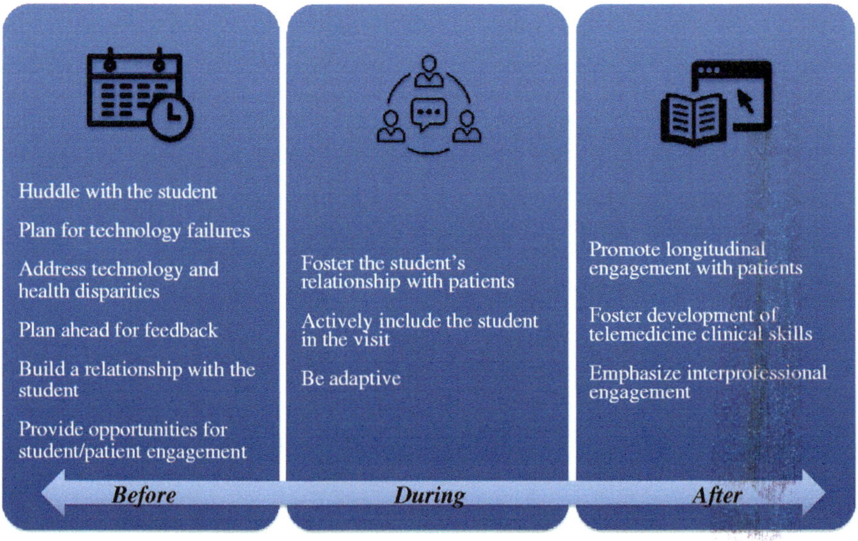

Fig. 14.2 Teaching learners using telemedicine patient visits: before, during, and after the visit. Originally published in Hovaguimian et al. (2021). Twelve tips for clinical teaching with telemedicine visits. Medical Teacher. 2021; 44 (1) 19–25. doi: 10.1080/0142159X.2021.1880558. Taylor &Francis Ltd. www.tandfonline.com [10].

Preparing learners for a telemedicine visit through a framework anchored around the patient helps minimize distractions caused by technology. A useful framework for teaching patient-centered virtual practices to trainees is the "TELEMEDS" model. Based on the review of literature and contributions from key stakeholders, Alkureishi et al. (2021) proposed this framework for faculty educating trainees and students on patient-centered virtual telemedicine practices. Figure 14.3 outlines this framework and serves as a useful visual aid for faculty embarking on teaching patient-centered virtual care [11–15].

T	Test it out first	Prior to the visit, **practice** using your virtual visit platform. Check audio & video. Test mute & screen share. Practice **splitting the screen** to allow you to see your patient & the EHR at the same time.
E	Evaluate your schedule	Identify patients that **should not** have virtual visits. Proactively **anticipate** needs for the visit (outside records, translation services, etc).
L	Layout an agenda	**Contextualize** your visit agenda by reviewing your patient's interval history (last note, labs, etc). Note any outstanding orders or preventative health needs that should be addressed.
E	Establish visit rules	**Introduce** yourself, team members & verify your patient. Determine a technical **back-up** plan. Identify your patient's **goals** for the visit & balance those with your agenda items.
M	Modify your speech	**Vary** tone & inflection. Speak **slowly** to allow for buffering & lag. **Pause** for questions often. Check for understanding.
E	Encourage patient engagement	Look for **opportunities** to educate patients using **screen share** - demonstrate websites, review EHR information. Engage patients in **note writing** when appropriate and jointly create an **after visit summary** to reinforce the plan.
D	Demonstrate positive nonverbal communication	Maintain good **eye** contact. Smile or express concern when appropriate. Signal **active listening** by nodding or shaking your head.
S	Summarize next steps	Be specific about **when & how** to follow up. Encourage **patient portal** use to review their after visit summary & chart updates for reference. Elicit direct patient **feedback**.

© Alkureishi ML, Lenti G, Weyer G, Castaneda J, Choo Z, Oyler J, Lee W. April 2020

Fig. 14.3 TELEMEDS tips to optimize virtual visits. Copyright ©Maria Alcocer Alkureishi, Gena Lenti, Zi-Yi Choo, Jason Castaneda, George Weyer, Julie Oyler, Wei Wei Lee. Originally published in JMIR Medical Education (https://mededu.jmir.org), 29.04.2021

Tailoring the Undergraduate Medical Education Experience

Medical schools are refining and implementing telemedicine curricula for their students, and the academic medical practice serves a key function in the clinical translation of this curricula [16]. Faculty should provide a pre-clinic huddle with the medical student to demonstrate the use of telemedicine technology and discuss their communication methods for the student outside of the virtual exam room. We recommend faculty and medical students jointly review tier 1 of the AAMC Telehealth Competencies and identify educational goals for the telemedicine clinic session. Fostering a connection between the student and patient is especially important given the challenges in creating a humanistic connection in the virtual world. Faculty can give this special attention at the start of a virtual visit to clearly identify the role of the student and explain to the patient what to expect [17].

During the telemedicine visit, faculty can choose to virtually supervise the student at an alternate workstation or join the learner in the same physical space to review the history, confirm physical examination findings, and discuss assessment and plan with the student and patient jointly. If faculty choose to virtually supervise the student for the duration of the telemedicine visit, faculty should turn off their own camera and audio to minimize interruption of the student and patient during the initial interview [9].

Telemedicine also offers a unique opportunity for students to engage in virtual care across different specialties. When possible, faculty should encourage students to participate in subspecialty telemedicine visits for patients whose care they are involved with. This will allow the student to benefit from ongoing experiential learning [17].

Tailoring the Graduate Medical Education Experience

Residents likely will arrive to their residency programs with some prior exposure to telemedicine [11, 18]. Knowing this, faculty can expect to tailor the telemedicine training to the expertise level of the resident using the TELEMEDS framework. As residents move forward through telemedicine clinic experiences, faculty should engage them in active learning through and experiential and reflective process in the framework of Kolb's experiential learning cycle [19]. Constructing a learning environment for residents that offers them legitimate participation and permits them to learn will enhance their telemedicine clinic experience. For telemedicine-specific feedback, faculty should reference ACGME digital health competency milestones (Fig. 14.1) and tier two of the AAMC telehealth competencies [2, 4].

Scheduling Spectrum of Telemedicine Clinics

Incorporating learners into telemedicine clinics adds additional complexity that requires thoughtful planning. The scheduling of telemedicine visits may exist as "***100% virtual visits***" or telemedicine visits may be interwoven in a traditional clinic schedule, which we term as "***hybrid clinics***."

The attending physician is charged with ensuring that the same standard of care can be delivered via telemedicine as an in-person evaluation based upon the chief concern of the patient [20]. Each clinical practice should develop scheduling protocols that streamline appropriate usage of telemedicine based upon the chief concern of the patient. In preparation for telemedicine visits, attending physicians can review learners' schedules and ensure that the type of visit scheduled is appropriate for the chief concern visit.

Hybrid Schedule: Face-to-Face and Virtual Visits

Practices commonly implement a hybrid scheduling model where telemedicine visits are interspersed with traditional face-to-face visits. This hybrid approach is flexible for patient scheduling needs. However, this approach is challenging to the clinical workflow as it divides the attention of faculty and staff between the virtual patients and in-person patients. This can disorient learners and highlights the importance of the pre-clinic huddle.

When resident telemedicine visits utilize the hybrid clinic approach, preceptors' attention is significantly divided. This is especially challenging in resident hybrid clinics that require direct supervision. In these circumstances, a staggered schedule blocking alternating resident appointment times can be considered. This allows faculty adequate time to transfer between telemedicine technology and in-person visits to directly supervise resident care.

100% Virtual Schedule

Practices can also designate specific clinic sessions solely for telemedicine visits. A 100% virtual schedule can improve workflows since residents and staff are not dividing their attention between the virtual environment and the physical clinic environment. Similarly, the preceptor workflow is simplified. Additionally, virtual clinics specifically designated for upper respiratory infection chief concerns may mitigate infectious disease spread to patients and staff.

Equitable and Inclusive Telemedicine

Telemedicine has the potential to both exacerbate and alleviate preexisting healthcare inequities. Disparities of geographical locations of clinics in underserved urban areas and rural areas can theoretically be bridged with telemedicine. However, the penetration of broadband and cellular plan access in the USA is not universal [21]. The challenges posed by restricted access to health care, limited broadband and cellular coverage, digital illiteracy, and generational divide are significant. Yet, these challenges must be separated from faculty and learners' preconceived bias regarding which populations can access telemedicine. Faculty should guide learners to address social determinants of health that pertain to telemedicine access and identify ways to best mitigate barriers.

Special Consideration: Trauma-Informed Care Telehealth Strategies

Telemedicine provides a unique picture of a patient's life, and residents should be aware that having a clinician remotely enter their home may trigger strong emotions for patients, especially those who have experienced past trauma. Trauma is defined by the Substance Abuse and Mental Health Services Administration (SAMHSA) as resulting from "an event, series of events, or set of circumstances that is experienced by an individual as physically or emotionally harmful or life threatening and that has lasting adverse effects on the individual's functioning and mental, physical, social, emotional, or spiritual well-being" [22]. Faculty need to understand how to handle these situations and be available for the learners should issues arise. Trauma-informed care principles, as defined by SAMHSA, can strengthen telemedicine encounters by promoting safe and collaborative exchanges between patients and the health care team including the learner (Table 14.3) [23].

Table 14.3 Trauma-informed telehealth strategies based on SAMHSA principles

Principles	Strategies
Safety	• Verify the patient's location/contact information at the beginning of the encounter. • Ensure that the patient's physical and virtual environments are secure and private, including from other family/household members. • Obtain informed consent for the visit. • Use headphones to ensure patient confidentiality unless you are in a private space. • Proceed according to patient comfort level; obtain consent for examinations, minimize removal of clothing, and proceed with follow-up discussions once the patient is clothed. • During an examination, avoid personalizing language such as "[instruction] for me" or "show me your [body part]." consider instead: "In order to help us treat you, it would be useful for me to examine the arm. Would you mind rolling up the sleeve so that I can see the rash?" • Provide education/information on safety resources that can be accessed virtually (e.g., crisis hot lines).
Trustworthiness and transparency	• Actively listen to the patient's concerns about their health and/or the telehealth environment. • Alert the patient to possible ambient noises. • Sit far enough from the screen that the patient can see your body language, which also helps to ensure the appearance of better eye contact through the camera. • Provide the patient with time to adapt to the telehealth environment. • Provide clear information on changes to scheduling, access, and contact process. • Dress professionally for the visit and avoid busy, unprofessional backdrops.

(continued)

Table 14.3 (continued)

Principles	Strategies
Peer support	• Consider developing and/or referring to telehealth groups (e.g., PTSD, DM support groups). • Provide information on virtual peer support.
Collaboration and mutuality	• Thank the patient for connecting with their medical team using this care modality. • Collaboratively identify and develop an agenda for the visit. • Partner with the patient to attain goals and mitigate treatment challenges.
Empowerment, voice, and choice	• Follow patient preferences regarding the extent of the visit; some may prefer to just talk or test the connection for their first appointment. • Assure the patient that they may choose to end the visit at any point. • Allow the patient to choose the room where the visit takes place. • Emphasize that the topic of discussion can change, even abruptly, when needed.
Cultural, historical, and gender issues	• Use gender-affirming language (including patient's pronouns). • Encourage/praise the patient's willingness to try this care modality. • Consider social determinants of health during the visit (e.g., housing stability, food insecurity, impact of racism). • Be sensitive to the patient's feelings in revealing their personal space during the visit; refrain from comment about their home/living space. • Seek ways to make telehealth accessible to those who lack devices/internet access or need an interpreter.

Abbreviations: *DM* Diabetes mellitus, *PTSD* Post-traumatic stress disorder, *SAMHSA* Substance Abuse and Mental Health Services Administration
Reproduced with permission from Trauma-Informed Telehealth in the COVID 19 Era and Beyond. Gerber et al. (2020) [23]

Conclusion

Telemedicine use has increased exponentially. Competency in telemedicine is now considered an expectation by the AAMC and the ACGME. The leaders of academic medical practices need to support telemedicine clinical experiences for medical students and residents that ensure that they are meeting expected competencies. Clinical experiences that provide learners meaningful participation in telemedicine clinical care ensure active learning. We recommend the following tips to optimize learner's telemedicine clinical experience:

- Provide faculty development both in telemedicine skills and teaching
- Establish scheduling and clinical workflows that minimize disruptions

- Promote a telemedicine-specific preclinic huddle between faculty and learners
- Provide hands-on orientation to clinic-specific telemedicine technology
- Utilize TELEMEDS to optimize virtual visits
- Review AAMC and ACGME competencies to guide education goal setting and provide tailored feedback to learners

References

1. AAMC. Our Work on Competency-Based Medical Education (CBME). https://www.aamc.org/about-us/mission-areas/medical-education/cbme. Accessed 20 Nov 2022.
2. AAMC. Telehealth competencies across the learning continuum. AAMC new and emerging areas in medicine series. Washington, DC: AAMC; 2021.
3. ACGME. The milestones guidebook; 2020.
4. ACGME. Internal Medicine Milestones; 2021. p. 29.
5. ACGME Common Program Requirements Section VI with Background and Intent, VI.A.2.c).(1); 2017.
6. Specialty-Specific Program Requirements: Direct Supervision Using Telecommunication Technology, VI.A.2.B.(1). a (2021).
7. ACGME. ACGME Response to COVID-19: Clarification regarding Telemedicine and ACGME Surveys; 2020.
8. Stovel RG, Gabarin N, Cavalcanti RB, Abrams H. Curricular needs for training telemedicine physicians: a scoping review. Med Teach. 2020;42(11):1234–42. https://doi.org/10.1080/0142159X.2020.1799959.
9. Zickuhr L, Kolfenbach J, Bolster MB. Applying educational theory to optimize trainee education in the ambulatory virtual Care environment. Med. Sci Educ. 2021;31:1715. https://doi.org/10.1007/s40670-021-01365-0.
10. Hovaguimian A, Joshi A, Onorato S, Schwartz AW, Frankl S. Twelve tips for clinical teaching with telemedicine visits. Med Teach 2021:1–7. doi:https://doi.org/10.1080/0142159X.2021.1880558, 44, 19.
11. Alcocer Alkureishi M, Lenti G, Choo ZY, Castaneda J, Weyer G, Oyler J, et al. Teaching telemedicine: the next frontier for medical educators. JMIR Med Educ. 2021;7(2):e29099. https://doi.org/10.2196/29099.
12. Zulman D, Verghese A. Tele PRESENCE 5 by Stanford Medicine; 2020.
13. Zulman DM, Haverfield MC, Shaw JG, Brown-Johnson CG, Schwartz R, Tierney AA, et al. Practices to Foster physician presence and connection with patients in the clinical encounter. JAMA. 2020;323(1):70–81. https://doi.org/10.1001/jama.2019.19003.
14. Ansary AM, Martinez JN, Scott JD. The virtual physical exam in the 21st century. J Telemed Telecare. 2021;27(6):382–92. https://doi.org/10.1177/1357633X19878330.
15. Benziger CP, Huffman MD, Sweis RN, Stone NJ. The telehealth ten: a guide for a patient-assisted virtual physical examination. Am J Med. 2021;134(1):48–51. https://doi.org/10.1016/j.amjmed.2020.06.015.
16. Waseh S, Dicker AP. Telemedicine training in undergraduate medical education: mixed-methods review. JMIR Med Educ. 2019;5(1):e12515. https://doi.org/10.2196/12515.
17. Wamsley M, Cornejo L, Kryzhanovskaya I, Lin BW, Sullivan J, Yoder J, et al. Best practices for integrating medical students into telehealth visits. JMIR Med Educ. 2021;7(2):e27877. https://doi.org/10.2196/27877.
18. Pourmand A, Ghassemi M, Sumon K, Amini SB, Hood C, Sikka N. Lack of telemedicine training in academic medicine: are we preparing the next generation? Telemed J E Health. 2021;27(1):62–7. https://doi.org/10.1089/tmj.2019.0287.

19. Schultz K, McEwen L, Griffiths J. Applying Kolb's learning cycle to competency-based residency education. Acad Med. 2016;91(2):284. https://doi.org/10.1097/01.ACM.0000479943.21563.6f.
20. Care Ct. Telehealth for Providers: What You Need to Know. CMS.gov2021. p. 4.
21. Commission FC. 2020 Broadband Deployment Report; 2020.
22. Initiative SsTaJS. SAMHSA's concept of trauma and guidance for a trauma-informed approach; 2014.
23. Gerber MR, Elisseou S, Sager ZS, Keith JA. Trauma-informed telehealth in the COVID-19 era and beyond. Fed Pract. 2020;37(7):302–8.

Part V
Pain and Substance Use Disorders

Chapter 15
Establishing an Integrative Chronic Pain Management Clinic Within an Academic Medical Practice

Meroë B. Morse, Alicia Carrasco, and Daniel G. Tobin

Introduction

Chronic non-cancer pain (CNCP) is the most common presenting complaint to primary care physicians (PCPs) in the outpatient setting, generates rates of high frustration and low satisfaction by both patients and PCPs, and leads to greater overall healthcare utilization compared to patients without chronic non-cancer pain. Pain is a multifaceted issue influenced by physical, biochemical, neurological, nutritional, and psychosocial components. Historically, the medical model approaches pain management from a *biomedical* perspective, with medications and procedural interventions as the primary therapeutic recommendations. Ongoing research now supports a *biopsychosocial* approach to pain management with integrative, multimodal therapies. The twenty-first-century opioid epidemic and scant research on non-opioid and nonpharmacologic therapies for pain exposed deficiencies in knowledge,

M. B. Morse (✉)
Integrative Medicine Program, Department of Palliative Care, Rehabilitation, & Integrative Medicine, The University of Texas MD Anderson Cancer Center, Houston, TX, USA

Baylor College of Medicine, Houston, TX, USA
e-mail: MBMorse@mdanderson.org

A. Carrasco
University of Washington School of Medicine, Seattle, WA, USA

Boise VA Medical Center, Boise, ID, USA
e-mail: alicia.carrasco@va.gov

D. G. Tobin
Yale University School of Medicine, New Haven, CT, USA

Adult Medicine, New Haven Primary Care Consortium, Cornell Scott Hill Health Center, New Haven, CT, USA
e-mail: daniel.tobin@yale.edu

L. B. Lu et al. (eds.), *Leading an Academic Medical Practice*,
https://doi.org/10.1007/978-3-031-40273-9_15

training, and resources to effectively address CNCP conditions. Medical directors of academic medical practices can narrow this gap through the development of an integrative pain management infrastructure, transform trainee education, and enhance the delivery for patients of a biopsychosocial model of CNCP care. This chapter serves as a road map for the medical director to assess each clinic's needs, enhance clinician expertise, and implement evidence-based integrative pain management programming.

Outline
- Terminology
- Role of a faculty champion
- Chronic pain impacts on an academic medical practice
  - Standardizing education for trainees
  - Patient engagement
- Nonpharmacologic approaches to chronic non-cancer pain
- Lifestyle modification
- Behavioral health interventions/mind-body therapies
- Movement therapies
- Manual therapies
- Topical pharmacologic therapy
- Systemic non-opioid pharmacologic therapy for chronic pain
- Financing and affordability for integrative chronic pain therapies
- Practice level solutions
  - Case reviews
  - Roleplaying
  - Templates
  - Macros
- Treatment options
- Patient resources
- Conclusion

Terminology

Given the expanding landscape of pain neuroscience and evolving therapeutic approaches for pain management, a brief description of terms and care delivery systems commonly used in the biopsychosocial approach to chronic pain management is shown in Table 15.1.

Table 15.1 Glossary of terms for multidisciplinary approaches to chronic pain management

Complementary and alternative medicine (CAM)	Complementary therapy is a nonmainstream approach used *together* with conventional medicine.Alternative therapy is a nonmainstream approach used *in place* of conventional medicine [1].
Group medical visits/ shared medical appointments	Clinicians see patients in a voluntary group setting for follow-up or routine care to provide a more efficient and effective care delivery system. These visits provide a secure and interactive setting between physicians, peers, and additional members of a healthcare team.
Integrated behavioral health care (IBHC)	The care a patient experiences because of a team of primary care and behavioral health clinicians working together with patients and families, using a systematic and cost-effective approach to provide patient-centered care for a defined population. This care may address mental health and substance use disorders, health behaviors (including their contribution to chronic medical illnesses), life stressors and crises, stress-related physical symptoms, and ineffective healthcare utilization patterns [2].
Integrative medicine	The practice of medicine that reaffirms the importance of the relationship between practitioner and patient, focuses on the whole person, is informed by evidence, and makes use of all appropriate therapeutic approaches, healthcare professionals, and disciplines to achieve optimal health and healing [3, 4].
Multidisciplinary care teams	A group of healthcare professionals with different areas of expertise who unite to treat complex medical conditions [5].
Pain neuroscience education (PNE)	A patient education technique that incorporates the complexity of a pain experience and helps patients rethink pain through understanding the multiple neurophysiological, neurobiological, sociological, and physical components that may be involved in their individual pain experience [6].
Standard (usual) medical care for pain	Treatment that medical experts accept as a proper treatment for pain and that is widely used by healthcare professionals.

Role of a Faculty Champion

A wide spectrum of CNCP management infrastructure exists across academic medical practices across the USA. Some academic medical clinics may already have well-established programs for offering and teaching integrative pain management strategies, while other clinics may be in the nascent stages of innovation and change. A key factor for successfully and sustainably introducing foundational changes will be the identification of a faculty champion by the medical director. Ideally, this faculty champion is well versed with a biopsychosocial model of care to support the trainees' learning about CNCP and apply the concepts of pain neuroscience to patient care. This champion should serve as the point person for remaining up to date with the evidence, standardizing efforts across the clinic, and assisting in implementing best practices to manage CNCP. Additionally, the identified faculty champion may use this focus area to engage in scholarly activity and quality improvement initiatives within their respective residency programs and health systems.

How Patients with Chronic Pain Impact an Academic Medical Practice

CNCP is one of the most common indications for patients to seek medical care and incurs an expense to society of approximately $560 billion annually in direct medical costs, lost productivity, and disability programs [7]. Patients with CNCP challenge academic medical practices, which often have a high turnover of learners and educators. Variable clinician continuity and inadequate pain management training hinder many aspects of successful CNCP management: frequency of visits, consistency of patient-clinician relationship, uniformity of management plans, use of patient-centered language, provision of CNCP patient education, and standardized opioid prescribing practices. To improve ambulatory clinic continuity hurdles, the medical director can work with their respective training programs to leverage ambulatory block scheduling templates and team-based care models. To maintain consistent prescribing practices, the medical director/faculty champion can develop protocols and policies for prescribing controlled substances. The medical director/faculty champion can outline a referral network of ancillary services and clinicians to support patients with CNCP. Additionally, the medical director/faculty champion can create a list of integrative resources for clinicians and patients to use to manage CNCP conditions (see suggested national resource list below).

Standardizing Education for Trainees

Ensuring a foundation of knowledge about pain education and CNCP management is essential for trainees working in an academic medical clinic. CNCP education should be prioritized in the curriculum for trainees and offered across multiple levels of training to ensure that the knowledge remains updated and woven into trainees' clinical practice. Medical directors can discuss with those who develop the trainees' educational programming to prioritize didactics on integrative CNCP management. For internal medicine residency programs, the Accreditation Council for Graduate Medical Education (ACGME) identified a core value that "the program must provide instruction and experience in pain management if applicable for the specialty, including recognition of the signs of addiction" [8]. Identifying faculty to lead in the instruction and outsourcing already established course material are initiatives academic programs can take to educate learners about CNCP. Examples of high-quality, accessible course material are detailed in Table 15.2.

Table 15.2 Web-based resources for chronic pain management education for clinicians

Course material in chronic pain management	URL
American College of Physicians (ACP)	https://www.acponline.org/clinical-information/clinical-resources-products/pain-management-learning-hub
Andrew Weil Center for Integrative Medicine: Integrative Pain Management Series	https://integrativemedicine.arizona.edu/online_courses/pain_series.html
Project Extension for Community Health Outcomes (Project ECHO) - Chronic Pain	https://hsc.unm.edu/echo/partner-portal/echos-initiatives/opioid.html
International Association for the Study of Pain: Curriculum Outline on Pain for Medicine	https://www.iasp-pain.org/education/curricula/iasp-curriculum-outline-on-pain-for-medicine/

Patient Engagement

Just as patients' emotions influence pain, patients' expectations also influence the pain experience [9]. Similarly, setting clear expectations on the first visit will help establish a solid foundation for the patient and clinician to work together towards helping the patient with their pain.

In a busy primary care practice, clinicians have limited time to teach their patients about the complexity of CNCP. However, informing patients about the complexities of CNCP using basic concepts of pain neuroscience education, effective treatment modalities, and relapsing and remitting nature of CNCP can improve engagement in pain management plans and reduce fear-avoidance behaviors and catastrophizing [10, 11]. Patient education reduces the frequency of primary care visits for low back pain compared to usual care [12]. The faculty champion can develop a list of resources available for patients to learn about CNCP outside the time allocated for each medical visit.

Clinicians should specifically address the following when setting expectations with a new patient with CNCP:

- Clinic policies (if opioids will be prescribed)
- Evidence supporting the efficacy of multimodal care
- Frequency of visits expected to develop a CNCP management plan
- Care escalation plans
- Management principles
- Resource availability
- Reaffirmation/education about the relapsing and remitting nature of CNCP

Nonpharmacologic Approaches to Chronic Non-cancer Pain

Nonpharmacologic approaches to CNCP encompass lifestyle modifications, mind-body therapies, movement therapies, and manual manipulation. Understanding the pain reduction mechanism behind each of these modalities is outside this chapter's scope. It is important for clinicians to become familiar with pain neuroscience research in support of these nonpharmacologic approaches to pain. This chapter lists the recommended approaches to be integrated into each patient's care plan for comprehensive CNCP management.

Lifestyle Modifications

- *Nutrition and weight management*
- *Sleep hygiene*
- *Smoking cessation*

While lifestyle and behavior changes are challenging at baseline, *small yet measurable* modifications in eating, activity, sleeping, and substance use patterns can contribute to meaningful change in the pain experience for patients. Examples of recommendations include substituting high-calorie sodas and juices with water, taking stairs instead of elevators to encourage activity, improving sleep routines, and supporting nicotine cessation.

The medical director can take a role in facilitating the ease of referrals and patient access to dieticians, physical therapists, or group exercise classes. The medical director can also compile a list for their clinicians detailing referral resources for the lifestyle interventions detailed below. Similarly, the medical director may be able to work with their electronic medical record (EMR) and information technology (IT) departments to create convenient EMR-based mechanisms to choose from a list of lifestyle-based interventions to ease the referral process for clinicians. The clinician should highlight to patients how certain lifestyle changes have improved pain symptoms. Table 15.3 details resources for patients on various lifestyle modifications that have been proven effective in reducing pain.

Behavioral Health Interventions/Mind-Body Therapies

- *Cognitive behavioral therapy (CBT)*
- *Mindfulness-based stress reduction (MBSR)*
- *Mindfulness-based cognitive therapy (MBCT)*
- *Acceptance commitment therapy (ACT)*
- *Therapeutic breathwork and relaxation techniques*

Table 15.3 Lifestyle modification resources for patients

Nutrition	
The anti-inflammatory diet	https://www.va.gov/WHOLEHEALTH/veteran-handouts/docs/EatReduceInflam__Final508__07-25-2019.pdf
The Mediterranean diet	https://www.nutrition.va.gov/docs/UpdatedPatientEd/Mediterraneandiet.pdf
Kaiser Permanente plant-based eating pattern	https://www1.villanova.edu/content/dam/villanova/dining/documents/Nutrition/Plant%20Based%20Diet%20Booklet.pdf
Sleep hygiene	
Healthy sleep habits	https://sleepeducation.org/healthy-sleep/healthy-sleep-habits/
University of Wisconsin Family Medicine Sleep Handout	https://www.fammed.wisc.edu/files/webfm-uploads/documents/outreach/im/handout_sleep.pdf
Smoking cessation	
Smokefree.gov	http://www.smokefree.gov/
The Centers for Disease Control and Prevention	http://www.cdc.gov/TOBACCO/quit_smoking/how_to_quit/
The American Lung Association	http://www.lung.org/stop-smoking/how-to-quit/
Free quit hotlines:	• English: 1-800-QUIT-NOW (1-800-784-8669) • Spanish: 1-855-DÉJELO-YA (1-855-335-3569) • Mandarin and/or Cantonese: 1-800-838-8917 • Korean: 1-800-556-5564 • Vietnamese: 1-800-778-8440

This section details the evidence-based behavioral, mind-body, and manual therapies that improve pain and function in patients with chronic pain. The section "Paying for integrative therapies for chronic pain" details more about therapy payments. Other than some behavioral therapies, most insurance companies do not cover these services listed below. Patients with Health Savings Accounts (HSAs) and Flexible Spending Accounts (FSAs) may submit a bill to be reimbursed for the service provided. Some patients will not be able to pay for these therapies, and the medical director can play an influential role in compiling a list of low-cost and free resources for patients to obtain mind-body therapies.

Mind-body therapies emphasize the interplay between the brain, rest of the body, mind, and behavior, including how emotional, social, spiritual, experiential, and behavioral factors can directly affect health. Mind-body therapies include mindfulness and meditation, relaxation techniques (including breathing exercises), biofeedback, guided imagery and hypnosis, and laughter therapy. The most robust evidence about CNCP management exists for cognitive behavioral therapy (CBT). The medical director can compile a list for clinicians detailing various behavioral health and mind-body therapies, available locally, web based, and app based, to address CNCP. Similarly, the medical director may work with their EMR and IT departments to create convenient EMR-based mechanisms such as macro phrases or referral bundles to choose from a list of evidence-based mind-body interventions described in Table 15.4.

Table 15.4 Behavioral health resources for patients

Cognitive behavioral therapy	***Website***
Psychology Today	https://www.psychologytoday.com/us/therapists/cognitive-behavioral-cbt
Mindfulness	***Website***
UMass Memorial Health Center for Mindfulness	https://www.ummhealth.org/center-mindfulness
The Center for Mind-Body Medicine	https://cmbm.org/
Palouse Mindfulness	https://palousemindfulness.com/
Center For Mindfulness—University of California San Diego	https://cih.ucsd.edu/mindfulness
University of Wisconsin Department of Family Medicine - Patient Meditation Resource (Spanish)	(Español) https://www.fammed.wisc.edu/files/webfm-uploads/documents/outreach/im/module_meditation_patient_sp.pdf
Therapeutic breathwork	***Website***
Dr. Andrew Weil—Three Breathing Exercises	https://www.drweil.com/health-wellness/body-mind-spirit/stress-anxiety/breathing-three-exercises/
Elfenworks Breathing Butterfly™ (Available in 23 languages)	https://elffound.org/butterfly.php

Movement Therapies

- *Therapeutic exercises*
- *Tai chi*
- *Yoga*

While American College of Physician (ACP) guidelines suggest no superiority of one movement therapy over another to treat CNCP, high-quality evidence shows that the use of movement therapy as part of the biopsychosocial approach improves physical function and helps patients overcome pain-related anxiety and kinesiophobia [13]. Having a resource list for clinicians and patients is important, detailing the local and online resources to engage in various movement therapies (Table 15.5). Clinicians and trainees can help empower their patients to choose the best therapies, as described below, for each patient's needs based on access, ability, and efficacy.

Manual Therapies

- *Acupressure (self-administered)*
- *Acupuncture*
- *Massage*

Acupressure and acupuncture are traditional Chinese medicine (TCM) techniques of applying physical pressure (in the case of acupressure) or inserting a needle into the skin (in the case of acupuncture) to a point along the meridian of the

Table 15.5 Movement resources for patients

Tai chi	***Website***
American Tai Chi and Qigong Association	http://www.americantaichi.net/
National Center for Complementary and Integrative Health—Tai Chi	https://nccih.nih.gov/health/taichi/introduction.htm
Tai chi for beginners (with Dr. Paul Lam)	https://www.youtube.com/watch?v=hIOHGrYCEJ4&t=153s
Tai chi for arthritis (with Dr. Paul Lam)	https://www.youtube.com/watch?v=tAOuEpa01j4
Yoga (free)	***Website***
Yoga Green Book—affirming and empowering yoga for people of color	https://www.youtube.com/c/YogaGreenBook/featured
Yoga with Adriene—for beginners	https://www.youtube.com/watch?v=v7AYKMP6rOE
Chair yoga—Yoga with Adriene	https://www.youtube.com/watch?v=-Ts01MC2mIo
Chair yoga—Veterans Affairs Administration	https://www.youtube.com/watch?v=pLVgrHzCTOg
Brenda Medina Yoga en Español	https://www.youtube.com/user/brendamedinayoga
Xuan Lan Yoga en Español	https://www.youtube.com/watch?v=WamU36hXiNw
Cosmic yoga—Kid-friendly yoga	https://www.youtube.com/user/CosmicKidsYoga
Give Back Yoga	https://www.givebackyoga.org

body to alter the energy (known in China as "qi") and thereby relieve pain. Both acupressure and acupuncture have proven beneficial in treating pain and anxiety. Three million Americans seek out acupuncture services annually [14], with pain being the most common reason acupuncture is used (World Health Organization). Considered to be extremely minimal risk when done by a trained practitioner, many national agencies now broadly recommend acupuncture as first-line therapy for CNCP (Army Surgeon General Pain Task Force, American College of Physicians (ACP), the US Agency for Health Care Research and Quality (AHRQ), the National Institutes of Health (NIH), the National Academy of Medicine (NAM), and the Joint Commission (TJC)).

Massage, defined as soft tissue manipulation using the hands or a mechanical device, exists in multiple forms and has been shown to improve subacute and chronic low back pain for short periods. While further research is needed to establish strength in the current research, the evidence for the role of massage therapy in reducing pain is preliminarily positive. While acupuncture and massage therapy can be cost-prohibitive for under-resourced patients, collaboration with local acupuncture and massage therapy schools to bring these low-cost therapies to the clinics is advisable. Self-administered acupressure is a low-cost alternative approach for patients with resource limitations. Patient resources for manual therapies are detailed in Table 15.6.

Table 15.6 Manual therapy resources for patients (from U.S. Department of Veterans Affairs)

Acupressure	*Website*
Acupressure for stress relief	https://www.youtube.com/watch?v=9755-VnnQFM
Acupressure for neck pain	https://www.youtube.com/watch?v=BCqGsDdH1g0
Acupressure for low back pain	https://www.youtube.com/watch?v=ijclWX702mU
Acupressure for headache	https://www.youtube.com/watch?v=Ngq-Y1JH-QA
Acupressure for sleep	https://www.youtube.com/watch?v=2yu4GPwmrF0

Topical Pharmacologic Therapy

Topical agents, when applied as directed over intact skin, are an excellent option to treat chronic musculoskeletal and neuropathic pain due to minimal systemic absorption. The medical director can compile a list for clinicians detailing formulary options for topical pain therapies. Similarly, the medical director may be able to work with their EMR and IT departments to create convenient EMR-based mechanisms to choose from a list of topical pain-reducing agents. When choosing a topical therapy, essential considerations include an indication, carrier, concentration, and cost.

Systemic Non-opioid Pharmacologic Therapy for Chronic Pain

The combination of nonpharmacologic and pharmacologic therapies benefits patients with CNCP. A resource list of low-risk oral and topical non-opioid pharmacologic options can be embedded as a macro phrase in the EMR for ease of use to include common formularies. Formularies will vary across insurance payors and health systems. Clinicians must review the risks and benefits of each medication with the patient and use a shared decision-making process before initiating pharmacotherapy.

For comprehensive information about pharmacologic therapies, including topical and non-opioid pharmacotherapy for chronic pain, the American Chronic Pain Association (ACPA)-Stanford Resource Guide to Chronic Pain Management (2021 Edition) [15] is a valuable and evidence-based resource.

Financing and Affordability for Integrative Chronic Pain Therapies

One in three adults uses complementary services each year [14], and national research has shown that the type of insurance a person has dictates what services a person uses [16]. Thirty billion dollars, out of pocket, are spent annually on complementary services and products, with $12.8 billion in costs on non-vitamin, non-mineral supplements, and $14.7 billion on nonpharmacologic therapies such as osteopathic manipulation, yoga, meditation, and massage [17]. While many can afford to pay for these services out of pocket, under-resourced and underinsured patients lack the financial resources to obtain integrative care. Even those who have insurance that covers some of these services report that coverage is only partial [14]. It is recommended for clinics to mobilize free technology using apps and websites and identify free or low-cost resources within each community to share with clinicians and patients.

Patients may be able to use their FSA or HSA to pay for complementary, integrative services.

Table 15.7 details integrative services at the time of publication covered by the Centers for Medicare & Medicaid Services (CMS).

Table 15.7 Medicare insurance coverage information for nonpharmacologic interventions (from medicare.gov)

Lifestyle modifications	
Nutrition	Medicare Part B members with body mass index (BMI) of ≥30 receive coverage for obesity screenings and behavioral counseling to help with weight loss through diet and exercise when delivered by a primary care physician or another qualified clinician. There is no cost to patients for this service in Medicare Parts A and B [18]. Medicare Part B members with diabetes and/or chronic kidney disease can receive medical nutrition therapy (MNT) services at no additional cost [19].
Sleep hygiene	Medicare Part B covers type I, II, III, and IV sleep tests and devices for patients with clinical signs and symptoms of sleep apnea. Original Medicare members pay 20% of the Medicare-approved amount after meeting the Part B deductible [20].
Smoking cessation	Medicare Part B covers, at no cost, up to 8 visits of smoking and tobacco-use cessation counseling visits in a 12-month period for members who use tobacco [21].

(continued)

Table 15.7 (continued)

Lifestyle modifications	
Mind-body therapies	
Mindfulness meditation	Not covered
Therapeutic breathwork	Not covered
Behavioral health interventions	
Cognitive behavioral therapy (CBT)	Medicare Part B covers the following outpatient mental health services: • One depression screening annually, performed from a primary care doctor's office or primary care clinic that can provide follow-up treatment and referrals. • Individual and group psychotherapy with licensed professionals allowed by the state where services are rendered. • Family counseling, if related to treatment. • Psychiatric evaluation. • Medication management. • Prescription drugs administered by a clinic. • Diagnostic tests. • Partial hospitalization. • A one-time "Welcome to Medicare" preventive visit. • A yearly "Wellness" visit. Part B also covers outpatient mental health services to treat inappropriate alcohol and drug use. Annual depression screening is included in Medicare membership coverage. Members pay 20% of the Medicare-approved amount for visits to the healthcare provider to diagnose or treat the condition. The Part B deductible applies. Additional copayment or coinsurance payments may apply for services rendered in a hospital or outpatient hospital center [22].
Acceptance commitment therapy (ACT)	Not covered
Movement therapies	
Tai chi	Not covered
Yoga	Not covered
Therapeutic exercises	Medicare Part B covers medically necessary outpatient physical and occupational therapy. Original Medicare members pay 20% of the Medicare-approved amount, and the Part B deductible applies. Note: Medicare law no longer limits how much it pays for medically necessary outpatient therapy services in one calendar year [23].
Other	
Acupuncture	Medicare Part B covers up to 12 acupuncture visits in 90 days for chronic low back pain. An additional eight sessions will be covered if improvement is shown. No more than 20 acupuncture treatments can be given yearly. Note: Medicare does not cover acupuncture (including dry needling) for any condition other than chronic low back pain [24].

Table 15.7 (continued)

Lifestyle modifications	
Acupressure	Not covered
Manipulation therapies/massage	Medicare Part B covers manual manipulation of the spine by a chiropractor or other qualified provider if medically necessary to correct subluxation. Medicare does not cover other services or tests, including X-rays, massage therapy, and acupuncture (other than for low back pain). Original Medicare members pay 20% of the Medicare-approved amount, and the Part B deductible applies [25].
Biofeedback	Not covered
Heat/ice/compression/TENS	Not covered

Practice-Level Solutions

Managing CNCP in a non-specialty setting can be daunting. Physicians feel ill-equipped to manage CNCP in the clinic. Lack of resources and support leads to physician burnout, career choices outside of the primary care settings, and patient dissatisfaction [26–29]. The medical director plays an influential role in developing comprehensive practice-level solutions and providing guidance to help standardize the approaches used by residents and faculty to evaluate and manage CNCP. Local practice patterns and resources vary widely, so individualization for your region will be essential. There is no substitute for experience and individualized mentorship, and faculty must balance this with the recognition that inconsistent and conflicting approaches between preceptors can be disorienting to trainees [30].

Comfort in treating CNCP can develop over time, and active coaching and guidance improve the rate at which resident physicians feel comfortable managing these conditions [31]. This section aims to cover the anticipated needs of faculty and trainees to increase their comfort in leading discussions about pain, use tips to establish and maintain patient rapport, and utilize best-practice pain management approaches. Some of the most shared challenges primary care clinicians and trainees face and the practical options and solutions are discussed in this section.

Case Reviews

Case reviews provide an opportunity to discuss ideas, approaches, and local resources. Faculty are encouraged to model the use of patient-centered language when talking about patient cases. These forums can help support residents who may have negative attitudes towards managing patients with CNCP and experience perceived roadblocks in caring for these patients. Case reviews are an opportune time to discuss implicit biases and the potential impact these biases can have on the diagnostics and treatments offered [31].

Case review: Chronic abdominal pain
Chris is a 38-year-old nurse who had recently been laid off from their[a] job. After the layoff, their intermittent abdominal pain became more frequent and severe. Chris has tried many prescribed medications without improvement. An extensive medical workup was unable to pinpoint an organic etiology, and Chris was given the diagnosis of functional abdominal pain. Chris' symptoms continued to worsen, resulting in weekly emergency department visits for symptom control. The emergency room staff labeled them drug-seeking, and Chris felt hostility from the care team.
During their next visit, Chris and their primary care physician (PCP) discussed the frequent emergency department visits. Chris stated that the pain was disabling and sought the emergency department as the only option. The PCP and Chris identified that coping skills could help prevent emergency department visits and added that to their care plan.
Chris engaged with behavioral health and learned strategies to cope with their pain. Chris sought out complementary medicine services, including acupuncture and massage. Chris' PCP prescribed ketorolac injections in the clinic when severe pain flares.
Over the next several months, Chris required fewer and fewer clinic visits for pain flares, and emergency department visits ceased. Chris continues to have bouts of severe abdominal pain, yet the frequency has decreased, and the pain is no longer disabling.

[a]To promote diversity and inclusion throughout medical academic literature, a gender-neutral pronoun is used in this case review.

Role-Playing

Role-playing exercises can prepare residents to identify and address common patient behaviors or thought patterns that may hinder progress [31]. Motivational interviewing principles in a controlled setting prepare clinicians for challenging patient encounters.

Sample responses that can be adapted and adjusted to each patient's needs are detailed in Table 15.8.

Templates

The medical director can guide the development of a standardized template for residents and faculty to use when managing patients with CNCP conditions. Residents are well versed in collecting history of pain qualifiers, such as location, severity, and nature of pain. These skills are essential in the initial workup of pain complaints when the diagnostic and treatment focus is on finding and treating reversible causes. Once the pain becomes a pathologic entity, the discussion should shift from a "diagnose and treat" approach to one of "management" [32].

Table 15.8 Sample responses to common patient behaviors (developed for this chapter by Alicia Carrasco, MD)

Patient behavior	Responses
Passive	"Getting control of your pain is going to take a lot of work on your part. I will not be able to fix it for you, but I can help support you." "Tell me about what you are doing to manage your pain."
Resistant to active modalities	"Not all physical therapists are the same. If you have tried one before and it did not help, let us try another therapist." "Just because you tried physical therapy in the past without success does not mean yoga/tai chi/paced activity will not work. Every person responds differently to various movement therapies, and we know movement is effective for helping with chronic pain."
Focus on opioids	"I am worried about using opioids to treat your pain because I think they could cause a dangerous interaction with your other medications. Could we explore non-opioid treatments to reduce risk and maximize benefit? "Your medical conditions make opioids too dangerous to try. We need to focus on other ways to control your pain." "We only use opioid medications for chronic non-cancer pain when we have tried and failed all our other, safer options. Luckily, we still have many options we have not tried." "Opioids can be helpful for a few days, but in the long term, they may worsen the pain."
Perseveration on a cure	"When you have had pain for this long, there is no easy fix. Your body will signal pain even if the original problem is gone." "*There may be no cure for your type of chronic pain.* We can do many things to reduce its impact on your life."
Catastrophizing	"Let's try to balance those negative thoughts with other ones." "Tell me about how you keep going."

The management of CNCP requires a different approach from treating acute pain. Those residents guided to shift from questions about the quality of the pain to questions related to function and impact will benefit.

Faculty can educate residents on motivational interviewing techniques and "Specific, Measurable, Achievable, Relevant, and Timely (SMART)" goals [33] to empower patients to discover self-management strategies for their pain. Templates are a valuable tool to cue residents to ask pertinent questions and maintain a consistent care plan when multiple residents see the patient longitudinally in a clinic. An example of a CNCP template follows.

Template: Integrative chronic pain plan (Adapted from "Chronic Pain Management: Addressing Physician Knowledge and Confidence," Triozzi J, McDermott L, Morse M, Baylor College of Medicine Department of Medicine Housestaff Research Symposium, April 2020)

The following management items for chronic pain have been addressed, when indicated:

Pain description

- Location of pain:
- Duration of pain:
- Pain character/description:
- Exacerbating factors:
- Alleviating factors:

Pain, enjoyment, general activity (PEG) score:
Functional goal/SMART goal:
Coping mechanisms:
Imaging:
Consults:
Surgeries (previous/planned):
Physical therapy:
Lifestyle modifications:

- Healthy eating:
- Healthy movement/physical activity:
- Sleep hygiene:
- Breathwork exercises:

Integrative therapies:
Manipulation:
Massage:
Movement therapies (i.e., yoga/tai chi)
Acupuncture/acupressure:
Other:
Medications trialed:

- Topical analgesics:
- Acetaminophen:
- NSAIDs:
- Anticonvulsant/neuropathic medications:
- Antispasmodic medications:

Macros

Most EMRs allow for macros. Providing the residents with pre-built text early on in their careers improves documentation while also guiding them through questions and discussions. The following are examples of macros that can be adapted to the clinic's needs.

*...**Avoiding opioids***: We discussed the evidence for opioid treatment in chronic pain, namely that most patients do not find long-term benefits in pain or function with opioid initiation. We reviewed CDC guidelines emphasizing non-opioid pain control strategies and risks of opioid therapy. Given the unlikely benefit and potential for harm, we opted to avoid opioid initiation.

*...**Chronic pain treatment***: We discussed that effective management of chronic pain requires a multimodal approach. We discussed the options available to the

patient, and I recommended they try at least one type of treatment from each modality.

...Paced activity: We spoke about the importance of pacing activities and alternating periods of activity with periods of rest. Specifically, we discussed ways to avoid the pain cycle, including not overdoing activities on "good" days or avoiding all activities on "bad days." I provided the patient with the following paced activity handout: https://www.mentalhealth.va.gov/coe/cesamh/docs/Activity_Pacing-patients.pdf

...Sleep pain: We discussed the importance of sleep in the management of chronic pain. We discussed sleep hygiene, including maintaining regular sleep/wake hours, using the bed only for sleep and sex, avoiding TV/computers before bed, and limiting caffeine intake after 2 pm. We discussed techniques to help relieve pressure points when in bed.

...Cannabis pain: I counseled the patient on the lack of evidence related to the use of cannabinoids for chronic pain conditions and the risk for adverse side effects from the use of cannabis products.

Treatment Options

Leverage the EMR to facilitate multimodal treatments for CNCP. Collocation within a single order set is ideal and should include medication orders, behavioral health referrals, active modalities, and complementary medicine. Collocation facilitates ease of ordering and provides treatment ideas.

A sample order set is listed below:

Pain order set
Medications
• Topical analgesics
• Acetaminophen [not to exceed 2 g daily if hepatic dysfunction; 3gm daily for others]
• Nonsteroidal anti-inflammatories [lack of response to one agent does not predict response to another]
• Anticonvulsant/neuropathic medications
• Antidepressants (TCA/SNRI)
• Antispasmodic medications
Supplies
• TENS unit and leads
• Braces and splints
• Traction devices
Referrals
• Physiatrist/Physical Medicine & Rehabilitation
• Physical and occupational therapy
• Behavioral health
• Dietician
• Chiropractor
• Orthopedics
• Pain medicine/interventional procedures

Patient Resources

A multimodal approach is critical to effective pain management. The resources available within a community and to an individual patient vary widely depending on a patient's rurality, financial resources, and insurance status [28]. Delegating a team member to keep an updated list ensures an updated resource. Many complementary and alternative medicine practitioners provide sliding-scale services, and training institutions may provide free and low-cost care. Some community clinics often keep lists of resources to help patients navigate a costly healthcare system and are willing to share.

In the document, try to provide the following information:

- Name of business and contact information
- Location (include the distance from your clinic and public transportation options)
- Cost/payment options
- Additional information (i.e., discounts for seniors and students)

Consider listing local options for the following resources:

- Acupuncture
- Chiropractors
- Behavioral health providers
- Gymnasiums/pools
- Massage
- Tai chi
- Yoga

A list of patient resources is available in Table 15.9.

Patient Education Resources

Apps

Apps provide a free or low-cost way for patients to track or manage their pain. This list is not comprehensive but provides a starting point for the clinic champion to update. The authors have no financial interest in any of the following apps:

- **Curable™** guides patients through a biopsychosocial approach to managing their pain. It includes exercises and meditations that aim to empower patients to take control of their pain. The free version has introductory lessons, and a paid subscription provides more in-depth content.
- **Branch™** is free of charge and uses its network to link patients to a supportive community. Patients track and record their experience and treatment. The app provides cognitive behavior-based techniques.

Table 15.9 Patient resources

Websites		
Oregon Pain Guidance	https://www.oregonpainguidance.org/paineducationtoolkit/	This user-friendly website has information on managing pain. Information is broken up into small, focused sections. Each section has videos, patient handouts, and links to more resources.
Veteran Affairs Pain Management Resources	https://www.va.gov/PAINMANAGEMENT/Veteran_Public/index.asp	Full of many excellent resources to help patients understand and manage persistent pain.
Videos		
"Tame The Beast" Video by Lorimer Moseley	https://www.tamethebeast.org/#tame-the-beast	A 5-min animated feature created by Australian neuroscientist and physiotherapist Lorimer Moseley, Ph.D., that describes the differences between acute and persistent pain and encourages patients to think about their pain differently.
"The mysterious science of pain" by Joshua Pate	https://www.youtube.com/watch?v=eakyDiXX6Uc	A 5-min animated feature that goes into more detail about biological reasons for chronic pain.
"A Car With 4 Flat Tires"	https://youtu.be/5RIii6OUK2A	This video uses metaphor to stress the need for a multimodal approach to pain management. This cartoon emphasizes the importance of an active patient as the driver in their care.
Support groups		
Pain Connection National Support Groups	https://painconnection.org/support-groups/national/	Online community with support groups for patients with persistent pain.
Mindfulness resource		
Free Mindfulness Project	https://www.freemindfulness.org/download	This UK-based website provides free guided audio and imagery meditations in addition to scheduled mindfulness sessions.

- **FlowLy™** uses biofeedback to modulate breathing and improve self-regulation. There are some free modules, but the mainstay of the app is a subscription-based service. iPhone only.
- **What's Up? A Mental Health App™** uses acceptance and commitment therapy (ACT) to help clients understand their situation. Using ACT and CBT, this app helps patients find and change unhealthy thinking patterns; there is also a forum to connect with other users.
- **Headspace™** provides guided meditation, sleep meditation, and breathing exercises of varying lengths. There is a free version, but most services are subscription based.

Conclusion

The clinic medical director is uniquely suited to define the mission and vision of CNCP management for the clinic and adapt to the evolving landscape of care surrounding comprehensive, quality therapies for CNCP management. As complementary and alternative therapies' efficacy and safety knowledge gaps narrow, clinicians are choosing to prioritize integrative, low-risk, evidence-based modalities over higher risk pharmacologic and interventional procedures. Patients are seeking complementary therapies to address their pain needs. To meet this demand, medical directors should implement robust integrative pain care models in their respective academic medical practices. While payment for integrative modalities will continue to be a challenge, clinic medical directors can advance the mission by using proper billing codes, collaborating with behavioral health and physical therapy teams, partnering with allied health training programs to bring low-cost therapies to the clinics, and engaging with administrative leadership for support and resources.

References

1. National Center for Complementary and Integrative Health [Internet]. 2022 [cited 27 September 2022]. https://www.nccih.nih.gov/
2. Agency for Healthcare Research and Quality (AHRQ) [Internet]. Ahrq.gov. 2022 [cited 27 September 2022]. https://www.ahrq.gov/
3. Integrative Medicine Board Certification I ABPS [Internet]. American Board of Physician Specialties; 2022 [cited 27 September 2022]. https://www.abpsus.org/specializations/integrative-medicine/
4. Academic Consortium for Integrative Medicine and Health [Internet]. Academic Consortium for Integrative Medicine and Health; 2022 [cited 27 September 2022]. https://imconsortium.org/
5. Concise Medical Dictionary (8 ed.) [Internet]. Concise Medical Dictionary. Oxford University Press; 2010 [cited 2022 Sep 27]. https://www.oxfordreference.com/view/10.1093/acref/9780199557141.001.0001/acref-9780199557141
6. Moseley GL. Reconceptualising pain according to modern pain science. Physical Therapy Reviews [Internet]. 2007;12(3):169–78. http://www.tandfonline.com/doi/full/10.1179/108331907X223010. [cited 2022 Sep 25].
7. Institute of Medicine (US) Committee on Advancing Pain Research, Care, and Education. Relieving Pain in America: A Blueprint for Transforming Prevention, Care, Education, and Research [Internet]. Washington (DC): National Academies Press (US); 2011 [Cited 2022 Sep 25]. (The National Academies Collection: Reports funded by National Institutes of Health). http://www.ncbi.nlm.nih.gov/books/NBK91497/.
8. ACGME Internal Medicine Program Requirements 2020 [Internet]. https://www.acgme.org/globalassets/pfassets/programrequirements/140_internalmedicine_2020.pdf
9. Shih YW, Tsai HY, Lin FS, Lin YH, Chiang CY, Lu ZL, et al. Effects of positive and negative expectations on human pain perception engage separate but interrelated and dependently regulated cerebral mechanisms. J Neurosci [Internet]. 2019;39(7):1261–74. [cited 2022 Sep 25]. https://www.jneurosci.org/lookup/doi/10.1523/JNEUROSCI.2154-18.2018
10. Malfliet A, Kregel J, Meeus M, Danneels L, Cagnie B, Roussel N, et al. Patients with chronic spinal pain benefit from pain neuroscience education regardless the self-reported signs of

central sensitization: secondary analysis of a randomized controlled multicenter trial. PM R. 2018;10(12):1330–1343.e1.
11. García-Ríos MC, Navarro-Ledesma S, Tapia-Haro RM, Toledano-Moreno S, Casas-Barragán A, Correa-Rodríguez M, et al. Effectiveness of health education in patients with fibromyalgia: a systematic review. Eur J Phys Rehabil Med. 2019;55(2):301–13.
12. Traeger AC, Hübscher M, Henschke N, Moseley GL, Lee H, McAuley JH. Effect of primary care-based education on reassurance in patients with acute low Back pain: systematic review and meta-analysis. JAMA Intern Med. 2015;175(5):733–43.
13. Booth J, Moseley GL, Schiltenwolf M, Cashin A, Davies M, Hübscher M. Exercise for chronic musculoskeletal pain: a biopsychosocial approach. Musculoskeletal Care [Internet]. 2017;15(4):413–21. [cited 2022 Sep 25]. https://onlinelibrary.wiley.com/doi/10.1002/msc.1191
14. Clarke TC, Black LI, Stussman BJ, Barnes PM, Nahin RL. Trends in the use of complementary health approaches among adults: United States, 2002-2012. Natl Health Stat Report. 2015;79:1–16.
15. Patient Resources [Internet]. Division of Pain Medicine. 2022 [cited 27 September 2022]. https://med.stanford.edu/pain/patients/patient-resources.html
16. Lafferty WE, Tyree PT, Bellas AS, Watts CA, Lind BK, Sherman KJ, et al. Insurance coverage and subsequent utilization of complementary and alternative medicine providers. Am J Manag Care. 2006;12(7):397–404.
17. Nahin RL, Barnes PM, Stussman BJ. Expenditures on complementary health approaches: United States, 2012. Natl Health Stat Report. 2016;95:1–11.
18. Obesity Screening Coverage [Internet]. Medicare.gov. 2022 [cited 27 September 2022]. https://www.medicare.gov/coverage/obesity-behavioral-therapy
19. Medical Nutrition Therapy Insurance Coverage [Internet]. Medicare.gov. 2022 [cited 27 September 2022]. https://www.medicare.gov/coverage/nutrition-therapy-services
20. Sleep Study Coverage [Internet]. Medicare.gov. 2022 [cited 27 September 2022]. https://www.medicare.gov/coverage/sleep-studies
21. Smoking Cessation Counseling Coverage [Internet]. Medicaregov 2022 [cited 27 September 2022]. https://www.medicare.gov/coverage/counseling-to-prevent-tobacco-use-tobacco-caused-disease
22. Outpatient Mental Health Coverage [Internet]. Medicare.gov. 2022 [cited 27 September 2022]. https://www.medicare.gov/coverage/mental-health-care-outpatient
23. Physical Therapy Coverage [Internet]. Medicare.gov. 2022 [cited 27 September 2022]. https://www.medicare.gov/coverage/physical-therapy
24. Acupuncture coverage [Internet]. Medicare.gov. 2022 [cited 27 September 2022]. https://www.medicare.gov/coverage/acupuncture
25. Coverage for Chiropractic Services [Internet]. Medicare.gov. 2022 [cited 27 September 2022]. https://www.medicare.gov/coverage/chiropractic-services
26. Jamison RN, Sheehan KA, Scanlan E, Matthews M, Ross EL. Beliefs and attitudes about opioid prescribing and chronic pain management: survey of primary care providers. J Opioid Manag. 2014;10(6):375–82.
27. Upshur CC, Luckmann RS, Savageau JA. Primary care provider concerns about management of chronic pain in community clinic populations. J Gen Intern Med. 2006;21(6):652–5.
28. Purcell N, Zamora K, Tighe J, Li Y, Douraghi M, Seal K. The integrated pain team: a mixed-methods evaluation of the impact of an embedded interdisciplinary pain care intervention on primary care team satisfaction, confidence, and perceptions of care effectiveness. Pain Med [Internet]. 2018;19(9):1748–63. https://doi.org/10.1093/pm/pnx254. [cited 2022 Sep 25].
29. Garcia J, Ohanisian L, Sidley A, Ferris A, Luck G, Basich G, et al. Resident knowledge and perception of pain management. Cureus. 2019;11(11):e6107.
30. Regunath H, Cochran K, Cornell K, Shortridge J, Do D, Kim S, et al. Is it painful to manage chronic pain? A cross-sectional study of physicians in-training in a university program. Mo Med. 2016;113:72–8.

31. Ruff AL, Alford DP, Butler R, Isaacson JH. Training internal medicine residents to manage chronic pain and prescription opioid misuse. Subst Abus. 2017;38(2):200–4.
32. Schneiderhan J, Clauw D, Schwenk TL. Primary care of patients with chronic pain. JAMA. 2017;317(23):2367–8.
33. Doran G. There's a S.M.A.R.T. way to write Management's goals and objectives. Manag Rev. 1981;70:35–6.

Chapter 16
Safe Opioid Prescribing and Controlled Substance Policies

Daniel G. Tobin and Ernie-Paul Barrette

Introduction

The analgesic and "narcotic" properties of opioids have been recognized for hundreds if not thousands of years [1], but a full appreciation of their potential risks is a much more recent phenomenon. Appropriately, as the risks of overdose, addiction, and other adverse effects become clearer, the opioid prescribing regulatory landscape has become more restrictive. And yet, there are some patients who do benefit from opioid prescribing, and they should not be withheld when their potential benefits clearly outweigh potential harms for an individual patient. It is important for the primary care physician and, by extension, the medical residency continuity clinic to recognize this equipoise and approach opioid prescribing deliberately, rationally, and in a manner that prioritizes safety. In this chapter, we will explore this in more depth and guide the clinic director through this challenge.

Outline
- Background
- The role of opioids in the management of chronic pain
- Principles of safe opioid prescribing

D. G. Tobin (✉)
Yale University School of Medicine, New Haven, CT, USA

Adult Medicine, New Haven Primary Care Consortium, Cornell Scott Hill Health Center, New Haven, CT, USA
e-mail: daniel.tobin@yale.edu

E.-P. Barrette
Washington University School of Medicine, St. Louis, MO, USA
e-mail: ernie-paulbarrette@wustl.edu

L. B. Lu et al. (eds.), *Leading an Academic Medical Practice*,
https://doi.org/10.1007/978-3-031-40273-9_16

- Safety monitoring
- Special considerations for the academic medical practice
- Conclusion

Background

Prevalence and Impact of Chronic Pain

An estimated 20% of American adults suffer from chronic pain [2], resulting in hundreds of billions of dollars each year in lost wages, reduced productivity, and medical expenses [3]. Moderate-to-severe pain is also one of the most common chief complaints in primary care [4]. As a result, evaluating chronic pain is a part of everyday practice, and its management is extremely important to the functionality and well-being of our patients. This is particularly true since patients with chronic pain are frequently subjected to social stigma and discrimination [5]. The wise clinic director will anticipate this need and leverage clinical and community resources to benefit the practice.

The Competing Epidemics of Pain and Addiction

The suffering from severe pain can be profound, but so is the impact of opioid misuse, diversion, and addiction. In a systematic review of 38 studies, 26% from primary care settings and 53% from pain clinics, opioid misuse (defined as using an opioid in a manner other than that intended by the prescriber) was found to have an incidence of 21–29% ([95% CI] 13–38%) [6]. In the same study, opioid use disorder (compulsive drug seeking and use despite harmful consequences) had an incidence of 8–12% ([95% CI] 3–17%). The data on overdose deaths is even more profound; from May 2020 to April 2021, 75,673 people died from an opioid overdose, equating to over 200 overdose deaths every day [7]. Misuse, diversion, and addiction have dramatic negative consequences, and physicians must consider these potential harms before prescribing opioids. Here too, the clinic director must anticipate this challenge and gather resources to help their teams diagnose and manage substance use disorders when they occur.

This Historical Impact of Overprescribing

Overprescribing fueled the opioid epidemic in the USA. As the prevalence and impact of chronic pain became better understood in the early 1990s, well-intentioned but misguided efforts such as the "Pain as the 5th Vital Sign" campaign promoted by the American Pain Society and later adopted as a matter of policy by the

Veterans Health Administration drove opioid prescribing [8]. This worsened in 2001 when the Joint Commission on Accreditation of Healthcare Organizations (JCAHO) released new pain management standards, further promoting the concept and again in 2006 when the Centers for Medicare Services (CMS) linked reimbursement to patients' satisfaction with pain management in their Hospital Consumer Assessment of Healthcare Providers and Systems survey (HCAHPS) [9]. This problem was compounded by poorly trained prescribers and insufficient access to pain specialists; in 2011, only 5 of the 133 medical schools had a mandatory course on pain [10], and nationally there are only four board-certified pain specialists for every 100,000 patients suffering from chronic pain [11]. In addition, pharmaceutical companies such as Purdue Pharma promoted opioid analgesics to prescribers as "nonaddictive" or illegally pushed their use, further driving overprescribing [12]. By 2012, clinicians wrote 259 million prescriptions for opioid pain medication, enough for every adult in the USA to have their own bottle of pills [13]. These factors increased the risk of diversion, fueled the prevalence of addiction, and led to hundreds of thousands of preventable deaths across America.

The Impact of Pain and Addiction on an Academic Medical Practice

It is extremely likely that academic medical practices will encounter patients suffering from chronic pain and addiction, sometimes concurrently. The relief of suffering is a core principle of medicine, and academic practices often have limited access to pain specialists, so they must learn to manage this themselves. In addition to being in short supply, many pain specialists limit referrals to privately insured patients or to procedural interventions only [11]. Compounding this, as previously noted, most medical students graduate without any formal training in pain management [10, 14]. The high incidence of pain and addiction, along with lack of training and access to resources, can lead to chaos and dysfunction unless the clinic director makes sure that trainees and faculty have the appropriate education, tools, and support needed to treat chronic pain and addiction safely and rationally.

The Role of Opioids in the Management of Chronic Pain

Mechanism, Efficacy, and Indications

The analgesic effect from opioid agonists results primarily through stimulation of G protein-coupled receptors—mainly the μ-opioid receptor but also other opioid receptors (κ-opioid and δ-opioid) and the nociceptin receptor (ORL1), which impact drug pharmacodynamics [15]. Through these receptors, opioids inhibit activation of peripheral nociceptors, reduce the ascending transmission of pain signals from the spinal cord to the brain, and activate the descending inhibition of pain signaling from the periaqueductal gray matter of the midbrain back down the spinal cord.

For acute severe pain that does not respond sufficiently to non-opioid analgesics (e.g., acute femur fracture managed in the emergency room), opioids can be highly effective. However, when used for chronic non-cancer pain, the efficacy data is much less compelling [16], and there is precious little data studying their efficacy when used for more than 6 months. The Agency for Healthcare Research and Quality (AHRQ) continues to update the evidence on opioids for chronic non-cancer pain. Their conclusion remains: "At short-term follow up … opioids are associated with small beneficial effects versus placebo but are associated with increased risk of short-term harms and do not appear to be superior to nonopioid therapy. Evidence on intermediate-term and long-term benefits remains very limited, and additional evidence confirms an association between opioids and increased risk of serious harms that appears to be dose-dependent" [16]. Yet, there are some patients who do exhibit sustained benefit, and opioids remain an important part of our analgesic armamentarium.

Although the data on efficacy for chronic opioid therapy is sparse, there are many well-established and sometimes serious harms associated with opioid use, including not only addiction, diversion, and overdose death, but also a plethora of potential adverse effects ranging from constipation to sexual dysfunction. As a result, the risk-benefit assessment is not always clear, and physicians should prescribe opioids sparingly and with great caution.

For chronic non-cancer pain, opioids are only indicated for patients with severe disabling pain that results from a potentially opioid-responsive diagnosis (i.e., not fibromyalgia, chronic headaches, or other pain syndromes for which there is little to no evidence that opioids are efficacious) that cannot be sufficiently controlled with non-opioid treatment alone including a combination of behavioral therapy, physical therapy, and multimodal pharmacotherapy. Even then, opioids should generally be avoided when contraindications are present (e.g., active untreated opioid use disorder). A full discussion of the potential risks and benefits of opioids is beyond the scope of this chapter, but there are several validated risk tools that can be used to help determine the relative risk of opioid use in an individual (e.g., the Revised Opioid Risk Took [ORT-R] [17] and the Screener and Opioid Assessment for Patients with Pain-Revised [SOAPP-R] [18]).

Treatment Goal Setting

Before initiating opioid treatment for chronic pain, treatment goals should be discussed. Improvement of pain is important, but an appropriate treatment objective should include improvement in function. The more objective and specific the goal, the better to assess if a patient is showing improvement with opioid therapy. For example, a patient may identify being able to go for a walk or do simple house chores or babysitting as stated objectives. Identifying *SMART* goals which are specific, measurable, achievable, relevant, and time-bound is a good approach. It is also important to educate patients that while opioids may improve pain severity, they cannot safely eliminate it completely. Living without pain cannot be the objective. Rather, living and functioning well *despite* the presence of pain is a much more realistic target.

To assess the baseline and subsequent impact of chronic pain once treatment is initiated, it can be helpful to use a validated tool to standardize the assessment. For example, the PEG score (pain average, interference with enjoyment and life, and interference with general activity) is short and easy to incorporate in practice [19]. This tool can help the clinician assess for and quantify improvement in pain and function. We recommend that the clinic director make this a practice-wide expectation.

Informed Consent and Controlled Substance Agreements

Patients must be counseled about the potential risks and benefits of opioids prior to the first prescription. Expectation setting is important; patients need to be informed that not all chronic pain is responsive to opioids and that they will not be continued in the absence of demonstrated benefit. The paucity of efficacy data, while sobering, should be shared as well.

Relatedly, the many potential risks of opioid use need to be discussed in depth so that shared decision-making can take place. Many patients are already aware of the more common potential side effects such as constipation, nausea, itching, and sedation, but the risk of falls, impaired driving, sleep-disordered breathing, and sexual dysfunction should be discussed as well. Discussing the risk of addiction and overdose is of paramount importance, and patients must know that the risk for sedation and overdose death increases as the daily total morphine milligram equivalent (MME) dose increases [20], and when opioids are mixed with other potentially sedating medications, such as benzodiazepines [21]. If a patient is already on benzodiazepine therapy, the perils of using these drugs in combination need to be carefully considered.

Patients may also confuse physical dependence for addiction, so it is prudent to counsel them about how they differ. The risk for withdrawal with a sudden decrease in opioid use should be part of an informed consent discussion and can segue nicely into counseling about never using more opioid than prescribed and never giving or selling their medication to another person. Safe storage and disposal of opioids, as well as the need to inform all treating clinicians (e.g., specialists, emergency room personnel) that opioids are prescribed, are an important part of safety counseling as well.

Use of a controlled substance agreement (CSA), often erroneously and coercively framed as a "narcotic contract," can be helpful since the elements of informed consent can easily be incorporated into the form. These tools are recommended by most professional societies and practice guidelines, are mandated in some states, and are used in most academic medical practices. To be useful, the agreement must be written in plain language that patients can understand and should be framed as a device intended to promote shared decision-making and informed consent while simultaneously emphasizing the shared responsibilities of both the patient and the prescriber to ensure safe use [22]. The document can and should clearly spell out office policies regarding refills, communication, safety monitoring (e.g., urine drug testing), and conditions under which opioids may need to be discontinued, but should not threaten discharge from the practice should the patient lose control over safe opioid use [23]. The clinician and the patient should review the CSA together and scan a signed copy into the medical record. An example of a controlled substance agreement, developed by one of the authors and adapted for use in their health system, is included at the end of this chapter as Appendix.

Before the First Prescription

In addition to assessing whether chronic opioid therapy is potentially indicated, taking a thorough history to assess for contraindications (including an assessment for unstable psychiatric disease or a history of unsafe use of drugs and alcohol), establishing SMART goals, and fully engaging in the informed consent process, there are several other safety measures to implement before writing the first prescription. Firstly, it is important to recognize that patients suffering from opioid use disorder or who divert prescription opioids for personal gain may have a stronger relationship with the opioid than they do with you [24], and thus may not be forthcoming with their history. Before writing the first prescription, it is prudent to review prior medical records, query the state prescription drug monitoring program (PDMP), and perform a urine drug test to assess whether there may be undisclosed controlled substances already in the patient's system that would present a safety risk. Depending on the place in which you practice, some or all these interventions may already be regulatory requirements. Some PDMPs can query records from other states, and each of these tools provides some degree of objective data to guide medial decision-making.

Principles of Safe Opioid Prescribing

The First Prescription: Quantity

The initiation of opioid therapy for chronic pain should be considered as a therapeutic trial that is only continued when the benefits clearly outweigh the risks. To minimize those risks, a good mantra is to "start low and go slow," which in practice means to start with a short-acting opioid at the lowest potentially effective treatment dose while performing frequent reassessments. The first prescription need not be for

30-days; an initial 1–2-week supply to assess for unexpected harm is a safe and sometimes mandated approach; several states legally limit the first prescription of new opioid therapy to no more than a 7-day (or fewer) supply [25]. Once a decision is made to continue opioid therapy, the wise prescriber will consider giving a 28-day supply rather than 30; a 28-day supply will always need to be refilled on the same predicable day of the week, thus empowering both the patient and the prescriber to more easily know when the next refill is due.

The First Prescription: Short Acting Only

For opioid-naïve patients, a low dose of a short-acting opioid is recommended. Extended-release formulations and long-acting (ER/LA) opioids are available and can be a valuable tool in the management of chronic pain, especially in the management of patients in hospice or with cancer-associated pain syndromes. However, even the lowest dose of most ER/LA opioids can be too much for opioid-naïve patients, and there is an increased risk for overdose when they are used early in therapy [26]. ER/LA formulations should only be used when higher doses of opioids are necessary, when tolerance to opioids is present, and when the patient is suffering from "around-the-clock" pain that is not intermittent in nature.

The First Prescription: Opioid Choice

Due to polymorphisms of the opioid receptor as well as individual differences in metabolism, it can be difficult to predict which opioid will work best for an individual. Asking for a specific opioid by name can be a "yellow flag" for opioid misuse, but a patient who has required opioid therapy before may also simply know what works best for them. That said, it is prudent to start with a lower potency opioid first, such as tramadol or hydrocodone, unless drug-drug interactions or other contraindications exist. If the total daily MME dose is low, short-acting morphine or oxycodone may be reasonable as well depending on the clinical situation. Transdermal buprenorphine, as a partial opioid agonist, has a favorable safety profile and may also be considered in opioid-naïve patients with severe chronic pain. In contrast, highly potent or metabolically complex opioids can be dangerous to prescribe and medications such as hydromorphone, fentanyl, and methadone should rarely if ever be used when starting opioid therapy. Due to methadone's cardiac risks, potential drug-drug interactions, and complicated metabolism, those considering prescribing methadone for chronic pain should seek additional guidance [27]. A full accounting of the nuances of which opioid to choose is beyond the scope of this chapter, but many excellent resources exist on this topic.

The First Prescription: Opioid Dose

While no dose of opioids is clearly safe, the higher the daily opioid dose, the greater the risk of an overdose. There is compelling evidence that the risk of an overdose rises 1.9- to 4.6-fold for those taking 50–99 mg MME/day, and those on >100 MME/day have a risk 2- to 8.9-fold higher than those on 1 to <20 MME/day [28]. The lower the dose, the safer the regimen. The CDC guidelines of 2016 state, "Most experts agreed that, in general, increasing dosages to 50 or more MME/day increases overdose risk without necessarily adding benefits for pain control or function and that clinicians should carefully reassess evidence of individual benefits and risks when considering increasing opioid dosages to ≥50 MME/day" [28]. Importantly, the updated 2022 CDC Clinical Practice Guideline for Prescribing Opioids for Pain no longer defines specific dosing recommendations but instead calls for an individualized assessment of benefits and harms when increasing or adjusting opioid dosing [29].

Ongoing Opioid Prescribing

For those on chronic opioids, follow-up visits should generally occur no less often than every 3 months, and more frequently when opioids are started or changed or aberrant drug use behaviors arise. Safety monitoring will be discussed more fully in the sections below, but indications and potential contraindications should be reviewed at each office visit and the safe storage and disposal of opioids should be periodically reemphasized. Repeatedly claiming that prescriptions were lost or stolen should raise concern for misuse or diversion, and a pattern of early refill requests suggests a safety concern that should prompt evaluation for opioid use disorder and possible medication discontinuation.

If pain remains severe despite opioid use, the clinician should consider increasing the dose or changing the opioid but should also assess whether the patient may have a pain syndrome that is either unresponsive to opioids or worsened by them (e.g., opioid-induced hyperalgesia). Dose increases should be made carefully, gradually, and with attention to the increased risks that accompany higher MME doses. Some patients will ultimately require high-dose opioid therapy, but in general, doses higher than 90 MME are rarely more effective than lower doses but are associated with significantly higher risk. Changing from one opioid to another can be effective but is also fraught with risk; differences in receptor affinity and metabolism lead to incomplete cross-tolerance, and thus a 1:1 equianalgesic dose conversion can lead to overdose. Instead, the calculated equianalgesic dose should be reduced by 25% or more to reduce this risk (many experts recommend a 30–50% initial dose reduction) and can then be increased later if needed [30].

For patients who are also taking other sedating medications, are on 50 MME/day or more of opioid therapy, or have other risks for overdose (e.g., untreated sleep apnea, history of prior overdose, history of substance use disorders), naloxone should be co-prescribed [29]. This lifesaving medication can quickly reverse an overdose and should be easily accessible to both the patient and their family or loved ones. Many electronic health record (EHR) systems have reminders for naloxone when opioids are ordered, and we encourage practices to leverage this functionality when it is available. In some states, naloxone may also be prescribed directly by the pharmacist without an order from a physician or other practitioner, and on March 29, 2023 the US Food and Drug Administration approved Narcan 4 mg (naloxone hydrochloride) nasal spray for over-the-counter use, although it was not yet widely available without a prescription at the time this chapter was written.

New Patients Already on Chronic Opioid Therapy

New patients who are already on chronic opioid therapy from a prior prescriber deserve special mention. Regardless of the prescribing history, the new physician has an obligation to reassess the indications, contraindications, and risk-benefit profile of opioids before continuing the prescription. Reviewing the PDMP to verify the prescription refill history, obtaining outside medical records to understand the prior clinical decision-making, and UDS testing are all important and prudent steps to take before continuing chronic opioid therapy. However, it can take time to obtain outside records, and an inadvertent prescribing gap can result in severe withdrawal and exacerbation of pain. Further, abrupt discontinuation of opioid therapy is associated with an increased rate of suicide [31]. In the absence of unambiguous evidence of misuse, offering a short-term refill (e.g., a few days) while verifying outside information can be acceptable.

Discontinuing Opioid Therapy

Opioids should be discontinued when the benefits of opioid therapy no longer outweigh their risks for an individual patient. Triggering factors could include insufficient analgesic benefit, severe side effects that cannot be effectively managed, unsafe opioid use, evidence of diversion, or new comorbidities (including addiction) that contraindicate ongoing prescribing. Whether opioids are slowly tapered off or stopped more quickly depends on the reason they are being discontinued and the risks associated with ongoing use. For example, if there is concern for diversion and UDS testing is negative for the prescribed opioid, it may be appropriate to discontinue opioids without a taper. However, a slow taper to minimize the risk of withdrawal is prudent if the opioid is being discontinued because of changing patient preference or lack of clinical benefit.

Treating Opioid Use Disorder

When chronic opioid use devolves into addiction or another substance use disorder is identified, the primary care physician must be able to screen for the problem, make the diagnosis, and refer the patient for treatment. Addiction is a brain disease, not a moral failing, and the presence of this diagnosis should not result in termination from the medical practice [23]. Instead, the treating physician should work with the patient to direct them to further care. The clinic director can gather information about community and specialty resources to empower the physicians in the practice and facilitate the referral process. Ideally, the practice should also be able to directly manage opioid use disorder with the use of buprenorphine, prescribed from the primary care setting. Until recently, physicians were required to complete an 8-h waiver training course before they could apply for a waiver (an "X number") from the Drug Enforcement Administration (DEA) to prescribe buprenorphine. However, recent policy changes by the Department of Health and Human Services have relaxed the prescribing requirements. Initially, physicians were required to file a Notice of Intent (NOI) with the Substance Abuse and Mental Health Services Administration (SAMHSA) which, after approval, allowed for buprenorphine treatment of up to 30 patients with opioid use disorder without additional training [32]. More recently, the buprenorphine-specific requirements were eliminated altogether; as of June 27, 2023 the DEA only requires a one-time attestation during controlled substance registration or renewal that prescribers have completed 8 hours of training on the management of patients with opioid or other substance use disorders. With these changes, the barrier to managing opioid use disorder in primary care has been significantly reduced, and there is little justification not to offer this service.

Safety Monitoring

Collateral Information

Protecting a patient's privacy and safeguarding their protected health information are critically important and a legal requirement. However, collateral information from family, friends, and other clinicians can be informative and helpful. Obtaining consent to reach out to significant others can facilitate communication, and the prescriber should be receptive to input from others when it can be obtained in a HIPAA-compliant way. Unsolicited concerns from family and friends should be considered carefully (while also remaining vigilant for the possibility of secondary gain), and outreach from other health professionals (e.g., the pharmacist) should be taken very seriously.

Prescription Drug Monitoring Programs (PDMPs)

Reviewing your state's PDMP prior to providing the first prescription and before issuing refills can provide essential safety data and is legally required in some states. This tool can help to detect concerning substance use behaviors such as early refills, outside prescribers, use of multiple pharmacies, and other evidence of "doctor shopping." In some states, the PDMP can be accessed on the prescriber's behalf by a clinical surrogate (e.g., nurse), and some health systems have worked with their state to allow for PDMP access directly through their electronic medical record via a single sign-on. The few moments it takes to gather this data is an important investment in patient safety, but practices should endeavor to access this resource efficiently and leverage the use of surrogates and support staff to minimize the associated burden on physician time [33]. Of note, not every controlled substance will show up in the PDMP. For example, methadone will not typically be visible when it is dispensed from a drug treatment program (i.e., not filled at a pharmacy).

Pill Counts

Periodically, and when concern for aberrant drug use behavior arises, it is prudent to ask the patient to bring their medication into the office for a pill count. If the patient is not able to account for missing medication, it suggests that the patient is either taking more of the medication than prescribed or diverting the medication elsewhere. In either case, this should prompt further assessment of the safety of ongoing opioid prescribing. Notably, asking patients to come to the office for pill counts can be inconvenient, and patients may interpret the request as a lack of trust. For these reasons, we advise clinicians to counsel patients about the potential need for this monitoring before the first prescription (e.g., in the CSA) and to standardize the practice as a routine part of safety monitoring.

Urine Drug Screening

Urine drug screening (UDS) should be part of the safety monitoring plan, and several excellent resources exist that outline best practices [34, 35]. Although UDS has several limitations (described below), it can provide objective data as to whether the patient is taking the prescribed medication and/or using non-prescribed or illegal substances, and this monitoring is part of the standard of care. When the need for UDS is disclosed up front and done routinely in a uniform safety-driven manner, potential stigma can be greatly reduced.

Although blood, hair, and nail testing can be used in some circumstances, urine is typically the most convenient and helpful substrate to test at the point of care. Depending on the assay, most controlled substances can be detected in the urine for

3 days or longer after last use, so it is important to ask the patient when they last took their medication before collecting urine for testing. If there is concern that the urine was adulterated, urine temperature, color, urinalysis, and/or urine creatinine can be used to verify the validity of the sample and detect dilution.

Interpreting UDS results requires an understanding of the assay used for testing and what medications your patient is taking. Immunoassays are good qualitative screening tests as they are inexpensive and result quickly, but they can be confounded by both false-positive and false-negative results. For example, a false negative may result if the patient is taking the medication as prescribed, but the measured value is just below the reporting threshold. Similarly, if your patient is taking a semisynthetic opioid such as oxycodone, it may not show up on an "opiate" immunoassay, which usually screens only for drugs that metabolize to morphine or codeine; in that case, it would need to be ordered separately. It is critically important to know what test you are ordering to understand what the results mean.

Unexpected results should be tested further with a confirmatory test (e.g., gas chromatography/mass spectrometry) on the same sample whenever possible. Many labs allow for reflex confirmatory testing, which can facilitate this process. These confirmatory tests are highly specific and quantitative, although slower to result and more expensive than screening immunoassays. Here, a knowledge of drug metabolism is extremely important. For example, if the prescriber is not aware that a small portion of hydrocodone is metabolized to hydromorphone and that substance is detected, they may mistakenly conclude that non-prescribed hydromorphone was being used. When in doubt, have a low threshold to reach out to your institution's toxicologist and lab specialists for further guidance on how to interpret a sample.

How often to test should depend on the clinician's assessment of risk. Getting a UDS before the first prescription is important for the reasons described previously, and UDS testing should then be done "periodically," but at least annually. We recommend urine drug testing on a quarterly basis and whenever the clinician suspects aberrant drug use behavior. Patient refusal to provide a urine sample for testing should be considered a red flag and warrants a careful reassessment as to whether opioids can continue to be safely prescribed.

The confirmed presence of an illegal or non-prescribed controlled substance in the urine should prompt a discussion and not an immediate termination of the drug and/or the patient. Additionally, cannabinoids have been legalized in many states (not federally) for medical and recreational use, so their presence needs to be considered within the regulatory framework of the state in which the physician is practicing. Cannabinoids may help with chronic pain management and can have an opioid-sparing effect, although a new meta-analysis published in November 2022 found the analgesic efficacy to be equivalent to placebo [36]; the medical use of cannabinoids is an area of active study and evolving regulatory changes. Of note, regular cannabinoid use can result in a persistently positive UDS for weeks to months after they are stopped, so this needs to be considered as well when interpreting the results of a UDS [37].

In contrast, the presence of a higher risk substance such as cocaine or methamphetamine represents a more immediate safety concern and may contraindicate the ongoing prescription of opioids if the patient is unable to refrain from future use. As always, the assessment of the best next step in these cases should be personalized, based on clinical judgment, and should prioritize safety. Patients with an active untreated substance use disorder may certainly have coexisting chronic pain, but opioid prescribing is rarely safe or appropriate in this circumstance. Repeatedly abnormal UDSs that demonstrate the presence of an illegal or non-prescribed controlled substance suggest that the patient has lost control over their prescription and substance use and addiction is likely. Opioids prescribed for analgesia should be tapered or discontinued, depending on the circumstances, and the patient should be treated (or referred) for addiction, as necessary. Importantly, a decision to discontinue opioid therapy should not equate to a decision to terminate the patient from the practice; a patient with a newly diagnosed substance use disorder needs ongoing care, and termination from the practice solely for this reason should be considered a form of patient abandonment [23].

Transparent, honest, and safety-focused communication is key when treating patients with chronic pain. Often, patients suffering from chronic pain—especially those on chronic opioid therapy—encounter stigma and discrimination during their care and may be "primed" to expect that you will discount their pain or look for a reason to discontinue their opioids. The wise prescriber will remain alert to the possibility of a scam (e.g., a patient who diverts most of their opioids for financial gain but saves a couple of doses to take before an anticipated UDS) but must also endeavor to remain sensitive to the many challenges patients face. The decision to prescribe or discontinue opioid therapy should be based on a rational and evidence-based assessment of the clinical circumstances, not on presumptions or countertransference.

Special Considerations for the Academic Medical Practice

Training

In an academic medical practice, physicians of variable experience and educational status share responsibility for the patients under their care. Without appropriate training and role modeling from attending physicians, patient safety can be jeopardized. Further, insufficient education will significantly disrupt resident confidence in how to prescribe opioids appropriately and safely in the ambulatory setting and may result in both overprescribing and underprescribing. To address this, we urge residency programs and academic medical practices to include dedicated training on safe opioid use early in the intern year, ideally during intern orientation. This should be supplemented by periodic faculty development and, when possible, availability of a local expert who can offer guidance to colleagues and trainees when complex cases arise. Additionally, the clinic director should prepare a summary of local clinic policies and regulatory requirements that is available for easy review.

We also recommend that the clinic director periodically audit the opioid prescribing patterns of their clinicians to identify the need for more training; use of chronic opioid registries or similar tools embedded within the EHR can facilitate this review. Opioids should be prescribed based on accepted medical principles and personalized to the clinical needs of the patient, so while there may be some variability, extremes in opioid prescribing suggest the need for additional education. Practices with some physicians who never prescribe opioids and others who do so very liberally should engage in reflection as to why this may be the case and look for opportunities to enhance training and standardization of care.

Standardizing Workflows

The importance of standardizing workflows cannot be overstated, especially in a busy resident clinic. When the approach to opioid prescribing varies significantly across the practice, the clinic can rapidly devolve into chaos, especially if there is inconsistency with how refills are handled.

For example, many residency programs function on a block schedule where residents periodically rotate in and out of the clinic setting, necessitating refills to be managed by colleagues. The academic medical practice should have a clearly defined approach to how refill requests are processed when the primary prescriber is on a nonambulatory rotation. Some clinics handle these refills via a "team resident" approach where a defined team of house staff and attendings manage a shared patient panel to preserve continuity. Other clinics utilize a rotating and less targeted "doc-of-the-day" approach. Still others ask the supervising attending to manage opioid refills in the resident's absence. Although unavoidable, prescribers should be aware that some PDMP systems may see multiple prescribers and inaccurately assign a patient a higher risk profile in their reports. Regardless of the approach the practice adopts, it should be deployed uniformly so that refill requests do not linger in an absent clinician's electronic in-basket, unseen and unfilled.

Relatedly, it is important to define how and when refill requests can be processed. For example, an academic medical practice should have a clear policy on whether controlled substance refills will be managed after hours or on weekends to minimize miscommunication and to preserve the sanity of the on-call physician. We strongly encourage clinics to adopt a policy that restricts opioid refills to normal business hours so that the treating physician can have sufficient time to review the refill request for safety.

There should also be a standardized workflow on how to handle early refill requests. If the request comes earlier than expected, is there a process by which the clinical support team communicates with the patient or pharmacy to determine why? Can the EHR be set up so that early requests are automatically flagged for review? Some patients may have previously encountered difficulty getting their refills handled in a timely way, so they may request refills early for fear that the prescription will not be processed in time. Having an organized, consistent, and logical process for managing refill requests benefits both patients and prescribers.

In addition to refill requests, academic medical practices should also standardize safety monitoring processes. Depending on the state, clinical support staff (e.g., RNs) may be able to access the PDMP on behalf of the prescriber, which can improve physician efficiency while enhancing safety. The clinical support team can also operationalize pill counts, UDS testing, and questionnaires to evaluate pain and to screen for opioid misuse (e.g., the Current Opioid Misuse Measure) [38] at defined intervals for an "average-risk" patient. We urge the clinic leadership to work with their teams so that everyone works to the top of their training and coordinates their efforts to improve opioid prescribing safety.

Institutional Drug Enforcement Administration (DEA) Number Use

Residents practicing in their sponsoring hospital's on-site clinic may be permitted to prescribe controlled substances to patients of the practice using the hospital's site-specific institutional DEA number, with an assigned suffix, as outlined by 21 CFR 1301.22 from the Code of Federal Regulations [39]. However, the DEA currently takes the position that residents practicing off-site at nonhospital-owned practices may *not* use the hospital's site-specific institutional DEA number for patients of the practice. Instead, the DEA requires the house staff either use that institution's own institutional DEA number—if they have one—or that controlled substances be prescribed only by clinicians assigned their own individual DEA number. In practice, this means that residents are not allowed to prescribe controlled substances at all in that practice setting. This is unfortunate as it negatively impacts residents' medical education; residents must learn to prescribe controlled substances safely, and this shortsighted stance deprives them of the ability to do so under supervision. Additionally, forbidding residents from prescribing controlled substances in an academic medical practice also impairs the clinic's ability to provide timely patient care. With this restriction in place, prescriptions cannot be filled by the patient's resident primary care provider but instead need to be passed along to other physicians for additional review, adding complexity and delay to what should be a straightforward process. Furthermore, Section IV.C.3.g(7) of the Accreditation Council for Graduate Medical Education (ACGME) Program Requirements for Graduate Medical Education specifically states: "residents must write all orders for patients under their care, with appropriate supervision by the attending physician ...," so this DEA prohibition violates that requirement. For all these reasons, several institutions are contesting the DEA's stance. However, until and unless things change, practices must ensure that processes are in place to prevent residents from prescribing opioids or any other controlled substance while working in those settings.

Treating Opioid Use Disorder

As previously detailed, safe opioid prescribing also requires the clinician to know when opioids are no longer safe to use and when the patient has developed an opioid use disorder. The academic medical practice can address this by incorporating training about buprenorphine prescribing and substance use disorder management into the educational curriculum. Several functional models for enhancing resident training in opioid use disorder exist, and we encourage the clinic director to take a leadership role in organizing this effort [40, 41].

Monitoring Best Practices and Quality Improvement

The ACGME Common Program Requirements prioritize quality improvement, practice-based learning, and faculty development as core objectives [42]. Academic medical practices are well positioned to implement initiatives to meet these goals with a focus on opioid safety. For example, the clinic director can partner with core faculty and practice management to audit opioid use and assess for adherence to best practices (e.g., controlled substance agreements, naloxone co-prescribing, urine drug screen testing) or risky prescribing (e.g., high-dose opioids, benzodiazepine co-prescribing). As gaps are identified, quality improvement initiatives as well as focused training (see prior section) can be implemented with the dual objectives of improving patient safety and enhancing medical education.

Conclusion

The evaluation and management of pain are unavoidable in primary care, and opioid therapy continues to play an important—although increasingly limited—treatment role. As potentially helpful but dangerous medications, the regulatory landscape of opioid prescribing continues to tighten and medical education on safe opioid prescribing is more important than ever. The academic medical practice stands at the intersection of care delivery and ambulatory medical education, so it is critical for the clinic director and the residency program to develop educational and opioid-related practice standards to protect patients and to guarantee that the next generation of prescribers will be able to prescribe opioids as safely and effectively as possible.

Appendix

Delivery Network/Location NAME: BIRTH DATE: MRN: DOS: (If handwritten, patient name, MRN, birth date, and DOS)	**Patient-Clinician Agreement for the Safe Use of Controlled Substances**

Your clinician has recommended a medication to treat your pain or anxiety called a "controlled substance". Common examples include opioids (sometimes called "narcotics") and sedatives.

These medications can be very helpful, but they can also be very dangerous. This agreement explains possible benefits and risks to help you decide if this kind of medication is best for you.

To use these medications, you must also agree to follow our office rules and expectations for your safety. If we can't prescribe them to you safely, we can't prescribe them to you at all.

Safety monitoring is for everyone. We monitor every patient receiving opioids or sedatives from our practice for their safety.

Possible benefits of opioids or sedatives:

- May improve your function both at home and at work
- May improve your pain or anxiety, although this may wear off over time. Opioids will probably not make your pain go away completely
- May improve your sleep by managing your pain and anxiety
- May help you to take better care of yourself by reducing your pain and anxiety
- May let your clinician spend more time helping you with your other medical problems by reducing your pain and anxiety
- May improve your quality of life overall

Possible risks of opioids or sedatives:

- May cause overdose, especially if the medication is not taken as directed or the dose is too high. Overdose can cause you to stop breathing which may be life threatening
- May cause your body to become physically dependent on these medications if they are used regularly for longer than one week. If this happens and the medication is stopped suddenly, you may have withdrawal and feel sick (flu-like symptoms, tremor, increased pain). If a sedative is stopped suddenly, it can cause seizures and can rarely be life threatening
- May cause addiction in some people. Overdose and addiction are more likely when opioids or sedatives are mixed with each other, alcohol, illegal drugs, or other controlled substances
- May cause confusion, sleepiness, and falls. Your driving may also be impaired, even if you don't realize it, which can lead to motor vehicle accidents
- May cause side effects including nausea, vomiting, constipation, itching, problems with erections and sexual function
- May hide the symptoms of other serious medical problems. Sometimes opioids can also cause your pain to get worse over time
- May increase your risk for theft or assault if people know you have these medications
- May cause serious harm or death to other people if they use your medications. All controlled substances need to be stored and disposed of safely

Safety and informed consent:

If you and your clinician agree that the possible benefits of these medications are greater than their risks at this time, you must follow our office rules for your safety. **Your clinician must stop prescribing these medications if they cannot be sure they are safe for you.**

Delivery Network/Location
NAME:
BIRTH DATE:
MRN:
DOS:
(If handwritten, patient name, MRN, birth date, and DOS)

Patient-Clinician Agreement for the Safe Use of Controlled Substances

Our office rules and requirements:

- All of our clinicians will monitor the safe use of these medications
- Only your clinician's team can give you these medicines. They cannot be prescribed to you from another medical office
- We cannot refill your controlled substance medications early. If your medication is lost, stolen, or used up sooner than expected we will not be able to replace it
- Refills take time to do safely. We can't refill controlled medications urgently or at the end of the day
- Our on-call clinicians cannot prescribe opioids or sedatives after-hours or on weekends
- You must keep your appointments with us for refills and monitoring
- If you do not give us an adequate urine sample for drug testing or bring in your pills when we ask you to, we will not be able to give you a refill of your medication at that time
- We prescribe generic (non-brand name) medications whenever possible
- For safety, we need to communicate with your other medical team members. We will not be able to prescribe controlled medications if you don't allow us to do this
- Violent, threatening, or disruptive behavior in our waiting room or our office must never happen, will not be tolerated, and may force us to discharge you from our practice

Your responsibilities: For your safety, we expect you to agree to the following:

- I will fill my medications at one pharmacy only. My pharmacy is:____________________
- I will tell all of my clinicians that you are giving me these medications, including the emergency room if I go there. I will not accept controlled substance prescriptions from another clinician unless they have spoken to your team
- I will let you know what other medications I am taking and if they change
- I will let you speak with my other clinicians and members of my family about my use of pain and sedative medications if needed for my safety
- I will use my medications only as directed. I won't take extra doses or change them on my own
- I will never give or sell my medications to anyone else for any reason
- I will not use anyone else's medications, even if they take the same medication I do
- I will lock up my medications somewhere safe and hide them from strangers and children
- I will safely dispose of my unused medications as instructed by my clinician or pharmacist. I will not save or store unused or expired controlled substance medications
- I will bring my pill bottles with me to my appointments if asked to
- I will tell you if I have any side effects or if the medications aren't working
- I will not use illegal drugs (cocaine, heroin, LSD, PCP, etc.) and I will avoid heavy alcohol or cannabis (marijuana) use. I know this mix is very dangerous
- I will keep my appointments with you and the specialists you refer me to
- I will not wait until the last minute to ask for a refill or walk-in to ask for a medication
- I will let you know if I am pregnant or if I am trying to get pregnant. I know you want to keep me and my baby safe

Our commitment to you:

- We will help you understand the possible benefits and risks of taking these useful but dangerous medications
- We will monitor your safety. This will include:
  - Randomly testing your urine for medications and other drugs,
  - Regularly reviewing your medical, pharmacy, and refill records,
  - Counting the number of pills you have left in each bottle, sometimes between visits,
  - Monitoring the Prescription Monitoring and Reporting System (legally required in our state)

Page 2 of 3

Delivery Network/Location
NAME:
BIRTH DATE:
MRN:
DOS:
(If handwritten, patient name, MRN, birth date, and DOS)

Patient-Clinician Agreement for the Safe Use of Controlled Substances

- We will not use these medications by themselves. They will be prescribed only with other helpful treatments (such as physical therapy) as part of a treatment plan
- We will ask for help when we need it. We may refer you to a specialist (such as a neurologist, orthopedist, or psychiatrist) if necessary
- We will keep up to date with new ways to treat pain and anxiety
- We will help you get the care you need, including treatment for addiction and mental health problems if necessary
- We will still treat your pain and anxiety in other ways if we decide that controlled substances are no longer safe or working for you and need to be stopped
- **We will not continue to prescribe opioids or sedatives if we don't think they are safe or helping you anymore**

By signing below, my clinician and I confirm that we spoke about these possible risks and benefits and how to use these medications safely. I understand the agreement, agree with the office rules, and had all of my questions answered.

Patient Signature

Time ________ Date ________ Patient's Signature ________________ Patient's Printed Name ________________

Authorized Patient's Representative Signature

To be used if patient is a minor, or otherwise lacking in decision making capacity:

Time ________ Date ________ Signature of Authorized Patient's Representative ________________ Printed Name of Authorized Patient's Representative ________________

I, ______________________ (Name) the ______________________ (Relationship to patient) hereby give consent on his/her behalf

Prescriber Signature

Time ________ Date ________ Prescriber's Signature / Title ________________ Prescriber's Printed Name / Title ________________

Interpretation Services (if necessary): An interpreter facilitated the communication between the health care provider(s) and the patient or person authorized to consent for the patient in ______________________ (language) to assist in obtaining informed consent.

The interpreter conveyed the content of the original information expressed by and for both parties.

Time: __________ AM/PM Date: ______________

Check here if: ☐ Telephone ☐ Video Interpreter ☐ Interpreter ☐ Bilingual Competency Program

ID Number (telephone/video only): ______________________

Print Name of Interpreter ______________________ Signature of **Interpreter (face to face only)** ______________________

Page 3 of 3

References

1. Macht DI. The history of opium and some of its preparations and alkaloids. J Am Med Assoc. 1915;LXIV(6):477–81.
2. Zelaya CE, Dahlhamer JM, Lucas JW, Connor EM. Chronic Pain and High-impact Chronic Pain Among U.S. Adults, 2019. NCHS Data Brief 2020(390):1–8.
3. Institute of Medicine (U.S.). Committee on Advancing Pain Research Care and Education. Relieving pain in America a blueprint for transforming prevention, care, education, and research. Washington, D.C.: National Academies Press; 2011. http://www.nap.edu/openbook.php?record_id=13172.
4. Mills S, Torrance N, Smith BH. Identification and Management of Chronic Pain in primary care: a review. Curr Psychiatry Rep. 2016;18(2):22.
5. Karos K. Discrimination as one of the social plights facing people with pain. Pain. 2022;163(2):e149–e50.
6. Vowles KE, McEntee ML, Julnes PS, Frohe T, Ney JP, van der Goes DN. Rates of opioid misuse, abuse, and addiction in chronic pain: a systematic review and data synthesis. Pain. 2015;156(4):569–76.
7. Centers for Disease Control and Prevention. Drug Overdose Deaths in the U.S. Top 100,000 Annually. National Center for Health Statistics. https://www.cdc.gov/nchs/pressroom/nchs_press_releases/2021/20211117.htm#:~:text=The%20new%20data%20documents%20that%20estimated%20overdose%20deaths,in%20the%2012-month%20period%20ending%20in%20April%202021. Accessed 7 May 2022.
8. Jones MR, Viswanath O, Peck J, Kaye AD, Gill JS, Simopoulos TT. A brief history of the opioid epidemic and strategies for pain medicine. Pain Ther. 2018;7(1):13–21.
9. Rummans TA, Burton MC, Dawson NL. How good intentions contributed to bad outcomes: the opioid crisis. Mayo Clin Proc. 2018;93(3):344–50.
10. Roehr B. US needs new strategy to help 116 million patients in chronic pain. BMJ. 2011;343:d4206.
11. Breuer B, Pappagallo M, Tai JY, Portenoy RK. U.S. board-certified pain physician practices: uniformity and census data of their locations. J Pain. 2007;8(3):244–50.
12. Van Zee A. The promotion and marketing of oxycontin: commercial triumph, public health tragedy. Am J Public Health. 2009;99(2):221–7.
13. Centers for Disease Control and Prevention. Opioid painkiller prescribing, where you live makes a difference. Atlanta, GA: Centers for Disease Control and Prevention; 2014. http://www.cdc.gov/vitalsigns/opioid-prescribing/. Accessed 7 May 2022.
14. Shipton EE, Bate F, Garrick R, Steketee C, Shipton EA, Visser EJ. Systematic review of pain medicine content, teaching, and assessment in medical school curricula internationally. Pain Ther. 2018;7(2):139–61.
15. Gudin J, Fudin J. A narrative pharmacological review of buprenorphine: a unique opioid for the treatment of chronic pain. Pain Ther. 2020;9(1):41–54.
16. Chou R, Hartung D, Turner J, Blazina I, Chan B, Levander X, et al. Opioid treatments for chronic pain. AHRQ comparative effectiveness reviews. Rockville, MD; 2020.
17. Cheatle MD, Compton PA, Dhingra L, Wasser TE, O'Brien CP. Development of the revised opioid risk tool to predict opioid use disorder in patients with chronic nonmalignant pain. J Pain. 2019;20(7):842–51.
18. Moore TM, Jones T, Browder JH, Daffron S, Passik SD. A comparison of common screening methods for predicting aberrant drug-related behavior among patients receiving opioids for chronic pain management. Pain Med (Malden, Mass). 2009;10(8):1426–33.
19. Krebs EE, Lorenz KA, Bair MJ, Damush TM, Wu J, Sutherland JM, et al. Development and initial validation of the PEG, a three-item scale assessing pain intensity and interference. J Gen Intern Med. 2009;24(6):733–8.

20. Bohnert AB, Valenstein M, Bair MJ, et al. ASsociation between opioid prescribing patterns and opioid overdose-related deaths. JAMA. 2011;305(13):1315–21.
21. Dasgupta N, Funk MJ, Proescholdbell S, Hirsch A, Ribisl KM, Marshall S. Cohort study of the impact of high-dose opioid analgesics on overdose mortality. Pain Med (Malden, Mass). 2016;17(1):85–98.
22. Tobin DG, Keough Forte K, Johnson MGS. Breaking the pain contract: a better controlled-substance agreement for patients on chronic opioid therapy. Cleve Clin J Med. 2016;83(11):827–35.
23. Tobin DG, Holt SR, Doolittle BR. Responding to unsafe opioid use: abandon the drug, not the patient. J Gen Intern Med. 2021;36(3):790–1.
24. Tobin DG, Andrews R, Becker WC. Prescribing opioids in primary care: safely starting, monitoring, and stopping. Cleve Clin J Med. 2016;83(3):207–15.
25. Zhang H, Tallavajhala S, Kapadia SN, Jeng PJ, Shi Y, Wen H, et al. State opioid limits and volume of opioid prescriptions received by medicaid patients. Med Care. 2020;58(12):1111–5.
26. Miller M, Barber CW, Leatherman S, Fonda J, Hermos JA, Cho K, et al. Prescription opioid duration of action and the risk of unintentional overdose among patients receiving opioid therapy. JAMA Intern Med. 2015;175(4):608–15.
27. Chou R, Cruciani RA, Fiellin DA, Compton P, Farrar JT, Haigney MC, et al. Methadone safety: a clinical practice guideline from the American Pain Society and College on problems of drug dependence, in collaboration with the Heart Rhythm Society. J Pain. 2014;15(4):321–37.
28. Dowell D, Haegerich TM, Chou R. CDC guideline for prescribing opioids for chronic pain—United States, 2016. JAMA. 2016;315(15):1624–45.
29. Dowell D, Ragan KR, Jones CM, Baldwin GT, Chou R. CDC clinical practice guideline for prescribing opioids for pain—United States, 2022. MMWR Recomm Rep. 2022;71(3):1–95.
30. Pereira J, Lawlor P, Vigano A, Dorgan M, Bruera E. Equianalgesic dose ratios for opioids. A critical review and proposals for long-term dosing. J Pain Symptom Manag. 2001;22(2):672–87.
31. Oliva EM, Bowe T, Manhapra A, Kertesz S, Hah JM, Henderson P, et al. Associations between stopping prescriptions for opioids, length of opioid treatment, and overdose or suicide deaths in US veterans: observational evaluation. BMJ. 2020;368:m283.
32. Department of Health and Human Services. Practice guidelines for the administration of buprenorphine for treating opioid use disorder. Federal Register, 2021. 86(80):22,439–40. [pdf]. https://www.govinfo.gov/content/pkg/FR-2021-04-28/pdf/2021-08961.pdf. Accessed 8 May 2022.
33. Tobin DG. A balance of burdens: pain, opioids, and the cost of prescription drug monitoring. Pain Med (Malden, Mass). 2018;19(10):1905–6.
34. Jannetto PJ, Langman LJ. Using clinical laboratory tests to monitor drug therapy in pain management patients. J Appl Labor Med. 2019;2(4):471–2.
35. Argoff CE, Alford DP, Fudin J, Adler JA, Bair MJ, Dart RC, et al. Rational urine drug monitoring in patients receiving opioids for chronic pain: consensus recommendations. Pain Med (Malden, Mass). 2018;19(1):97–117.
36. Gedin F, Blome S, Ponten M, Lalouni M, Fust J, Raquette A, et al. Placebo response and media attention in randomized clinical trials assessing cannabis-based therapies for pain: a systematic review and meta-analysis. JAMA Netw Open. 2022;5(11):e2243848.
37. Lowe RH, Abraham TT, Darwin WD, Herning R, Cadet JL, Huestis MA. Extended urinary Delta9-tetrahydrocannabinol excretion in chronic cannabis users precludes use as a biomarker of new drug exposure. Drug Alcohol Depend. 2009;105(1–2):24–32.
38. Butler SF, Budman SH, Fernandez KC, Houle B, Benoit C, Katz N, et al. Development and validation of the current opioid misuse measure. Pain. 2007;130(1–2):144–56.
39. National Archives. Code of Federal Regulations. Title 21, Chapter II, Part 1301. § 1301.22 Exemption of agents and employees; affiliated practitioners. https://www.ecfr.gov/current/title-21/chapter-II/part-1301/subject-group-ECFRa5bd18e3d01cd02/section-1301.22. Accessed 8 May 2022.

40. Graddy R, Accurso AJ, Nandiwada DR, Shalaby M, Holt SR. Models of resident physician training in opioid use disorders. Curr Addict Rep. 2019;6(4):355–64.
41. Holt SR, Segar N, Cavallo DA, Tetrault JM. The addiction recovery clinic: a novel, primary-care-based approach to teaching addiction medicine. Acad Med. 2017;92(5):680–3.
42. Accreditation Council for Graduate Medical Education. Common program requirements (Residency); 2020. https://www.acgme.org/globalassets/PFAssets/ProgramRequirements/CPRResidency2021.pdf. Accessed 8 May 2022.

Chapter 17
Leading a Substance Use Disorder Clinic

Carolyn A. Chan, Jeanette M. Tetrault, and Stephen R. Holt

Abbreviations

ACGME	Accreditation Council for Graduate Medical Education
AUD	Alcohol use disorder
CM	Contingency management
CME	Continuing medical education
DEA	Drug Enforcement Administration
GME	Graduate medical education
OBOT	Office-based opioid treatment
OTP	Opioid treatment program
OUD	Opioid use disorder
SAMHSA	Substance Abuse and Mental Health Services
SUD	Substance use disorder
UDT	Urine drug testing
UME	Undergraduate medical education
XR-BUP	Extended-release buprenorphine
XR-NTX	Ext5ended-release naltrexone

C. A. Chan
Division of General Internal Medicine, Department of Internal Medicine, University of Cincinnati Medical Center, Cincinnati, Ohio, USA
e-mail: chancl@ucmail.uc.edu

J. M. Tetrault · S. R. Holt (✉)
Program in Addiction Medicine, Section of General Internal Medicine, Department of Medicine, Yale School of Medicine, New Haven, CT, USA
e-mail: Jeanette.Tetrault@yale.edu; Stephen.Holt@yale.edu

L. B. Lu et al. (eds.), *Leading an Academic Medical Practice*,
https://doi.org/10.1007/978-3-031-40273-9_17

Introduction

Substance use disorders (SUDs) are widespread and are urgent public health issues that must be addressed within academic medicine. This chapter outlines a series of practical steps and considerations to develop a dedicated SUD clinic within an academic medical practice. Topics covered in this chapter include a stepwise approach to the development of such a clinic: defining clinic goals, defining a curricular approach, exploring institutional support, establishing clinic logistics, and "taking it to the next level" by expanding clinical and educational initiatives. To address the alarming rates of overdose deaths due to opioids and other substances, there is a critical need for academic medical centers to expand access to addiction treatment services within their departments.

Outline

- Overview
- Steps to setting up a substance use disorder clinic within a residency program primary care practice
  - Step one: define goals
  - Step two: define curricular approach
  - Step three: institutional support
  - Step four: patient and population considerations
  - Step five: clinic logistics
  - Step six: taking it to the next level
- Clinical initiatives
- Educational initiatives
- Conclusion

Part I: Overview

Substance use disorder (SUD) remains a prominent public health issue that has resulted in alarming rates of opioid, stimulant, and polysubstance overdose deaths [1]. The COVID-19 pandemic has only exacerbated the overdose crisis, as well as increased adult alcohol use [1, 2]. SUD's consequences extend beyond overdose deaths to include negative impacts on individual relationships, financial well-being, family stability, and risk for significant medical complications such as severe infection [3, 4]. Expanding access to addiction treatment services is paramount. In 2020, among individuals aged 12 years and older with an SUD in the past year, only an estimated 6.5% (2.6 million people) received any substance use treatment in the past year in the United States [5]. To address this crisis and decrease overdose-related deaths, internists must play an active role in helping to close the gap in screening, identification, and treatment of SUD.

This wide gap exists in part due to stigma and misconceptions around SUD, as well as a lack of SUD training in the primary care workforce at undergraduate medical education (UME), graduate medical education (GME), and continuing medical education (CME), as well as other health professional trainees and practitioners including physician assistants and advanced nurse practitioners [6]. Many highly effective medications used for the treatment of SUD remain underutilized in all medical settings. For example, it has been over 20 years since the passage of the Drug Addiction Treatment Act of 2000 (DATA 2000), which made it possible for clinicians to prescribe office-based buprenorphine for the treatment of opioid use disorder (OUD); yet, among those who have a waiver to prescribe buprenorphine, only about 51% reported writing at least one buprenorphine prescription in the past 22 months [7]. A survey of primary care physicians (PCPs) found that only 36% of participants reported feeling comfortable treating OUD with medications, with only 10% of PCPs reporting that they had the necessary waiver to prescribe buprenorphine for the treatment of OUD [8]. To expand access to lifesaving medications for addiction treatment, such as buprenorphine, residency programs must provide meaningful didactic and clinical training in addiction medicine. One way to do so is to establish a dedicated SUD clinical and learning experience within a residency program.

Currently, addiction medicine curricular content within medical schools' standard UME and GME training remains sparse. Throughout 4 years of UME education, an average of only 12 hours of curricular time is devoted to the topic of SUD [9]. This education tends to vary in content and teaching intensity, with a range of topics taught such as brief intervention and referral to treatment (SBIRT), opioid overdose response, and medication management of OUD with buprenorphine [10]. Within GME education, a national survey of internal medicine (IM) residency programs in 2019 reported that 71% of programs required a didactic for treating OUD, yet only 11.7% offered an ambulatory addiction medicine clinic rotation [11]. Even fewer programs offered addiction consult services (4.6%), and only 0.3% of residents completed buprenorphine training [11]. Notably, in a review of training modules to teach resident physicians to care for those with OUD, less than half of the interventions involved direct patient care [12]. Effective on July first, 2022, the ACGME requires IM programs to provide instruction within the multidisciplinary subspecialty of addiction medicine in their core educational content [13].

Investment in addiction medicine education involving direct patient care is likely to promote interest within the field. Educational interventions involving patient care have been noted to lead to residency graduates obtaining a DATA 2000 waiver to prescribe buprenorphine and prescribing the medication, which at this time is the gold standard in the care of patients with OUD treated in general medical settings [14]. Furthermore, residents have reported a desire to obtain education in prescribing buprenorphine if offered by their program [15]. Several programs have successfully created clinical sites to care for patients with SUD [16, 17]. Residency programs that have adopted robust, required, patient-centered, experiential addiction medicine training opportunities have successfully fostered an interest in treating patients with SUD [17]. Therefore, we suggest a series of steps (Fig. 17.1) that may be useful in developing and implementing an SUD clinic within a longitudinal residency practice. We recognize, in practice, that not all steps will be feasible or necessary depending on local resources (e.g., faculty with clinical expertise in addiction or the ability of the clinic to provide injectable medications). Of note, in this chapter, we focus on substances other than tobacco/nicotine, yet encourage clinics to include smoking cessation counseling and pharmacotherapy as a component of their primary care clinical practice. Likewise, while cannabis is not a focus of this chapter, certain clinics may elect to provide evidence-based treatment based on their preferences and local needs.

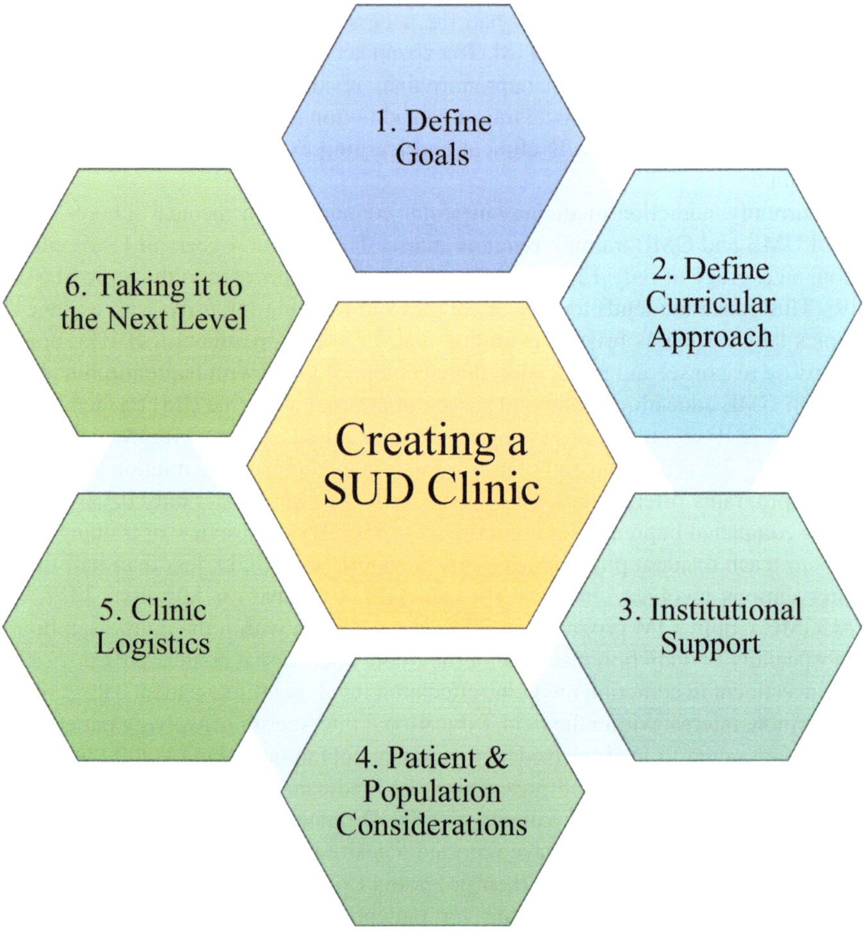

Fig. 17.1 A series of six suggested steps we have found helpful in developing and implementing a SUD clinic within a residency longitudinal practice. In practice, not all steps will be feasible or necessary depending on local circumstances

Part II: Steps to Setting up a Substance Use Disorder Clinic within a Residency Program Primary Care Practice

Step 1: Define Goals

The initial step in developing an outpatient SUD clinic integrated within a residency program is to define goals. An SUD clinic for residents can have a broad spectrum of goals and offer a variety of services. The purpose of the clinic may range from a straightforward assessment and referral to treatment for individuals with substance use to comprehensive on-site treatment that includes treating individuals with medications for all SUDs (opioid, benzodiazepine, alcohol, nicotine, stimulant, and cannabis use disorders) with the integration of behavioral care in the clinic (Fig. 17.2). Based on local needs, some clinics may opt to focus on a subset of disorders such as

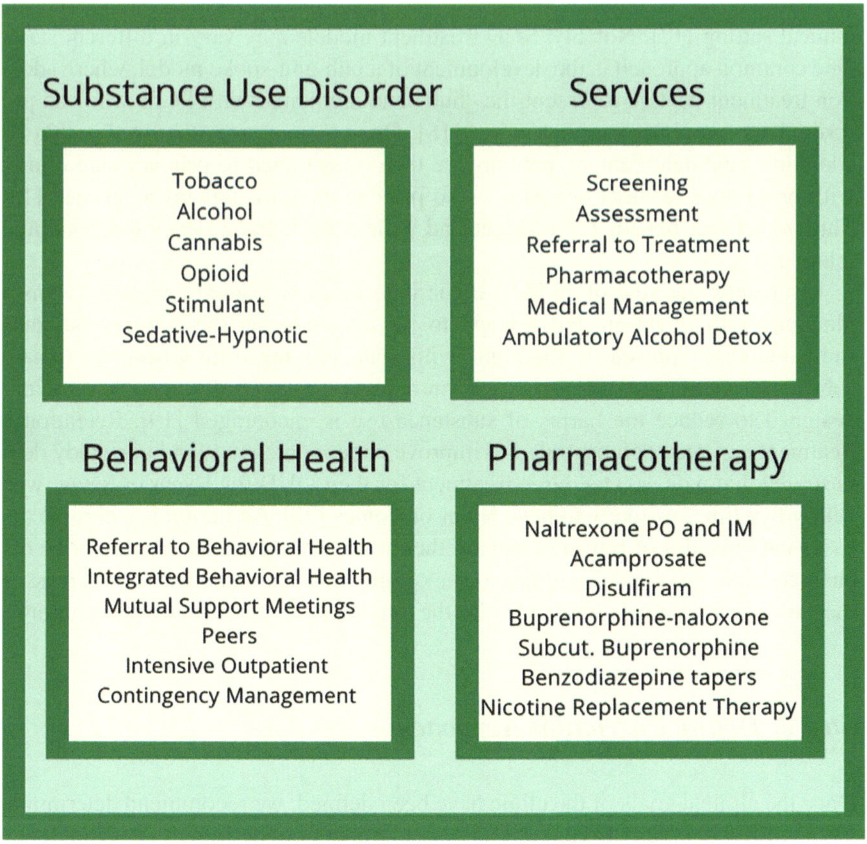

Fig. 17.2 Defining goals

alcohol use disorder (AUD) or OUD alone. Core components may include an array of options such as medications for opioid use disorder (MOUD), AUD pharmacotherapy, and a modicum of behavioral health support such as group visits or peer support. Figure 17.2 outlines several categories that one may consider when defining clinic goals.

To aid this effort, a targeted needs assessment should be performed to determine what current clinical and educational opportunities exist at your institution. This includes looking at addiction electives, or other specialties currently offering addiction services including psychiatry, family medicine, addiction psychiatry, addiction medicine, correctional medication electives, and high-risk obstetrics. In addition, obtaining information on local didactics such as DATA 2000 waiver trainings, lectures, and academic half-day content on SUD can be helpful in defining the scope of the curriculum. This will help create a balance of meeting the local clinical need for these services, as well as the educational need of the residents.

A helpful step in the needs assessment might include visiting another program to observe the implementation of goals and integrated core components within the clinical setting [12]. Notably, SUD treatment models may vary in different states. One common approach is the development of a hub-and-spoke model, where addiction treatment centers represent the "hub" and are paired with PCPs who can prescribe buprenorphine as the "spoke" [18]. Once patients are stabilized within the addiction treatment centers, patients are then transitioned to primary care clinics, with or without resident providers, who provide ongoing support as needed [18]. This model can benefit the resident and patient by helping develop a continuity relationship.

Ultimately, the goal of an SUD clinic is to focus on patient-centered treatment planning with retention and linkage to ongoing care as the primary outcome. Individuals may present to the clinic with goals ranging from abstinence to safer substance use practices. Embracing harm reduction as a set of pragmatic principles designed to reduce the harms of substance use is encouraged [19]. Retention in treatment has been demonstrated to improve patient outcomes, and one study demonstrated that patients staying in treatment for their OUD for 1 year or longer were nearly five times as likely to have better outcomes [20]. Addiction is a chronic disease, and episodes of return to use are the norm. Thus, patients should not be discharged from the clinic if a return to use occurs; instead, clinicians should reassess the patient's individual goals and tailor the treatment recommendations accordingly.

Step 2: Define Curricular Approach

Once the clinical goals of the clinic have been defined, we recommend determining the educational goals of the clinic. A key component underlying the curriculum is ensuring that the clinic adopts the use of accurate, non-stigmatizing medical terminology when discussing addiction medicine topics with leadership, staff, learners, patients, and families [21]. The use of language such as "abuse," "addict," "alcoholic," and "clean or dirty urine" should be avoided and replaced with person-first language, such as replacing the term "addict" with "patient with an SUD." Research suggests that stigmatizing language can negatively impact patient care [22]. Clinic staff modeling person-first language will help decrease stigma towards individuals with SUDs [22–24]. Training faculty and staff on the use of preferred terminology for individuals with SUD should be a component of developing your clinic.

The structure and delivery of addiction medicine education may vary, and the 2022 ACGME common program requirements have included addiction as the core content for internal medicine residency programs. Ideally, all residents will have some form of clinical experience providing assessment and treatment to individuals with SUDs. For example, an addiction subspeciality clinic could be created where trainees can rotate to learn how to assess and initiate treatment, while more stable patients with SUD can be cared for in primary care [18]. Depending on the ability of faculty to provide supervision in the management of SUD (i.e., buprenorphine for treatment of OUD, or familiarity with using medications for treatment of AUD), some programs may need to link learner curricula to faculty development activities [17]. Lastly, efforts should be made to maximize continuity for residents so they can gain experience in SUD chronic disease management.

In addition to addiction medicine clinical experiences, due to the heterogeneity of addiction education at the UME level, developing standard teaching content is necessary, so individuals will develop knowledge of medications and psychosocial interventions for SUD. Preclinic teaching, delivered immediately before the dedicated half-day SUD clinic sessions, is one method that may be used, so learners can immediately apply new knowledge in the context of direct patient care [17]. For programs that elect to integrate addiction experiences within a resident continuity panel, care should be taken to ensure that *all* residents receive core didactic and skill-based training in the diagnosis, assessment, and treatment of SUD.

Step 3: Institutional Support

Identifying local clinical champions as well as securing both institutional and educational support is an important step in establishing and sustaining an SUD clinic. For those developing a half-day SUD clinic, arranging a meeting with department and residency program leadership will be important to develop an attending staffing model. For example, one program created an attending staffing model utilizing 0.1 full-time equivalents for one half-day of precepting time in such a clinic [17]. When integrating addiction treatment, such as office-based opioid treatment (OBOT) within a residency continuity clinic, one should discuss at the leadership meeting how to ensure that residents will be paired with a consistent faculty member that feels comfortable prescribing buprenorphine for the treatment of OUD [18]. Recruiting new faculty, or providing faculty development for existing faculty, may be necessary [16]. In addition, consider seeking support for multidisciplinary staff such as APRNs or PAs, clinical psychologists, and licensed clinical social workers to integrate within your clinic site.

Step 4: Patient and Population Considerations

To provide care for individuals with SUD, we recommend clarifying insurance coverage for relevant medications (e.g., buprenorphine-naloxone formulations) and office visits, particularly for Medicaid/Medicare-covered individuals. Prior authorizations or annual limits may be imposed based on Medicaid formularies in certain states. Notably, states with Medicaid prior authorization requirements have been linked to lower odds of buprenorphine provision among addiction treatment programs [25]. Understanding state Medicaid coverage will assist with providing seamless evidence-based treatment as well as improve clinic efficiency.

Next steps include identifying referral sources for patients. Some examples may include the emergency department, a primary care practice, inpatient referrals, intensive outpatient programs, halfway houses, "hub-and-spoke model" [18], or inpatient addiction treatment service referrals. Factors to consider when eliciting referrals may include EMR integration, volume of referrals, geographic location, and community need. Depending on the referral source, an addiction medicine clinic may expect a range of show rates. For example, in our experience, patients referred internally from within our primary care practice have a higher show rate than individuals referred from the emergency department.

In addition to seeking referral sources, identifying and partnering with local community resources as well as with interprofessional team members are crucial to the success of a clinic. Many individuals will benefit from the addition of psychosocial interventions to their treatment plan. Knowing how to refer to intensive outpatient programs, psychologists, recovery coaches, peers, and mutual self-help groups is beneficial. Furthermore, as addiction is a chronic relapsing-remitting disease, individuals may, at times, require additional support beyond the outpatient clinic, such as detoxification or residential treatment. The American Society of Addiction Medicine (ASAM) has developed formal criteria for the level of care of treatment programs, which range from early intervention (level 0.5) to medically managed intensive treatment programs (level 4.0) [26]. Identifying local resources and the level of care they provide, as well as understanding the details of how to refer to these facilities, insurance coverage constraints, and overall availability, is crucial to the success of a nascent addiction clinic.

Beyond referral sources, to protect individuals with SUDs against discrimination, additional privacy regulations apply in certain conditions. These are defined by federal privacy regulation under 42 code of federal regulations Part 2 (42 CFR part 2) [27]. It requires that clinics whose primary function is providing addiction treatment (e.g., addiction specialty clinics) must have written consent before releasing SUD treatment information [27]. In contrast, 42 CFR Part 2 does not apply to clinicians who are providing SUD treatment within a primary care setting or integrated care setting (e.g., PCP prescribing buprenorphine to their longitudinal patient) [27]. How an addiction medicine clinic is integrated into a health care system, as well as the staffing model, will determine whether 42 CFR Part 2 privacy regulations will apply. We recommend meeting with your institution's compliance officer to assist with this determination.

Step 5: Clinic Logistics

Once the above issues have been worked out, there remain several practical considerations to address, particularly with regard to the use of OBOT. While providers previously needed to complete DATA waiver training (informally called the X-waiver), this requirement was eliminated on December 29, 2022 with President Biden's signing of the Consolidation Appropriations Act of 2023, which contained the Mainstreaming Addition Treatment Act. Currently, any individual with a DEA license can prescribe buprenorphine for the treatment of OUD in accordance with their state's scope of practice. Faculty who previously were not prescribing buprenorphine may require additional training or support as they gain comfort and familiarity with prescribing this medication.

Methadone for the treatment of OUD, in contrast to buprenorphine, is not an option for most residency-based SUD clinics, as federal regulations require that methadone for the treatment of OUD can only be provided via federally licensed methadone opioid treatment program (OTP) (i.e., methadone cannot be prescribed for OUD in primary care settings) [28].

The remaining medications for treating SUD, e.g., naltrexone for OUD or AUD, acamprosate for AUD, and disulfiram for AUD, require no special licensure or training and can be prescribed by any provider. Additionally, prescribing naloxone for overdose prevention does not require any special licensure or training. Logistical concerns regarding injectable medications, e.g., intramuscular naltrexone, are discussed below. While the focus in a substance use clinic may be the provision of OBOT, harm reduction strategies are no less important. In particular, patients should be co-prescribed naloxone with all opioid prescriptions, including medications for OUD, and those on long-term opioid treatment for pain [29]. If available, sharps disposal kits, needles, syringes, cookers, and other sterile supplies can be offered on-site or through referral to a syringe exchange program [30].

Successful implementation of a novel clinical service requires thoughtful attention to how that service is maintained during nonbusiness hours. This is particularly true of nascent buprenorphine treatment programs, which may be run by a sole individual who is comfortable prescribing buprenorphine. While additional training is no longer required to prescribe buprenorphine, prescribers will need to determine whether or not their clinical partners are willing to prescribe this medication during non-business hours. Until this sole clinician identifies a clinical partner to share weekend and after-hours coverage, they will be obligated to think creatively about how their patients will be cared for in their absence. Some providers may partner with other local clinical sites to share call responsibilities. In general, with buprenorphine's long half-life, most refill issues can be deferred until the next business day without complication. In contrast, patients experiencing opioid withdrawal resulting from a complicated home induction typically require the guidance of a trained buprenorphine prescriber. As such, a threshold minimum of two providers sharing clinical duties is recommended.

Ultimately, the goal of an addiction treatment clinic is to stabilize patients' substance use behaviors with pharmacotherapy and with adjunctive behavioral support to the point that they are no longer routinely using non-prescribed drugs or alcohol, are adhering to a stable medication regimen, and no longer need the weekly/monthly return to use prevention support of a dedicated addiction program. Such patients should ideally be transitioned back into primary care, with the caveat that both patient and primary care provider know to reach back out to the addiction clinic should the need arise. Transitioning stable patients who are prescribed buprenorphine, in particular, back to primary care serves to (1) ensure that access to the addiction clinic is maximally utilized; (2) maintain that the educational mission of the addiction clinic—to learn how to stabilize/manage unstable SUD in the primary care setting—is preserved; (3) encourage other core faculty to obtain their buprenorphine waivers, to aid in "reabsorbing" stable patients prescribed buprenorphine; and (4) foster the idea that treating addiction in primary care settings, especially for stable patients, should be considered a routine aspect of primary care medicine.

With the rapid turnover of residents rotating through a dedicated addiction clinic, it is fruitful to create note templates within one's EMR, geared towards ensuring consistency in documentation, while also cueing learners regarding what should be covered in a typical visit. For example, a template that includes question prompts, e.g., "Have you had any cravings since the last visit?" and clinical reminders, e.g., "Review of recent UDS results?" and "Patient prescribed naloxone and educated on its use?", ensures that important items are not neglected. See Appendix for examples of note templates.

Just as the standard care of patients with hypertension and diabetes requires routinely obtaining blood pressure, blood glucose, and urinalysis data, patients with SUD will also require a strategy for monitoring treatment. Principally, treatment monitoring heavily relies upon patient assessment and urine drug testing (UDT) [31]. While there may be regional variations, a UDT should generally include opiates, benzodiazepines, amphetamine/methamphetamine, cannabis, PCP, barbiturates, oxycodone, cocaine, and methadone. In light of the expansion of fentanyl and other high-potency synthetic opioid use across the United States, adding urine fentanyl may also be appropriate [32]. Lastly, urine buprenorphine and norbuprenorphine testing should be added for patients prescribed buprenorphine and should be interpreted with care. For patients undergoing a benzodiazepine or opioid taper, quantitative analysis may be useful [33]. UDT should be ordered with reflex confirmation testing.

In terms of timing, UDT should be ordered for all new patients, and regularly throughout treatment, for monitoring but not diagnostic purposes [31]. Patients with isolated AUD can be screened less often, though clinic leaders might consider obtaining an in-clinic breathalyzer as well. Most importantly, UDT should only be viewed as a measure of treatment success or the need for treatment plan adjustment, and unexpected findings should engender conversations with the patient regarding potential modifications to the treatment plan [34]. Lastly, providers should educate themselves regarding the accurate interpretation of UDT. Consider also identifying a liaison in laboratory medicine to help with interpretation, as needed.

Taking It to the Next Level

Once a residency-based addiction clinic has developed some momentum and is successfully implementing many of the policies and procedures outlined above, clinic leaders may wish to "take it to the next level," by incorporating some of the clinical and educational initiatives outlined in Fig. 17.3.

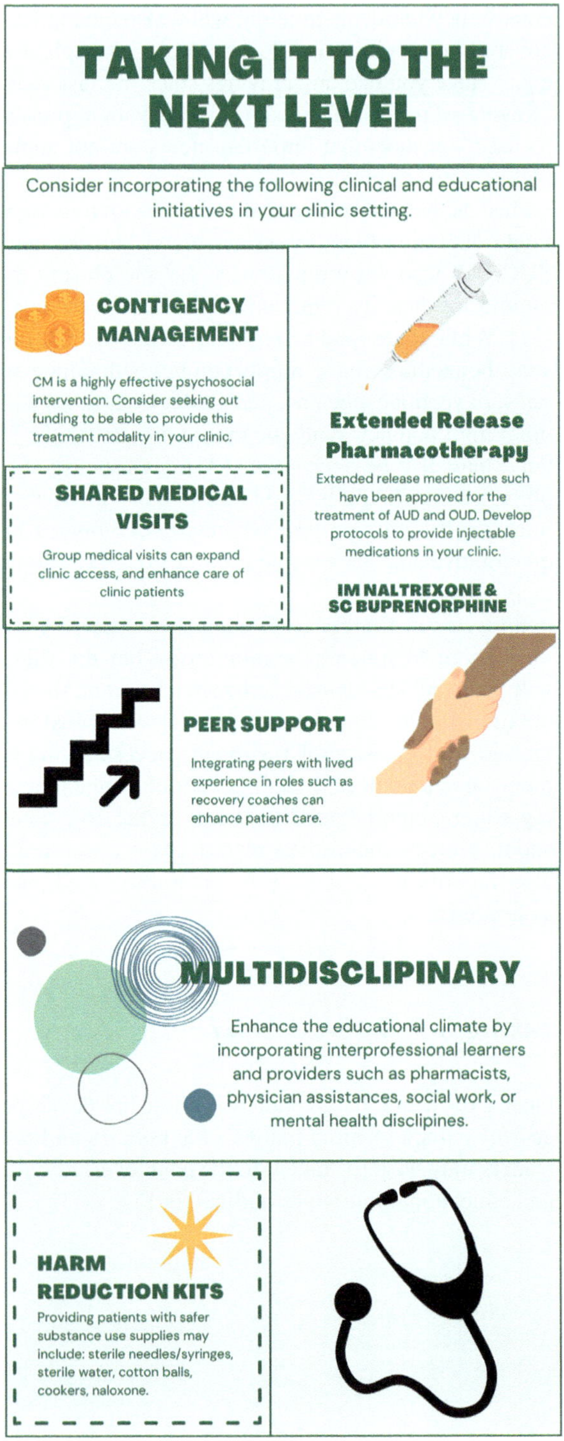

Fig. 17.3 The clinical and educational initiatives

Part III: Clinical Initiatives

While providing sublingual buprenorphine-naloxone to patients with OUD is already a first step in narrowing the addiction treatment gap, there are other treatment modalities to consider that provide additional options to patients. In particular, the long-acting injectable formulations of naltrexone for the treatment of AUD or OUD and buprenorphine for the treatment of OUD are excellent tools that, while necessitating a few logistical considerations, can aid in tailoring the right treatment to the individual patient [35]. Intramuscular extended-release naltrexone (XR-NTX), administered monthly as a 4 cc injection into the upper outer quadrant of the buttock, is FDA approved for both OUD and AUD and can be readily administered in the primary care setting with minimal training. It is helpful to partner with a single pharmacy that is willing to deliver XR-NTX to the practice before scheduled visits, where doses need to be refrigerated (for up to 6 months) before administration. While it is useful to train residents on how to administer XR-NTX, bear in mind that this medication can also be administered by nursing staff.

Extended-release buprenorphine (XR-BUP), administered monthly as a subcutaneous injection into the abdomen, is an excellent alternative to SL buprenorphine-naloxone, whether the patient is stable or unstable [36]. Like all buprenorphine formulations, the prescribing of XR-BUP no longer requires any formal training. As a controlled substance, unlike XR-NTX, XR-BUP must be kept in a locked refrigerator and must be administered by a health care provider. Similar to XR-NTX, it is useful to partner with a specific pharmacy, often a "specialty" pharmacy, that regularly dispenses XR-BUP and can consistently deliver it to the practice before patient visits.

While the treatment of both OUD and AUD benefits from evidence-based, FDA-approved pharmacotherapies, the treatment options for stimulant use disorders are considerably more limited. Nonetheless, the literature does support the use of contingency management (CM) programs for stimulant use disorders, which can be readily adopted in a residency-based substance use clinic, at a relatively low cost [37]. Obtaining a small grant (e.g., $5000) from the hospital or other local resource may be sufficient to run a CM program for months to years, if enrollment is limited to a half-day substance use clinic, and if only for patients with ongoing stimulant use disorder. Ideally, patients present to the clinic once or twice weekly for UDT, with monetary payouts of increasing value with each subsequent stimulant-negative urine, over 12 weeks.

While one-on-one encounters with patients form the bedrock of treatment for patients in a substance use clinic, added value can be gained by incorporating shared medical visits into this treatment setting [38, 39]. Shared medical visits can help to expand clinic access to more patients, expand learning opportunities for residents, and enhance the care of clinic patients by facilitating shared learning among those with lived experience while also maximizing billing potential for the practice. These appointments are best run by someone with experience in group visit facilitation, with physician involvement as needed to meet the individual needs of patients [40].

Special attention should be paid to the billing and coding requirements at the institution level to ensure that the service is financially viable.

In a similar vein, clinic services can be enhanced by the addition of peer support such as recovery coaches (individuals with lived experience and formal training) to the treatment team [41]. One might even consider creating a Patient Advisory Council to more explicitly solicit input from patients.

Part IV: Educational Initiatives

As one's substance use clinic grows in terms of services provided, patient volume, and resources available, numerous additional opportunities should be considered. First, one might consider enhancing the educational climate of the practice by inviting/incorporating interprofessional learners and providers. These might include students from pharmacy, physician assistants, nurse practitioner schools, or mental health and social work disciplines. Second, to ensure a basic fund of knowledge of OBOT, in particular, for all residents, many programs have incorporated buprenorphine training into the standard GME curriculum—ideally at new resident orientation. Lastly, looking more broadly at the residency program itself, one might consider developing a dedicated addiction medicine track within the residency program, as interest grows [42]. While providing a strong foundation in addiction medicine exposure for all residents is essential to residency training, a dedicated training track allows individual learners to further tailor their experience, potentially serving as a pipeline for addiction medicine fellowships.

Part V. Conclusion

SUD is a widely prevalent condition encountered by trainees in inpatient and outpatient settings that is affected by a significant treatment gap. Pervasive stigma and misconceptions about SUD threaten the delivery of evidence-based treatment. Additionally, trainees are disproportionately exposed to individuals presenting for complications of SUD or during times of crisis, rather than learning how to care for patients within the longitudinal, chronic disease model. Both stigma and lack of training at the undergraduate health profession education, GME, and CME levels lead to this treatment gap. Improvements in both didactic and clinical training are required to address this gap. Designing longitudinal, clinical training experiences as part of residency education is one initiative to increase the workforce of providers trained to care for patients with SUD. To achieve this aim, clinical and educational leaders should define the clinic's goals, define the curricular approach, establish institutional support through stakeholder engagement, consider the needs of the local patient population, and address clinic logistics. These foundational steps can then be built upon to further address the needs of the local population and the internal medicine resident learners.

Importantly, creating an embedded, residency program addiction clinical experience starts by recruiting a single patient or a small number of patients. Several freely accessible, unbiased, existing resources may be incorporated into the established curriculum. These include, but are not limited to, the American Academy of Addiction Psychiatry Providers Clinical Support System SUD 101 curriculum [43], the Association of Program Directors in Internal Medicine Primary Care Toolkit [44], the Coursera Addiction and its Treatment Course [45], and offerings provided by the American College of Academic Addiction Medicine including a high-yield yearly weekly didactic series [43], the American Society of Addiction Medicine [46], and the Association for Multidisciplinary Education in Substance Use and Addiction [47]. Additional materials to supplement and enhance learning include efforts such as the Curbsiders Addiction Medicine Podcast series, which is freely available [48]. Implementing a dual clinical and educational SUD clinic within an outpatient residency practice will increase the workforce of adequately trained physicians prepared to address one of the most pressing public health issues of our time.

Appendix

This appendix contains 3-sample note templates: (1) New Patient Visit (2) Assessment (3) Follow-up Visit

Template A: Sample New Patient Visit Template

ADDICTION RECOVERY CLINIC (ARC) NEW PATIENT VISIT NOTE

NAME presents today for evaluation and management of: ***

Primary substance use history (i.e. reason for referral, age of first use, last use, current use pattern and route of administration, etc): ***

Current withdrawal symptoms, if appropriate (e.g. CIWA for alcohol, COWS for opioids. Sx of opioid withdrawal may include arthralgias, insomnia, restlessness, yawning, diarrhea, piloerection, nausea): ***

Overdose events? ***

IVDU hx (ever shared needles?): ***

Longest time abstinent from substance in recent past: ***

Findings on CT-PMP (Prescription Monitoring Program)? ***

Other substance use history: (E.g. age of first use, last use, route, freq, amount)

Opioids-

Cocaine-

Crack-

Marijuana-

Benzodiazepines-
ETOH-
TOB-
Other-
Substance use treatment history: ***
Screen for complications of addictive disorders (e.g. Legal, Medical, Social, Employment): ***
Psychiatric Hx: ***
Relevant additional screening info:

Support systems (family, friends, faith community):
Family planning:
Hepatitis/HIV:
STIs:
Violence/Home safety:

Current Medications
Physical exam

Template B: Sample Assessment Template

Assessment:

1. Opioid Use Disorder, [severity?] ***

A minimum of 2–3 criteria is required for a mild substance use disorder diagnosis, while 4–5 is moderate, and 6–7 is severe (APA, 2013).

- Taking the substance in larger amounts and for longer than intended
- Wanting to cut down or quit but not being able to do it
- Spending a lot of time obtaining the substance
- Craving or a strong desire to use substance
- Repeatedly unable to carry out major obligations at work, school, or home due to substance use
- Continued use despite persistent or recurring social or interpersonal problems caused or made worse by substance use
- Stopping or reducing important social, occupational, or recreational activities due to substance use
- Recurrent use of substance in physically hazardous situations
- Consistent use of substance despite acknowledgment of persistent or recurrent physical or psychological difficulties from using substance
- *Tolerance as defined by either a need for markedly increased amounts to achieve intoxication or desired effect or markedly diminished effect with continued use of the same amount. (Does not apply for diminished effect when used appropriately under medical supervision)

- *Withdrawal manifesting as either characteristic syndrome or the substance is used to avoid withdrawal (Does not apply when used appropriately under medical supervision)

Plan:
1. Admit to Suboxone Maintenance/Opioid detoxification
Start at Suboxone at *** mg
Check UDS-9, urine bup
Behavioral component? ***
12-step programs? ***
Meet with Social Work?
Instruct patient to bring empty foil packets back to clinic at each visit.
Give copy of Buprenorphine Treatment Agreement for review and sign at next visit.
2. Additional Reminders/Things to consider:
Relevant Health Maintenance Issues?
Smoking cessation
Lab work—LFTs, HIV elisa and HCV ab today
Family Planning Issues (pregnancy testing, inquire re: infants/children in home, safe storage of buprenorphine…)
Overdose education and prescription for Naloxone Kit
Last PPD?
Follow-up plan and SPECIFIC GOALS FOR NEXT SESSION: *

Template C: Sample Follow-up Visit Template

ADDICTION RECOVERY CLINIC (ARC) FOLLOW-UP VISIT NOTE
Name is presenting for follow-up of *** use disorder.
Recent Urine drug screen results: ***
Drug or alcohol use since last visit? ***
Participation in 12-step groups or IOP since last visit? ***
Since last visit, any new problems with the following?

- Psychiatric: ***
- Medical: ***
- Employment: ***
- Social/Family: ***
- Legal: ***

Other new Issues?
Current Medication
Physical Exam
1. *** Use Disorder
Pharmacotherapy: ***

Order UDS-9

Behavioral component?

- 12-step programs?
- Relapse prevention counseling?

Meet with Social Work?

Follow-up plan?

Next week will be week *** of initial 8 weeks ARC follow-up.

2. Additional Reminders / Things to consider:

Relevant Health Maintenance Issues (See "problem overview" for any delinquent items)

Lab work—LFTs

Family Planning Issues (pregnancy testing, inquire re: infants/children in home)

Follow-up plan and SPECIFIC GOALS FOR NEXT SESSION: *

References

1. Ciccarone D. The rise of illicit fentanyls, stimulants and the fourth wave of the opioid overdose crisis. Curr Opin Psychiatry. 2021;34(4):344–50.
2. Pollard MS, Tucker JS, Green HD Jr. Changes in adult alcohol use and consequences during the COVID-19 pandemic in the US. JAMA Netw Open. 2020;3(9):e2022942-e.
3. Marks LR, Nolan NS, Liang SY, Durkin MJ, Weimer MB. Infectious complications of injection drug use. Med Clin N Am. 2022;106(1):187–200.
4. Daley DC. Family and social aspects of substance use disorders and treatment. J Food Drug Anal. 2013;21(4):S73–S6.
5. SAMHSA. Key substance use and mental health indicators in the United States: results from the 2019 National Survey on Drug Use and Health. Quality CfBHSa, editor. Rockville, MD; 2020.
6. Yoast RA, Wilford BB, Hayashi SW. Encouraging physicians to screen for and intervene in substance use disorders: obstacles and strategies for change. J Addict Dis. 2008;27(3):77–97.
7. Duncan A, Anderman J, Deseran T, Reynolds I, Stein BD. Monthly patient volumes of buprenorphine-waivered clinicians in the US. JAMA Netw Open. 2020;3(8):e2014045.
8. Foti K, Heyward J, Tajanlangit M, Meek K, Jones C, Kolodny A, et al. Primary care physicians' preparedness to treat opioid use disorder in the United States: a cross-sectional survey. Drug Alcohol Depend. 2021;225:108811.
9. Miller NS, Sheppard LM, Colenda CC, Magen J. Why physicians are unprepared to treat patients who have alcohol- and drug-related disorders. Acad Med. 2001;76(5):410–8.
10. Morford KL, Falker CG, Tetrault JM. Training medical students, residents, and fellows in opioid use disorder treatment. In: Wakeman SE, Rich JD, editors. Treating opioid use disorder in general medical settings. Cham: Springer International Publishing; 2021. p. 161–71.
11. Windish DM, Catalanotti JS, Zaas A, Kisielewski M, Moriarty JP. Training in safe opioid prescribing and treatment of opioid use disorder in internal medicine residencies: a National Survey of Program Directors. J Gen Intern Med. 2021:1–11.
12. Graddy R, Accurso AJ, Nandiwada DR, Shalaby M, Holt SR. Models of resident physician training in opioid use disorders. Curr Addict Rep. 2019;6(4):355–64.
13. ACGME. ACGME Program Requirements for Graduate Medical Education in Internal Medicine https://www.acgme.org/globalassets/PFAssets/ProgramRequirements/140_

InternalMedicine_2022.pdf?ver=2021-02-19-152614-193&ver=2021-02-19-152614-1932021 [updated 7 Feb 2021].
14. Kunins HV, Sohler NL, Giovanniello A, Thompson D, Cunningham CO. A buprenorphine education and training program for primary care residents: implementation and evaluation. Subst Abus. 2013;34(3):242–7.
15. Shuey B, Lee D, Ugalde I, Borgan S, Bresnan C, Qureshi M, et al. Evaluation of resident physicians' knowledge of and attitudes towards prescribing buprenorphine for patients with opioid use disorder. J Addict Med. 2021;15(3):219–25.
16. Pytell JD, Buresh ME, Graddy R. Outcomes of a novel office-based opioid treatment program in an internal medicine resident continuity practice. Addict Sci Clin Pract. 2019;14(1):1–7.
17. Holt SR, Segar N, Cavallo DA, Tetrault JM. The addiction recovery clinic: a novel, primary-care-based approach to teaching addiction medicine. Acad Med. 2017;92(5):680–3.
18. Sobel HG, Goedde M, Maruti S, Hadley-Strout E, Wahlberg E, Kennedy AG. Primary care residents delivering care: integration of office-based opioid treatment into an internal medicine residency curriculum. Acad Psychiatry. 2019;43(5):499–502.
19. Marlatt GA. Harm reduction: come as you are. Addict Behav. 1996;21(6):779–88.
20. Dwayne Simpson D, Joe GW, Rowan-Szal GA. Drug abuse treatment retention and process effects on follow-up outcomes1The interpretations and conclusions in this paper do not necessarily represent the position of NIDA or the Department of Health and Human Services.1. Drug Alcohol Depend. 1997;47(3):227–35.
21. Saitz R, Miller SC, Fiellin DA, Rosenthal RN. Recommended use of terminology in addiction medicine. J Addict Med. 2021;15(1):3–7.
22. Kelly JF, Westerhoff CM. Does it matter how we refer to individuals with substance-related conditions? A randomized study of two commonly used terms. Int J Drug Policy. 2010;21(3):202–7.
23. Kelly JF, Dow SJ, Westerhoff C. Does our choice of substance-related terms influence perceptions of treatment need? An empirical investigation with two commonly used terms. J Drug Issues. 2010;40(4):805–18.
24. Goddu P, O'Conor KJ, Lanzkron S, Saheed MO, Saha S, Peek ME, et al. Do words matter? Stigmatizing language and the transmission of bias in the medical record. J Gen Intern Med. 2018;33(5):685–91.
25. Andrews CM, Abraham AJ, Grogan CM, Westlake MA, Pollack HA, Friedmann PD. Impact of medicaid restrictions on availability of buprenorphine in addiction treatment programs. Am J Public Health. 2019;109(3):434–6.
26. Ries RK, Fiellin DA, Miller SC, Saitz R. The ASAM principles of addiction medicine. Lippincott Williams & Wilkins; 2014.
27. SAMHSA. Disclosure of substance use disorder patient records: does part 2 apply to me? https://www.samhsa.gov/sites/default/files/does-part2-apply.pdf.
28. SAMHSA. Federal Guidelines for Opioid Treatment Programs 2015 [updated March 2015]. https://store.samhsa.gov/product/Federal-Guidelines-for-Opioid-Treatment-Programs/PEP15-FEDGUIDEOTP.
29. FDA. New Recommendations for Naloxone 2020 [updated 7/23/2020]. https://www.fda.gov/drugs/drug-safety-and-availability/new-recommendations-naloxone.
30. Chan CA, Canver B, McNeil R, Sue KL. Harm reduction in health care settings. Med Clin. 2022;106(1):201–17.
31. Jarvis M, Williams J, Hurford M, Lindsay D, Lincoln P, Giles L, et al. Appropriate use of drug testing in clinical addiction medicine. J Addict Med. 2017;11(3):163–73.
32. Martinez S, Jones JD, Brandt L, Campbell ANC, Abbott R, Comer SD. The increasing prevalence of fentanyl: a urinalysis-based study among individuals with opioid use disorder in new York City. Am J Addict. 2021;30(1):65–71.
33. Donroe JH, Holt SR, O'Connor PG, Sukumar N, Tetrault JM. Interpreting quantitative urine buprenorphine and norbuprenorphine levels in office-based clinical practice. Drug Alcohol Depend. 2017;180:46–51.

34. Holt SR, Donroe JH, Cavallo DA, Tetrault JM. Addressing discordant quantitative urine buprenorphine and norbuprenorphine levels: case examples in opioid use disorder. Drug Alcohol Depend. 2018;186:171–4.
35. Gastfriend DR. Intramuscular extended-release naltrexone: current evidence. Ann N Y Acad Sci. 2011;1216(1):144–66.
36. Lofwall MR, Walsh SL, Nunes EV, Bailey GL, Sigmon SC, Kampman KM, et al. Weekly and monthly subcutaneous buprenorphine depot formulations vs daily sublingual buprenorphine with naloxone for treatment of opioid use disorder: a randomized clinical trial. JAMA Intern Med. 2018;178(6):764–73.
37. Prendergast M, Podus D, Finney J, Greenwell L, Roll J. Contingency management for treatment of substance use disorders: a meta-analysis. Addiction. 2006;101(11):1546–60.
38. Sokol R, LaVertu AE, Morrill D, Albanese C, Schuman-Olivier Z. Group-based treatment of opioid use disorder with buprenorphine: a systematic review. J Subst Abus Treat. 2018;84:78–87.
39. Sokol R, Albanese C, Chaponis D, Early J, Maxted G, Morrill D, et al. Why use group visits for opioid use disorder treatment in primary care? A patient-centered qualitative study. Subst Abuse. 2018;39(1):52–8.
40. Treatment; CfSA. Substance Abuse Treatment: Group Therapy. Treatment Improvement Protocol (TIP) Series, No. 41. Rockville, MD: Substance Abuse and Mental Health Services Administration; 2005.
41. Jack HE, Oller D, Kelly J, Magidson JF, Wakeman SE. Addressing substance use disorder in primary care: the role, integration, and impact of recovery coaches. Subst Abuse. 2018;39(3):307–14.
42. Kenneth L. Morford, Dana Cavallo, John Encandela, Rebecca Minahan-Rowley. Developing resident CHAMP-ions to practice behavioral health and addiction medicine in primary care. Poster presentation. AMERSA Annual Meeting; November 2020; Virtual2020.
43. The American Academy of Addiction Psychiatry Providers Clinical Support System SUD 101 curriculum https://pcssnow.org/education-training/sud-core-curriculum/.
44. Forum APC. The Association of Program Directors in Internal Medicine Primary Care Toolkit2005 [cited 2021 12/11]. https://higherlogicdownload.s3.amazonaws.com/IM/fecab58a-0e31-416b-8e56-46fc9eda5c37/UploadedImages/Documents/resources/Primary_Care_Toolkit_Second_Edition.pdf.
45. Tetrault JMK, Robert; Roessler, Elizabeth; Heimer, Robert; Powell, Mary Lindsay; Drew, Shannon; Edens, Ellen. Coursera course: addiction treatment: clinical skills for healthcare providers https://www.coursera.org/learn/addiction-treatment#reviews.
46. American Society of Addiction Medicine E-Learning Center. https://elearning.asam.org/.
47. Association for Multidisciplinary Education in Substance Use and Addiction (AMERSA). https://amersa.org/.
48. Chan CA, Cohen S, Stahl N, Morford KL. The curbsiders addiction medicine Podcast [Internet]; 2022. Podcast. https://thecurbsiders.com/addiction

Part VI
Curriculum, Education, and Scholarship

Chapter 18
Ambulatory Curriculum Design and Delivery for Internal Medicine Residents

Margaret C. Lo, Alia Chisty, and Emily Mullen

Introduction

The Accreditation Council for Graduate Medical Education (ACGME) issued significant changes in the common program requirements effective July 2022 for 10 months of residency training to occur in the ambulatory setting [1]. The Alliance for Academic Internal Medicine (AAIM) and ACGME have long advocated for decreasing the conflict between inpatient and outpatient experiences [1, 2]. These changes emphasize the need for the graduate medical education (GME) system to revitalize residents' ambulatory education.

Reform of ambulatory training in internal medicine is twofold. First, it requires improving the system infrastructure of clinic itself, and secondly, it mandates enhancing the educational experience of residents within the clinic [3]. Part of that movement includes a longitudinal ambulatory curricular design that enhances the resident continuity clinic experience and provides residents with a foundation for learning ambulatory medicine. Most ambulatory medical education is delivered into three clinic models—ambulatory block rotations (typically referred to as X + Y

M. C. Lo (✉)
Department of Medicine, Division of Internal Medicine, University of Florida College of Medicine, Gainesveille, FL, USA
e-mail: Margaret.lo@medicine.ufl.edu

A. Chisty
Department of Medicine, Division of General Internal Medicine, Penn State Health Milton S. Hershey Medical Center/Penn State College of Medicine, Hershey, PA, USA
e-mail: achisty@pennstatehealth.psu.edu

E. Mullen
Department of Internal Medicine, Cone Health Internal Medicine Residency Program, Moses H. Cone Health Systems, Greensboro, NC, USA
e-mail: emily.mullen@conehealth.com

L. B. Lu et al. (eds.), *Leading an Academic Medical Practice*,
https://doi.org/10.1007/978-3-031-40273-9_18

model), longitudinal continuity clinics, and ambulatory long blocks. Many resident continuity clinics provide some type of on-site instructional modality, usually as a preclinical conference or an ambulatory case-based discussion, to disseminate a core curricular thread of high-yield ambulatory topics [3]. The COVID-19 pandemic has elevated the need for instructions in digital learning and telemedicine education in the ambulatory curriculum. Residency clinic directors and program leadership have a responsibility to ensure a well-rounded longitudinal ambulatory experience focused on achievable learning objectives.

Outline

- Educational principles and steps in ambulatory medicine curriculum design
- Ambulatory curriculum delivery
- Ambulatory curricular design and venue
- Developing an ambulatory curriculum in one's own academic clinic
- Conclusion

Educational Principles and Steps in Ambulatory Medicine Curriculum Design

A variety of textbooks and online resources exist to guide faculty in the development of medical education curriculum. Three noteworthy books are "Curriculum Development for Medical Education: A Six-Step Approach" by Thomas et al. [4], "Teaching in Your Office, 2nd Edition: A Guide to Instructing Medical Students and Residents" by the American College of Physicians [5], and "The Toolkit Series: A Textbook for Internal Medicine Education Programs" by the Alliance for Academic Internal Medicine [6]. Online resources on curriculum development are available in three major categories—topic-specific online resources (e.g., MedEdPORTAL), resources within medical education journals, and resources from medical accrediting organizations [e.g., Association of American Medical Colleges (AAMC), Alliance for Academic Internal Medicine (AAIM), and Accreditation Council for Graduate Medical Education (ACGME)] [7, 8].

Six key principles and steps are essential in the planning of ambulatory educational curriculum, as detailed below and in Sect. V.

Curriculum Steering Committee for Educational Planning and Problem Identification

The first key step is to identify one faculty individual to oversee the ambulatory curriculum development process. Alternatively, a couple of individuals can share this role, such as the associate program director and clinic director. This person(s) is responsible for the day-to-day logistical planning of the curriculum. This includes scheduling the curriculum in residents' continuity clinics, recruiting faculty presenters, and ensuring content collection and aggregation of curriculum evaluation.

Creation of a curriculum steering committee with key ambulatory stakeholders can then provide input and identify deficits or problems in the ambulatory curriculum. This committee must continually review and update the curricular content at least annually to improve the ambulatory curriculum. This committee is distinct from the Program Evaluation Committee whose role focuses on continuous evaluation of the program and oversight of the entire curriculum development within the program. Key stakeholders should include the residency clinic directors, clinic preceptors, ambulatory chief resident, and residency program director or associate program director. The latter three individuals make certain that the clinic curriculum aligns with ACGME requirements and integrates well into the residency program.

General and Targeted Educational Needs Assessment

The needs assessment process is an important step to inform on relevant curricular content and design. This step must involve not only a general analysis of the institution's educational and programmatic needs but also a targeted assessment of learners' needs [4, 8]. It ensures alignment of the program's curriculum to ACGME/ABIM requirements and expert recommendations from major medical education organizations. Both general and targeted needs assessment can be done through various methods including, but not limited to, stakeholders' surveys, town hall meetings, focus group discussions, individualized faculty or resident interviews, in-training exam (ITE) performance on ambulatory topics, direct observation of learners' skills, and audits of current stakeholders' performance. The curriculum needs assessments must conclude with a review of the literature for related ambulatory education curriculum and a collection of all the available resources. Appendixes A and B provide sample templates of general and targeted needs-assessments for ambulatory curriculum development.

Goals and Objectives for Continuity Clinics in Relationship to ACGME Competencies

ACGME requires all training programs to develop specific goals and objectives for their educational curricula. Goals and objectives help to convey learning expectations, prioritize curricular content, tailor the individual clinic learning, and allow for curriculum evaluation [7]. Goals are set in SMART format—*s*pecific, *m*easurable, *a*ttainable, *r*elevant, and *t*imely [9, 10]. Learning objectives should follow Bloom's taxonomy, as illustrated in Table 18.1 [12, 13].

Goals and objectives for any ambulatory clinic curriculum must reflect the six domains of the ACGME Milestones 2.0 competencies [14]—patient care, medical knowledge, practice-based learning and improvement, interpersonal skills and communication, professionalism, and systems-based practice. Residents and preceptors should review these educational goals and objectives on at least a semiannual basis. Residency program directors need to verify residents' clinical competence and performance trajectory in the six Milestones core competencies within ambulatory

Table 18.1 Types of learning objectives [11]

Types of objectives	Definition	Sample learning objective for the professionalism competency
Learner focused	Cognitive (knowledge based) Affective (attitude based) Psychomotor (skill based, behavioral based)	By the end of the year, residents will be able to list five different personal, psychological, and/or physical limitations that may affect professional performance By the end of the year, residents will have rated more highly their empathy and compassion towards their primary care patients with chronic pain issues By the end of the year, residents will be able to demonstrate competency in providing support (physical, psychological, social, and spiritual) for dying patients and their families
Process focused	Curriculum implementation measures	By the end of the year, residents will review three mini-CEX sessions with faculty preceptor for feedback on professional interaction with patients
Outcome focused	Patient-related outcomes Healthcare outcomes Career choices	Three months into the academic year, a higher percentage of residents' primary care patients will report increased satisfaction in their interaction with their resident physician

education. The ACGME website (http://www.acgme.org/What-We-Do/Accreditation/Milestones/Overview) publishes Milestones 2.0 guidebooks and developmental toolkits in competency-based medical education for any program to adapt accordingly.

Educational Strategies: Structured Core Curricular Content and Delivery Strategies

A core curricular thread of supplemental teaching modalities is a fundamental component of any ambulatory medicine curriculum. This core thread helps to consolidate ambulatory concepts with learning in the clinical setting, promote self-directed learning beyond patient cases seen, and solidify clinical practice with evidence-based medicine [15–20]. There should be a balance of experiential training from direct patient care (e.g., acute care, chronic disease management, office-based procedures), formal educational instruction (e.g., teaching conferences, case-based small-group sessions, Web-based modules), and resident-driven learning strategies (e.g., problem-based learning, team-based learning, QI mini-projects, resident-led workshops, flipped classroom model).

The teaching pedagogies must focus on critical reasoning and active adult learning in small-group settings; ambulatory curriculum has shifted away from traditional lecture-based teaching to problem-based learning [21, 22]. Core curricular contents can be delivered in a variety of effective pedagogical modalities including, but not limited to, ambulatory conference series, ambulatory medicine morning report, ambulatory medicine journal clubs, synchronous virtual platforms, asynchronous online learning modules, and patient simulation exercises. Each instructional modality needs clear, achievable learning objectives, and its curricular contents need to be updated at least annually.

Implementation with Bidirectional Evaluation and Feedback

Implementation of any ambulatory curriculum must first address barriers, identify resources, and garner appropriate support. A rigorous evaluation system can then be established to routinely gauge its educational programming and primary stakeholders (i.e., residents, clinic staff, and faculty preceptors). Curricular measures reflect outcome-focused learning objectives and assess the level of Milestones-specific competencies acquired by residents in the longitudinal care of their primary care patients [8]. Semiannual internal evaluation of the ambulatory curriculum allows for timely improvements to the overall program.

Bidirectional evaluation of both residents and faculty preceptors is integral to the continual improvement of any ambulatory curriculum. Resident performance data can originate from a variety of ambulatory evaluation sources including, but not limited to, direct observation of patient encounters, mini-Clinical Evaluation Exercise (mini-CEX), Objective Structured Clinical Examination (OSCE), chart-simulated recall, and multisource feedback. These formative evaluations of residents are continuous throughout the academic year. To inform the Clinical Competency Committee (CCC) report to ACGME, faculty preceptors must complete a summative evaluation quarterly of their clinic residents' global performance in ambulatory Milestones 2.0 competencies. For reciprocity, faculty evaluation data should ideally be collected from residents' and peers' confidential and/or anonymous feedback of teaching performance. ACGME Common Program Requirements stipulate at minimum a yearly evaluation of faculty performance and include "review of the faculty member's clinical teaching abilities, engagement with the educational program, participation in faculty development related to their skills as an educator, clinical performance, professionalism, and scholarly activities" [1]. The individual responsible for these yearly faculty evaluations is usually the ambulatory APD, the residency clinic director, or a similar faculty leader who oversees the ambulatory curriculum (see Chap. 10—Resident Milestones, Assessments, and Feedback in the Continuity Clinic).

Ambulatory Faculty Development Needs

Every successful ambulatory curriculum capitalizes on the clinical and teaching skills of the ambulatory faculty, but this requires a well-structured plan to encourage and support ambulatory faculty development. Ambulatory preceptors must be able to skillfully diagnose patients' complaints while assessing and teaching their learners' needs. To do so, educational programs need to gauge the faculty development needs of their clinic preceptors and provide education on a variety of ambulatory teaching skills and instructional pedagogies. These include faculty training in effective ambulatory teaching models such as the One Minute Preceptor and SNAPPS (*S*ummarize, *N*arrow, *A*nalyze, *P*robe, *P*lan, and *S*elect) [23–26]. These validated models help to extract the highest-yield ambulatory concepts for learners in the busy ambulatory setting. See Chap. 19, Students in Clinic, for further details. ACP, SGIM, and AAIM all advocate for a "core faculty" group of master clinician educators with protected time, salary support, and organizational resources to teach learners and/or peer faculty [27–30] (see Chap. 2, Supervising and Supporting Faculty, and Chap. 3, Faculty Recruitment and Retention, for more details).

Ambulatory Curriculum Delivery

Core Curricular Content

Clinic time constraints and varying clinical experiences make learning from direct patient care insufficient to cover the breadth of knowledge in ambulatory medicine. Longitudinal ambulatory didactics are essential to solidify key ambulatory concepts beyond specific patient encounters. Curricular content must incorporate evidence-based medicine for high-quality care and lifelong learning [15, 16].

The standard curriculum must teach residents the core ambulatory contents commonly seen and managed in the clinical practice of outpatient medicine, whether primary care or subspecialty specific [31]. Academic institutions can further individualize certain ambulatory contents to their own clinical experiences. Preventive medicine is a key component of primary care, and residents must learn guidelines and evidence-based preventative care measures. Residents should receive longitudinal instructions in the panel management of their patient population, either as a cohort or alongside interprofessional team members [32–36]. See Chap. 24, Population Health and Quality, for further details. Core curricula should further include topics on outpatient billing and coding, transitions of care, team-based care, telemedicine care delivery, chronic disease management, quality improvement/patient safety, high-value care, electronic medical record navigation, and patient-physician communication including shared decision-making [37–39]. Additionally, ACGME requires clinical instruction in geriatrics, palliative medicine, hospice care, chronic pain, and addiction medicine [40]. These topics are very relevant and appropriate for the ambulatory curricula. The COVID-19 pandemic also escalated the need for ambulatory core curricula to teach fundamental competencies and skills in digital health so that residents can conduct effective telemedicine visits (Savage, BMJ Postgraduate Medical Journal, 2021) (Wong, JGME, 2020) [41, 42]. Depending on institutional needs and interests, programs may consider specialized topics addressing social determinants of health, health disparities, cultural competency, immigrant or refugee health, transgender health, LGBTQI+ care, or point-of-care ultrasound (POCUS) skills. Maintaining a 12-month to 36-month core curricular thread of these ambulatory topics either in a traditional half-day clinic model, x + y model, or academic half-day model will ensure a well-structured and well-balanced educational experience for residents (Appendix 18C).

Teaching Methods and Instructional Strategies: Formal Instruction

Small-Group Sessions

Small-group sessions in the ambulatory setting are a valuable tool to enhance outpatient learning. The small group allows for learner engagement, interactive didactics, and a forum to cover many broad clinical topics that are not commonly present in the clinic. Small groups can be utilized within the construct of a larger curriculum, e.g., Yale Office Based Curriculum [43], or can be learner directed [44] in the clinic. Small groups can focus on specific skill teaching [45] or work to improve soft skills such as patient interviewing [46]. These small-group sessions are particularly useful to teach any specific gaps in education identified by the program.

Ambulatory Morning Report

Morning report is a classic educational model that is easily adaptable to the ambulatory setting. Traditional morning report consists of case-based education where learners and teachers interact in a dynamic process to discuss patient care [47, 48]. However, there is no formal definition and no one effective format noted in the literature [47]. Ambulatory morning report is an excellent venue to introduce common outpatient medical problems and share experiences among a larger group of residents [49]. A few studies noted that the topics presented in ambulatory morning reports are more general and more practical than inpatient topics [49, 50].

Residency programs with an established inpatient morning report can adjust this educational modality to ambulatory topics. The key step is faculty and resident buy-in to ensure that the sessions are interactive and supported by faculty presence. Interactive facilitated discussions during morning report would then occur with the chief resident or attending input. Despite being called "morning" report, there is no best time or frequency for morning report, as long as resident attendance can be ensured [47]. Ambulatory morning report is suitable for teaching evidence-based medicine [51], morbidity and mortality [52], and more [47].

Evidence-Based Learning

Evidence-based medicine (EBM) uses current best scientific evidence to guide patient care decisions for management. Evidence-based learning consists of a four-step process [53]:

1. Formulate a clear clinical question from a patient problem.
2. Search the literature for relevant clinical articles.
3. Critically appraise the evidence for its validity and usefulness.
4. Implement useful findings in clinical practice.

With the six Milestones 2.0 competency domains, ACGME requires programs to train residents not only in clinical skills and medical knowledge, but also in quality, patient safety, EBM, and cost-effective care [54]. Residency programs should address residents' barriers to practicing EBM including limited time, lack of experience in EBM, influences from other team members, e.g., faculty role models, and their self-perceived inferiority and inertia to influence system-based change [55]. To surmount these barriers, ambulatory curricula must incorporate EBM teaching to promote residents' practice-based learning skills and lifelong learning.

Ambulatory Journal Club

Journal clubs are a popular modality to teach physicians how to critically appraise medical literature and stay current with new evidence. Journal club discussions that are small group, structured, and facilitated by faculty can lead to an increase in resident knowledge of critical appraisal and clinical epidemiology [56]. Systematic reviews found that journal clubs can overall enhance residents' knowledge of epidemiology, biostatistics, reading habits, and references to medical literature [57]. Further studies are still needed to determine if journal clubs improve clinical behavior. Nonetheless, ambulatory journal club is a vital instructional modality in any ambulatory curriculum to promote academic rigor and EBM practice among residents and faculty [58]. It can easily engage millennial learner by creating teams and fostering competition between teams to answer questions [59] or to the virtual space [60].

PICO Reports

Critical to practicing EBM is asking the right clinical question. Questions should be as specific as possible, including distinct patient characteristics, clinical intervention being considered, and desired outcome [53]. The PICO format helps to design such clinical questions to include the *P*atient or *P*roblem, the *I*ntervention, the *C*omparison group (usually the standard of care or main alternative), and the *O*utcome [61]. The PICO report provides a template for clinicians to build a specific clinical question and a search strategy to determine the main concepts of the article and answer the question posed. It prompts residents to research a specific clinical question during an actual patient care encounter. House staff presentations can apply the PICO format to complement ambulatory journal clubs. Residents can present the relevant article(s) and apply them appropriately in the clinical decision-making process. The University of Kentucky successfully adapted the PICO format into their "Ambulatory Teaching Minute," a curricular innovation presenting a case and a relevant article to answer the clinical question raised by the case. This format allows busy preceptors to review and engage their residents in EBM topics during real-time clinic encounters [62].

Structured Clinical Observations

Mini-Clinical Evaluation Exercises (Mini-CEX)

The mini-CEX, as defined by the ABIM, consists of 10–20 min of direct assessment by a clinical faculty member. It allows for a quick view or "snapshot" into a resident's competence. This, in turn, helps faculty teach any resident's learning deficits in a certain clinical area or topic. The mini-CEX is not intended to be a comprehensive assessment of a full patient encounter but rather serves as a focused assessment of a resident's competence in a key encounter element (e.g., history-gathering, physical examination skills, counseling, or procedural skills). Appendix 18D provides a sample mini-CEX for a GYN examination. The ABIM website encourages faculty to perform at least one mini-CEX per clinical rotation. After such an interaction, faculty should provide timely and specific feedback [63].

The mini-CEX format is reproducible and feasible and provides reliable results [64]. A major benefit is its ability to provide immediate feedback to the learner and tailor teaching of specific clinical areas based on mini-CEX performance. Educators find this valuable given the lack of time for administrative, clinical, and teaching responsibilities [65, 66]. Mini-CEXs also provide an aspect of realism to the encounter that can be lost in other educational models such as an OSCE [66]. Since residents interact with patients on a daily basis, it is simple to carve time out within the academic year for this type of instructional modality.

The mini-CEX is a perfect tool to assist in documenting resident advancement along the ACGME Milestones 2.0 trajectory, whether it be for patient care 1 (PC1) on history-taking or interpersonal and communication skills 1 (ICS1) on developing a therapeutic relationship with a patient. Yet, little publications exist to date around connecting mini-CEX evaluations to the residency milestones; however, appropriate changes to the feedback structure could pave a way to assess residents' achievement of specific milestones [67].

Some pitfalls of the mini-CEX tool include the need for faculty development and rater training [65, 66]. Depending on the type of model implemented and the level of faculty expertise, a significant amount of faculty training may be required to limit the inter-rater variation and increase the value of the feedback/rating gathered. Choosing high-yield areas of evaluation (i.e., breaking bad news, communication

Table 18.2 Steps in the development and implementation of a mini-CEX for a residency program

1st: Convene a group of faculty educators vested in mini-CEX development and participation.
2nd: Identify a list of competencies and skills that are conducive to mini-CEX assessment and important to be evaluated in the residency program.
3rd: Decide on the minimum competency requirements needed to be achieved for each resident contingent to his/her training level.
4th: Determine the role of the mini-CEX, i.e., educational only vs. formative feedback vs. both.
5th: Determine the number of mini-CEX assessments needed for each PGY level.
6th: Develop a mini-CEX assessment form appropriate to your program. See ABIM website for a sample direct observation mini-CEX template.
7th: Disseminate the mini-CEX form to clinical sites which are easily accessible and well known to all faculty and learners.
8th: Be sure to assess residents routinely and regularly throughout the academic year.
9th: Be sure to document every mini-CEX assessment encounter.
10th: Provide immediate, specific feedback to the resident during the mini-CEX encounter.
11th: Designate one faculty at each clinical site to take responsibility for disseminating and collecting mini-CEX forms.
12th: Analyze all mini-CEX results in a timely manner based on curricular goals.

Adapted from Liao K, Pu S, Liu M, Yang C, Kuo H. Development and implementation of a mini-Clinical Evaluation Exercise (mini-CEX) program to assess the clinical competencies of internal medicine residents: from faculty development to curriculum evaluation. BMC Med Educ 2013;13 [31]

skills) can help to mitigate this issue since these areas are already linked to other curricular goals [65]. Time is another concern of the mini-CEX tool. Several studies note that faculty time commitment can range between 19 min and 31 min including feedback time [68, 69].

The ABIM website provides a generic template for the development and implementation of a mini-CEX tool into a residency program (Table 18.2) [70]. The form is modifiable to the needs of a residency program. One can denote on this form the level of satisfaction with the mini-CEX experience, which is useful for faculty development. Programs can also develop their own forms based on the clinical skills involved. Further research should focus on linking specific evaluations to the ACGME milestones.

Direct Observation of Procedural Skills (DOPS)

The classic teaching adage of *See One, Do One, Teach One* may not be the best way to ensure appropriate training around procedural skills. In fact, literature reveals heterogeneity across programs in the method of training in procedures and the outcome measures for residents. This leads to inconsistency in competency around procedures for graduating residents [71]. Hospital privileges across the country, in turn, lack a consistent or updated approach to credentialing bedside procedures [72]. Similar to the mini-CEX, the direct observation of procedural skills (DOPS) can provide a standardized instructional method for procedural skills. This type of assessment differs from the mini-CEX in that procedural skills are the sole focus. The DOPS can assess residents' understanding of the indications for a procedure, knowledge of the appropriate anatomy, communication skills about the procedure, and professionalism during the procedure [73].

Literature suggests that the DOPS has more educational impact than the mini-CEX due to its assessment of a pre-specified procedure, whereas the mini-CEX can sometimes have vague or generalized outcomes [73]. A pilot study of 60 residents demonstrated success with a standardized simulation-based curriculum in invasive bedside procedural skills, including those in the ambulatory setting, e.g., knee arthrocentesis. This curriculum served as proof of concept for the DOPS instructional method to standardize training around procedural skills [74].

The DOPS instruction is more commonly utilized in procedural based specialties such as surgery and nursing. Publications are sparse on its use in internal medicine education. Further research needs to investigate the value of DOPS to teach outpatient skills such as arthrocentesis and skin biopsies.

Patient Simulation Exercises in Clinic

Most residency programs use patient simulation exercises to teach emerging clinical scenarios such as "rapid response" and/or cardiopulmonary arrest ("Code Blue") situations. Simulation modalities also help to teach both inpatient and outpatient procedural skills such as central line placements, paracentesis, and arthrocentesis. Simulations ensure that residents receive high-yield experiences (e.g., mock exercises related to patient safety) and improve practical clinical skills that may be difficult to achieve during an 80-h workweek. Simulation can apply to a variety of clinical scenarios, ranging from management of a specific medical issue (e.g., back pain in the clinic) to crisis management (e.g., acutely ill or medically unstable patient in the clinic) [75, 76]. An added advantage of the simulation modality is its removal of risk associated with learning a procedure on an actual patient [75]. It allows deliberate practice to occur with immediate feedback available [76] and increases competence in clinical skills as an outcome [77]. However, further research is needed on how to best adapt this type of instructional modality in ambulatory internal medicine.

Point-of-Care Ultrasound in the Ambulatory Setting

Point-of-care ultrasound (POCUS) is a growing area of clinical interest in internal medicine. It is useful in the primary assessment of acutely ill patients and helps to increase patient safety in the performance of both inpatient and outpatient procedures [78, 79]. Technological advances have made ultrasound technology more accessible to the bedside or the clinic setting and capable for real-time, point-of-care use [80]. Clinic-based procedures improved by POCUS include abdominal paracentesis [78], arthrocentesis of multiple joints, and abscess drainage.

A well-defined POCUS curriculum will require residents to be competent in its use for clinical care [78]. Educational directors should consider coupling the POCUS curriculum with direct observation of procedural skills or mini-CEX instructional tools. Educational models around POCUS are well defined in emergency medicine and are being defined in internal medicine [78].

Digital Health Instruction

Panel Management and Electronic Health Record Skill Development

ACGME requires programs to educate residents on health promotions and chronic care management utilizing population-based health data. Several studies highlight the use of panel management curricula to teach a variety of clinical experiences: management of one or two specific chronic medical conditions [32, 81], collaborative team-based care with other interprofessional members on chronic care needs [34, 82], inbox management and expectations [83], management of electronic health records (EHR) before and during the visit [84], and skills in intervisit patient care [84, 85]. Please see Chaps. 6 and 13 for further details. Most studies suggest that panel management interventions primarily enhance residents' perception of improved patient care or increase their confidence in EHR use but do not improve clinical or practice-based outcomes [34, 81, 84]. Implementation of a merit-based incentive payment system may be effective to motivate residents to practice value-based care in the management of their patient panel, as demonstrated by one study with team improvement in average HbA1c outcomes [83]. Another population health care model within a Seattle VA interprofessional team showed trends towards improvement in HbA1c and blood pressure goals, increase in opiate prescription monitoring, and reduction in ED visits for nonacute concerns [82].

Telemedicine Curriculum and Telehealth OSCEs

With the advent of COVID-19 pandemic, residency continuity clinics had to adapt rapidly to delivery of patient care via virtual platforms. Telemedicine curricula have emerged to train residents in general telehealth skills for virtual video and phone clinic visits [41, 86], telehealth communication tools [41], and e-messaging/coordination of interdisciplinary care post-visit [42]. The Medical University of South Carolina initiated a robust 3-year longitudinal curriculum prior to the pandemic that included in-person and online learning for remote management of chronic diseases [87]. Following implementation of these curricula, residents perceived more effective use of telehealth in their clinical practice [41, 42, 86, 87]. Cleveland Clinic's telemedicine curriculum included faculty preceptor training in proper supervision of telehealth visits and provided a mini-CEX tool for direct feedback to residents on their telemedicine performance [41].

In addition to the mini-CEX, video OSCEs (VOSCEs) are another tool to provide feedback to residents and allow for the practice of virtual visit skills, specifically around transitions of care for recently discharged patient [88] or in triaging skills [89]. Findings demonstrate that residents excelled at information gathering, relationship development, and patient education/counseling [88]. Strengths of VOSCEs were comparable to those of in-person OSCEs the year prior [90]. An area in need of improvement and additional teaching was leveraging the video platform to complete a virtual physical exam [88, 89].

Digital Clinical Resources

With the emerging use of digital smart technology for clinical care and patient well-being (e.g., smart phone/watch for heart rate monitoring), educational directors must develop ambulatory curricula to train residents on how to use, comprehend, and leverage these digital clinical resources. One study found that very few responding residency programs teach learners about continuous glucose monitoring or time-in-range for diabetes management. Respondents were "somewhat familiar" with these technologies with varied implementation at their institutions [91]. With increasing clinical use of smart technologies, ambulatory curricula should begin incorporating this important educational need for our trainees. Formal instructional modalities can include preclinic small-group conferences, mini-CEX sessions, and/or patient simulation exercises in the clinic.

Teaching Methods and Instructional Strategies: Resident-Directed Learning

Team-Based Learning

Initially developed by Larry Michaelson [92, 93], team-based learning (TBL) is an adult learning pedagogy that uses small-group instruction, problem-solving, and a knowledge application process for residents to be active participants in their learning. There is a specific sequence of events, starting with an individual pre-class preparation, and then individual and group testing based on the pre-class reading known as the Readiness Assurance Process, followed by a team-based application exercise and feedback. TBL is successful in undergraduate medical education [94] with increasing use in graduate medical education, especially in the ambulatory setting. Given the considerable faculty investment, sustainability of TBL instructions in the ambulatory setting often requires close partnership with program leadership and ongoing support from the chief resident(s). At Northwell Health, faculty converted all their ambulatory didactics to a modified TBL pedagogy. They found that the use of TBL pedagogy increased resident engagement, facilitated group learning, and had higher preference by residents and faculty over traditional didactic lectures

[95]. Similar results were found at Rutgers New Jersey Medical School [96]. A meta-analysis of seven unique TBL curricula in a variety of GME programs noted higher levels of learner engagement and positive or neutral responses by learners of the TBL pedagogy. However, many faculty reported increased time investment for developing TBL curricula. Despite reported knowledge gains, it is unclear how TBL compares to traditional instructional models in terms of content retention and faculty time investment [97]. A comprehensive TBL curriculum for internal medicine residents at Albany Medical College found high faculty and learner satisfaction despite increased preparation time needed by faculty [98].

Problem-Based Learning

Interdisciplinary medical education has incorporated problem-based learning (PBL) for the last 40 years [99]. PBL is an active, learner-centered educational strategy focused on a specific problem, whether it is a clinical, scientific, or a community-based problem. Residents use the problem as a starting point to guide their individual learning needs [99]. Unlike TBL, learners are presented with a problem with no pre-work or preparation. They work either individually or in small groups through the case scenario and identify unfamiliar terms or concepts. The group determines underlying mechanisms and formulates potential explanations for the problem scenario. The group identifies learning issues associated with the clinical encounter and related to the learning objectives as identified by faculty. Following this stage is a period for individual study for accessing a range of educational resources. The group then reconvenes to share what they have learned and apply the learning to the problem scenario. This stage may uncover new learning points that require further individualized study. The final stage is to generalize the learning to the knowledge, skills, or attitudes of other relevant scenarios [99]. PBL has been studied extensively in the undergraduate medical literature, and unfortunately review of the literature suggests no substantial evidence that PBL improves clinical performance or increases medical knowledge base; however, students and faculty find greater satisfaction in learning and teaching in this format [100].

Flipped Classroom

Flipped classroom reverses the traditional educational arrangement by delivering instructional content outside the teaching session. Successful implementation requires a focus on learner-driven learning, faculty adaptability in teaching, and emphasis on knowledge application over fact acquisition. Flipped classroom redefines in-class activities to include a pre-application activity, traditionally considered "homework." The contents are in the form of audio, video, text, or images, which learners review prior to the in-class session. The learners then gather together and engage in a learner-centered activity (e.g., case-based discussions, problem-solving exercises) to apply the knowledge acquired from the pre-work. This strategy requires the learner to be an active participant in acquiring knowledge, evaluating self-performance, and reflecting on peer feedback. Application of knowledge can occur in interactive formats, such as traditional PBL or TBL, or involve simulation activities, role-play, patient encounters, interactive quizzes, or debates [101–104]. Faculty educators take on the role of facilitator rather than lecturer. They organize interactive experiences, challenge students to think creatively, and provide expert insight and feedback. The instruction is less didactic and more personalized to the learners [105]. Flipped classroom remains a viable strategy in the age of distance learning and virtual education. Its blend of asynchronous and synchronous learning leverages technology to meet the educational needs of learners and allows online access to the material for knowledge mastery [106–108]. Chats, breakout rooms, virtual polls, and gamification (e.g., Kahoot) on the digital platform offer interactivity to apply the knowledge during the face-to-screen teaching session. Residency programs [109–114] and health professional schools have adapted the flipped classroom pedagogy with some success [105, 115]. One institution utilized a flipped classroom approach in the ambulatory teaching of cardiovascular prevention and found greater immediate knowledge acquisition with sustained retention at 6 months. Challenges included increased preparation time for residents [114].

Quality Improvement Instruction and Application

Quality improvement (QI) and patient safety (PS) education is an essential component of ambulatory education for programs to meet specific ACGME milestones in resident QI/PS skills. Training residents in QI/PS also gives residents experiential learning in QI/PS issues encountered in independent practice. It is important to integrate ambulatory QI projects into the resident continuity clinic experience to not only develop fundamental skills in QI and panel management but also drive residents' investment and engagement in their primary care clinics. One educational innovation to consider for teaching ambulatory patient safety is the Graduation Clinic Hand-Off. Literature reports that some of these innovations incorporate patients directly into the handoff process or involve dedicated handoff sessions from a senior resident to a junior resident on his/her clinic patient panel [116, 117]. For more information on ambulatory QI curriculum, please refer to Chap. 17 on quality improvement.

Digital Learning

Asynchronous Web-Based Learning

Educational tools that utilize Web-based learning (also known as e-learning) are useful to augment any ambulatory curriculum, especially in the pandemic era. E-learning modules help mitigate work-hour constraints and present general information regardless of the expertise of the teaching faculty. The Web-based module format is effective in teaching a variety of topics to learners, with improved knowledge [118, 119] and communication skills [120]. Many educational models use e-learning as an adjunct to well-established ambulatory curricula. The major advantages of Web-based learning include the portability of knowledge through a universal digital access point and its adaptability to many levels of learners. This instructional modality does not increase the attending workload and is sustainable with little maintenance [121]. Literature has further cited residents' preference for and satisfaction with Web-based learning compared to print materials [122]. Multiple teaching models of e-learning exist in the literature and include education in end-of-life and palliative care [121], nephrology at the point of care [123], education about diabetic ketoacidosis [124], dermatology [125], and cultural competency [126]. Many e-modules also focus on specific topics available to health systems and universities. These include the Institute for Healthcare Improvement's Open School [127], Centers to Advance Palliative Care Modules [128], and American Academy of Dermatology Basic Dermatology Curriculum [129]. In addition, many apps exist for mobile devices to supplement in-person ambulatory instructions on a variety of clinical topics and skills. These apps are best suited for just-in-time clinical teaching moments. Some popular apps for acquisition of clinical knowledge and evidence-based medicine include MDCalc medical calculator, Epocrates, DynaMed, USPSTF Prevention Task Force, ACP Clinical Guidelines, and Journal Club Medicine. Some well-known skill-building apps include Aquifer Clinical Learning for clinical reasoning and communication skills, HumanDx and Prognosis for clinical diagnosis, VirtualDx for clinical decision-making support, and Butterfly iQ for POCUS skills. With available technical support, residency programs can create their own e-learning tools that directly complement established education in the clinic.

Use of Social Media

Emerging literature in emergency medicine, psychiatry, and general medical education touts the influence of social media, in particular Medical Twitter, in clinical teaching and learning. One study demonstrated an increase in the percentage of residents and frequency of social media use for educational purposes when the residency program established a Twitter page. The majority of residents perceived social media as a useful tool for education [130]. Another study on chief resident tweets also showed that residents felt that Twitter enhanced their overall education in residency [131]. Literature review found no specific studies on the use of social media in ambulatory medicine or as an adjunct teaching tool in ambulatory curricula for internal medicine residency programs. This is an area for further medical educational research.

Synchronous Virtual Learning

The COVID-19 pandemic forced many academic programs to pivot to digital methods of teaching. Fortunately, a significant number of free or inexpensive options exist for synchronous/real-time virtual learning. A popular option includes adapting the pre-pandemic learning tools onto a virtual platform such as Zoom, Microsoft TEAMS, or WebEx. This is an easy-to-use option and requires only appropriate audiovisual equipment. Online chats, polls, and breakout rooms are features in the digital platform to promote engagement and interactivity among participants. Other instructional options include virtual white boards such as Google Jamboard, Miro, and Explain Everything. These white boards allow participants to interact with the subject and develop projects together virtually. Educators can also utilize gamification to teach certain ambulatory subjects. Many gamification products are available, such as Poll Everywhere, Kahoot, and online Jeopardy games, to assist faculty in the development of fun and interactive online teaching modalities. Literature review on synchronous virtual education reveals many programs developing unique interactive instructions and a wide variety of ambulatory content that is conducive to virtual learning. These include team-based learning [132], motivational interviewing [133], preclinical didactics [134], and clinical skills [135]. Educational programs should gauge the time and ability of the faculty to develop new virtual teaching tools with the adaptability of existing tools to digital platforms. Educational directors ultimately need to decide the most cost-effective instructional modalities for their ambulatory training.

Ambulatory Curricular Design and Venue

Delivery of ambulatory medicine education to residents occurs through two major clinic designs—longitudinal continuity clinics and ambulatory block rotations, which includes the X + Y burst model [136, 137]. Longitudinal continuity clinics allow residents to manage a panel of patients on a weekly basis over the entire training period. Ambulatory blocks arranged in an X + Y model provide a variation of 1–4-week concentrated clinic experience in primary care and various ambulatory disciplines. Ambulatory long blocks are a third unique design to entrench residents in a year-long dedicated ambulatory clinical experience [138]. Most recently, the emergence of primary care immersion blocks [139] and ambulatory boot camps [140] offers shorter but more intensive curricular designs to prepare residents for ambulatory medicine. Clinical experiential training remains the crux of all these curricular designs. Embedded within these curricular designs are various instructional venues to allow for dedicated time blocks for formal ambulatory teaching with no patient care obligations. These include academic half-days, pre-clinic or post-clinic conferences, and daily protected didactics, e.g., ambulatory morning reports and noon conferences. These supplementary educational venues consolidate the experiential learning, extend the curriculum beyond clinical cases, and connect clinical practice with evidence-based medicine [15, 16]. See Chap. 4 for more information on the various academic scheduling models.

Developing an Ambulatory Curriculum in One's Own Academic Clinic

Step-by-Step Guide of Essential Elements in Developing an Ambulatory Curriculum

The design and delivery of an ambulatory curriculum involve six key steps for successful implementation (Fig. 18.1). The process starts with assembling a dedicated team to address the ambulatory educational needs and goals for residents and concludes with establishing a forum for feedback, assessment, and faculty development. Appendix 18.E provides educational directors with a systematic checklist for curriculum development.

Existing Ambulatory Curricula

Well-established ambulatory curricula are available for purchase to facilitate the development of a program's ambulatory curriculum. The two most popular curricula are the Internal Medicine Ambulatory Care Curriculum offered through Johns Hopkins and the Yale Office-Based Medicine Curriculum. The Internal Medicine Ambulatory Care Curriculum through the Physician Education and Assessment Center (PEAC) at Johns Hopkins consists of 43 modules relevant to outpatient medicine (https://www.peaconline.org/). Topics are in a case-based format with a pretest and posttest to assess resident knowledge. Each module has links to relevant journal articles, abstracts, images, and videos [141]. This curriculum can help complement the core residency ambulatory content and fulfill any clinical knowledge gaps at any institution. Over 180 residency programs have subscribed to this curriculum. Alternatively, the Yale Office Based Curriculum is available to help house staff assess and manage common ambulatory problems through an evidence-based syllabus. It covers 3 years of ambulatory training with over 144 clinical cases with case-related questions. There are two formal guides: a house staff guide composed of the case, clinical questions, and key references, and a faculty guide composed of teaching points with answers. The Yale Office Based Curriculum is used by over 245 internal medicine, nursing, medicine-pediatrics, and family medicine residency programs, medical schools, and individuals (https://medicine.yale.edu/intmed/obm/) [43]. Both of these curricula have an annual subscription fee for institutions or individuals to purchase. Residency programs can also use the ACP "In the Clinic" series to provide foundational teaching in core ambulatory clinical topics such as type 2 diabetes, obesity medicine, hypertension, and heart failure. Each topic article offers a comprehensive review of the evidence for diagnosis, evaluation, and treatment and concludes with MKSAP questions to solidify knowledge. This series is purchasable from ACP and is a monthly feature of the Annals of Internal Medicine journal (https://www.acpjournals.org/topic/category/in-the-clinic).

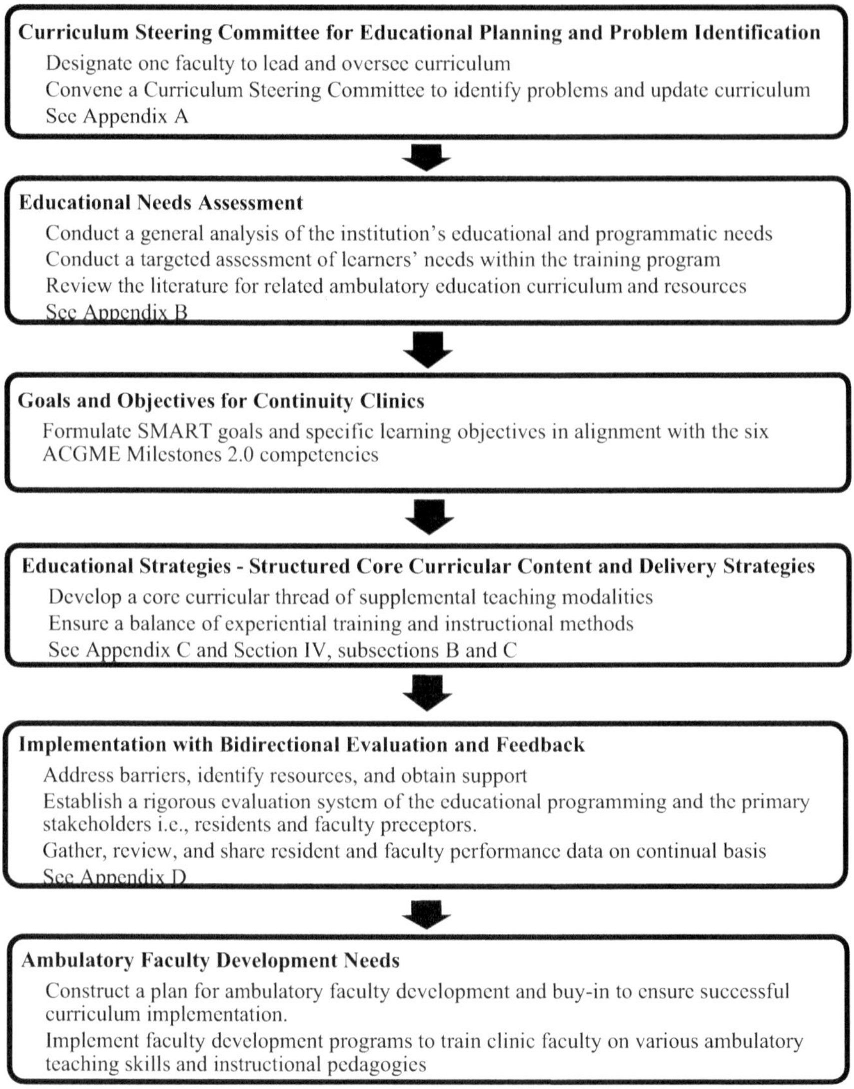

Fig. 18.1 Step-by-step guide in developing an ambulatory curriculum. **Adapted from** Thomas PA, Kern DE, Hughes MT, Chen. Curriculum Development for Medical Education: A Six-Step Approach. Third Edition. Johns Hopkins University Press, 2015

Conclusion

The revised ACGME Common Program Requirements in July 2022 dictate ambulatory education to make up 10 months of total residency time. Therefore, ambulatory experiential training needs to be supplemented by a structured core curricular thread. This curricular thread guides the educational needs of both the learners and institutions, has achievable learning objectives specific to ACGME Milestones 2.0 competencies, and teaches foundational outpatient skills such as electronic health record management, chronic disease management, telehealth technologies, and team-based care. Most medicine graduates will practice in the outpatient setting after residency or fellowship and require these core ambulatory skills for success. A variety of instructional modalities, ranging from formal programmatic instructions and digital resources to resident-directed learning methods, can help address the diverse learning styles of learners, harness existing technological tools, and leverage unique teaching techniques used by faculty.

Appendix A: A General Needs Assessment of Ambulatory Medicine Curriculum

Problem Identification - What is current approach? Barriers to implementation?	**Ideal Approach?**	**Goals & Objectives**	**Resources needed for implementation?**

Appendix B: Targeted Needs Assessment of Learners

Key Learners	Impact of Curriculum	Relevant Info needed from Learners	Methods for Learner Needs Assessment	Resources needed for Implementation

Appendix C: Sample 18-month curriculum for X+Y clinic design, repeated twice over residency

Block	Theme
1	Introduction to office-based practice I
2	Screening, prevention, population health
3	Pain management/musculoskeletal
4	Cardiology
5	Psychiatric disease
6	Pulmonary
7	Infectious disease/HIV
8	Endocrine
9	Gastroenterology
10	Renal
11	Geriatrics
12	Women's health
13	Neurology/dermatology
14	ENT/ophthalmology/hematology
15	Palliative
16	High-value cost-conscious care
17	Urban curriculum
18	Career development and wellness

Sample 36-Month Curriculum for Traditional or Hybrid Weekly Half-Day Clinic Design

Month	Topics		
	Year 1	Year 2	Year 3
July	Billing and coding	Billing and coding	Billing and coding
August	Preventative services: Vaccine/cancer screen	Preventative services: Vaccine/cancer screen	Preventative services: Vaccine/cancer screen
September	Type 2 diabetes mellitus	Preoperative evaluation	Sexually transmitted diseases
October	Hypertension	Coronary artery disease	Geriatric wellness
November	Hyperlipidemia	Obesity	Congestive heart failure
December	Panel management	Panel management	Panel management
January	Depression/anxiety	Hypogonadism and erectile dysfunction	Chronic pelvic pain and dysmenorrhea
February	Chronic pain syndrome	Gout vs. osteoarthritis	Women's health
March	URI vs. sinusitis	Fibromyalgia	Hepatitis C
April	Asthma and COPD	CVA/TIA	Atrial fibrillation
May	Thyroid disease: hypo/ hyperthyroidism	GERD	Community-acquired pneumonia vs. influenza
June	Transitions of care	Migraines vs. tension headaches	Osteoporosis and vitamin D deficiency

Sample Schedule for Academic Half-Day Design

8:30–8:45	**Medicine in the news, EBM quiz:** Learning based on medical issues reported in the media as well as published studies
8:45–9:15	**Ambulatory morning report:** PGY1 residents on ambulatory block present an outpatient case for discussion
9:15–9:30	**Board review questions** focused on ambulatory medicine topics
9:30–10:00	**Problem-based learning** directed by an attending, covering chronic disease management, acute disease management in the outpatient setting, preventive medicine and immunizations, women's health, laboratory testing, medication management, etc.
10:00–10:15	**Break**
10:15–10:45	**Residents as teachers:** PGY2 residents on ambulatory block discuss outpatient medicine topics based on educational prescriptions
10:45–11:15	**Introduction to EBM, basic principles, and literature search strategies:** We will utilize teaching scripts based on patient encounters, to teach EBM concepts and promote lifelong learning behaviors. EBM sessions alternate with the **ACP high-value cost-conscious curriculum (HVCC)** as it pertains to outpatient care
11:15–11:45	**Residents as teachers:** PGY3 residents present an EBM consult (literature review to answer a clinical question) based on educational prescription
11:45–12:00	**QI project review and progress**

Appendix D: Sample Mini-CEX for Gynecological Examination

Resident: ______________________________
Date: ______________________________
Supervisor: ____________________________
Please rate the resident on the following criteria:

	Poor/not done	Minimal/ adequate	Excellent
1. Proper patient positioning	1	2	3
2. Communication with patient during exam	1	2	3
3. Inspection of the external genitalia	1	2	3
4. Use of speculum (insertion and removal)	1	2	3
5. Inspection of vaginal walls and cervix	1	2	3
6. Obtained sample for PAP smear and/or wet mount/culture	1	2	3
7. Bimanual examination	1	2	3
8. Examination for inguinal adenopathy	1	2	3
9. Overall rating	1	2	3

Do you feel this resident is competent in performance of the pelvic exam? Yes No

Please provide any additional comments below:

Appendix E: Checklist for Curriculum Implementation

- Identify resources
  - Personnel required: faculty, staff, other
  - Time: faculty, learners, support staff
  - Facilities: space, equipment, sites
  - Funding/costs: direct and indirect costs
- Obtain support
  - Internal: program director, department chair, learners, faculty
  - External: professional societies, if applicable (e.g., SGIM, AAIM)
- Develop administrative mechanisms to support the curriculum
  - Administrative structure of team

    Necessary for delineating responsibilities and decision-making

- Communication

  Content to learners and faculty: includes goals and objectives, information about curriculum, facilities, scheduling, changes, evaluation results
  Mechanisms: email, meetings, website, etc.

- Operations

  Preparation and distribution of schedules and curricular materials
  Method of collecting, collating, and distributing evaluation data
  Process for revisions

• Anticipate and address barriers

  - Financial
  - Competing demands
  - People: attitudes of learners and faculty, faculty without enough time, authority, etc.

• Introduce curriculum in stepwise fashion

  - Pilot project
  - Phase-in
  - Full implementation

Adapted from Kern DE, et al.: Curriculum Development for Medical Education – A Six-Step Approach, 2nd edition. Baltimore: The Johns Hopkins Univ. Press. 2009

References

1. Accreditation Council for Graduate Medical Education. ACGME common program requirements. 2021. https://www.acgme.org/what-we-do/accreditation/common-program-requirements/. Accessed 14 Nov 2021.
2. Meyers FJ, Weinberger SE, Fitzgibbons JP, Glassroth J, Duffy FD, Clayton CP, et al. Redesigning residency training in internal medicine: the consensus report of the Alliance for Academic Internal Medicine Education Redesign Task Force. Acad Med. 2007;82(12):1211–9.
3. Nadkarni M, Reddy S, Bates CK, Fosburgh B, Babbott S, Holmboe E. Ambulatory-based education in internal medicine: current organization and implications for transformation. Results of a national survey of resident continuity clinic directors. J Gen Intern Med. 2011;26(1):16–20.
4. Thomas PA, Kern DE, Hughes MT, Chen. Curriculum development for medical education: a six-step approach. 3rd ed. Baltimore, MD: Johns Hopkins University Press; 2015.
5. Alguire PC, DeWitt DE, Pinsky LE, Ferenchick GS. Teaching in your office: a guide to instructing medical students and residents. 2nd ed. Philadelphia, PA: American College of Physicians; 2008.
6. Colbert C, Costa ST, Garcia M, Kothari N, Krikorian A, Mortley A, Pindiprolu S, et al. Developing a Curriculum. In: Williams FK, Wininger DA, editors. The toolkit series: a textbook for internal medicine education programs. 12th ed. Alliance for Academic Internal Medicine; 2017.

7. Schneiderhan J, Guetterman TC, Dobson ML. Curriculum development: a how to primer. Fam Med Com Health. 2019;7:e000046. https://doi.org/10.1136/fmch-2018-000046.
8. Green ML. Identifying, appraising, and implementing medical education curricula: a guide for medical educators. Ann Intern Med. 2001;135(10):889–96.
9. Doran GT. There's a S.M.A.R.T. way to write management's goals and objectives. Man Rev. 1981;70:35–6.
10. Meyer PJ. Attitude is everything: if you want to succeed above and beyond. Waco, TX: Meyer Resource Group; 2003.
11. Johns Hopkins School of Medicine. Writing better objective. http://www.hopkinscme.edu/Uploads/StaticFiles/WritingBetterObjectives.pdf. Accessed 13 Aug 2016.
12. Armstrong P. Bloom's taxonomy. Vanderbilt University Center for Teaching; 2010. https://cft.vanderbilt.edu/guides-sub-pages/blooms-taxonomy/.
13. Bloom BS, et al. Taxonomy of educational objectives: Handbook 1: cognitive domain. London: Longman Publishing Group; 1984.
14. Accreditation Council for Graduate Medical Education. ACGME Milestones. http://www.acgme.org/What-We-Do/Accreditation/Milestones/Overview. Accessed 14 Nov 2021.
15. Irby DM. Teaching and learning in ambulatory care settings: a thematic review of the literature. Acad Med. 1995;70(10):898–931.
16. Bowen JL, Irby DM. Assessing quality and costs of education in the ambulatory setting: a review of the literature. Acad Med. 2002;77(7):621–80.
17. Lesky LG, Borkan SC. Strategies to improve teaching in the ambulatory medicine setting. Arch Intern Med. 1990;150(10):2133–7.
18. Skeff KM. Enhancing teaching effectiveness and vitality in the ambulatory setting. J Gen Intern Med. 1988;3(2 Suppl):S26–33.
19. Holmboe ES, Bowen JL, Green M, Gregg J, DiFrancesco L, Reynolds E, et al. Reforming internal medicine residency training. A report from the Society of General Internal Medicine's task force for residency reform. J Gen Intern Med. 2005;20(12):1165–72.
20. Lesky LG, Hershman WY. Practical approaches to a major educational challenge. Training students in the ambulatory setting. Arch Intern Med. 1995;155(9):897–904.
21. Laidley TL, Braddock CH. Role of adult learning theory in evaluating and designing strategies for teaching residents in ambulatory settings. Adv Health Sci Educ Theory Pract. 2000;5:43–54. https://doi.org/10.1023/A:1009863211233.
22. Taylor DCM, Hamdy H. Adult learning theories: Implications for learning and teaching in medical education: AMEE Guide No. 83. Med Teach. 2013;35(11):e1561–72. https://doi.org/10.3109/0142159X.2013.828153.
23. Furney SL, Orsini AN, Orsetti KE, Stern DT, Gruppen LD, Irby DM. Teaching the one-minute preceptor. A randomized controlled trial. J Gen Intern Med. 2001;16(9):620–4.
24. Wolpaw TM, Wolpaw DR, Papp KK. SNAPPS: a learner-centered model for outpatient education. Acad Med. 2003;78(9):893–8.
25. Aagaard E, Teherani A, Irby DM. Effectiveness of the one-minute preceptor model for diagnosing the patient and the learner: proof of concept. Acad Med. 2004;79(1):42–9.
26. Irby DM, Aagaard E, Teherani A. Teaching points identified by preceptors observing one-minute preceptor and traditional preceptor encounters. Acad Med. 2004;79(1):50–5.
27. Lo MC, Tolentino J, Fazio SB, Vinciguerra S, Amin AN, Dentino A, Hingle ST, Palamara K, Modak I, Kisielewski M, Moriarty JP. Identifying solutions to ambulatory faculty recruitment, retention, and remuneration in graduate medical education: an AAIM position paper. Am J Med. 2020;133(3):386–94. https://doi.org/10.1016/j.amjmed.2019.11.001. Epub 2019 Nov 9.
28. Fazio SB, Chheda S, Hingle S, Lo MC, Meade L, Blanchard M, Hoellein A, Brandenburg S, Denton GD. The challenges of teaching ambulatory internal medicine: faculty recruitment, retention, and development: an AAIM/SGIM position paper. Am J Med. 2017;130(1):105–10. https://doi.org/10.1016/j.amjmed.2016.09.004. Epub 2016 Oct 1.

29. Denton GD, Lo MC, Brandenburg S, Hingle S, Meade L, Chheda S, Fazio SB, Blanchard M, Hoellein A. Solutions to common problems in training learners in general internal medicine ambulatory settings. Am J Med. 2015;128(10):1152–7. https://doi.org/10.1016/j.amjmed.2015.05.023. Epub 2015 Jun 10.
30. Weinberger SE, Smith LG, Collier VU, et al. Redesigning training for internal medicine. Ann Intern Med. 2006;144(12):927–32. https://doi.org/10.7326/0003-4819-144-12-200606200-00124. Epub 2006 Apr 6.
31. Bharel M, Jain S, Hollander H. Comprehensive ambulatory medicine training for categorical internal medicine residents. J Gen Intern Med. 2003;18(4):288–93.
32. Hadley Strout EK, Landrey AR, MacLean CD, Sobel HG. Internal medicine resident experiences with a 5-month ambulatory panel management curriculum. J Grad Med Educ. 2018;10(5):559–65. https://doi.org/10.4300/JGME-D-18-00172.1.
33. Dulay M, Bowen JL, Weppner WG, Eastburn A, Poppe AP, Spanos P, Wojtaszek D, Printz D, Kaminetzky CP. Interprofessional population health advocacy: developing and implementing a panel management curriculum in five Veterans Administration primary care practices. J Interprof Care. 2018:1–11. https://doi.org/10.1080/13561820.2018.1469476.
34. Kaminetzky CP, Beste LA, Poppe AP, Doan DB, Mun HK, Woods NF, Wipf JE. Implementation of a novel population panel management curriculum among interprofessional health care trainees. BMC Med Educ. 2017;17(1):264. https://doi.org/10.1186/s12909-017-1093-y.
35. Khera SP, Chung JJ, Daw M, Kaminski MA. A framework and curriculum for training residents in population health. Popul Health Manag. 2021;25(1):57–64. https://doi.org/10.1089/pop.2021.0079.
36. Bodenheimer T, Syer S, Fair M, Shipman S. Teaching residents population health management. November 2019. Association of American Medical Colleges. https://store.aamc.org/downloadable/download/sample/sample_id/311/. Accessed 3 Oct 2021.
37. Gupta R, Dubé K, Bodenheimer T. The road to excellence for primary care resident teaching clinics. Academic Med. 2016;91(4):458–61. https://doi.org/10.1097/ACM.0000000000001100.
38. Holt SR, Tobin DG, Whitman L, Ellman M, Moriarty JP, Doolittle B. Creating a satisfying continuity clinic experience for primary care trainees. Am J Med. 2021;134(4):547–53. https://doi.org/10.1016/j.amjmed.2020.12.005. Epub 2020 Dec 30.
39. Rusiecki J, Schell J, Rothenberger S, Merriam S, McNeil M, Spagnoletti C. An innovative shared decision-making curriculum for internal medicine residents: findings from the University of Pittsburgh medical center. Acad Med. 2018;93(6):937–42. https://doi.org/10.1097/ACM.0000000000001967.
40. Accreditation Council for Graduate Medical Education (ACGME). https://www.acgme.org/specialties/internal-medicine/program-requirements-and-faqs-and-applications/ Accessed 3 Oct 2021.
41. Savage DJ, Gutierrez O, Montané BE, Singh AD, Yudelevich E, Mahar J, Brateanu A, Khatri L, Fleisher C, Jolly SE. Implementing a telemedicine curriculum for internal medicine residents during a pandemic: the Cleveland Clinic experience. Postgrad Med J. 2022;98(1161):487–91. https://doi.org/10.1136/postgradmedj-2020-139228. Epub ahead of print. PMID: 33692154; PMCID: PMC7948159.
42. Wong R, Ng P, Spinnato T, Taub E, Kaushal A, Lerman M, Fernan A, Dainer E, Noel K. Expanding telehealth competencies in primary care: a longitudinal interdisciplinary simulation to train internal medicine residents in complex patient care. J Grad Med Educ. 2020;12(6):745–52. https://doi.org/10.4300/JGME-D-20-00030.1. Epub 2020 Dec 4. PMID: 33391599; PMCID: PMC7771597.
43. Yale University. Yale office-based medicine curriculum. 2022. https://medicine.yale.edu/intmed/obm/about/. Accessed February 2022.
44. Kernan WN, Quagliarello V, Green ML. Student faculty rounds: a peer-mediated learning activity for internal medicine clerkships. Med Teach. 2005;27(2):140–4.

45. Leung J, Bhutani M, Leigh R, Pelletier D, Good C, Sin DD. Empowering family physicians to impart proper inhaler teaching to patients with chronic obstructive pulmonary disease and asthma. Can Respir J. 2015;22(5):266.
46. Chou C, Lee K. Improving residents' interviewing skills by group videotape review. Acad Med. 2002;77(7):744.
47. McNeill M, Ali SK, Banks DE, Mansi IA. Morning report: can an established medical education tradition be validated? J Grad Med Ed. 2013;5(3):374.
48. Demopoulos B, Pelzman F, Wenderoth S. Ambulatory morning report: an underutilized educational modality. Teach Learn Med. 2001;13(1):49–52.
49. Spickard A 3rd, Hales JB, Ellis S. Outpatient morning report: a new educational venue. Acad Med. 2000;75(2):197.
50. Malone ML, Jackson TC. Educational characteristics of ambulatory morning report. J Gen Int Med. 1993;8(9):512.
51. Luciano GL, Visintainer PF, Kleppel R, Rothberg MB. Ambulatory morning report: a case-based method of teaching EBM through experiential learning. South Med J. 2016;109(2):108.
52. Wong C, Evans G. The ambulatory morbidity and mortality conference meets the morning report. Med Ed. 2012;46:501.
53. Rosenberg W, Donald A. Evidence based medicine: an approach to clinical problem-solving. BMJ. 1995;310(6987):1122–6.
54. Fazio SB, Steinmann AF. A new era for residency training in internal medicine. JAMA Intern Med. 2016;176(2):161–2.
55. van Dijk N, Hooft L, Wieringa-de WM. What are the barriers to residents' practicing evidence-based medicine? A systematic review. Acad Med. 2010;85(7):1163–70.
56. Green ML. Graduate medical education training in clinical epidemiology, critical appraisal, and evidence-based medicine: a critical review of curricula. Acad Med. 1999;74(6):686–94.
57. Ebbert JO, Montori VM, Schultz HJ. The journal club in postgraduate medical education: a systematic review. Med Teach. 2001;23(5):455–61.
58. DaRosa DA, Dunnington GL, Stearns J, Ferenchick G, Bowen JL, Simpson DE. Ambulatory teaching "lite": less clinic time, more educationally fulfilling. Acad Med. 1997;72(5):358–61.
59. Rodriguez RG, Hawley-Molloy JS. Revamping journal club for the millennial learner. J Grad Med Educ. 2017;9(3):377–8. https://doi.org/10.4300/JGME-D-16-00667.1. PMID: 28638526; PMCID: PMC5476397.
60. Chetlen AL, Dell CM, Solberg AO, Otero HJ, Burton KR, Heller MT, Lakomkin N, Desouches SL, Smith SE. Another time, another space: the evolution of the virtual journal club. Acad Radiol. 2017;24(3):273–85. https://doi.org/10.1016/j.acra.2016.08.030. Epub 2016 Dec 1.
61. Richardson WS, Wilson MC, Nishikawa J, Hayward RS. The well-built clinical question: a key to evidence-based decisions. ACP J Club. 1995;123(3):A12–3.
62. Oller D. The ambulatory teaching minute: development of brief, case-based, evidence-based medicine exercises for the internal medicine resident continuity clinic. MedEdPORTAL. 2020;16:10909. https://doi.org/10.15766/mep_2374-8265.10909. PMID: 32656330; PMCID: PMC7331953.
63. ABIM Website. abim.org. Accessed November 2021.
64. Pelgrim EA, Kramer AW, Mokkink HG, van den Elsen L, Grol RP, van der Vleuten CP. In-training assessment using direct observation of single-patient encounters: a literature review. Adv Health Sci Educ Theory Pract. 2011;16(1):131–42. https://doi.org/10.1007/s10459-010-9235-6. Epub 2010 Jun 18. PMID: 20559868; PMCID: PMC3074070.
65. Liao KC, Pu SJ, Liu MS, Yang CW, Kuo HP. Development and implementation of a mini-Clinical Evaluation Exercise (mini-CEX) program to assess the clinical competencies of internal medicine residents: from faculty development to curriculum evaluation. BMC Med Educ. 2013;13:31. https://doi.org/10.1186/1472-6920-13-31. PMID: 23442216; PMCID: PMC3599226.

66. Alves de Lima AE, Conde D, Aldunate L, van der Vleuten CPM. Teachers' experiences of the role and function of the mini clinical evaluation exercise in post-graduate training. Int J Med Ed. 2010;1:68–73.
67. Johnson NR, Pelletier A, Berkowitz LR. Mini-clinical evaluation exercise in the era of milestones and entrustable professional activities in obstetrics and gynaecology: resume or reform? J Obstet Gynaecol Can. 2020;42(6):718–25. https://doi.org/10.1016/j.jogc.2019.10.002. Epub 2019 Dec 25.
68. Kogan JR, Bellini LM, Shea JA. Feasibility, reliability, and validity of the mini-clinical evaluation exercise (mCEX) in a medicine core clerkship. Acad Med. 2003;78(10 Suppl):S33–5. https://doi.org/10.1097/00001888-200310001-00011.
69. Hauer KE. Enhancing feedback to students using the mini-CEX (Clinical Evaluation Exercise). Acad Med. 2000;75(5):524. https://doi.org/10.1097/00001888-200005000-00046.
70. American Board of Internal Medicine. Mini-CEX clinical evaluation for trainees: direct observation assessment tool. 2016. http://www.abim.org/program-directors-administrators/assessment-tools/mini-cex.aspx. Accessed Nov 2021.
71. Brydges R, Stroud L, Wong BM, Holmboe ES, Imrie K, Hatala R. Core competencies or a competent core? a scoping review and realist synthesis of invasive bedside procedural skills training in internal medicine. Acad Med. 2017;92(11):1632–43. https://doi.org/10.1097/ACM.0000000000001726.
72. Jensen TP, Soni NJ, Tierney DM, Lucas BP. Hospital privileging practices for bedside procedures: a survey of hospitalist experts. J Hosp Med. 2017;12(10):836–9. https://doi.org/10.12788/jhm.2837. Epub 2017 Sep 6.
73. Lörwald AC, Lahner FM, Nouns ZM, Berendonk C, Norcini J, Greif R, Huwendiek S. The educational impact of Mini-Clinical Evaluation Exercise (Mini-CEX) and Direct Observation of Procedural Skills (DOPS) and its association with implementation: A systematic review and meta-analysis. PLoS One. 2018;13(6):e0198009. https://doi.org/10.1371/journal.pone.0198009. PMID: 29864130; PMCID: PMC5986126.
74. Lenchus JD. End of the "see one, do one, teach one" era: the next generation of invasive bedside procedural instruction. J Am Osteopath Assoc. 2010;110(6):340–6.
75. McLaughlin S, Fitch MT, Goyal DG, Hayden E, Kauh CY, Laack TA, Nowicki T, Okuda Y, Palm K, Pozner CN, Vozenilek J, Wang E, Gordon JA, et al. Simulation in graduate medical education 2008: a review for emergency medicine. Acad Emerg Med. 2008;15(11):1117–29. https://doi.org/10.1111/j.1553-2712.2008.00188.x. Epub 2008 Jul 14.
76. Gaba DM. The future vision of simulation in healthcare. Qual Saf Health Care. 2004;13(Suppl 1):i2.
77. Offiah G, Ekpotu LP, Murphy S, Kane D, Gordon A, O'Sullivan M, Sharifuddin SF, Hill ADK, Condron CM. Evaluation of medical student retention of clinical skills following simulation training. BMC Med Educ. 2019;19(1):263. https://doi.org/10.1186/s12909-019-1663-2. PMID: 31311546; PMCID: PMC6632214.
78. Olgers TJ, Azizi N, Blans MJ, Bosch FH, Gans ROB, Ter Maaten JC. Point-of-care Ultrasound (PoCUS) for the internist in acute medicine: a uniform curriculum. Neth J Med. 2019;77(5):168–76.
79. Guidelines U. Emergency, point-of-care and clinical ultrasound guidelines in medicine. Ann Emerg Med. 2017;69(5):e27–54. https://doi.org/10.1016/j.annemergmed.2016.08.457.
80. Bhagra A, Tierney DM, Sekiguchi H, Soni NJ. Point-of-Care ultrasonography for primary care physicians and general internists. Mayo Clin Proc. 2016;91(12):1811–27. https://doi.org/10.1016/j.mayocp.2016.08.023. Epub 2016 Nov 5.
81. Haynes C, Yamamoto M, Dashiell-Earp C, Gunawardena D, Gupta R, Simon W. Continuity clinic practice feedback curriculum for residents: a model for ambulatory education. J Grad Med Educ. 2019;11(2):189–95. https://doi.org/10.4300/JGME-D-18-00714.1. PMID: 31024652; PMCID: PMC6476079.
82. Gardner AL, Kaminetzky CP, Poppe AP, Wipf JE. Interprofessional academic patient aligned care team panel management model. Fed Pract. 2019;36(6):278–83. PMID: 31258321; PMCID: PMC6590949.

83. Bolyard J, Viswanathan V, Fribourg D, Narayanan R. MIPS in residency? a look at merit-based incentives in an internal medicine residency outpatient practice. J Grad Med Educ. 2019;11(1):79–84. https://doi.org/10.4300/JGME-D-18-00239.2. PMID: 30805102; PMCID: PMC6375335.
84. Nikiforova T, Spagnoletti CL, Rothenberger SD, Jeong K, Hariharan J. Peers know best: a novel curriculum for onboarding interns' electronic health record skills in continuity clinic. J Gen Intern Med. 2021. doi: https://doi.org/10.1007/s11606-021-06796-4.
85. Hom J, Richman I, Chen JH, Singh B, Crump C, Chi J. Fulfilling outpatient medicine responsibilities during internal medicine residency: a quantitative study of housestaff participation with between visit tasks. BMC Med Educ. 2016;16:139. https://doi.org/10.1186/s12909-016-0665-6. PMID: 27160008; PMCID: PMC4862079.
86. Keyserling K, Janetos E, Sprague C. Teaching telehealth during a pandemic and beyond: an intern's survival guide for virtual medicine. J Gen Intern Med. 2021;36(10):3219–23. https://doi.org/10.1007/s11606-021-07009-8. Epub 2021 Jul 21. PMID: 34287776; PMCID: PMC8294316.
87. Kirkland EB, DuBose-Morris R, Duckett A. Telehealth for the internal medicine resident: A 3-year longitudinal curriculum. J Telemed Telecare. 2021;27(9):599–605. https://doi.org/10.1177/1357633X19896683. Epub 2019 Dec 31.
88. Sartori DJ, Hayes RW, Horlick M, Adams JG, Zabar SR. The TeleHealth OSCE: preparing trainees to use telemedicine as a tool for transitions of care. J Grad Med Educ. 2020;12(6):764–8. https://doi.org/10.4300/JGME-D-20-00039.1. Epub 2020 Dec 2. PMID: 33391602; PMCID: PMC7771608.
89. Haidet P, Hempel EV, Louw BC, Chisty A. Virtual decisions: using a telehealth OSCE to enhance trainees' triage skills. Med Educ. 2021;55(5):659. https://doi.org/10.1111/medu.14493. Epub 2021 Mar 17. PMID: 33733539; PMCID: PMC8250726.
90. Boardman D, Wilhite JA, Adams J, Sartori D, Greene R, Hanley K, Zabar S. Telemedicine training in the COVID era: revamping a routine OSCE to prepare medicine residents for virtual care. J Med Educ Curric Dev. 2021;8:23821205211024076. https://doi.org/10.1177/23821205211024076. PMID: 34189270; PMCID: PMC8212360.
91. Morales J, Kuritzky L, Lavernia F, Santiago M. Are residents receiving the training needed within their residency programs to optimally manage patients with diabetes? Postgrad Med. 2021;133(4):388–94. https://doi.org/10.1080/00325481.2020.1857603. Epub 2020 Dec 17.
92. Parmelee D, Michaelsen LK, Cook S, Hudes PD. Team-based learning: a practical guide: AMEE guide no. 65. Med Teach. 2012;34(5):e275–87.
93. Parmelee DX, Michaelsen LK. Twelve tips for doing effective Team-Based Learning (TBL). Med Teach. 2010;32(2):118–22.
94. Searle NS, Haidet P, Kelly PA, Schneider VF, Seidel CL, Richards BF. Team learning in medical education: initial experiences at ten institutions. Acad Med. 2003;78(10 Suppl):S55–8.
95. Balwan S, Fornari A, DiMarzio P, Verbsky J, Pekmezaris R, Stein J, et al. Use of team-based learning pedagogy for internal medicine ambulatory resident teaching. J Grad Med Educ. 2015;7(4):643–8.
96. Feurdean M, Matassa D, Kang M, Matthews G, Kothari N. A modified team based learning approach to enhance resident education in outpatient internal medicine. MedEdPublish. 2017;6(4):1–11. https://doi.org/10.15694/mep.2017.000176.
97. Poeppelman RS, Liebert CA, Vegas DB, Germann CA, Volerman A. A narrative review and novel framework for application of team-based learning in graduate medical education. J Grad Med Educ. 2016;8(4):510–7.
98. Schynoll G, Irish E, Wayne J, Smith R. Feasibility of a comprehensive medical knowledge curriculum in internal medicine using team-based learning. J Grad Med Educ. 2018;10(1):78–83. https://doi.org/10.4300/JGME-D-17-00465.1. PMID: 29467978; PMCID: PMC5821028.
99. Davis MH. AMEE medical education guide No. 15: problem-based learning: a practical guide. Med Teach. 1999;21(2):130–40.
100. Dolmans D, Michaelsen L, van Merrienboer J, van der Vleuten C. Should we choose between problem-based learning and team-based learning? No, combine the best of both worlds! Med Teach. 2015;37(4):354–9.

101. Prober CG, Khan S. Medical education reimagined: a call to action. Acad Med. 2013;88(10):1407–10.
102. Ding C, Wang Q, Zou J, Zhu K. Implementation of flipped classroom combined with case- and team-based learning in residency training. Adv Physiol Educ. 2021;45(1):77–83. https://doi.org/10.1152/advan.00022.2020.
103. Hu X, Zhang H, Song Y, Wu C, Yang Q, Shi Z, Zhang X, Chen W. Implementation of flipped classroom combined with problem-based learning: an approach to promote learning about hyperthyroidism in the endocrinology internship. BMC Med Educ. 2019;19(1):290. https://doi.org/10.1186/s12909-019-1714-8. PMID: 31362729; PMCID: PMC6668058.
104. van Alten D, Phielix C, Janssen J, Kester L. Effects of flipping the classroom on learning outcomes and satisfaction: A meta-analysis. Educ Res Rev. 2019;28:1–18. https://doi.org/10.1016/j.edurev.2019.05.003.
105. McLaughlin JE, Roth MT, Glatt DM, Gharkholonarehe N, Davidson CA, Griffin LM, et al. The flipped classroom: a course redesign to foster learning and engagement in a health professions school. Acad Med. 2014;89(2):236–43.
106. Patel B, Taggar JS. Virtual teaching of undergraduate primary care small groups during Covid-19. Educ Prim Care. 2021;32(5):296–302. https://doi.org/10.1080/14739879.2021.1920475. Epub 2021 Jun 28.
107. Lichvar AB, Hedges A, Benedict NJ, Donihi AC. Combination of a flipped classroom format and a virtual patient case to enhance active learning in a required therapeutics course. Am J Pharm Educ. 2016;80(10):175. https://doi.org/10.5688/ajpe8010175. PMID: 28179724; PMCID: PMC5289731.
108. Wade SD, Freed JA, Kyttaris VC, Saunders S, Hausmann JS. Implementing a virtual flipped classroom in a rheumatology fellowship program. Arthritis Care Res (Hoboken). 2021;75(3):634–9. https://doi.org/10.1002/acr.24791. Epub ahead of print.
109. Young TP, Bailey CJ, Guptill M, Thorp AW, Thomas TL. The flipped classroom: a modality for mixed asynchronous and synchronous learning in a residency program. West J Emerg Med. 2014;15(7):938–44.
110. Grant LL, Opperman MJ, Schiller B, Chastain J, Richardson JD, Eckel C, Plawecki MH. Medical student engagement in a virtual learning environment positively correlates with course performance and satisfaction in psychiatry. Med Sci Educ. 2021;31(3):1–8. https://doi.org/10.1007/s40670-021-01287-x. Epub ahead of print. PMID: 33868773; PMCID: PMC8041389.
111. Kurup V, Sendlewski G. The feasibility of incorporating a flipped classroom model in an anesthesia residency curriculum-pilot study. Yale J Biol Med. 2020;93(3):411–7. PMID: 32874146; PMCID: PMC7448396.
112. Pontius LN, Hooten J, Lesesky E, Rao C, Nicholas M, Bialas R, Liu B, Green CL, Atwater AR. A comparison of knowledge acquisition and perceived efficacy of a traditional vs flipped classroom-based dermatology residency curriculum. Cutis. 2020;105(1):36–9.
113. Sivarajah RT, Curci NE, Johnson EM, Lam DL, Lee JT, Richardson ML. A review of innovative teaching methods. Acad Radiol. 2019;26(1):101–13. https://doi.org/10.1016/j.acra.2018.03.025. Epub 2018 May 9.
114. Graham KL, Cohen A, Reynolds EE, Huang GC. Effect of a flipped classroom on knowledge acquisition and retention in an internal medicine residency program. J Grad Med Educ. 2019;11(1):92–7. https://doi.org/10.4300/JGME-D-18-00536.1. PMID: 30805104; PMCID: PMC6375314.
115. Hew KF, Lo CK. Flipped classroom improves student learning in health professions education: a meta-analysis. BMC Med Educ. 2018;18(1):38. https://doi.org/10.1186/s12909-018-1144-z. PMID: 29544495; PMCID: PMC5855972.
116. Phillips E, Harris C, Lee WW, Pincavage AT, Ouchida K, Miller RK, Chaudhry S, Arora VM. Year-end clinic handoffs: a national survey of academic internal medicine programs. J Gen Intern Med. 2017;32(6):667–72. https://doi.org/10.1007/s11606-017-4005-2. Epub 2017 Feb 14. PMID: 28197967; PMCID: PMC5442016.

117. Pincavage AT, Lee WW, Beiting KJ, Arora VM. What do patients think about year-end resident continuity clinic handoffs? A qualitative study. J Gen Intern Med. 2013;28(8):999–1007. https://doi.org/10.1007/s11606-013-2395-3. PMID: 23595932; PMCID: PMC3710383.
118. Truncali A, Lee JD, Ark TK, Gillespie C, Triola M, Hanley K, et al. Teaching physicians to address unhealthy alcohol use: a randomized controlled trial assessing the effect of a Web-based module on medical student performance. J Subst Abuse Treat. 2011;40(2):203.
119. Desai T, Stankeyeva D, Chapman A, Bailey J. Nephrology fellows show consistent use of, and improved knowledge from, a nephrologist-programmed teaching instrument. J Nephrol. 2011;24(3):345.
120. Lee CA, Chang A, Chou CL, Boscardin C, Hauer KE. Standardized patient-narrated web-based learning modules improve students' communication skills on a high-stakes clinical skills examination. J Gen Int Med. 2011;26(11):1374.
121. Ross DD, Shpritz DW, Wolfsthal SD, Zimrin AB, Keay TJ, Fang H, et al. Creative solution for implementation of experiential competency-based palliative care training for internal medicine residents. J Canc Educ. 2011;26:436.
122. Bell DS, Fonarow GC, Hays RD, Mangione CM. Self-Study from web-based and printed guideline materials. A randomized controlled trial among resident physicians. Ann Intern Med. 2000;132(12):938.
123. William JH, Huang GC. How we make nephrology easier to learn: Computer-based modules at the point-of-care. Med Teach. 2014;36:13.
124. Yu CH, Straus S, Brydges R. The ABCs of DKA: development and validation of a computer-based simulator and scoring system. J Gen Intern Med. 2015;30(9):1319.
125. McCleskey PE. Clinic teaching made easy: a prospective study of the American Academy of Dermatology core curriculum in primary care learners. J Am Acad Dermatol. 2013;69(2):273.
126. Staton LJ, Estrada C, Panda M, Ortiz D, Roddy D. A multimethod approach for cross-cultural training in an internal medicine residency program. Med Educ Online. 2013;18:20352.
127. Institute for Healthcare Improvement. IHI Open School Courses. 2016. http://www.ihi.org/education/ihiopenschool/courses/Pages/default.aspx. Accessed 1 Sep 2016.
128. Centers to Advance Palliative Care. CAPC CME courses. https://www.capc.org/. Accessed 1 Sep 2016.
129. American Academy of Dermatology. Basic Dermatology Curriculum. 2016. https://www.aad.org/education/basic-derm-curriculum. Accessed 1 Sep 2016.
130. Galiatsatos P, Porto-Carreiro F, Hayashi J, Zakaria S, Christmas C. The use of social media to supplement resident medical education - the SMART-ME initiative. Med Educ Online. 2016;21:29332. https://doi.org/10.3402/meo.v21.29332. PMID: 26750511; PMCID: PMC4707390.
131. Bergl PA, Narang A, Arora VM. Maintaining a twitter feed to advance an internal medicine residency program's educational mission. JMIR Med Educ. 2015;1(2):e5. https://doi.org/10.2196/mededu.4434. PMID: 27731845; PMCID: PMC5041360.
132. Cross CE, Robinson C, Todd E. Development and implementation of a synchronous online TBL using microsoft forms. Med Sci Educ. 2020;31(1):11–3. https://doi.org/10.1007/s40670-020-01133-6. PMID: 33133755; PMCID: PMC7584486.
133. Bryan JL, Saxon LC, Mesidor MM, Asghar-Ali AA. Virtual synchronous motivational interviewing training for geographically dispersed interprofessional learners. J Contin Educ Health Prof. 2021;41(3):226–9. https://doi.org/10.1097/CEH.0000000000000356.
134. Khalil R, Mansour AE, Fadda WA, Almisnid K, Aldamegh M, Al-Nafeesah A, Alkhalifah A, Al-Wutayd O. The sudden transition to synchronized online learning during the COVID-19 pandemic in Saudi Arabia: a qualitative study exploring medical students' perspectives. BMC Med Educ. 2020;20(1):285. https://doi.org/10.1186/s12909-020-02208-z. PMID: 32859188; PMCID: PMC7453686.
135. Domb S, Manly E, Elman D. Pandemic patch-up: Using Zoom™ videoconferencing software to create a virtual teaching clinic. Can Fam Physician. 2021;67(1):65–8. https://doi.org/10.46747/cfp.670165. PMID: 33483398; PMCID: PMC7822599.

136. Shalaby M, Yaich S, Donnelly J, Chippendale R, De Oliveira MC, Noronha C. X + Y scheduling models for internal medicine residency programs-a look back and a look forward. J Grad Med Educ. 2014;6(4):639–42. https://doi.org/10.4300/JGME-D-14-00034.1. PMID: 26140111; PMCID: PMC4477545.
137. Ray A, Jones D, Palamara K, Overland M, Steinberg KP. Improving ambulatory training in internal medicine: X+Y (or why not?). J Gen Intern Med. 2016;31(12):1519–22. https://doi.org/10.1007/s11606-016-3808-x. Epub 2016 Jul 20. PMID: 27439977; PMCID: PMC5130949.
138. Warm EJ, Schauer DP, Diers T, Mathis BR, Neirouz Y, Boex JR, Rouan GW. The ambulatory long-block: an accreditation council for graduate medical education (ACGME) educational innovations project (EIP). J Gen Intern Med. 2008;23(7):921–6. https://doi.org/10.1007/s11606-008-0588-y. PMID: 18612718; PMCID: PMC2517908.
139. Graham KL, Glassman AR, Davis RB, Ayub M, Libman H, Reynolds E. Effect of an immersive primary care training program on educational and clinical outcomes in an internal medicine residency training program: meeting the training needs of a modern-day physician workforce. J Gen Intern Med. 2021. doi: https://doi.org/10.1007/s11606-021-07101-z. Epub ahead of print.
140. Esch LM, Bird AN, Oyler JL, Lee WW, Shah SD, Pincavage AT. Preparing for the primary care clinic: an ambulatory boot camp for internal medicine interns. Med Educ Online. 2015;20:29702. https://doi.org/10.3402/meo.v20.29702. PMID: 26609962; PMCID: PMC4660998.
141. Johns Hopkins University Physician Education and Assessment Center. Internal Medicine Curriculum. 2016. https://ilc.peaconline.org/. Accessed August 2021.

Chapter 19
Medical Students in Clinic

Kelly White, Achilia Morrow, and Marla Tschepikow

Introduction

Incorporating medical students into academic practices with resident clinics can present unique challenges for the learners and faculty. The goals of all stakeholders may not be aligned, and the unique time pressures of ambulatory clinic may present teaching and learning obstacles. Learners have different experience levels and distinct learning objectives. Faculty may not be equipped with adequate teaching skills for this setting. This chapter explores various teaching models in the ambulatory setting, describes faculty responsibilities, addresses common problems, and illustrates potential benefits for faculty and residents.

Outline
- Overview
- Learning goals for students
- System logistics and regulatory organizations
- Models of incorporating students into clinic and continuity
- Preceptor responsibilities
- Residents as teachers

K. White (✉)
Division of General Internal Medicine, University of Colorado School of Medicine, Aurora, CO, USA
e-mail: kelly.white@cuanschutz.edu

A. Morrow
DE&I, Internal Medicine Residency, Department of Medicine, Baylor College of Medicine, Houston, TX, USA
e-mail: achilia.morrow@bcm.edu

M. Tschepikow
United Health Group, Minnetonka, MN, USA

L. B. Lu et al. (eds.), *Leading an Academic Medical Practice*,
https://doi.org/10.1007/978-3-031-40273-9_19

- Faculty benefits
- Troubleshooting common problems
- Conclusion

Overview

Academic practices are often closely aligned to medical schools; thus, medical students will often be present in academic affiliated clinics. Medical students may participate in clinic at various levels of their training including longitudinal experiences, block clerkships, and ambulatory electives. Resident clinics often have students as well, as evidenced in the 2019–2020 Medical Resident Clinic Director Interest Group (MRCDIG) Surveys, where 78–88% of respondents reported that they had medical students in their clinics [1, 2]. As a result, it is likely that part of the responsibility as clinic director will be integrating and providing a learning experience for medical students. This can create unique challenges as follows:

- Faculty must meet goals as set forth by governing bodies and associated medical schools.
- Increasing productivity pressures for faculty affect their availability to teach and the ability to recruit faculty who want to teach.
- Faculty need resources to continue to learn and improve their teaching and feedback and assessment skills.
- Faculty need resources to provide support for students in clinic to have successful learning experiences.
- When residents are present, their schedules are often not aligned with the students, making it more difficult to integrate both groups of learners into the clinic.

This chapter focuses on the logistics of having medical students in clinic, addressing the challenges listed above, and providing a rewarding experience for students, faculty, and residents.

Learning Goals for Students

The clerkship or rotation director will likely distribute information to the clinic director regarding learning goals and objectives for the students. Learning goals and objectives for students in the ambulatory setting are guided by the Liaison Committee on Medical Education (LCME), the accrediting body for degree programs leading to an MD. For students, the CDIM-SGIM Core Medicine Clerkship Curriculum Guide Fourth Edition provides additional guidance on content for students [3] (CDIM = Clerkship Directors in Internal Medicine, SGIM = Society of General Internal Medicine). The guide includes sections on diagnoses and core clinical conditions (Part I) and core competencies (Part II). The guide also provides end-of-clerkship goals (Table 19.1).

Table 19.1 CDIM-SGIM training problems for students [3]

Diagnoses	Clinical conditions	Core competencies
Acute coronary syndrome	Abdominal pain	Advanced imaging
Chronic kidney disease	Acid-base	Basic labs
Chronic obstructive pulmonary disease	Acute kidney injury	Case presentation
Cirrhosis	Altered mental status	Chest radiograph interpretation
Congestive heart failure	Anemia	Collaboration
Coronary artery disease	Back pain	Diagnostic decision-making
Dementia	Cancer screening	ECG interpretation
Depression	Chest pain	Electronic health records
Diabetes	Constipation	Health equity and social determinants of health
Dyslipidemia	Cough	History
Gastroesophageal reflux	Diarrhea	Information mastery
Hypertension	Dyspnea	Palliative care
Hyperthyroidism	Edema	Patient-centered care
Hypothyroidism	Fatigue	Patient notes
Osteoporosis	Fever	Personal development and wellness
Pancreatitis	Gastrointestinal bleed	Physical examination
Pneumonia	Headache	Point-of-care ultrasound
Substance use	Hyponatremia	Professionalism
Tobacco use	Joint pain	Self-directed learning
Upper respiratory tract infection	Knee pain	Systems-based practice
Urinary tract infection	Nosocomial infections	Therapeutic decision-making
Venous thromboembolism	Obesity	–
–	Skin and soft tissue infections	–
–	Skin lesions	–
–	Syncope	–
–	Unintentional weight loss	–

The Association of American Medical Colleges (AAMC) also discusses medical student education. In 2014, the AAMC developed the "Core Entrustable Professional Activities for Entering Residency" (EPAs) that every student should be able to perform with supervision when they graduate [4]. Educators also working with residents will note that the EPAs align with the Accreditation Council for Graduate Medical Education (ACGME) Milestones. Below are the EPAs with ACGME Milestones 2.0 listed beside them (if applicable) [4, 5] (Table 19.2).

Thus, for those already working with residents in clinic, accomplishing the goals and objectives for students should not be "additional work" but reflect what is already occurring.

Based on AAMC's EPAs, students will be working towards being able to perform their goals with supervision (i.e., being ready for internship). Specific goals will also vary depending on when a student has his or her ambulatory experience.

Table 19.2 AAMC EPAs and corresponding ACGME milestones

EPA	ACGME milestones
EPA 1: Gather a history and perform a physical examination	PC1 PC2
EPA 2: Prioritize a differential diagnosis following a clinical encounter	PC3
EPA 3: Recommend and interpret common diagnostic and screening tests	MK3
EPA 4: Enter and discuss orders and prescriptions	PC6
EPA 5: Document a clinical encounter in the patient record	ICS3
EPA 6: Provide an oral presentation of a clinical encounter	ICS2
EPA 7: Form clinical questions and retrieve evidence to advance patient care	PBLI1
EPA 8: Give or receive patient handover transition care responsibility	SBP2
EPA 9: Collaborate as a member of an interprofessional team	SBP2
EPA 10: Recognize a patient requiring urgent or emergent care and initiate evaluation and management	PC5
EPA 11: Obtain informed consent for tests and/or procedures	ICS1
EPA 12: Perform general procedures of a physician	
EPA 13: Identify system failures and contribute to a culture of safety and improvement	SBP2

PC patient care, *MK* medical knowledge, *ICS* interpersonal communication skills, *SBP* systems-based practice, *PBLI* problem-based learning and improvement

For example, second- or early third-year students may be focused on accurately collecting and organizing information, while more advanced students will be expected to interpret results and perhaps suggest management plans. The RIME method, described in a later section, can be helpful in describing the goals a student is expected to achieve while on the ambulatory rotation.

System Logistics-Regulatory Organizations

The LCME requires those supervising or teaching medical students, regardless of setting, to be familiar with the learning objectives of the course and to be prepared for their role in teaching and assessment [6]. All providers involved in teaching students in clinic should have access to the course learning objectives, including residents, fellows, and other faculty or instructors involved in teaching. In addition, the LCME requires that the supervising clinicians need to provide appropriate supervision of the students in the clinic setting and be comfortable with providing both formative and summative feedback during the rotation. Supervising faculty must be aware of and willing to employ various tools of measurement of students' achievement of course objectives by means such as direct observation according to the schools' requirements. At the end of the rotation, a timely evaluation should be completed including a narrative summary of the students' performance.

In addition to LCME requirements, the school of medicine may have specific requirements for teaching students. For example, the University of Colorado SOM requires all faculty who are involved in teaching and assessing medical students to have a faculty appointment with the School of Medicine. Additionally, many schools may require specific faculty development focusing on feedback and assessment of students. Being aware of the schools' requirements and appropriately training faculty will be essential for success. The hospital or hospital organization may have additional rules regarding students in the clinical setting. They may require proof of immunizations (including COVID), drug testing, EMR training, a letter of good standing, or other documentation. Often, this can be handled by the student, the clerkship coordinator, or the school, but an awareness of the rules can help a clinic director appropriately guide the students. Depending on the clinic's affiliation with a hospital, the Joint Commission on Accreditation of Healthcare Organizations (JACHO) standards may also apply. According to the JACHO, a medical student has no legal status as a provider of healthcare services, which may have a direct effect on the role that student can take in delivering healthcare and documenting in the EMR [7]. Awareness of Medicare billing rules is equally important. Medicare rules state that any student contribution to a billable service must be performed in the physical presence of a faculty or resident. Prior to March 5, 2018, students could document in the medical record; however, the teaching faculty had to re-document everything for billing purposes except for review of systems (ROS) and past social and/or family history (PSFH) [8]. However, CMS rules changed in 2018 to "allow the teaching physician to verify in the medical record any student documentation of E/M services, rather than re-documenting the work (March 2018 MLN)." The University of Kentucky has produced a video available on YouTube that discusses how to incorporate these guidelines into actual practice [9, 10]. Despite the changes, several institutions and hospitals have not yet adopted these guidelines. Clinic directors should work with their local compliance and legal departments before implementing these guidelines or modifying their billing practices. Having knowledge of the expectations of the various governing bodies, both national and local and incorporating these into the orientation and structure of the clinical experience will help promote success.

If residents are present, incorporating students into resident clinic requires awareness of the different regulatory associations' rules and regulations. The ACGME program requirements state that the learner (residents and students)-to-faculty ratio in resident clinic cannot exceed 4:1, so this will need to be considered when adding students [11]. Faculty must also not have other patient care responsibilities if supervising more than two learners or faculty also cannot see patients independently if supervising more than two learners. The LCME standards expect that residents be prepared for their roles in terms of teaching and evaluation of students. The LCME standards also expect that these residents be familiar with the specific course (clerkship, rotation) goals and objectives [6]. Adequate preparation of the residents is essential and may benefit from good communication between clerkship directors and clinic directors.

Models of Incorporating Students into Clinic and Continuity

Models include the following:

1. *Attending-student clinic*: In this model, the student sees patients on the faculty's private panel. This may occur in a private practice clinic or an academic center with a pairing of one student to one attending. Advantages include that the fac-

ulty knows the patients and can better select which ones are to be seen by students. For efficiency, at least two rooms are needed if possible. This allows the student to see one patient while the preceptor may see up to three patients in the other room (wave scheduling). This process is described in more detail in Alguirre's chapter on "Patient Scheduling" in his 2008 book and allows the student more time to see the patient without delaying clinic flow [12].

2. *Learner clinics (fellows, residents)*: This describes clinics where multiple learners are being precepted by supervising faculty. Students can be added to the clinic as additional learners as long as the learner-to-faculty ratio remains 4:1. The director and precepting faculty will need to make a decision whether the student has their own patients and presents directly to the preceptor or is paired with an upper level learner. This latter method allows the resident to do initial precepting and direct teaching before the patient is presented and can make documentation easier on faculty. Students may be paired with one resident per session or work with different residents based on patient and resident interest and availability.
3. *Incorporate students into clinic teams*: In this model, students are incorporated into clinic teams to improve continuity, inter-professional collaboration, and efficiency of patient care. This can represent a combination of any of the other models, with the idea that the student remains on the same team in clinic, whether they are working with faculty individually or with residents or seeing their own student panel with the faculty. Students can function on different inter-professional levels, working with medical assistants to room patients, obtain vital signs, and perform medication reconciliation, as permitted by the individual institution. This increases students' autonomy and perceived value to the team and can improve efficiency of patient care.
4. *Student-only clinic*: In this model, faculty precept only students. Panels of patients are created for students to see. This model may work best as a longitudinal model. In this model, it is vital that preceptors are knowledgeable of the student billing guidelines of their institution.

Continuity

Clinic directors will need to decide on priorities for providing continuity: student-faculty continuity, student-resident continuity, student-patient continuity, or exposure to a variety of teaching styles. What is feasible will also depend on faculty available to precept and how often students will attend clinic. If present, the ability to involve residents, and whether student and resident schedules are aligned (e.g., X + 1, longitudinal), will also affect feasibility. As many residency programs move towards block scheduling (e.g., X + Y), many medical schools are incorporating longitudinal clerkship experiences in different years. Discussions with the rotation director and faculty to review the proposed method for integrating the student will ensure that the experience meets the learning objectives of the rotation.

Preceptor Responsibilities

Orientation to the Clinic and the Team

Although students may receive an overall orientation at the beginning of their rotation, it is important that each student be oriented to each specific clinic as well. This will often need to be done by the clinic director or their designee. The purpose of the orientation is to:

Familiarize students with the clinic. This includes informing students where things are physically located. It includes how are patient rooms structured, where supplies are kept, and where physicians, nurses, and other staff sit. Even things like the location of bathrooms will be useful to students. This will be their medical home for the next few weeks to months, and it is helpful to know where things are.

Introduce them to the team. This is an excellent time for students to be made aware of the importance of everyone in the clinic; medicine is increasingly becoming an inter-professional discipline. Explain the roles and job of various personnel, especially those they will be working with closely. In addition, if the clinic director is the primary preceptor, it is a good time to explain the role and the journey to become a primary care physician. Ambulatory rotations will hopefully persuade more students to consider primary care as they meet role models they want to emulate.

Explain clinic flow. Describe the process of how things work from the time a patient checks in to the time a patient checks out. They will also need to know their role in this process.

Setting Goals and Expectations

Students

Clinic directors should discuss learning goals and expectations for the rotation with the student during orientation or shortly afterwards. Overall learning goals are covered earlier in the chapter. Directors will want to review these as well as goals and information specific to the clinic, student goals, and other important logistics.

Clinic goals. Specific patient populations may lend themselves to specific goals not covered in the overall goals. For example, for students working in a women's health clinic, the goals might include diagnosis and management of amenorrhea and/or management of menopausal symptoms.

Student goals. The student may have their own learning goals and expectations. Eliciting these objectives from the learner at the beginning of the rotation will help faculty develop an individualized educational plan that will make the student's experience more rewarding.

Logistical information. This includes detailed information pertaining to the organization of the clinic, clinic volume, and documentation. A few examples of such information include:

1. Clarifying the number of patients the student is expected to see (e.g., 2–4 patients in ½-day session)
2. Confirming that the student has an active username and password for accessing EMR
3. Introducing students to various templates to be used in the EMR (if applicable)
4. Demonstrating an approach to the patient chart
5. Reviewing different types of patient visits (e.g., new, urgent, follow-up)
6. Describing the telehealth process (if applicable)

Faculty, Residents, and Staff

Faculty and residents working with the students must also know the learning goals and expectations listed above. Although residents may have experience working with students in the inpatient setting, they may not have worked with students in the ambulatory setting. Thus, faculty should clearly define the role the residents will have in supervising the student in the clinic setting. The students likely will be performing the history and physical exam and may be responsible for documentation. Identifying how faculty and resident feedback will be included in the student's evaluation will also be important.

Clinic staff members can be an integral part of the student's learning experience. Typical responsibilities for staff members include patient introductions, assisting with basic skill training and student evaluations. Clinic directors should clearly define expectations for staff interactions with the student prior to the rotation. It is important to remember that it is often difficult to juggle regular patient care duties and the needs of early learners. Communicating with staff members on a regular basis about their own experience will help ensure that staff are not overwhelmed and that the student has a positive learning environment.

Priming the Student

Depending on the time of year, or the structure of the medical school curriculum, many students may not have been in the ambulatory setting before. Even more experienced students may need specific instruction of what is expected of them. In "priming," the preceptor provides the student with information to make the encounter more successful, focused, and time efficient before the actual clinical encounter. Information imparted to the student may include:

Patient information. This can include both specifics about the patient (if known) and reasons for the visit. ("Mrs. Charlie is a 65 yo lady who I have been seeing for years. She is often accompanied by her daughter. Today she is here for a follow-up of her diabetes.") The chief complaint may also be discussed with the student prior to him or her entering the room.

The task. Describe what faculty would like the student to do and how much time is allotted to complete it. ("I would like you to take 3 minutes to review the chart, then take 10 minutes to do a focused history and physical on the patient. Please make sure to ask about her glycemic control and do a foot exam.")

Precepting encounter. Inform the learner what will be expected after the task is completed. Where they will meet and what information faculty will want to know should be answered. ("After you finish, meet me in the conference room and give me a 3-minute summary of history and physical findings. We will then discuss a plan for her diabetes and see the patient together.")

Teaching and Learning Models

How one teaches in the ambulatory setting is dependent on the level of learner, patient population, and time constraints. Compared to inpatient, there is a higher volume of patients seen in shorter periods of time in the outpatient setting. The challenge of allowing the student independence and time to learn is often balanced with the need for efficiency in a busy practice. Models of teaching that allow time efficiency, active learning, and focusing on specific teaching points have been developed. The list below is not exhaustive but represents some common methods of teaching/precepting in the outpatient setting.

"One-Minute Preceptor." This method allows preceptors to ask questions regarding the diagnosis and to probe the learner's thinking. (It "diagnoses the patient and the learner.") It consists of five steps and does not require the learner to know the method. Although originally designed to discuss diagnoses, it can be applied to other aspects of a patient presentation as well (e.g., history, interpretation of abnormal physical findings and labs, patient follow-up) [13] (Table 19.3).

SNAPPS. Originally described by Wolpaw in 2003, SNAPPS is a learner-centered model that focuses on differential diagnosis [14]. The learner must be

Table 19.3 One-minute preceptor skills and examples

Microskills step	Example
1. Get a commitment	"What do you think is the cause of his abdominal pain?"
2. Probe for supporting evidence	"Why do you think the patient has dyspepsia?"
3. Provide general rules	"Remember to always ask about weight loss when someone is presenting with chronic abdominal pain"
4. Reinforce what was done correctly	"You characterized the pain well including asking about quality, intensity, radiation, and alleviating and exacerbating factors"
5. Correct mistakes	"When pain is located on right side, need to consider gallbladder and liver etiologies of pain as well"

Table 19.4 SNAPPS model with corresponding learner action

SNAPPS model	Learner action
Summarize	The learner is asked to summarize the case
Narrow the differential	The learner presents 2–3 conditions in the differential diagnosis that can explain the condition of the patient
Analyze the differential	The learner explains what they think the actual diagnosis is and why
Probe the preceptor	The learner asks any specific question they have about the case
Plan management	The learner develops assessment and plan
Select a case-related issue for self-directed learning	The learner chooses an issue related to the case to explore further

trained in the model in order for it to be successful. As it requires higher level thinking, it can be challenging for early learners. The steps of the model are shown in Table 19.4.

The model assumes that the learner is already proficient at oral presentations as it focuses on the assessment and plan.

Reflections/educational prescriptions. This learning activity is centered on unanswered questions relevant to a patient seen. Students are asked to further explore a clinical question (e.g., "What can be done for treatment of a patient with fatty liver?") or reflect on a patient encounter ("What factors do you think might be affecting Mrs. S's ability to adhere to her medical regimen. What could be done to help?"). This method allows the student to continue thinking about the patient outside the patient encounter and can be reviewed at a later time [15–17].

Observation. This method can be used in several ways to encourage active learning by the student. Examples include having the learner observe and scribe while the preceptor performs the history and physical. To do this effectively, the student has to assimilate information in real time. Afterwards, the student and preceptor can generate a problem list and discuss the assessment and plan.

Traditional observation can be more active as well if planned. For example, the student can be asked to observe the preceptor performing a specific task. This can then be discussed and reviewed in detail. Finally, the preceptor can observe the student performing a specific skill. This can be taking a history, performing an exam, or counseling a patient. In general, observations eliminate the need for the preceptor to repeat portions of the history and exam separately from the student.

Teacher reflection and resources. One final important aspect of teaching is reflection by the teacher of what methods work well and why. If several faculty have teaching duties, consider sharing ideas and developing methods together.

More information about teaching in the ambulatory setting can be found in review articles, faculty development programs at the affiliated academic institution, sessions at regional and national meetings (including SGIM), and online modules such as this provided by Alliance of Academic Medicine (AAIM, https://hl.im.org/aaim/home).

Providing Useful Feedback

Feedback from clinical teachers is needed for learners to improve. Students should receive both formal and informal feedback from those involved in their education. Explicitly stating that feedback is being given can help learners realize that they are receiving information to improve their performance. Consider prefacing informal feedback with statements such as "I want to give you feedback about" or "Here is feedback regarding ...." Formal feedback sessions, which should happen at least twice during a rotation, should reference goals and objectives set at the beginning of the rotation. Setting aside time for the formal feedback sessions can be useful to ensure that they happen in an unrushed manner (and that they get done)!

Feedback should **be specific, be based on observable behaviors, be nonjudgmental, and include suggestions for improvement**. In addition, studies have shown that it is useful to have the student reflect upon his or her own performance first. There are several pneumonic, models, and tools to guide giving feedback including those in Table 19.5.

The authors of an article featured in Medical Teacher in 2012 noted that learners reported a lack of feedback in clinical settings [21]. They performed a literature review of feedback for graduate and undergraduate students and came up with 12 suggestions or "tips" for effective feedback. The tips and suggestions for implementation below are adapted from this article (Table 19.6).

Evaluation of the Student

Although many forms of evaluation may be used to give students a grade, the clinical preceptor evaluation is a significant component. When agreeing to take students in a clinic, it needs to be determined what is expected in terms of evaluation.

Logistics

What evaluation forms will need to be completed? In addition to a summative evaluation form, are there formative or additional ones, such as an observation form that needs to be done as well? Most traditional or block clerkships include midpoint

Table 19.5 Feedback methodologies

BOSS [18]	ARCH [19]	Modified feedback sandwich [20]
Brief	**A**llow/ask for self-assessment	Give positive feedback
Observations of learner actions	**R**einforce what is being done well	Discuss what can be improved
Significance of the feedback being given and why important	**C**onfirm what needs correction or improvement	Give specific suggestions for improvement
Suggestions for how to improve	**H**elp the learner with plans for improvement	

Table 19.6 Tips for effective feedback with implementation strategies

Tips for establishing effective feedback	Suggestions for implementation
Establish a respectful learning environment	If both parties feel comfortable, feedback will be easier. The learner should view feedback as a chance to reflect and improve, not just to be told what they are doing wrong
Communicate goals and objectives for feedback	Decide what should be the purpose or outcome of the conversation. Agenda setting can be done by the preceptor or the learner. Examples of goals can be how to improve an exam skill, discussing progress made towards goals set at the beginning of the rotation, or improving the formatting of notes
Base feedback on direct observation	Specific examples of what was done correctly or incorrectly should be used and given to the learner
Make feedback a timely and regular occurrence	Again, formal feedback sessions will be expected halfway through the rotation and at the end. However, informal feedback should happen throughout the rotation
Begin the session with the learner's self-assessment	Allow time for the learner to assess and verbalize how he thinks he is doing
Reinforce and correct observed behaviors	This is best done in a timely manner when possible
Use specific, neutral language to focus on performance	Be nonjudgmental
Confirm the learner's understanding and facilitate acceptance	Giving feedback requires the clinician to be "in tune" with the learner to ensure that the learner is "getting it"
Conclude with an action plan	A plan should be made that informs the learner of specific things that should be done to improve. "Reading the sections relevant to your patient's diagnosis in UpToDate after each patient encounter" is more useful than "read more"
Reflect on your feedback skills	Giving good and useful feedback is a skill that needs to be practiced. Allow time to determine what was done well and what needs to be improved
Create staff development opportunities	Faculty development opportunities may be available and/or can be developed for those who would like further information regarding giving feedback
Make feedback part of institutional culture	Faculty development opportunities may be available and/or can be developed for those who would like further information regarding giving feedback

feedback for students, while longitudinal clerkships may have multiple feedback sessions before the final evaluation, and faculty may be asked to complete these. It is important to review copies of the evaluation form beforehand.

Who is expected to complete the evaluation? Whether the evaluation will be summative from all those involved with the student or individual should be determined either by the rotation or by the clinic director. For example, if the student works with a resident, will both faculty and resident do an evaluation or will it be collective? This consideration may not be applicable in all situations.

Table 19.7 RIME framework

Reporter	Usually applies to early learners and describes a student who can gather and clearly communicate facts
Interpreter	Learners can now interpret data, prioritize problems, and offer a differential diagnosis based on data collected
Manager	In this stage, the learner is able to develop management plans for the patient. They function as the doctor and are able to explain these plans to patients and their families
Educator	In addition to being able to educate colleagues and students, learners in this stage continue to strive to practice evidence-based medicine. They seek answers to questions that cannot always be found in a textbook

Are evaluations criterion based or normative? Evaluations can be criterion based or normative based. In normative evaluations, learners are compared against those at a similar stage, whereas in criterion based, the same standards are used regardless of when a student rotates. Thus, students just starting their clinical rotations are likely to perform at a lower level (and receive a lower "score") than ones who are months away from graduation. Regardless, the same scale is used. Anchors for items to be evaluated can be used to guide the evaluator. If unclear, it is important to communicate with the clerkship/rotation director for instructions on how forms are to be completed.

Student evaluations have often mirrored resident evaluations in using the six core competencies. However, similar to resident evaluations, student evaluations are increasingly moving towards being milestone and competency based.

Comments and RIME

Comments can be a very useful part of the evaluation. Giving specifics and examples of what the student did well, how to improve, and concerns are invaluable for both evaluation and feedback. The RIME framework is a tool that many programs have integrated into evaluations (and feedback) to help specifically define what knowledge, skills, and attitudes the student has attained [22, 23]. The RIME framework is shown in Table 19.7.

The RIME framework has gained popularity in its ability to allow evaluators to come to the same conclusion regarding a student's clinical capabilities. As mentioned earlier, it can also be used to help set goals and expectations for students in clinic.

Observation

Stemming from LCME standard ED-27, programs now require students to be directly observed in patient interactions as part of their evaluation. Preceptors may be asked to complete a mini-CEX or other observation form. Again, it is helpful to have the form early in a rotation with a student, so it can be determined who will complete the observation and when. Other considerations include the following: Is the observation formative or summative? Do specific skills need to be observed, for example, physical exam, or patient education? Time allotted to observe and complete the form is also an excellent opportunity to give the student specific feedback on their performance.

Final Tips on Evaluation

- Obtain as much information as possible about the components of feedback and evaluation for which faculty and house staff will be responsible.
- If present, use anchoring statements on evaluations to guide as opposed to using a numerical score.
- If a faculty member cannot adequately assess an item on the evaluation, it is okay to mark "cannot assess" or its equivalent. For example, if a faculty member has never observed a student doing a physical exam, they cannot evaluate this item.
- Remember that evaluations are a summary of what is observed. There are other components, and the student's final grade will not be solely determined by one faculty member.
- Feedback and evaluation are often partners. When discussed, evaluations can serve as a tool to give specific feedback to residents.
- Implement faculty development on assessment and feedback of learners.

Evaluation of the Rotation, Faculty, and Residents by the Student

Students will have the opportunity to evaluate the clinic rotation, teaching faculty, and residents according to the evaluation process developed by the medical school. The students' evaluations are important for ongoing feedback regarding the rotation, so improvements can be made to optimize the student participation and learning. Students will also provide evaluations of the attendings and residents they work with during the rotation. Often, these evaluations are held until multiple evaluations have been completed in order to protect student anonymity. The students' completed evaluations of faculty may be released directly to the faculty members or may be given to a supervisor such as the division head or department leadership. Similarly, the resident evaluations may be released directly to the residents or given directly to the residency program director to review prior to distribution. Sharing completed student evaluations with supervising faculty provides an opportunity for faculty and resident feedback, recognition of teaching prowess, and remediation.

Residents as Teachers

Residents are responsible for teaching medical students in the clinical setting, and their teaching may be responsible for up to one-third of acquired medical knowledge [24]. Residents have been found to spend 20% of their time in direct teaching [25]. When provided with a curriculum aimed at improving teaching skills, residents are found to be more enthusiastic about teaching and report improvement in teaching skills and increased satisfaction [26]. Many residency training programs now include a formal teaching curriculum for residents, with varying topics, on instructional and evaluation methods [25]. These may include resident or intern orientations, electives, optional seminars, educator pathways, or other areas. A brief description of some previously described curriculum follows.

One-Minute Preceptor: A recent review suggests that the One-Minute Preceptor model continues to a commonly used and effective teaching strategy; however, the literature establishing effective teaching strategies in the clinical setting remains limited, and more research is needed to determine optimal teaching strategies, assessments, and measurement of outcomes [25, 27]. This teaching strategy, described previously, may be used to teach students, and as a model for designing residents as teachers curriculum. The time commitment required is relatively short, and existing curricula are well described.

AAIM Residents-as-Teachers online curriculum: This topic is of national interest, and CDIM and APDIM created the joint Residents-as-Teachers Task Force to provide program directors and clerkship directors with practical and efficient strategies to help residents become more effective teachers in the course of their normal work duties [20, 28]. This is available for all AAIM members and includes ten multimedia, evidence-based modules with topics ranging from oral presentations to clinical reasoning and professionalism. These tools may help faculty design their own curriculum and provide an excellent basis for a teaching program. Resident clinic directors may connect with local clerkship directors or residency leadership regarding AAIM membership.

Workshops and longitudinal curricula: Many different residents-as teachers curricula have been described in the literature, and their efficacy has been variously assessed [29]. Workshops range from just over an hour to more than 1 day, can occur singularly or longitudinally, and may be mandatory or voluntary based on scheduling. From the authors' perspective, these workshops seem to be most successful for upper level residents as opposed to interns. Teaching methods include seminars (virtual and in-person), PowerPoints, role-playing, reflections, observation and feedback, and electronic content delivery of key themes. Assessment of various teaching curricula does not support one method of delivery, leading experts to recommend ongoing research and developing programs, which adapt to the individual needs of the local institution.

Collaboration between clerkship directors and clinical leaders could result in improved teaching skills of residents and improved experiences for students in clinic. Similar curricula could be developed for residents in clinic teaching students, with a focus on ambulatory topics and primary care settings. Teaching curricula could parallel faculty development, with a focus on course objectives, feedback strategies, rules of documentation, and effective evaluations. Since residents are also learners, it is a crucial role of the clinic leadership and precepting faculty to provide feedback to them on their teaching skills, even if a formal curriculum does not exist.

Faculty Benefits

Many physicians teach for the joy of teaching—they enjoy imparting their clinical knowledge, perspective, and love of what they do to others. However, academic physicians often must balance the missions of clinical services, research, and teaching. Although participation in teaching of residents and medical students is often an expectation, compensation does not always reflect this. Compensation for physicians in the ambulatory setting is often based on clinical productivity (RVUs) or total number of visits. Thus, clinic directors must consider how to incentivize teaching and make it a realistic option for those who want to do it [30].

Monetary/time compensation. Education value units (eVus) have been described and implemented in various institutions to compensate teaching [31–33]. This system acknowledges that teaching takes time and clinical productivity will not be as high. Some institutions may also offer a monetary stipend to clinic preceptors. Georgia, Colorado, Hawaii, Maryland, and South Carolina offer tax credits or other financial incentives for qualifying clinicians who precept students; other states are considering this as well [34, 35]. If an institution has a method for compensating teaching, it is important to determine if precepting students will be considered in the calculation. Medical directors will need to consider if having students changes clinical duties for their faculty (i.e., number of patients they are to see, how many residents they are covering).

Consideration for promotion. More and more programs have well-developed clinician-educator pathways for promotion. Promotion along this pathway usually requires evidence of breadth, quantity, and quality of teaching. Evaluations from students can be part of the evidence of quality and can be added to teaching portfolios. Teaching students in addition to residents may increase breadth as well.

Eligibility for teaching awards. Institutions and professional societies have developed teaching awards. Receiving a teaching award can be through nomination or by application. In addition to recognition, receiving an award may lead to opportunities to apply for grants, support applications for promotion, as well as give faculty institution-wide recognition for their work.

Other options/benefits. If a clinic has volunteer faculty, some of the options above (desire for promotion) may not be an incentive to teach students. Having a school offer access to CME activities, faculty development retreats, faculty appointments, and medical library might be preferable options. Acknowledgment by plaque or certificate signed by the Department Chair of Medicine and/or Medical School Dean may also be valuable as a thank-you even when monetary compensation is not available.

Troubleshooting and Common Problems

This section addresses common scenarios when working with students in the ambulatory setting. Each begins with a brief vignette followed by suggestions, many of which are explained in detail in other parts of the chapter as well.

"Too Slow"

You enjoy having Student A, a third-year clerkship student, in your clinic. However, some of your patients have started to complain about having longer waits. Also, your morning clinic is going deep into your lunch hour. You want to continue teaching, and you want Student A to have a good experience, but you are becoming exhausted. How can you balance teaching with effective/efficient patient care?

- Use wave scheduling to stagger your patients and/or have multiple rooms available. This allows the faculty member to see one or two patients while the student is performing their H&P.
- If possible, preselect patients for the student to see. This allows faculty to prepare the patient for a longer visit with the student. It may also allow the student to read about the patient in advance.
- "Prime" the student. Setting clear expectations of what the faculty would like the student to do in the clinical encounter will help make the visit more efficient.
- Do not try to teach everything for every patient. Pick one or two teaching points on which to focus.
- Be familiar with various forms of time-effective methods of teaching including having the student present in the room, SNAPPS, and One-Minute Preceptor.

"More than Shadowing"

You have had students in your clinic over the past year. You are receiving feedback from the clerkship director regarding your evaluations. While students feel that you are very knowledgeable and compassionate towards your patients, many of them complain about "doing nothing" in your clinic but shadowing. They would like to be more involved in the patient's care. You have a very busy clinic and limited amount of space, but are open to the idea of giving the students more independence, but how?

- Even if only one room is available, have the student take a more active role. The student can perform as a scribe, lead the history or physical, place/place orders, check vital signs, provide patient education, communicate with team members, and/or provide patient instructions.
- Allow time for student to derive own assessment and plan. The faculty may perform other tasks (i.e., documentation) at this time.
- Try wave scheduling if not already implementing.

"Read More"

Student B, your student from 2 months ago, comes to you upset. This student received a "pass" from the rotation and is confused. During the rotation, you constantly told Student B that they were doing a good job and that they should just "read more." Student B would like more concrete information about what they could have done to receive a better grade.

First, students should direct concerns about their grades to the clerkship director unless instructed to do otherwise. In this case, it would be appropriate to ask the student to contact the clerkship director. Reflecting on what could have been done better to make the student more aware of her performance:

- Go over evaluation with the student at the end of the rotation.
- Set objectives at the beginning. Then review the objectives periodically, and discuss the progress the student is making.
- Give feedback in real time. After a presentation, and exam, let the student know "I want to give you feedback regarding …."
- Evaluating faculty can discuss a student's evaluation with the clerkship director to make sure that they are following the appropriate standards.

Conclusion

The majority of physicians will spend at least part of their career in the ambulatory setting. In order to prepare them for future practice, the time students spend in the ambulatory setting likewise has continued to grow. Meeting the needs of students and allowing faculty to still meet their clinical and educational goals are possible. Preparing faculty with course objectives and learning goals will help direct teaching. Both innovative scheduling and telemedicine offer opportunities for increased involvement of students in ambulatory care and maintaining continuity. Finally, various teaching models exist which can help preceptors manage time wisely while simultaneously providing students with increasing autonomy and learning experiences.

Teaching students in clinic is rewarding and can have many benefits. However, increasing pressure on primary care faculty to achieve clinical productivity goals can sometimes conflict with faculty desire for protected time for teaching students. Engaging hospital administration and academic leadership to provide support for teaching faculty will be essential in maintaining these models. Similarly, supporting faculty and resident time for education on course objectives and milestones will also be important. If we continue to work together to align goals of learners with those of hospital institutions and patient care, we can strive to build teaching models that will optimize these roles.

References

1. SGIM MRCDIG 2019 Annual survey results. Connect.SGIM.org.home.
2. SGIM MRCDIG 2020 Annual survey results. Connect.SGIM.org.home.
3. CDIM-SGIM Core Medicine Clerkship Curriculum Guide, 4th Edition AAIM : CDIM-SGIM Core Medicine Clerkship Curriculum.

4. Core EPA Faculty and Learner Guide. aamc.org.
5. ACGME milestones–InternalMedicineMilestones.pdf [Internet]. https://www.acgme.org/globalassets/pdfs/milestones/internalmedicinemilestones.pdf.
6. Standards, Publications, & Notification Forms | LCME [Internet]. 2016. Available from: http://lcme.org/publications/#Standards.
7. Standards FAQ Details.
8. Association of American Medical Colleges Compliance advisory: electronic health records (EHRs) in academic health centers [internet]. Association of American Medical Colleges; 2014.
9. Medicare Learning Network®. E/M service documentation provided by students (manual update). 2018b. https://www.cms.gov/Outreach-and-Education/Medicare-Learning-Network--MLN/MLNMattersArticles/Downloads/MM10412.pdf.
10. Using Student Documentation for Billing. 2018. https://www.youtube.com/watch?v=ENXEiHkLAdE.
11. ACGME Common program requirements (residency). https://www.acgme.org/globalassets/PFAssets/ProgramRequirements/CPRResidency2021.pdf.
12. Alguire PC, Dewitt DE, Pinsky LE, Ferenchick GS. Teaching in your office: a Guide to instructing medical students and residents. 2nd ed. Philadelphia, PA: American College of Physicians; 2008. p. 145.
13. Neher JO, Gordon KC, Meyer B, Stevens N. A five-step "microskills" model of clinical teaching. J Am Board Fam Pract. 1992;5(4):419–24.
14. Wolpaw TM, Wolpaw DR, Papp KK. SNAPPS: a learner-centered model for outpatient education. Acad Med. 2003;78(9):893–8.
15. Sandars J. The use of reflection in medical education: AMEE Guide no. 44. Med Teach. 2009;31(8):685–95.
16. Aronson L. Twelve tips for teaching reflection at all levels of medical education. Med Teach. 2011;33(3):200–5.
17. ktcclearinghouse. Centre for evidence-based medicine : educational prescriptions. 2016. http://ktclearinghouse.ca/cebm/practise/formulate/eduprescriptions.
18. AAIM Alliance for academic internal medicine: providing structure to written qualitative feedback: the BOSS framework–Alliance of academic internal Medicine. 2022. https://higherlogicdownload.s3.amazonaws.com/IM/fecab58a-0e31-416b-8e5646fc9eda5c37/UploadedImages/Documents/resources/Providing_Structure_to_Written_Qualitative_Feedback_The_Boss_Framework_.pdf.
19. Hayes JR, Zeman J, Johnston B, Cmpbell N. Outpatient teaching and feedback skills workshop for resident physicians. Med Ed Portal. 2020;16:10930.
20. AAIM Alliance for academic internal medicine: residents-as-teachers curriculum modules, "feedback on the Fly"–Alliance of academic internal Medicine [internet]. 2022. https://www.im.org/resources/resources-program/curriculum-resources/residents-as-teachers.
21. Ramani S, Krackov SK. Twelve tips for giving feedback effectively in the clinical environment. Med Teach. 2012;34(10):787–91.
22. Hemmer PA, Papp KK, Mechaber AJ, Durning SJ. Evaluation, grading, and use of the RIME vocabulary on internal Medicine clerkships: results of a National Survey and comparison to other clinical clerkships. Teach Learn Med. 2008;20(2):118–26.
23. Pangaro L. A new vocabulary and other innovations for improving descriptive in-training evaluations. Acad Med J Assoc Am Med Coll. 1999;74(11):1203–7.
24. Bing-You R, Sproul W. Medical students' perceptions of themselves and residents as teachers. Med Teach. 1992;14:133–8.
25. Post R, Quattlebaum R, Benich J 3rd. Residents-as-teachers curricula: a critical review. Acad Med. 2009;84(3):374–80.
26. Morrison E, Shapiro J, Harthill M. Resident doctors' understanding of their roles as clinical teachers. Med Educ. 2005;39:137–44.
27. Pierce C, Corral J, Aagaard E, Harnke B, Irby DM, Stickrath C. A BEME realist synthesis review of the effectiveness of teaching strategies used in the clinical setting on the development of clinical skills among health professionals: BEME Guide no. 61. Med Teach. 2020;42(6):604–15. https://doi.org/10.1080/0142159X.2019.1708294. Epub 2020 Jan 21.

28. AAIM Alliance for Academic Internal Medicine: Residents as Teachers Curriculum Modules. 2016. http://www.im.org/p/cm/ld/fid=401.
29. Dannaway J, Ng H, Schoo A. Literature review of teaching skills programs for junior medical officers. Int J Med Educ. 2016;31(7):25–31.
30. Teachingphysician Incentives for Precepting. (2020). https://www.teachingphysician.org/become-a-preceptor/incentives-for-precepting-2019.
31. Nutter DO, Bond JS, Coller BS, D'Alessandri RM, Gewertz BL, Nora LM, et al. Measuring faculty effort and contributions in medical education. Acad Med J Assoc Am Med Coll. 2000;75(2):199–207.
32. Watson RT, Romrell LJ. Mission-based budgeting: removing a graveyard. Acad Med J Assoc Am Med Coll. 1999;74(6):627–40.
33. Stites S, Vansaghi L, Pingleton S, Cox G, Paolo A. Aligning compensation with education: design and implementation of the educational value unit (EVU) system in an academic internal medicine department. Acad Med J Assoc Am Med Coll. 2005;80(12):1100–6.
34. augusta.edu Preceptor tax incentive program [internet]. Preceptor tax incentive Program 2016. http://www.augusta.edu/ahec/ptip/index.php.
35. Rutter, A., Biehle, Ryan, Wimmer, Becky, Fulton, Fay, Withy, Kelley, & Pabst, Kathy. (n.d.). Tax incentives for precepting: how do they work and are they making a difference?

Chapter 20
Scholarship in Clinic

Louisa Whitesides and Jillian Catalanotti

Introduction

Scholarship plays a key role in guiding the day-to-day practice of evidence-based medicine. In addition to understanding how to stay abreast of new treatments and guidelines by being consumers of the medical literature, physicians should learn how to contribute to the ever-growing body of medical knowledge. In fact, the Accreditation Council for Graduate Medical Education (ACGME) requires internal medicine residency programs to "facilitate resident and faculty involvement in scholarly activities" and to "advance residents' knowledge and practice of the scholarly approach to evidence-based patient care" [1]. Scholarship in the medical field generally implies dissemination of knowledge, whether institutionally, regionally, nationally, or internationally, through oral presentations, posters, written abstracts, or manuscripts.

By undertaking the art of inquiry and writing, learners grow in a multitude of ways. For residents, the act of completing and publishing research can be a source of personal accomplishment. Finishing one project can open doors to further research [2]. For faculty, the act of mentoring trainees on discrete scholarly projects can be gratifying, and successful publication may contribute to academic promotion. For both, discovering answers to clinical questions can improve patient outcomes and can further resident and faculty career development by establishing a successful record of publication or presentation to disseminate their work.

L. Whitesides (✉)
Department of Medicine, Division of Geriatrics and Palliative Care,
The George Washington University, Washington, DC, USA
e-mail: lwhitesides@mfa.gwu.edu

J. Catalanotti
Department of Medicine, Division of General Internal Medicine, The George Washington University, Washington, DC, USA
e-mail: jcatalanotti@mfa.gwu.edu

L. B. Lu et al. (eds.), *Leading an Academic Medical Practice*,
https://doi.org/10.1007/978-3-031-40273-9_20

This chapter seeks to provide guidance to attendings and trainees on the act of scholarship in the clinic.

Outline

- Role of the preceptor and clinic director
- Formulating an effective research question
- Types of scholarly research available to residents
- Choosing an appropriate venue for presentation and publication
- Writing for medical publications
- Continuing the research process
- Conclusion

What Is the Role of the Preceptor and Clinic Director?

Clinic preceptors and directors play key roles in encouraging inquisitive thought and guiding residents through the research process in ambulatory clinic. While most of their work with residents is in direct observation, active feedback, and collaboration for intervisit care [3], preceptors can also use these interactions to plant seeds for self-directed inquiry. For example, if a learner asks a question regarding a certain patient encounter, the preceptor may ask the learner to investigate the evidence behind the question, rather than simply providing an answer. If this research leads to further investigation, the preceptor can either provide mentorship through the research process or direct the trainee to an appropriate guide. Frequently, patients who seek care at academic medical centers have complex medical problems that may be appropriate not only for learning but also for dissemination of knowledge through publication in the form of case reports or clinical vignettes.

Clinic directors have opportunities to promote and mentor scholarly work as well. They are uniquely situated to identify areas of need across the entire residency clinic experience and may serve to propose, coordinate, or guide more global projects that are inspired not by just one patient but by the entire clinic experience. In addition to mentoring scholarly projects that may impact patient care or clinic operations, due to their key role as medical educators, residency clinic directors may also design and study educational initiatives for their residents in the ambulatory curriculum. Clinic directors can also promote the scholarship of others by acting as a connector to direct interested learners to preceptors with aligning interests and serving as a resource for mentor-mentee relationships.

Preceptors and residency clinic directors must develop specific skills to provide active research mentorship. They may play important roles in every step of the research process by assisting residents to (1) focus their research questions; (2) choose a type of scholarship (e.g., clinical vignette, QI, clinical study); (3) select a venue for submission; (4) progress through the writing and editing process; and (5) continue the line of research after the initial project has been submitted.

How to Formulate an Effective Research Question

Learners are often curious but lack the skills and experience to articulate and narrow research questions. Guidance from a preceptor, mentor, and/or formal curriculum in this area is paramount to ensure a resident's success in developing a project. Many residency programs have piloted structured research electives to provide dedicated time to support resident inquiry and scholarship [4, 5]. At least one curriculum designed to improve writing skills is available on MedEdPORTAL [6]. Other sources, such as the Academic Alliance of Internal Medicine (AAIM), have short presentations that can be used to teach residents the steps in research design [6].

Whether it be from a structured program or mentor, trainees must learn the steps to formulate a research question: perform background research, narrow the focus of the question, and determine the best type of research for the question. Once residents have chosen a topic, they should carry out a cursory literature review to answer the following questions: Is there comprehensive information available on this topic? What questions have been left unanswered? These questions should guide residents to frame their formal research question, which should be as precise and narrowly worded as possible and fill a gap in the medical literature. At some institutions, research librarians may be available for assistance with performing literature searches. Finally, determining the overall type of study—observational or interventional—as well as the appropriate scholarly approach for the question at hand—for example, clinical vignette, quality improvement, chart review, survey, or clinical study—is helpful to place the question into context and understand the scope of the project [7]. We will discuss these types of research projects further in our next section.

What Are the Various Types of Scholarly Research Available to Residents?

When developing a research project, residents can choose from many categories of scholarship. Below is a list of these genres and their definitions. It is important to remember that while residents may believe that their projects are best suited to a certain research category, their time in training is limited. If they aspire to finish the project prior to graduation, it is more reasonable for them to pursue one of the first three types, which require less time rather than to undertake a prospective study. The later type of project will likely not be completed within a 2- to 3-year time frame. In that case, residents may work together or pass on projects to more junior learners depending on the length and scope of the project. The different types of research projects that residents may pursue, also summarized in Table 20.1, are as follows:

1. Clinical vignette: Describes an interesting case or clinical dilemma that the author personally encountered. These writings are typically abstract length and are submitted to conferences as posters or oral presentations [8]. Consider

Table 20.1 Example opportunities for residents seeking to present or publish scholarly activity

Type of scholarship	Description	Example places to publish/present	Helpful resources
Clinical vignette	Abstract-length submission for oral or poster presentation at a conference describing a case the author has seen personally	Institutional research days, regional or national SGIM, ACP meetings	American College of Physicians. Writing a clinical vignette (case report) abstract. https://www.acponline.org/membership/residents/competitions-awards/acp-national-abstract-competitions/guide-to-preparing-for-the-abstract-competition/writing-a-clinical-vignette-case-report-abstract
Case report or case series	Manuscript submitted to a journal describing a case(s) the author has seen personally	Various medical journals that accept case reports (*JAMA Internal Medicine* Teachable Moments section specifically for trainee authors)	Moore K. A medical writing curriculum for internal medicine residents: Using adult learning theory to teach formal medical writing and publication of case reports. MedEdPORTAL. May 1, 2015. https://doi.org/10.15766/mep_2374-8265.10073 Sun Z. (2013). Tips for writing a case report for the novice author. J Med Rad Sci, 60(3), 108–113. https://doi.org/10.1002/jmrs.18
Quality improvement project	Data-guided activities to cause immediate improvements in patient care; often faster than traditional research and performed without significance testing	*American Journal of Medical Quality* (Q-TIP section specifically for trainee authors); IHI conference; ACC quality summit; institutional, regional, and national meetings	Wong BM, Sullivan GM. How to write up your quality improvement initiatives for publication. J Grad Med Educ. 2016;8(2):128–133. Doi:10.4300/JGME-D-16-00086.1 Institute for Healthcare Improvement. Where to submit your writing: Journals publishing QI work. http://www.ihi.org/education/ihiopenschool/resources/pages/wheretosubmityourwritingqifriendlypeerreviewedjournals.aspx
Observational study	Commonly utilize chart review or surveys/interviews to answer clinical or medical educational questions		Vassar M, Holzmann M. The retrospective chart review: important methodological considerations. J Educ Eval Health Prof. 2013;10:12. Published 2013 Nov 30. doi:10.3352/jeehp.2013.10.12 Panacek E. Performing chart review studies. Air Med J. Sept 2007. 26(5):206–10. doi: https://doi.org/10.1016/j.amj.2007.06.007

Interventional study	Study the impact of an educational or clinical intervention Randomized controlled studies may require more time and/or finances	Clinical journals in various fields; Medical education-focused journals (e.g., *Academic Medicine; Medical Education; Journal of Graduate Medical Education, Teaching and Learning in Medicine; Journal of General Internal Medicine*); MedEdPORTAL for original curricula at https://www.mededportal.org	Aggarwal R, Ranganathan P. study designs: Part 5 - interventional studies (II). Perspect Clin Res. 2019;10(4):183–186. Doi:10.4103/PICR.PICR_138_19 Magee C, Rickards G, A Byars L, Artino AR Jr. tracing the steps of survey design: a graduate medical education research example. J Grad Med Educ. 2013 Mar;5(1):1–5. Doi: 10.4300/JGME-D-12-00364.1. PMID: 24404217; PMCID: PMC3613291 Atluru A, Wadhwani A, Maurer K, Kochar A, London D, Kane E, Spear K. AAMC OSR Medical Education Committee. Research in Medical Education: A primer for medical students. April 2015. https://www.aamc.org/media/24771/download

SGIM Society of General Internal Medicine, *ACP* American College of Physicians, *JAMA* Journal of the American Medical Association, *IHI* Institute for Healthcare Improvement, *ACC* American College of Cardiology general medicine regional or national conferences, in addition to conferences of specialty societies.

2. Case report or series: Describes a case or group of cases that the author has seen. These writings are typically in manuscript format and are submitted to a journal for publication [9]. Note that many journals require a publication fee for these types of publications, and most require written patient consent.
3. Quality improvement study: Recounts data-guided interventions that immediately improve patient care. These studies are often IRB exempt, are completed faster than traditional research, and can be carried out without significance testing. They can be submitted in abstract or manuscript forms to either general medicine conferences or journals or quality-focused conferences or journals [10, 11].
4. Observational study: Analyzes data through chart review, surveys, or interviews to answer clinical questions. Depending on the topic studied, those surveyed may include patients, learners, providers, or others who interact with the resident clinic experience. Data analysis may be quantitative or qualitative. Observational studies are typically submitted as manuscripts but may be presented as posters as well [12, 13]. These studies require review by your organization's Institutional Review Board (IRB) before being carried out.
5. Interventional study: Describes the impact of a clinical or educational intervention performed by the learner and/or mentor. These studies are prospective and may require more time and finances to complete. As with observational studies, data analysis may be qualitative or quantitative. Common approaches to quantifying impact include showing change in attitudes or beliefs on surveys, in clinical outcome metrics using chart review or data analytics, or in scores on knowledge exams before and after the intervention. Like observational studies, these projects are often submitted in manuscript form to journals and may also be presented as posters [14, 15]. These projects typically also require review by your organization's IRB before they can be begun.

Figure 20.1 illustrates the different types of research that may stem from seeing a patient with diabetes in continuity clinic. As illustrated, a single patient seen in clinic can lead to a multitude of questions, resulting in very different scholarly projects. It is important to assist learners to identify which category they wish to pursue and to clarify the scope of the question once articulated.

A note about clinical vignettes or case reports: when choosing a case for a clinical vignette or case report, remember that a case need not be a "zebra" or very rare diagnosis to be suitable for presentation or publication in the medical literature. Other great cases may illustrate uncommon presentations of common illnesses, diagnostic dilemmas, "don't miss" diagnoses, or novel or nuanced therapeutic approaches. Often, general medicine conferences also accept clinical vignettes about important, though not necessarily uncommon, diagnoses or situations as teaching tools. Learners often need guidance from faculty to identify the 1–2 learning objectives that will be illustrated by the case. These should be used to guide the entirety of the work to remain focused. Often learners need to shorten the case

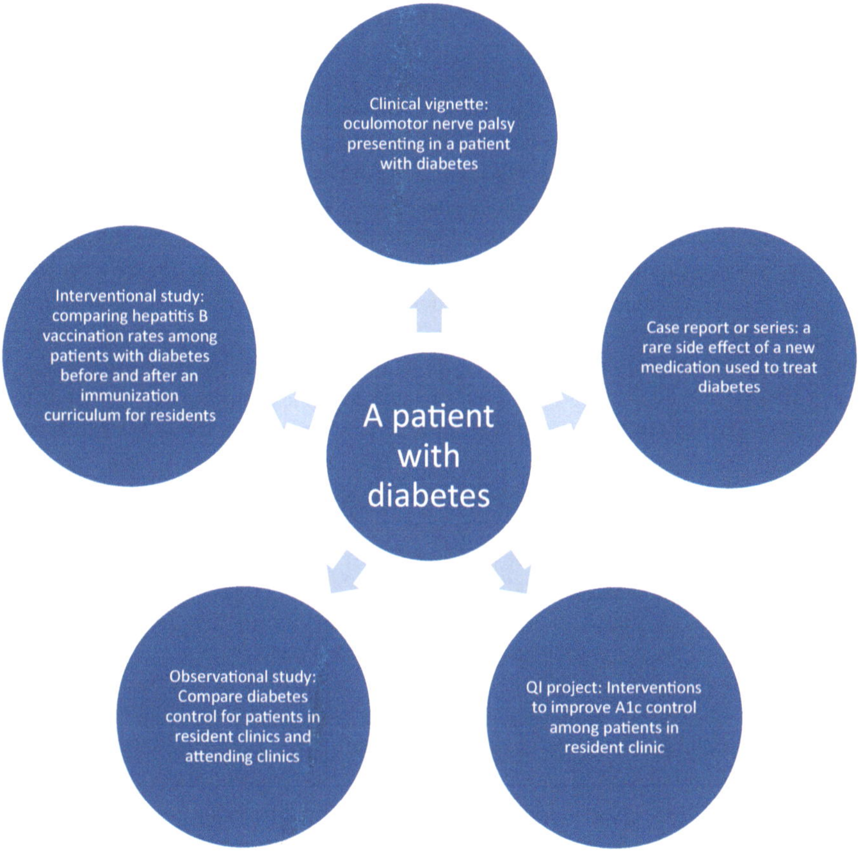

Fig. 20.1 Seeing a patient(s) with diabetes in resident may inspire several different forms of scholarship. Some examples are shown here

presentation section of these projects and lengthen the discussion section; the case should be thought of as a launching point so that the discussion section can achieve the learning objectives.

How to Choose an Appropriate Venue for Presentation and Publication

In determining the scope of a scholarly project, it is helpful to discuss what formal works should come about and where to submit them. In general, smaller projects are more suitable for abstracts and poster presentations at the institutional, regional or national level, while larger more in-depth projects may be able to support manuscript format. This section outlines the initial decisions and steps needed to create abstracts and manuscripts; our next section will review the writing processes for both.

Abstracts are shorter pieces of writing, often presented (once accepted) in poster format. They may be presented at various conferences throughout the year and may be published in conference reports. Some clinical inquiries and research endeavors are submitted only as abstracts; however, it is also acceptable to present an abstract on a research topic and then follow with a more complete manuscript later [16].

Several general medicine conferences accept abstracts from trainees every year, including Society of General Internal Medicine (SGIM), American College of Physicians (ACP), and AAIM. Each of these conference websites provides information on how to write an abstract, what types of abstracts are accepted, and instructions for submission. Given its academic mission, AAIM can be a great place to present research evaluating the impact of educational initiatives. SGIM and ACP typically also accept abstract submissions for regional meetings, which provide more opportunities for presenting smaller scale or early-stage research. For some conferences, organizations may specify that submitted work must include trainee or student authors. Finally, depending on the topic of research, specialty-focused conferences may be a good fit for presentation. For example, if a learner would like to write an abstract addressing diabetes mellitus, in addition to conferences of generalist organizations, conferences on diabetes or for an endocrinology professional society may also accept trainee submissions and be suitable.

There are several reasons why submitting abstracts is beneficial to residents. First, these projects are more reasonable in scope for residents with busy schedules and limited dedicated research time. Many residents can complete multiple abstracts during their training. In addition, since these abstracts are submitted to conferences, if accepted, residents can attend them, sometimes with funding from their program or the organization. At these conferences, residents can network with future colleagues and mentors and share their findings with other possible collaborators. Finally, many residents can develop manuscripts from an initial abstract, serving as a starting point for future publications.

Some resident research projects may be suitable for manuscript submission. When these situations arise, it is important to help the trainees develop the papers in systematic ways. Table 20.1 provides multiple sources that can guide both mentors and learners in the writing process for the different types of research projects. As with all scholarship, the first step is to perform a thorough literature search as described above to better identify the gap in the literature to be filled by the project. We recommend creating an annotated bibliography to which all authors may refer to be reminded of the main findings of each reference reviewed. While not necessary, using citation software can be an easy way to keep track of references, and "libraries" of citations can often be shared between authors. At this point, the mentor and trainee should together create a timeline that is attainable for both parties.

Next, the mentor should guide the trainee in identifying a target journal that matches scope, impact, and readership for their research. Although trainees may only be familiar with the most popular journals, not all submissions are appropriate for *New England Journal of Medicine*, for example. While it can be appropriate to choose a publication with a high Impact Factor as a starting point, there are many journals with narrowed scopes that may be more reasonable options. By choosing the publication up front, the trainee can tailor and format the paper according to the journal's standards. We strongly recommend that faculty mentors meet with the trainee author to compose and agree upon an outline for the piece, including major discussion points or objectives, before more detailed writing is begun by the trainee. Doing so ensures that trainees are headed in the right direction, exposes questions to be further searched in the literature, and saves time in the writing phase.

One other topic to discuss early is authorship, especially if there are multiple trainees or students involved with the project. If the resident does most of the work and/or writes the first draft, then that resident should be offered first author position. Other researchers and coordinators should fall in order behind, and the mentor should typically be listed as the last author, a position typically reserved for the mentor for the project. For faculty, although having first or second authorship on some projects may be important for their own academic promotion pursuits, last author positions are typically also viewed favorably by institutional promotion committees as a demonstration of mentorship.

How to Write for Medical Publications

Medical writing can be difficult, and many trainees need sufficient guidance in the process. The art of writing for medical publications is not taught in depth at many institutions [17]. Some researchers in medical education have created guidelines that can be used to develop such curricula [15, 18]. Mentors should start by gaining an understanding of their learners' experience and training in this field. If the mentor does not have experience in research or medical writing, many institutions provide internal faculty development opportunities that address these gaps. Sometimes, university writing tutors or similar programs may be available to faculty or trainees to review or edit written drafts. As previously stated, conference and journal websites can provide helpful guidelines for organization, scope, length, and timelines.

Abstracts should be written in a compelling way and in accordance with conference guidelines; however, they will ultimately be presented in poster format. Some residency programs may develop templates for residents to use that to serve as a launch point for presenting their research. Pictures and graphics are always more meaningful than words. There is also an increasing push in the scientific community to format research posters using significantly less text, writing the key takeaway in large letters at the center, and providing a QR code for interested conference attendees to seek further information, such as the full text of the abstract, related resources, or type of materials typically found in an appendix (e.g., survey tools and more extensive data tables) [19]. Mentors should also encourage residents to create an "elevator talk" that succinctly summarizes the project for viewers in under 5 min. When residents have the opportunity to present at conferences, consider recommending they bring business cards (if furnished by your residency program) for networking purposes and advising them to take written notes on questions they receive from visitors to their posters so that they can learn from and incorporate that information into any future iterations of the project, such as a subsequent manuscript submission.

Manuscripts may require more collaboration between mentor and trainee depending on the trainee's experience with the writing process. One other source that may be helpful for residents when writing manuscripts is your institution's library, if available. Both library websites and librarians can provide guidance in collecting background sources and tools for medical writing. As much as possible, mentors should direct their learners in this way. Regardless of the state of the initial draft, many manuscripts require multiple iterations before reaching a final product, and residents should be counseled throughout the editing process.

Despite careful writing and editing, manuscripts are often rejected. Many publications must be submitted to multiple journals before achieving acceptance for publication. Throughout this process, it is easy for learners to get discouraged. Mentors must bolster learners and teach them how to both respond to reviewer comments and improve their manuscript by using the input that they receive from reviewers along the way.

How to Continue the Research Process

Mentors and residents should always remember that a research project does not end once the abstract is presented or the manuscript is published. Research is ongoing, but only by identifying new questions from the previous project will the line of inquiry continue. It is helpful for mentor and trainee to meet after the final product has been accepted to discuss lessons learned from the experience and to develop new ideas from the initial work. By debriefing on the experience in an intentional way, residents can reflect and improve their research and writing techniques, as well as develop and carry out multiple projects during residency. If there are multiple residents working on a project, they can learn from each other through active discussion. More junior residents may be able to apply lessons learned to further iterations of the project.

Conclusion

Scholarly work allows for both preceptors and residents to explore and understand lines of inquiry that develop from the work that they do together in the clinical setting. Residents should learn how to research clinical questions effectively and to create meaningful products from the research that they do during their training. Collaboration between preceptors and resident learners on research projects can provide better patient care by disseminating answers to important clinical questions, improvements in medical education by studying curricula and educational programming, and professional development for residents and attendings alike.

By guiding residents effectively, preceptors and/or mentors can meet these goals. This guidance includes formulating good research questions; identifying the type of scholarly work and the appropriate venue for publication; assisting in writing and editing; and encouraging further research. Mentors can also direct trainees to rich resources through libraries and helpful online tools as illustrated in this chapter.

References

1. ACGME. Program requirements for graduate medical education in internal medicine. 2021. https://www.acgme.org/globalassets/pfassets/programrequirements/140_internalmedicine_2021.pdf. Accessed 27 Jan 2022.
2. Rivera JA, Levine RB, Wright SM. Brief report: completing a scholarly project during residency training. J Gen Intern Med. 2005;20:366–9.
3. Penner JC, Hauer KE, Julian KA, Sheu L. How preceptors develop trust in continuity clinic residents and how trust influences supervision: a qualitative study. Perspect Med Educ. 2021;11:73.
4. Parsonnet J, Gruppuso PA, Kanter SL, Boninger M. Required vs. elective research and in-depth scholarship programs in the medical student curriculum. Acad Med. 2010;85:405–8.
5. Stevenson MD, Smigielski EM, Naifeh MM, Abramson EL, Todd C, Li ST. Increasing scholarly activity productivity during residency: a systematic review. Acad Med. 2017;92:250–66.
6. Alliance for Academic Internal Medicine. https://hl.im.org/aaim/home. Accessed 14 Feb 2022.
7. Harvard Medical School. Trends in medicine: 3 steps to designing effective research questions and study methods. 2021. Harvard Medical School. https://postgraduateeducation.hms.harvard.edu/trends-medicine/3-steps-designing-effective-research-questions-study-methods. Accessed 22 Dec 2021.
8. American College of Physicians. https://www.acponline.org/?gclid=CjwKCAiAsNKQBhAPEiwAB-I5zXZdonvLYb3uTW3To5VWqhjKze8_EqLzezNX5pFDYsJxdybzEyJN_BoCowUQAvD_BwE&gclsrc=aw.ds. Accessed 14 Feb 2022.
9. Sun Z. Tips for writing a case report for the novice author. J Med Radiat Sci. 2013;60:108–13.
10. Wong BM, Sullivan GM. How to write up your quality improvement initiatives for publication. J Grad Med Educ. 2016;8:128–33.
11. Institute for Healthcare Improvement. Where to submit your writing: journals publishing QI work. http://www.ihi.org/education/IHIOpenSchool/resources/Pages/WhereToSubmitYourWritingQIFriendlyPeerReviewedJournals.aspx.
12. Vassar M, Holzmann M. The retrospective chart review: important methodological considerations. J Educ Eval Health Prof. 2013;10:12.
13. Panacek EA. Performing chart review studies. Air Med J. 2007;26:206–10.
14. Aggarwal R, Ranganathan P. Study designs: part 5- interventional studies (II). Perspect Clin Res. 2019;10:183–6.
15. Magee C, Rickards G, Byars LA, Artino AR. Tracing the steps of survey design: A graduate medical education research example. J Grad Med Educ. 2013;5:1–5.
16. SGIM. Getting your clinical vignette published in JGIM… or other journals: a step-by-step approach. Minnesota: SGIM Annual Meeting; 2010. https://www.sgim.org/File%20Library/SGIM/Resource%20Library/Meeting%20Handouts/SGIM/2010/WD13---Getting-Your-Vignette-Published.pdf

17. Yanoff KL, Burg FD. Types of medical writing and teaching of writing in U.S. medical schools. J Med Educ. 1988;63:30–7.
18. Moore K. A medical writing curriculum for internal medicine residents: using adult learning theory to teach formal medical writing and publication of case reports. Med Ed PORTAL. 2015;11:10073.
19. Morrison M. How to create a better research poster is less time. YouTube. 2019. https://www.youtube.com/watch?v=1RwJbhkCA58.

Part VII
Social Justices, Diversity, Bias, and Healthcare Advocacy

Chapter 21
Structural and Social Determinants of Health

Iman Hassan, Alia Chisty, and Thuy Bui

Introduction

Structural determinants of health (SDH) are defined by the World Health Organization (WHO) as the "conditions in which people are born, grow, live, work, and age" that "are shaped by the distribution of money, power, and resources at global, national, and local levels" [1]. The factors that shape SDH are termed the structural determinants of health and more specifically encompass "all social and political mechanisms that generate, configure, and maintain social hierarchies" such as our labor market, education system, political institutions, and cultural and social values. These mechanisms serve to generate social stratification, for instance along the lines of income, race/ethnicity, and gender [2]. The structural and social determinants of health (SSDH) together account for over half of population health outcomes and are the single greatest contributor to individual health, exceeding the impact of genetics and personal behavior [3]. Additionally, SSDH are responsible for health disparities, the preventable differences in disease, injury, and opportunities for health witnessed by socially disadvantaged groups [4]. The impact of SSDH has led a number of medical organizations to call for their explicit incorporation into clinical care and medical education [5–7]. Additionally, the Accreditation Council for Graduate Medical

I. Hassan (✉)
Albert Einstein College of Medicine, Montefiore Health System, Bronx, NY, USA
e-mail: ihassan@montefiore.org

A. Chisty
Penn State Health Milton S. Hershey Medical Center/Penn State College of Medicine, Hershey, PA, USA
e-mail: achisty@pennstatehealth.psu.edu

T. Bui
University of Pittsburgh School of Medicine, Pittsburgh, PA, USA
e-mail: buithuy@pitt.edu

L. B. Lu et al. (eds.), *Leading an Academic Medical Practice*,
https://doi.org/10.1007/978-3-031-40273-9_21

Education (ACGME) in its Common Goals of Residency Education has called on all residencies to train in healthcare disparities and incorporate activities aimed at reducing healthcare disparities [8]. SDH have also been acknowledged as a key component of health systems science, a conceptual framework for systems-based thinking that aligns with the ACGME milestone category of systems-based practice [9]. Despite this, medicine has historically incorporated little training in SSDH, and recent reviews have shown few published curricular studies in SDH and GME [10, 11]. In this chapter, we provide an introduction to conceptualizing SSDH using structural competency as a framework, including navigating anticipated challenges.

Outline

- Frameworks for structural and social determinants of health
- Incorporating structural competency into clinical care
- Incorporating systems-based practice into medical education
- Evaluating the impact of training in SSDH
- Conclusion

Frameworks for Structural and Social Determinants of Health

Several frameworks exist that discuss the impact of SSDH. The WHO Conceptual SDH framework demonstrates how social, economic, and political factors like income, education, occupation, gender, race, and ethnicity influence a person's socioeconomic position (Fig. 21.1). Socioeconomic position subsequently affects material circumstances such as living and working conditions and access to food, physical or behavioral factors like substance use, and mental health factors, all of

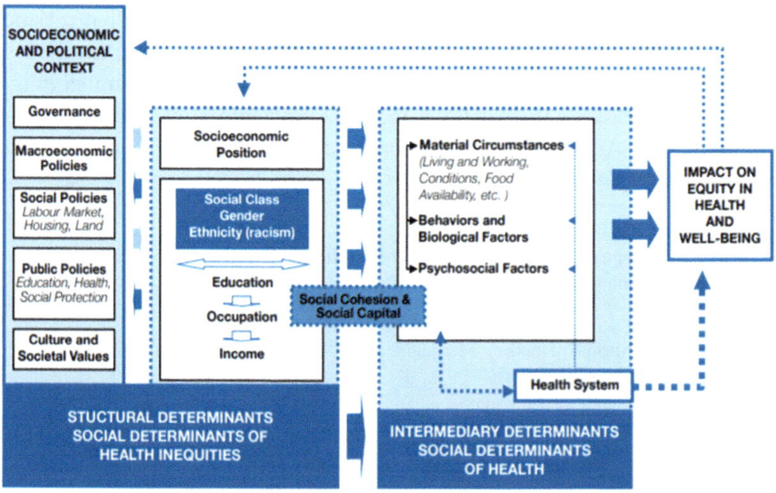

Fig. 21.1 WHO Framework for Structural and Social Determinants of Health. Source: Solar O, Irwin A. A conceptual framework for action on the social determinants of health. Social Determinants of Health Discussion Paper 2 (Policy and Practice). https://www.who.int/sdhconference/resources/ConceptualframeworkforactiononSDH_eng.pdf?ua=1. Accessed February 2, 2022

which ultimately impact health, equity, and well-being. Health, well-being, and equity then act as a feedback loop to the SSDH [2].

The Centers for Disease Control endorses the Healthy People 2030 proposed by the U.S. Department of Health and Human Services. They divide SDH into five domains: economic stability, education access and quality, healthcare access and quality, neighborhood and built environment, and social and community context (Fig. 21.2). Each of these factors plays an important role in affecting the health, well-being, and quality of life of individuals by impacting education, job opportunities, income, literacy skills, access to nutritious foods, safe housing, and transportation. SSDH contribute significantly to health disparities and inequities and require

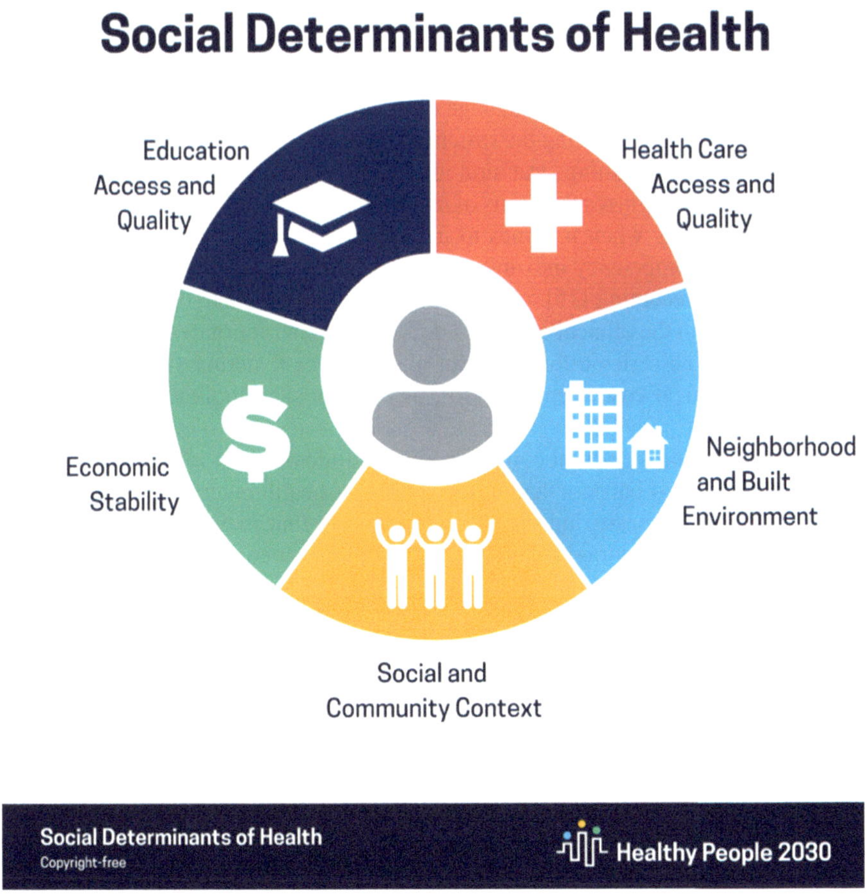

Fig. 21.2 Domains of Social Determinants of Health. Source: Healthy People 2030, U.S. Department of Health and Human Services, Office of Disease Prevention and Health Promotion. Retrieved [date graphic was accessed], from https://health.gov/healthypeople/objectives-and-data/social-determinants-health

partnering with sectors in education, transportation, and housing to impact meaningful change [12].

Understanding these frameworks helps to contextualize the impact of social, economic, political, and other factors that drive individual health behaviors and the overall health of the population. It is critical to understand the SSDH in order to address health disparities rooted in social and economic inequities.

Incorporating Structural Competency into Clinical Care

Structural competency, proposed by Drs. Helena Hansen and Jonathan Metzl in 2014, provides a powerful framework for the incorporation of SSDH into clinical practice. It has five major principles: (1) recognizing structures, including the upstream social, economic, and political forces, that shape behavior, illness, and health; (2) drawing on fields such as anthropology, urban planning, and economics to cultivate an "extra-clinical" language of structure; (3) rearticulating "culture" in structural terms by recognizing the structural forces that mediate "cultural" barriers; (4) observing and imagining structural interventions; and (5) developing structural humility, which recognizes the limits of medical expertise and actively decenters the clinician, especially when it comes to interventions [13]. Efforts to actively integrate structural competency into ambulatory teaching, for example, case-based sessions [14] and precepting [15], can serve as a road map to help operationalize this framework within the clinical context. The New England Journal of Medicine cases in social medicine series offer a helpful blueprint for fostering structural competency using clinical case scenarios [16], as do published toolkits [17] and curricula [18].

Operationalizing structural competency into clinical care starts with identifying structural and social barriers that influence patient health outcomes. Strategies for doing this include sensitizing clinicians to triggers that may indicate underlying social needs [19], encouraging all clinicians to obtain a comprehensive social history that incorporates identification of both social needs and individual and community assets [20], and universal screening for social needs [21]. Triggers for social needs are clinical clues that may serve to prompt clinicians to inquire further, using open-ended questions, about a wide range of underlying social needs. These triggers include, but are not limited to, not taking prescribed medications; uncontrolled chronic disease such as asthma, diabetes, and hypertension; frequent missed appointments or gaps in care; and frequent emergency room visits (Fig. 21.3). Triggers often represent more end-stage clinical manifestations of unmet social needs, and use of social history-gathering strategies and universal screening for social needs may allow for earlier detection. A number of social history-gathering tools including IHELP and the structural vulnerability checklist can allow clinicians to obtain a more detailed social history that goes beyond alcohol, tobacco, and other substance use, and also help gain important meaningful insights into patients' social needs [22, 23]. Additionally, taking a strength-based approach to history gathering

Trigger	What could be going on?
Frequent ED visits or hospitalizations	Homelessness/housing instability Lack of insurance Lack of access to primary care/healthcare
Missed appointments/ Gaps in care	Transportation barriers Lack of insurance/underinsurance Homelessness/housing instability Lack of childcare Financial insecurity/lack of job security
Uncontrolled disease (ex. asthma, diabetes, obesity, hypertension)	Mold, pests or other asthma triggers in the home Food insecurity Lack of spaces for exercise Inability to afford medications Lack of insurance/underinsurance
Medication non-adherence	Lack of insurance/underinsurance Inability to afford medications Financial insecurity

Fig. 21.3 Example triggers for potential underlying social needs

by explicitly asking about patients' sources of strengths, support systems, and resources allows clinicians to identify those factors which protect against poor health outcomes [24]. Finally, universal screening for social needs using validated social needs screening tools such as the Health Leads screening tool or the Accountable Health Communities Health-Related Social Needs Screening Tool is increasingly being utilized in healthcare settings to help identify individual-level needs for which intervention may result in improved outcomes [25, 26]. These screening tools can be incorporated into the electronic medical record (EMR) to facilitate the development of clinical workflows and the monitoring of progression towards impacting social needs (Fig. 21.4). Universally screening all individuals within the clinical setting has the benefit of avoiding assumptions about which patients may or may not be struggling with an unmet social need. Additionally, communication about social needs using a relationship-centered approach can help to mitigate the stereotype and stigma that may be associated with these conversations and help to foster structural humility [27]. Importantly, social history gathering and social needs must be contextualized within broader historical and structural narratives in order to begin to drive meaningful change beyond the level of the individual patient [28].

After identifying SSDH, clinicians should be encouraged to explicitly name unmet social needs and provide assessments for those social needs in the same way they might do so for traditional "clinical" problems [29]. The socio-ecological model can help to guide clinicians in addressing social needs and conceptualizing

Screening Tool	# of Items	Social Needs Domains Assessed	Reading Level	Languages other than English?
AAFP Tool	15	Childcare, Education, Employment, Financial Strain, Food Insecurity, Housing Insecurity, Housing Quality, Interpersonal Violence, Transportation, Utilities	7th grade	
Access Health: Spartanburg	38	Education, Employment, Food Insecurity, Healthcare, Income, Literacy, Veteran Status	5th grade	
AHC-Tool	27	Disabilities, Education, Employment, Financial Strain, Food Insecurity, Housing Insecurity, Housing Quality, Interpersonal Violence, Social Support, Stress, Transportation, Utilities	8th grade	
Arlington	11	Financial Strain, Food Insecurity, Housing Insecurity, Housing Quality, Interpersonal Violence, Social Support, Transportation, Utilities	10th grade	
BMC Thrive	11	Education, Employment, Food Insecurity, Healthcare, Housing Insecurity, Transportation, Utilities	7th grade	
HealthBegins	28	Civic engagement, Education, Employment, Financial Strain, Food Insecurity, Housing Insecurity, Housing Quality, Immigration, Interpersonal Violence, Neighborhood Safety, Social Support, Stress, Transportation	11th grade	
Health Leads	10	Childcare, Food Insecurity, Healthcare, Housing Insecurity, Literacy, Social Support, Transportation, Utilities	6th grade	
MLP IHELLP	10	Benefits, Education, Employment, Housing Insecurity, Housing Quality, Immigration, Income, Interpersonal Violence, Guardianship	8th grade	
Medicare Tool Health Assessment Questionnaire	39	Food Insecurity, Housing Insecurity, Housing Quality, Guardianship, Social Support, Stress	College	
NAM Domains	24	Education, Financial Strain, Income (geocoded), Interpersonal Violence, Social Support, Stress	6th grade	
NC Medicaid	11	Food Insecurity, Housing Insecurity, Interpersonal Violence, Transportation, Utilities	5th grade	Yes
PRAPARE	21	Childcare, Clothing, Education, Employment, Food Insecurity, Healthcare, Housing Insecurity, Immigration, Incarceration, Income, Interpersonal Violence, Neighborhood Safety, Social Support, Stress, Transportation, Utilities, Veteran Status	8th grade	Yes
Structural Vulnerability Assessment	43	Benefits, Discrimination, Education, Employment, Financial Strain, Food Insecurity, Housing Insecurity, Housing Quality, Immigration, Incarceration, Interpersonal Violence, Literacy, Neighborhood Safety, Social Support, Workplace Safety	6th grade	
WellRx	11	Childcare, Education, Employment, Food Insecurity, Housing Insecurity, Interpersonal Violence, Neighborhood Safety, Transportation, Utilities	2nd grade	Yes
Your Current Life Situation	29	Caregiver responsibilities, Childcare, Financial Strain, Food Insecurity, Healthcare, Housing Insecurity, Housing Quality, Interprofessional Violence, Literacy, Neighborhood Safety, Social Support, Stress, Transportation, Utilities	9th grade	

Fig. 21.4 Example screening tools for social risk and social needs in adults. Source: Social Needs Screening Tool Comparison Table. UCSF Social Interventions Research & Evaluation Network (SIREN). Accessed on February 13, 2022, at https://sirenetwork.ucsf.edu/tools-resources/resources/screening-tools-comparison

solutions for positively impacting SSDH. This model posits that interventions start at the individual level, having the smallest impact, and proceed to the health system, community, and ultimately policy levels [30]. Actively incorporating SSDH into clinical plans allows clinicians to generate concrete interventions and imagine broader structural solutions to social needs, which directly impact patient health. For example, when clinicians uncover social needs such as lack of health insurance, housing instability, or food insecurity, which actively contribute to uncontrolled diabetes, they can propose individual-level interventions such as referring to interdisciplinary team members (e.g., social workers, community health workers, or care managers), referring to medical-legal partnerships, and referring to community-based organizations. At the health system level, initiatives to screen for social needs or co-locate social services such as developing hospital-based food pantries can be proposed. At the community and health policy levels, initiatives to advocate alongside community organizations for universal healthcare access, healthier neighborhood food options, and more affordable housing can be extremely impactful. Recognition of how health systems, community-based advocacy, and health policy interface with individual-level health is important in fostering clinician activism and advocacy. Importantly, solutions should embrace structural humility in the recognition that physicians are not principally in charge of structural solutions, but instead serve to support and elevate larger interdisciplinary and community-led initiatives for social change [13].

Incorporating Systems-Based Practice into Medical Education

In July 2021, the ACGME provided updated Milestones 2.0 to use for resident assessment. They are meant to be developmental skills, knowledge, attitudes, and behaviors that help a resident physician work towards independent practice. In the new Milestones, SDH appear in several competencies, including patient care, medical knowledge, and systems-based practice (SBP) [31], with SBP having the greatest focus on providing high-value, high-quality care to patients within the context of the healthcare system. The ACGME defines the SBP competency as "an awareness of the responsiveness to the larger context and system of healthcare, including the social determinants of health, as well as the ability to call effectively on other resources to provide optimal health care" [32]. Core themes of the SBP competency include (1) patient safety and quality improvement, (2) navigation of the healthcare system for patient-centered care, and (3) the physician's role in the healthcare system [32, 33]. Although SBP Milestones 2.0 include attaining skills, knowledge, and attitudes on enhancing care on the institutional or community level, designing initiatives that optimize patient outcomes across delivery systems, advocating for communities with healthcare disparities, and possibly engaging in health policy to influence health systems, these behaviors are identified for the aspirational resident [30].

Health inequities that stem from systemic, structural, and social forces strongly impact the health and well-being of patients. By focusing on the currently existing healthcare systems, Castillo et al. argue that we are preparing physicians to work *for* the existing healthcare system instead of examining factors within the healthcare system that might perpetuate health inequities and individual health disparities. Using a health equity and social justice lens, they propose a new competency that would better encapsulate structural competency, health equity, and social responsibility [34].

SBP already encapsulates important themes including patient safety, quality improvement, cost containment, high-quality health care across domains, and team-based care. Despite having been introduced over 20 years ago, it is still inadequately incorporated into graduate medical education. Residents, program directors, and faculty have trouble conceptualizing SBP; there are limited formalized curricula to teach SBP concepts, few opportunities to directly observe these skills with residents, and no standardized teaching and evaluation methods [33, 35–38]. Adding SSDH into this competency assessment might require expanding the concept to health systems science and adopting a "systems thinking" mindset [39]. Residency programs can consider creating their own requirements of competency in the different aspects of the SSDH based on the patient populations they serve.

Evaluating the Impact of Training in SSDH

Evaluation is critical to demonstrating the value of teaching and addressing SDH. There is considerable variability in how trainees are taught about SDH. While some studies have shown that screening for and addressing social needs in the clinical setting can improve patient-level outcomes and decrease healthcare utilization [40, 41], there is currently a gap in evidence with regard to the impact of SDH educational interventions on the health or well-being of the community. Currently, there are no best practices in the assessment and evaluation of training on SDH. The National Collaborative for Education to Address the Social Determinants of Health (NCEAS) and other educational entities are working to establish criteria for SDH education effectiveness. They aim to develop a comprehensive and systematic approach to aligning criteria for SDH education effectiveness with specific indicators of achievement by adapting Kirkpatrick's four-level model of training criteria [42]. Selecting appropriate indicators of educational effectiveness of SDH education is a challenging task when criteria of SDH intervention effectiveness are not well defined. However, the structural competency framework, with its goal of achieving health equities and meeting community needs, provides an approach to learner assessment and evaluation of educational outcomes. Figure 21.5 has questions that can guide structural competency assessment of faculty and learners in the ambulatory setting.

Interviews and pre/post-surveys could elucidate learners' knowledge and attitudes, but assessment of behaviors through observation as well as feedback from patients, community members, and stakeholders are vital to evaluating educational effectiveness. Built-in EMR tools could aid in providing process measures such as use of social need screening tools, Z codes, and e-referrals and track the use of stigmatizing language and documentation of SSDH, along with interprofessional communication regarding care coordination. Readmissions by race/ethnicity and area deprivation index can additionally support quality improvement initiatives and system transformation. Ultimately, the goal is to assess the impact of SDH education on the organization and community in terms of decreasing health disparities and

A SSDH assessment of clinicians in ambulatory settings	YES	NO
Are trainees able to describe the root causes of health inequities?		
Do they recognize the structural factors that shape clinical interactions such as structural racism and the political economy of healthcare?		
Can they assess structural vulnerability in their patients?		
Can they integrate social needs and SSDH into their clinical reasoning?		
Do they utilize the clinic infrastructure (support staff, electronic health record systems) to screen for social needs and to track outcomes?		
Can they help patients navigate the healthcare system?		
Are they familiar with community resources and can they refer patients to appropriate resources in the community?		
Can they design or participate in an upstream health equity focused quality improvement project as part of an interprofessional team?		
Do they participate in advocacy initiatives to improve SSDH in collaboration with community partners or advocacy organizations?		

Fig. 21.5 Sample structural competency assessment of faculty and learners

improving health outcomes. Several organizations are working on health equity measures and guidance for healthcare organizations to improve health equity for the patients and communities they serve [43–45].

Community-oriented primary care (COPC) is a model that combines primary clinical care for individuals and families together with a public health focus on the community served when appraising needs, planning, and providing services. Although COPC is not based on a structural competency framework, lessons learned from this model could inform structurally competent training and practice. Evaluation methodologies of the COPC programs in US family medicine residencies since 1969 have included quasi-experimental control group study, pretests and posttests of knowledge and attitudes, focus groups, and semi-structured interviews. Reported outcomes include changes in residents' knowledge, attitudes, and behaviors; effect on graduates' career choice and future practice; and impact on patient care and community health [46, 47].

Conclusion

In effectively incorporating SSDH into academic clinical practice, it is important to ensure buy-in and participation from key stakeholders, including clinicians, educators, administrators, interdisciplinary team members such as social workers and community health workers, and the communities served. Integrating structural competency into clinical teaching and care involves a reimagining of current systems of practice and the explicit naming of SSDHs that impact patient care. Practices that actively incorporate workflows to screen for and address social needs, and those that utilize the COPC model, have already begun the work of incorporating SSDH. Importantly, academic practices should seek to promote interventions at all levels of the socio-ecological model, which necessitates that both providers and trainees are involved in advocacy to change practices and policies at the institutional, community, and societal levels. Faculty and trainees will quickly come to realize that practices and policies within their own academic medical institutions can serve to further health inequities. Incentives must therefore exist for healthcare administrators and leaders to address institutional barriers and enhance transparency. Vital to this effort are the development of evaluation tools that measure progress towards greater health equity and the cultivation of local expertise in structural competency through educational training initiatives.

References

1. World Health Organization. Social determinants of health. https://www.who.int/social_determinants/sdh_definition/en/Accessed April 1, 2019.
2. Solar O, Irwin A. A conceptual framework for action on the social determinants of health. Social Determinants of Health Discussion Paper 2 (Policy and Practice). https://www.who.int/sdhconference/resources/ConceptualframeworkforactiononSDH_eng.pdf?ua=1. Accessed 2 Feb 2022.
3. Hood CM, Gennuso KP, Swain GR, Catlin BB. County health rankings: relationships between determinant factors and health outcomes. Am J Prev Med. 2016;50(2):129–35. https://doi.org/10.1016/j.amepre.2015.08.024. Epub 2015 Oct 31.
4. CDC. Community health and Program services (CHAPS): health disparities among racial/ethnic populations. Atlanta: U.S. Department of Health and Human Services; 2008.
5. National Academies of Sciences Engineering Medicine. A framework for educating health professionals to address the social determinants of health. Washington (DC): National Academies Press; 2016.
6. Daniel H, Bornstein SS, Kane GC, et al. Addressing Social Determinants to Improve Patient Care and Promote Health Equity: An American College of Physicians Position Paper. Ann Intern Med. 2018;168:577–8. https://doi.org/10.7326/M17-2441.
7. Byhoff E, Kangovi S, Berkowitz SA, et al. A Society of General Internal Medicine position statement on the internists' role in social determinants of health. J Gen Intern Med. 2020;35:2721–7. https://doi.org/10.1007/s11606-020-05934-8.
8. Koh NJ, Wagner R, Newton RC, Kuhn CM, Co JPT, Weiss KB, et al. CLER National Report of findings 2021. Chicago, IL: Accreditation Council for Graduate Medical Education; 2021. https://doi.org/10.35425/ACGME.0008.
9. Gonzalo JD, Dekhtyar M, Starr SR, Borkan J, Brunett P, Fancher T, Green J, Grethlein SJ, Lai C, Lawson L, Monrad S, O'Sullivan P, Schwartz MD, Skochelak S. Health systems science curricula in undergraduate medical education: identifying and defining a potential curricular framework. Acad Med. 2017;92(1):123–31. https://doi.org/10.1097/ACM.0000000000001177.
10. Gard LA, et al. Social determinants of health training in U.S. primary care residency programs: a scoping review. Acad Med. 2019;94(1):135–43.

11. Hunter K, Thomson B. A scoping review of social determinants of health curricula in post-graduate medical education. Can Med Educ J. 2019;10(3):e61–71.
12. Health.Gov. Healthy People 2030. U.S. Department of Health and Human Services, Office of Disease Prevention and Health Promotion. https://health.gov/healthypeople/objectives-and-data/social-determinants-health. Accessed 9 Feb 2022.
13. Metzl JM, Hansen H. Structural competency: theorizing a new medical engagement with stigma and inequality. Soc Sci Med. 2014;103:126–33. https://doi.org/10.1016/j.socscimed.2013.06.032.
14. Krishnan A, Rabinowitz M, Ziminsky A, Scott SM, Chretien KC. Addressing race, culture, and structural inequality in medical education: a guide for revising teaching cases. Acad Med. 2019;94(4):550–5. https://doi.org/10.1097/ACM.0000000000002589.
15. Scott S and Hassan I. "Demystifying structural competency: promoting anti-racist training in ambulatory medical education" workshop. National Collaborative for Education to Address the Social Determinants of Health Conference, Virtual. 2021.
16. NEJM Group. Case studies in social medicine. New England Journal of Medicine. https://www.nejm.org/case-studies-in-social-medicine. Accessed 2 Feb 2022.
17. Hassan I, Abraham R, Bradley C, Mateja C. Subgroup 3: patient experience. Alliance for academic internal medicine health disparities collaborative learning community resources. https://www.im.org/resources/ume-gme-program-resources/resources-disparities Accessed 2 Feb 2022.
18. Neff J, Holmes SM, Knight KR, et al. Structural competency: curriculum for medical students, residents, and interprofessional teams on the structural factors that produce health disparities. MedEdPORTAL. 2020;16:10888. https://doi.org/10.15766/mep_2374-8265.10888.
19. Hassan I, Mansour M, Narayan L, Browder C, Patel VV, Lefrancois D, Shapiro L. Addressing social determinants of health in an ambulatory setting: quasi-experimental controlled study of a curricular intervention for residents. J Gen Intern Med. 2018;33(7):996–8. https://doi.org/10.1007/s11606-018-4427-5.
20. Behforouz HL, Drain PK, Rhatigan JJ. Rethinking the social history. N Engl J Med. 2014;371(14):1277–9. https://doi.org/10.1056/NEJMp1404846.
21. Garg A, Boynton-Jarrett R, Dworkin PH. Avoiding the unintended consequences of screening for social determinants of health. JAMA. 2016;316(8):813–4. https://doi.org/10.1001/jama.2016.9282.
22. Kenyon C, Sandel M, Silverstein M, Shakir A, Zuckerman B. Revisiting the social history for child health. Pediatrics. 2007;120(3):e734–8. https://doi.org/10.1542/peds.2006-2495.
23. Bourgois P, Holmes SM, Sue K, Quesada J. Structural vulnerability: operationalizing the concept to address health disparities in clinical care. Acad Med. 2017;92(3):299–307. https://doi.org/10.1097/ACM.0000000000001294. PMID: 27415443; PMCID: PMC5233668.
24. Boynton-Jarrett R, Flacks J. Strengths-based approaches to screening families for health-related social needs in the healthcare setting. Washington, DC; 2018.
25. Berkowitz SA, Hulberg AC, Hong C, Stowell BJ, Tirozzi KJ, Traore CY, Atlas SJ. Addressing basic resource needs to improve primary care quality: a community collaboration programme. BMJ Qual Saf. 2016;25(3):164–72. https://doi.org/10.1136/bmjqs-2015-004521. Epub 2015 Nov 30.
26. The Accountable Health Communities Health-Related Social Needs Screening Tool. https://innovation.cms.gov/files/worksheets/ahcm-screeningtool.pdf. Accessed 15 Feb 2022.
27. Schoenthaler A, Hassan I, Fiscella K. The time is now: fostering relationship-centered discussions about patients' social determinants of health. Patient Educ Couns. 2019;102(4):810–4. https://doi.org/10.1016/j.pec.2018.10.025. Epub 2018 Oct 29.
28. Seymour CK, Griffin C, Holmes SM, Martinez C. Structural differential – a 32-year-old man with persistent wrist pain. N Engl J Med. 2018;379(25):2385–8. https://doi.org/10.1056/NEJMp1811574.
29. Hassan IH, Bui T. Incorporating structurally competent clinical reasoning into case-based presentations. J Gen Intern Med. 2022;37(13):3465–70.

30. Dahlberg LL, Krug EG. Violence: a global public health problem. In: Krug E, Dahlberg LL, Mercy JA, Zwi AB, Lozano R, editors. World report on violence and health. Geneva: World Health Organization; 2002. p. 1–21.
31. ACGME Milestones 2.0. Internal medicine. https://www.acgme.org/globalassets/PDFs/Milestones/InternalMedicineMilestones2.0.pdf?ver=2020-12-02-140941-453&ver=2020-12-02-140941-453. Accessed 13 February 2022.
32. ACGME Common Program Requirements. https://www.acgme.org/globalassets/PFAssets/ProgramRequirements/CPRResidency2021.pdf. Accessed 13 Feb 2022.
33. Guralnick S, Fondahn E, Amin A, Bittner EA. Systems-based practice: time to finally adopt the orphan competency. J Grad Med Educ. 2021;13(2s):96–101. https://doi.org/10.4300/JGME-D-20-00839.1.
34. Castillo EG, Isom J, DeBonis KL, Jordan A, Braslow JT, Rohrbaugh R. Reconsidering systems-based practice: advancing structural competency, health equity, and social responsibility in graduate medical education. Acad Med. 2020;95(12):1817–22. https://doi.org/10.1097/ACM.0000000000003559.
35. Roberts SM, Jarvis-Selinger S, Pratt DD, Polonijo A, Stacy E, Wisener K, Black KP. Reshaping orthopaedic resident education in systems-based practice. J Bone Joint Surg Am. 2012;94(15):e1131–7. https://doi.org/10.2106/JBJS.K.00638. Erratum in: J Bone Joint Surg Am 2012 Sep 19;94(18):e141. Polinijo, Andrea [corrected to Polonijo, Andrea].
36. Delzell JE Jr, Ringdahl EN, Kruse RL. The ACGME core competencies: a national survey of family medicine program directors. Fam Med. 2005;37(8):576–80.
37. Englander R, Agostinucci W, Zalneraiti E, Carraccio CL. Teaching residents systems-based practice through a hospital cost-reduction program: a "win-win" situation. Teach Learn Med. 2006;18(2):150–2. https://doi.org/10.1207/s15328015tlm1802_10.
38. Chen EH, O'Sullivan PS, Pfennig CL, Leone K, Kessler CS. Assessing systems-based practice. Acad Emerg Med. 2012;19(12):1366–71. https://doi.org/10.1111/acem.12024. Epub 2012 Dec 13.
39. Borkan JM, Hammoud MM, Nelson E, Oyler J, Lawson L, Starr SR, Gonzalo JD. Health systems science education: the new post-Flexner professionalism for the 21st century. Med Teach. 2021;43(sup2):S25–31. https://doi.org/10.1080/0142159X.2021.1924366.
40. Beck AF, Cohen AJ, Colvin JD, et al. Perspectives from the society for pediatric research: interventions targeting social needs in pediatric clinical care. Pediatr Res. 2018;84(1):10–21. https://doi.org/10.1038/s41390-018-0012-1.
41. Kreuter MW, Thompson T, McQueen A, Garg R. Addressing social needs in health care settings: evidence, challenges, and opportunities for public health. Annu Rev Public Health. 2021;42:329–44. https://doi.org/10.1146/annurev-publhealth-090419-102204. Epub 2021 Dec 16. PMID: 33326298; PMCID: PMC8240195.
42. Developing an assessment and evaluation toolkit for social determinants of training in medical education and physician assistant education. National Collaborative for Education to Address the Social Determinants of Health. https://sdoheducation.org/research/developing-an-assessment-and-evaluation-toolkit-for-social-determinants-of-training-in-medical-education-and-physician-assistant-education/. Accessed 13 Feb 2022.
43. Wyatt R, Laderman M, Botwinick L, Mate K, Whittington J. Achieving health equity: a guide for health care organizations. IHI White Paper. Cambridge, Massachusetts: Institute for Healthcare Improvement; 2016. (Available at ihi.org).
44. Martino SC, Ahluwalia S, Harrison J, Kim A and Elliot MN. Developing health equity measures. RAND health care. Prepared for the Office of the Assistant Secretary for planning and evaluation (ASPE) at the U.S. Department of Health and Human Services. https://aspe.hhs.gov/reports/developing-health-equity-measures. Accessed 13 Feb 2022.
45. Agniel D, Martino SC, Burkhart Q, Hambarsoomian K, Orr N, Beckett MK, James C, Scholle SH, Wilson-Frederick S, Ng J, Elliott MN. Incentivizing excellent care to at-risk groups with a health equity summary score. J Gen Intern Med. 2021;36(7):1847–57. https://doi.org/10.1007/s11606-019-05473-x. Epub 2019 Nov 11. PMID: 31713030; PMCID: PMC8298664.

46. Institute of Medicine (US) division of health care services. Community oriented primary care: new directions for health services delivery. In: Connor E, Mullan F, editors. Community oriented primary care: meaning and scope. Washington (DC): National Academies Press; 1983. https://www.ncbi.nlm.nih.gov/books/NBK234632/.
47. Dobbie A, Kelly P, Sylvia E, Freeman J. Evaluating family medicine residency COPC programs: meeting the challenge. Fam Med. 2006;38(6):399–407.

Chapter 22
Institutional Racism

Thuy Bui and Alia Chisty

Introduction

Institutional racism is a set of practices and policies that disadvantage individuals not part of societies' dominant groups and result in racial disparities in outcomes [1]. Institutional racism, often indirect and unintentional, is caused by the processes, structure, and governance of an organization. There is well-documented discrimination, subjugation, and oppression of Black patients, patients of color, and uninsured and poor patients in our healthcare system. Moreover, personal racism is reinforced by institutional promotion of policies, behaviors, and attitudes, which advantage Whites to the detriment of other racial groups. Institutional racism also contributes to lack of diversity in the health professions, poor primary care, and specialty access for racial minority patients and lower quality of care [2, 3]. Healthcare in the USA is a business that utilizes exploitive practices seen in other industries. Most of the current institutional efforts are related to cultural competency and personal and interpersonal racism without attention to broader policies and practices. Implicit bias and cultural competency training are often mandated to shield upper management from the difficult task of addressing institutional racism. Healthcare organizations can start by examining all policies and practices for racial bias, embracing equity-centered design together with concerted efforts to recruit, retain, and promote clinicians and staff from underrepresented backgrounds.

T. Bui (✉)
Division of General Internal Medicine, University of Pittsburgh School of Medicine, Pittsburgh, PA, USA
e-mail: buit@upmc.edu

A. Chisty
Department of Medicine, Division of General Internal Medicine, Penn State Health Milton S. Hershey Medical Center/Penn State College of Medicine, Hershey, PA, USA
e-mail: achisty@pennstatehealth.psu.edu

L. B. Lu et al. (eds.), *Leading an Academic Medical Practice*,
https://doi.org/10.1007/978-3-031-40273-9_22

Outline

- Historical context
- Racism in medical training
- Stereotype, bias, microaggressions, the hidden curriculum, and interventions
- Segregation in health
- Race-based medicine
- Institutional practices that perpetuate health disparities
- Recommended interventions to address institutional racism in healthcare
- Conclusion

Historical Context

The Flexner Report, when it came out in 1910, was revolutionary for attempting to standardize the quality of medical education [4]. Unfortunately, it had extremely dire consequences, leading to closure of five out of seven historically Black medical schools when Black students were excluded from attending White medical schools [5]. Following Flexner, only Howard and Meharry continued but experienced fiscal challenges (Morehouse opened in 1978). Additionally, Black physicians were prevented from membership in professional societies or earning leadership roles [5]. In 1968, following *Brown v the Board of Education* (1954) and the Civil Rights Act (1964), the AAMC and the AMA endorsed expanding enrollment in medical schools in an effort to enroll more racial and ethnic minority students. At this point, due to racial segregation efforts, structural racism had already taken a toll with less investment in K-12 education for Black communities, which meant fewer students in the pipeline to pursue medical education. Different resources for Black compared to traditionally White medical schools and separate opportunities for Black physicians to gain leadership or continued education through professional societies led to a staggering disparity in the physician workforce.

The Medical College Admissions Test (MCAT), implemented in 1928 to assess aptitude, has historically been used as a tool by medical school admissions committees to guide applicant selection. Through older and newer versions of the MCAT exam, mean scores are lower for applicants from underrepresented in medicine (URiM) groups compared to groups well represented in the medical field [6–8]. Lucey et al. propose that MCAT is not necessarily a biased exam, but that structural racism and its effects on education, housing, and other factors contribute to the disparities seen [8].

Finally, affirmative action efforts in the 1970s and 1980s attempted to address parity in medical education. The seminal Supreme Court case to challenge affirmative action was the *Regents of the University of California v. Bakke* filed in 1974. Alan Bakke, a White man, was denied admissions to the University of California, Davis School of Medicine. Even though the court ruled in favor of Bakke, they did uphold the right of the schools to take race into consideration when choosing applicants [5, 9, 10].

Racism in Medical Training

Underrepresented in medicine (URiM) refers to the stark disparity between the representation of certain groups in the national population compared to the physician workforce. Traditionally, this includes individuals who identify as Black or African American, Hispanic or Latinx, Native American or Alaskan Native, and Native Hawaiian or other Pacific Islander. Despite efforts to improve the URiM physician workforce, disparities between representation of Black and Latinx groups in the national population compared to the physician workforce continue to exist. US Census data from 2021 illustrates that 13.4% of the total population identifies as Black or African American and 18.5% identifies as Latinx [11]. AAMC data from 2018–2019 demonstrate that only 7.1% of accepted students to US medical schools were Black or African American and only 6.2% were Hispanic, Latinx, or Spanish origin. The same year, only 6.2% of US medical school graduates identified as Black or African American, 5.3% identified as Latinx, and 54.6% were White (AAMC website) [12, 13]. In December 2021, the AAMC announced that Black/African American students made up 11.3% of matriculants to medical school and Hispanic/Latinx individuals made up 12.7% of first-year medical students. Unfortunately, American Indian or Alaskan Native first-year students declined by 8.5% and made up only 1% of matriculants to medical school. Overall, this trend signifies some improvements in trying to match the diversity of the physician workforce to the national population (AAMC press release Dec 2021) [14].

There is much evidence describing disparity in clerkship grades and narrative evaluations of URiM and other minority students compared to White students. When comparing non-URiM and URiM students, evaluations of URiM students were associated with fewer honors grades than evaluations of non-URiM students across all specialties. Furthermore, URiM students are more likely to be described by personality traits rather than competency [15]. In an analysis of Medical School Performance Evaluations (MSPEs), the most common word used for Black students was "competent," which carries a less positive connotation, compared to standout descriptors like "exceptional" or "outstanding" used to describe White learners [16]. Furthermore, when adjusting for USMLE step 1 scores, research productivity, community service, leadership activity, and Gold Humanism membership, Black and Asian American students were less likely to be members of the Alpha Omega Alpha medical honor society than White students [17]. Clerkship grades, MSPE evaluations, and AOA are all factors that heavily impact competitiveness for residency programs.

Racism and bias create a negative clinical learning environment for URiM students. Minority students are more likely to report that their race or ethnicity adversely affected their medical school experience and cite racial discrimination, prejudice, isolation, and different cultural expectations as the cause [18]. Minority students endorsing these experiences were also more likely to have burnout, depression, and lower quality-of-life scores [19]. Moreover, a greater proportion of URiM students are more likely to experience mistreatment based on race/ethnicity and experience two or more types of mistreatment compared to White counterparts [20, 21]. Persistent experiences of microaggressions by faculty, peers, and structural elements of the curricula contribute to URiM students feeling devalued, and these experiences negatively impact their academic performance and personal well-being [22]. Additionally, URiM residents have similar experiences. In a study of 232 internal medicine residents from two states, 45% of Black or Latinx residents experienced instances of explicit racial epithets, refusal of care, or request to change providers. Residents more often debriefed with family, friends, or team members but rarely reported these instances to the institution. Sometimes, they did not address specific instances and cited busy clinical days and futility of responding as the main drivers for why they might not have acted [23]. A mixed-methods analysis of faculty, trainees, staff, and students found that marginalized groups experienced greater infringements on their professional boundaries, increased scrutiny over their professional actions, and increased pressures to assimilate to an existing majority culture. In this study, gender identity and sexual minority groups and Black individuals were more likely to consider changing jobs due to unprofessional behavior experienced at work [24, 25].

Finally, the dearth of URiM faculty, who serve as important role models and mentors for URiM medical students [26], contributes to lack of mentorship for URiM students and residents. AAMC data from 2018 show that only 3.6% of full-time US medical school faculty identify as Black or African American and only 3.2% identify as Latinx [27]. URiM residents are significantly less likely to establish mentoring relationships compared to peers despite adjusting for demographics, career plans, and a personal history of mentorship in medical school or college. Interestingly, URiM residents were as likely to be satisfied with their mentoring relationship as their colleagues, and there were no differences in satisfaction of mentorship based on demographics of mentor including mentor's race/ethnicity, gender, or work setting [28]. A systematic review of mentoring programs for URiM faculty and trainees reports high satisfaction with mentoring programs [29].

The first step is increasing the recruitment and retention of URiM faculty. Higher rates of URiM faculty are linked to improved cultural competence in medical school graduates, more inclusive learning environments, more comprehensive research agendas, and improved patient care. But URiM faculty have lower rates of academic promotion and experience the "minority tax" where they are increasingly asked to promote diversity efforts that take time away from pursuits traditionally linked to academic promotion [30]. At the clinic level, we can extrapolate data from successful programs at academic medical centers that have led to absolute increases in recruitment and retention of URiM faculty. Successful recruitment strategies included mandatory implicit bias training for interviewers with standardized interview protocols and evaluation tools [31], broad dissemination of open positions [31], targeted outreach to URiM faculty [32], competitive compensation and professional development packages [32], committed stakeholders [33], dedicated diversity committees [31, 33], explicit timelines with financial backing [33], and integration of diversity into the overall mission of the institution [33]. One institution focused on improving the climate for faculty, which included regular measurement and distribution of demographic data, wide dissemination of policies and procedures, and investment in faculty development programs [34]. This led to a substantial increase in the percent of URiM faculty and matched URiM retention with non-URiM retention rates [34]. Higher retention rates among URiM faculty were seen when URiM faculty participated in career development programs [34]. Clinics at academic medical centers will need to approach recruitment, retention, and support with a multifaceted approach with leadership support, financial investment, and commitment from the institution to make diversity a priority. Aggressive recruitment of URiM faculty with faculty development programming will help URiM faculty achieve promotions, leadership positions, scholarly productivity, and, ultimately, institutional cultural change by embracing diversity efforts widely [35].

The LCME and ACGME have set forth several standards to focus on increasing diversity in the student and resident pool, respectively. Specifically, the ACGME has produced a framework for enhancing diversity in the trainee workforce that includes setting diversity as a priority, actively recruiting candidates through holistic review [36], implementing recruitment practices like implicit bias training for interviewers, providing microaggression and upstander training to support trainee success, and building a pipeline through collaboration with local schools and community outreach [37]. Medical students believe that diversity enhances their education experiences, including understanding of medical conditions [38]. Hearing perspectives of URiM students also allows students to better support their patients [39]. Some innovative structured curricula to specifically address structural racism and implicit bias have been developed such as the Health Equity Rounds, a longitudinal case-based conference series at Boston University which was developed by residents for interdisciplinary groups. Eighty-eight percent of respondents indicated that this curriculum fostered personal reflection on implicit bias, and 75% or more indicated that it would influence their clinical practice [40]. Moreover, given the high prevalence of burnout among resident physicians, higher rates of burnout were associated with higher rates of implicit and explicit racial bias. Therefore, addressing resident burnout can help reduce racial disparities in care provided by resident physicians [41].

Stereotype, Bias, Microaggressions, the Hidden Curriculum, and Interventions

The hidden curriculum affects teaching, learning, and assessment of patients, students, trainees, and faculty. Bias deeply affects the care of our patients as we inadvertently teach students and trainees that health inequities are the result of race or ethnicity, instead of deepening the understanding that health inequities experienced by racial or ethnic groups are the result of structural and social determinants of health that lead to disparate health outcomes. Healthcare professionals at all levels, from student to resident to attending, foster bias against Black, Latinx, and dark-skinned individuals and are more likely to associate them with "noncompliance" or less engagement in care. Latinx individuals were also associated with "risky behavior." There is mixed evidence on whether implicit bias affects health outcomes of our patients, with the greatest effect demonstrated in patient-physician relationships where patients of physicians with higher levels of bias felt less comfortable with their physician [42]. In one study, about 50% of White medical students and residents endorsed false beliefs of Black individuals (e.g., "Blacks have thicker skin and therefore feel less pain"), and these beliefs demonstrate racial bias in underassessing and undertreating pain [43]. Finally, we endorse the practice of evidence-based medicine by acknowledging that many research recommendations are based on trials that inadequately represent racial and ethnic minorities [44], which may lead to different qualities of medical care [45].

In order to address biases and more directly address the social constructs of disease, there are several suggestions from the literature. First, we can promote a "stop the line" culture against racism that is adopted from "stop the line" safety and quality measures used in industry. This can empower anyone who notices a problem to speak up to leaders, across patients, staff, learners, or physicians [46]. Next, community engagement through service-learning opportunities can increase knowledge among students and residents about the individual needs of the community they serve. At the University of Texas, Southwestern, a longitudinal community service-learning program increased self-reported knowledge in cultural competency, public health, community-based population research, population health, health promotion, health literacy, and social determinants of health. Objective skills improved in history taking, patient communication strategies, levels of prevention, and other important skills to engage physicians in the social and structural determinants of health [47]. Additionally, these programs rely on interdisciplinary teamwork and at their mission promote social justice [48]. Furthermore, these projects can directly address important community-based factors that heavily influence health like substance use disorder, violence prevention, stress management, and parent education workshops for adolescents [49]. Finally, service-learning opportunities can strengthen students' desires to continue community service work after medical school and preserve their intention for serving underserved communities in the future [50]. Also, as stated in the previous section, increasing the diversity of medical schools, trainees, and faculty is a necessary step in dismantling biases against racial and ethnic minority groups. Increasing the diversity of medical school classes has been associated with students feeling better prepared to care for minority populations with a strong attitude toward endorsing equitable access to care. URiM students are also more likely to plan to serve underserved communities [51]. Both the LCME and ACGME have endorsed policies to increase the number of URiM learners, but academic medical centers must also promote and embrace anti-racism policies [46] to ensure that students, residents, faculty, patients, and staff are nurtured in these environments.

Segregation in Healthcare

Residential segregation has been linked to higher mortality for Black populations and to specific health conditions [52–55]. With Title VI of the Civil Rights Act passed in 1964, Medicare forced the desegregation of every hospital in America. However, the legacy of racial segregation that resulted in residential segregation translates to hospital segregation with safety net hospitals disproportionally serving patients from communities of color [56]. Current hospital reimbursement and fee-for-service systems perpetuate hospital segregation where some hospitals disproportionately serve patients from Black and Brown communities and receive lower reimbursement and are more under-resourced, while other hospitals make more profits serving White and wealthier populations [57–59]. Medical mistrust and limited access to high-quality providers by residents in racially concentrated neighborhoods contribute to underutilization of primary care as their usual source of care compared to the emergency department [60]. Seven of the ten states with the highest Black populations chose not to expand Medicaid [61]. More than half of the people who are now categorically unable to access any affordable health coverage are people of color [62]. Neighborhood segregation is still correlated with the likelihood of hospital closings, and the safety-net hospitals that often serve Black people have been under extraordinary financial stress; their closure resulted in loss of residency training spots and lower quality of care [63, 64]. America's healthcare segregation problem will persist without investment in healthcare workforce, universal coverage, and social determinants of health. Academic primary care practices should recognize the impacts of residential segregation and do their parts to address mistrust and care quality while increasing workforce diversity and community engagement to improve health outcomes for underserved populations.

Race-Based Medicine

Race-based medicine is the system by which research characterizing race as an essential, biological variable is translated into clinical practice, leading to inequitable care [65]. Race is often learned or taught in medical schools as an independent risk factor for disease, rather than as a mediator of structural inequalities resulting from racist policies. Here are some examples of race-based medicine:

- Textbooks or images on the internet of skin conditions or manifestations of systemic disease often just highlight the conditions on lighter skin, but infectious disease conditions tend to be on darker skin patients [66, 67].
- The use of isosorbide dinitrate/hydralazine (marketed as BiDil) to treat congestive heart failure in African Americans: It was the first drug approved for a single racial group when the drugmaker showed decreased mortality in Black participants, but the original clinical trial actually failed to show efficacy for a multiracial population [68, 69].
- Because Asians have greater percent body fat than Caucasians for the same BMI, they are considered to be at risk for diabetes at lower body mass indices. More recent research suggests that the ethnic variation in susceptibility to metabolic syndrome may not arise from difference in body fat and the major determinants contributing to visceral adiposity in Asians are far from conclusive [70, 71].
- Research does show that Black patients of African origin have more severe and resistant hypertension, often because of genetically determined predisposition to

salt and water retention, with suppressed plasma renin activity [72]. Consequently, ACE-I is considered less effective in Black patients than in White patients, and they might not be prescribed to Black patients with hypertension [73]. It is also plausible that nongenetic factors such as diet, weight, and environmental factors are responsible for inter-individual variation in the drug pharmacokinetics [74].

Examples of race adjustments in clinical algorithms include the following:

- Race has been incorporated into the calculation of glomerular filtration rate (eGFR) because Black patients are presumed to have greater muscle mass than patients of other races, perpetuating the notion that black bodies are biologically different than white ones. Race-based eGFR calculation could adversely impact kidney transplantation evaluation and decisions related to living kidney donation [75]. Driven by student activism, a joint task force established by the National Kidney Foundations and the American Society of Nephrology in 2021 recommended the adoption of the new eGFR equation that estimates kidney function without a race variable [76]. In an academic practice, faculty and students should question the use of race as proxy for biology or genetics in clinical evaluation and management. We should also explore alternative indicators to race to stratify medical risk factors for disease states. When reviewing research studies, we should question the use of race as variables in the methodology and/or database and whether the results reflect racism rather than race.
- The Society for Maternal-Fetal Medicine endorses an algorithm for estimating the probability of successful vaginal birth for women underdoing trial of labor after cesarean, called vaginal birth after cesarean section (VBAC) calculator [77]. Predictions are heavily influenced by race and ethnicity without considering provider attitudes and institutional differences, and several authorities have started to challenge the use of race in the VBAC calculator as it might exacerbate racial disparities by not offering a trial of labor to African American or Hispanic mothers [78, 79].
- The standard practice in pulmonary function test is to adjust reference values for persons of African or African American ancestry, Hispanic ethnicity, or Asian ancestry. All racial-ethnic groups have lower lung volumes compared to their White counterparts [80]. Researchers have also documented other confounding factors to lung capacity such as socioeconomic status (SES), poverty, education, altitude, and chest dimensions [81]. During the COVID-19 pandemic, race adjustment in spirometry could lead to underdiagnosis of restrictive ventilatory dysfunction in Black patients resulting in fewer referrals to pulmonary rehabilitation [82].

Institutional Practices that Perpetuate Health Disparities

As we outlined above, decades of lack of funding for hospitals and clinics which serve racial/ethnic minority populations results in lower quality care for those patients. Lack of diversity in healthcare workforces at the physician and upper management level leads to marginalization of needs and services for communities of color. Market-driven "reforms" tend to exacerbate segregation and health disparities. Moreover, academic health centers traditionally focus on high-tech high-profit procedures to maintain its elitism, power, and privilege and are reluctant to change the dominant discourse to engage in anti-racist research and practice.

Here are some examples of discrimination and bias in policies and practices by US healthcare systems:

- Patients served by resident clinics affiliated with major academic medical centers were more likely to be uninsured or have Medicaid, be more diverse, be less likely to speak English as a primary language, and have higher rates of chronic disease, mental health conditions, and addiction. When measuring health outcomes, patients cared for by residents had lower rates of age-appropriate cancer screening and fewer patients meeting chronic disease metrics compared to patients cared for by attending physicians [83].
- Hospitals are increasingly forming their own private police departments. As a result, hospital-based academic practices will likely encounter police officers designed to protect workers from potentially hostile patients and family members. They might have a deterrent effect on crime and make staff and some patients feel safe. However, they are typically not required to answer to the public. Physicians and nurses are infrequent victims of hospital-related shootings, and in 23% of shootings within the ED, the weapon was a security officer's gun taken by the perpetrator [84]. Police officers are trained to use force, execute warrants, and make arrests. It is important that physicians, administrators, and staff have clear policy and procedure about police involvement to ensure accountability. In the George Floyd era, de-escalation training and crisis management were more important for police officers if they were to function as part of an interprofessional team to provide compassionate care, dignity, and respect to patients of any gender, race, and ethnicity.
- Patient satisfaction surveys are often used as a metric for quality-based financial incentives, but several studies suggest a potential bias toward underrepresented and female physicians [85]. Patient-physician racial-ethnic and gender discordance with Black and Asian patient race were both associated with lower patient experience ratings [86]. Patient satisfaction scores can be influenced by many policies and practices beyond the control of clinicians. Care must be taken when publicly reporting and/or using the Consumer Assessment of Healthcare Physician and Systems Clinician & Group Survey (CG-CAHPS) or Press Ganey scores to evaluate physicians on an individual level to provide financial incentive.
- Racism and bias may be communicated in the medical record and could potentially exacerbate racial and ethnic healthcare disparities [87]. A recent analysis of over 40,000 physician notes showed that compared with White patients, Black patients had 2.54 times the odds of having at least one negative descriptor in the history and physical notes such as nonadherent, aggressive, agitated, angry, challenging, combative, exaggerate, hysterical, unpleasant, noncompliant, refuse, and resist [87].

Structural racism in healthcare usually manifests through two main mechanisms—cost-containing measures and risk management—and most are combinations of both. Cost-containing measures include productivity targets that penalize providers caring for socially high-risk patients, inadequate interpretation services for patients with limited English proficiency, prioritization of quantity over quality, copayments, deductibles, fines for no-shows, and debt collection practice. Fragmentation of mental and behavioral healthcare systems is by design to minimize cost. Administrative burdens—filling out forms and lengthy wait "on hold"—are discriminating practices as they create barriers to access that disproportionately impact disabled, poor, and minority patients [88–90]. When it comes to new technology such as telemedicine and home monitoring devices, lack of health systems and lack of government funding and support for vulnerable patients, such as the elderly, those with low income and low digital literacy, and rural residents, have resulted in furthering the digital divide [91, 92].

The data-rich electronic medical records allow tools such as natural language processing and machine learning to inform risk management, resource allocation, and clinical decision-making, which are often fraught with bias. Obermeyer and colleagues identified a racial bias in a risk stratification algorithm that is used to prioritize patients for care management [93]. Other risk management strategies that disproportionately impact patients of color include rigid rules around treatment policies for those with mental illness and/or substance use disorder, terminating or firing patients, and quality improvement initiatives that fail to consider upstream factors such as systems and social determinants of health. QI interventions might actually worsen disparities if there is greater uptake or effectiveness of the intervention among patients with better outcomes at baseline.

Ambulatory practices that serve poor patients and patients of color fared worse under pay for performance (P4P). Research also suggests that much of the variation in performance is due to factors over which organizations have limited control. Incentive payment (or penalty) might exacerbate health disparities by rewarding the highest achievers with scarce resources taken from organization serving disadvantaged patients [94, 95].

Recommended Interventions to Address Institutional Racism in Healthcare

Institutional racism is commonly noted or experienced by minoritized populations in governance, policy implementation, service delivery, employment, and financial accountability. In their work with the Aboriginal and Torres Strait Islander people, Came and Humphries described five sites of institutional racism in health systems [96]:

1. Majoritarian decision-making or tyranny of the majority
2. Misuse of evidence (including biomedical evidence and excluding Indigenous evidence)
3. Culturally incompetent policy maker

4. Flawed consultation practices (asking the wrong questions of the wrong people)
5. Indigenous policy implementation requiring non-Indigenous agreement

Even though their work applied mainly to public health policy in New Zealand, we can derive valuable lessons to clinical practice. When working with marginalized members of a community or clinic staff, it is vital that their voices are elevated and incorporated into decision-making and that achieving consensus is not always the preferred or correct way to unravel institutional racism.

In their scoping review of anti-racism interventions in healthcare settings, Hassen and colleagues suggest the following foundational principles for anti-racism interventions [97]:

1. Clearly define a problem and set clear goals and objectives.
2. Incorporate explicit and shared anti-racism language.
3. Establish leadership buy-in and commitment.
4. Invest dedicated funding and resources.
5. Bring in the right support and expertise.
6. Establish ongoing, meaningful community and patient partnerships.

In order to implement and evaluate anti-racism strategies, the authors recommend a multi-level, long-term approach embedding racial equity policies and procedures (e.g., hiring, retention, and promotion), linking mandatory anti-racism work to broader systems of power, hierarchy, and dominance, and building in stop-and-reflect mechanisms in a cyclical process [97]. The work to dismantle institutional racism practice in the USA is still nascent. To tailor QI interventions to reduce rather than exacerbate disparities, the Institute for Healthcare Improvement (IHI) recommends six key activities that include collecting and analyzing data by race, ethnicity, and language and testing change ideas that address patients' social conditions and cultural influences [98]. In 2021, the American College of Physicians published a policy paper titled "Understanding and Addressing Disparities and Discrimination in Education and in the Physician Workforce," which offered recommendations to create safe, inclusive, and supportive educational and workplace environments [30].

We would like to offer some overarching approaches for directors of ambulatory practices as there is very limited work on effective anti-racism interventions in healthcare. To dismantle structural racism in healthcare, we would need a bottom-up as well as a top-down approach that goes beyond hosting training workshops and conferences. Top-down approaches include the following:

1. Increase diversity and representation of minoritized members at all levels of the workforce but particularly in leadership and upper level management. Institutions should focus on time-limited, goal-directed task forces rather than committees, which typically serve to preserve the status quo. Diversity metrics and dashboards that track the hiring and retention of diverse faculty and staff may also serve as surrogate markers of success for institutions. The ultimate goal is to decrease the power differential between institutional authorities, patients, staff, and trainees and to promote empowerment, allyship, and sustainability [99].

2. Implement quality improvement initiatives that promote community engagement and partnerships with community-based organizations that serve vulnerable communities. These upstream QI initiatives should be designed to address social needs and social determinants of health. Academic practices could also partner with FQHCs to leverage resources and support quality improvement initiatives. Healthcare providers need to recognize the resource and power differential inherent in the healthcare vs. social service systems and seek to support and integrate social service referrals and feedback in the routine workflow. We recognize that without more investment in social services and anti-poverty programs, healthcare-based social care will not result in better health outcomes.
3. Address health literacy, language, and cultural barriers. Besides offering translation and interpretation services, ambulatory practice should aim to hire navigators, community health workers, health educators, and/or social workers who are able to help patients with social needs and system navigation. Alternative payment models will be necessary to facilitate such teamwork and to make care more accessible and equitable.
4. Implement equity dashboards to understand disparities in patient outcomes and impacts of equity-focused interventions. Data collection that includes geographic mapping, socioeconomic status, housing conditions, and transportation use patterns could create a more comprehensive narrative about a patient's barriers to care and how the practice could better support their needs.
5. Make the reduction of healthcare segregation a goal. This is certainly not the responsibility of individual institutions nor is it feasible to achieve without an all-hands-on-deck approach. Minority-serving providers should be given more support and incentives to focus on preventative health, to manage chronic diseases, and to improve the quality of care they provide. We must include measures of segregation in the healthcare quality and disparity report cards of providers and plans regionally and nationally [100] as well as include such measures in regional planning.
6. Diversity and equity should be part of the annual goal setting, success metrics, and eligibility for promotion and bonuses. Concurrently, concrete goals about community engagement and partnerships should be clearly stated and monitored. The top-down approach requires legislative advocacy and substantial policy changes along the line of universal healthcare coverage as well as mental health and primary care integration.

Bottom-up strategies involve individual and small entities within the healthcare organization that are patient-facing, including our "essential" workers. Trainees, faculty, and staff need to question whether standard protocols are harmful for historically disenfranchised populations. Space and time should be reserved to evaluate all rules, guidelines, and policies for racist and disparity consequences whether intentional or not with organizational leadership committed to follow the recommendations of its most valued members. Input from frontline workers is critical to understand the intersectionality effects of each policy and practice on employees, trainees, and patients. Those who identify multiple factors of disadvantage include members of the LGBTQ+ community, people with disabilities, and/or older workers and people with caregiving responsibilities.

Equity training for clinical staff should include (1) historical context of racism in medicine, (2) racism and non-racism in scientific and health disparity research, and (3) strategies to address structural racism on individual and system levels. Antiracist training should be part of the institution's mission, vision, values, and priorities with the recognition that racism often occurs in tandem with other systems of oppression (e.g., sexism, classism, ableism, homophobia, transphobia). Training should include bystander response, confidential reporting mechanism, and valuing a culture in which racism is openly confronted and challenged. Some departments and organizations have adopted an Anti-Racist Code of Conduct [101, 102]. The purpose of a code of conduct against racism is to recognize speeches, actions, or procedures that may lead to discrimination of minoritized individuals and to take actions to prevent and counter racist incidents.

It is time to challenge traditional concepts of what constitutes professional behavior in medicine to include anti-racism as a professional competence. Professionalism must include advocacy, particularly advocacy for social justice and structural improvements for affected communities. For Internal Medicine Entrustable Professional Activities (EPAs), anti-racism competencies could be incorporated into EPA #13—Improve the quality of healthcare at both the individual and system level, 14—Advocate for individual patients, and 16—Demonstrate professional behavior [103]. These EPAs pertain to physicians' role in combating racism, discrimination, and other contributors to inequities among adult populations through advocacy, quality improvement methods, and population health strategies. As academic practice hosting students, preceptors should follow the recommendations to promote equity in internal medicine clerkship assessment and grading, including monitoring clerkship variables that relate to equity, such as gender and URiM status, mistreatment experiences reported by students, and student satisfaction in areas related to race, ethnicity, and gender [104].

There are often signs of institutional resistance to anti-racist work. Rather than acknowledging the difficult issue of racism, institutions talk instead about increasing diversity. Corporate leaders and management create endless number of committees and subcommittees who have limited power to address racist practices. They often cite the economic challenges and invoke crisis to divert attention from the issue at hand. They also spend more resources on messaging, public relations, and advertisement and less on making substantial differences in the lives of their members—staff, clinicians, nurses, and patients.

Conclusion

Institutional and structural racism is embedded in almost all policies and practices in healthcare settings, reflecting our racist history and the industry's capitalistic foundation. We can start to dismantle institutional racism by ensuring a diverse healthcare workforce and engaging vulnerable communities. Anti-racism principles need to be incorporated into training curriculum, continuing medical education, professionalism code, and competencies. We also need to continually identify guidelines, norms, and practices that promote inequities and reinforce structural racism. Organizational self-study and interprofessional solidarity are vital to counteract the profit-driven systems that harm poor, Black, and Brown patients and other minoritized groups.

References

1. Adkins-Jackson PB, Legha RK, Jones KA. How to measure racism in academic health centers. AMA J Ethics. 2021;23(2):E140–5. https://doi.org/10.1001/amajethics.2021.140.
2. Smedley BD, Stith AY, Colburn L, Evans CH, et al. The right thing to do, the smart thing to do: enhancing diversity in the health professions: summary of the symposium on diversity in health professions in honor of Herbert W.Nickens, M.D. Washington (DC): National Academies Press (US); 2001.
3. Mahajan S, Caraballo C, Lu Y, Valero-Elizondo J, Massey D, Annapureddy AR, Roy B, Riley C, Murugiah K, Onuma O, Nunez-Smith M, Forman HP, Nasir K, Herrin J, Krumholz HM. Trends in differences in health status and health care access and affordability by race and ethnicity in the United States, 1999-2018. JAMA. 2021;326(7):637–48. https://doi.org/10.1001/jama.2021.9907. PMID: 34402830; PMCID: PMC8371573.
4. Flexner A. Medical education in the United States and Canada: a report to the Carnegie Foundation for the Advancement of Teaching. Bulletin no. 4, vol. 32. Boston, Mass: Updyke; 1910. p. 41.
5. Steinecke A, Terrell C. Progress for whose future? The impact of the Flexner report on medical education for racial and ethnic minority physicians in the United States. Acad Med. 2010;85(2):236–45.
6. Davis D, Dorsey JK, Franks RD, Sackett PR, Searcy CA, Zhao X. Do racial and ethnic group differences in performance on the MCAT exam reflect test bias? Acad Med. 2013;88(5):593–602. https://doi.org/10.1097/ACM.0b013e318286803a.
7. Girotti JA, Chanatry JA, Clinchot DM, McClure SC, Swan Sein A, Walker IW, Searcy CA. Investigating group differences in examinee preparation for and performance on the new MCAT exam. Acad Med. 2020;95(3):365–74. https://doi.org/10.1097/ACM.0000000000002940.
8. Lucey CR, Saguil A. The consequences of structural racism on MCAT scores and medical school admissions: the past is prologue. Acad Med. 2020;95(3):351–6. https://doi.org/10.1097/ACM.0000000000002939.
9. Genao I, Gelman J. The MCA's restrictive effect on the minority physician pipeline: a legal perspective. Ann Intern Med. 2018;169(6):403–4. https://doi.org/10.7326/M18-0545. Epub 2018 Aug 28.
10. Institute of Medicine. The right thing to do, the smart thing to do: enhancing diversity in the health professions—Summary of the symposium on diversity in health professions in honor of Herbert W. Nickens, M.D. Washington, DC: The National Academies Press; 2001. https://www.nap.edu/catalog/10186/the-right-thing-to-do-the-smart-thing-to-do. opens in new tab.
11. United States Census Bureau Quick Facts. (https://www.census.gov/quickfacts/fact/table/US/PST045221). Accessed 12 June 2022.
12. Association of American Medical Colleges. Diversity in medicine: facts and figures 2019. https://www.aamc.org/data-reports/workforce/interactive-data/figure-8-percentage-

matriculants-us-medical-schools-race/ethnicity-alone-academic-year-2018-2019. Accessed 12 June 2022

13. Association of American Medical Colleges. Diversity in Medicine: Facts and Figures 2019. https://www.aamc.org/data-reports/workforce/interactive-data/figure-14-percentage-us-medical-school-graduates-sex-race/ethnicity-alone-and-us-citizen. Accessed 12 June 2022.
14. Associate of American Medical Colleges. Medical school enrollment more diverse in 2021. https://www.aamc.org/news-insights/press-releases/medical-school-enrollment-more-diverse-2021#:~:text=Diversity%20of%20the%202021%20entering%20medical%20school%20class&text=Black%20or%20African%20American%20studentsthis%20group%20increased%20by%2020.8%25. Accessed 12 June 2022.
15. Rojek AE, Khanna R, Yim JWL, Gardner R, Lisker S, Hauer KE, Lucey C, Sarkar U. Differences in narrative language in evaluations of medical students by gender and under-represented minority status. J Gen Intern Med. 2019;34(5):684–91. https://doi.org/10.1007/s11606-019-04889-9. PMID: 30993609; PMCID: PMC6502922.
16. Ross DA, Boatright D, Nunez-Smith M, Jordan A, Chekroud A, Moore EZ. Differences in words used to describe racial and gender groups in medical student performance evaluations. PLoS One. 2017;12(8):e0181659. https://doi.org/10.1371/journal.pone.0181659. PMID: 28792940; PMCID: PMC5549898.
17. Boatright D, Ross D, Connor P, Moore E, Nunez-Smith M. Racial disparities in medical student membership in the alpha omega alpha honor society. JAMA Intern Med. 2017;177(5):659–65. https://doi.org/10.1001/jamainternmed.2016.9623. PMID: 28264091; PMCID: PMC5818775.
18. Orom H, Semalulu T, Underwood W 3rd. The social and learning environments experienced by underrepresented minority medical students: a narrative review. Acad Med. 2013;88(11):1765–77. https://doi.org/10.1097/ACM.0b013e3182a7a3af.
19. Dyrbye LN, Thomas MR, Eacker A, Harper W, Massie FS Jr, Power DV, Huschka M, Novotny PJ, Sloan JA, Shanafelt TD. Race, ethnicity, and medical student well-being in the United States. Arch Intern Med. 2007;167(19):2103–9. https://doi.org/10.1001/archinte.167.19.2103.
20. Hill KA, Samuels EA, Gross CP, Desai MM, Sitkin Zelin N, Latimore D, Huot SJ, Cramer LD, Wong AH, Boatright D. Assessment of the prevalence of medical student mistreatment by sex, race/ethnicity, and sexual orientation. JAMA Intern Med. 2020;180(5):653–65. https://doi.org/10.1001/jamainternmed.2020.0030. PMID: 32091540; PMCID: PMC7042809.
21. Hariharan B, Quarshie LS, Amdahl C, Winterburn S, Offiah G. Experiencing racism within medical school curriculum: 2020 ICCH student symposium. Patient Educ Couns. 2021;105(7):2599–602. https://doi.org/10.1016/j.pec.2021.12.018. Epub ahead of print.
22. Ackerman-Barger K, Boatright D, Gonzalez-Colaso R, Orozco R, Latimore D. Seeking inclusion excellence: understanding racial microaggressions as experienced by underrepresented medical and nursing students. Acad Med. 2020;95(5):758–63. https://doi.org/10.1097/ACM.0000000000003077. PMID: 31725462; PMCID: PMC7185051.
23. de Bourmont SS, Burra A, Nouri SS, El-Farra N, Mohottige D, Sloan C, Schaeffer S, Friedman J, Fernandez A. Resident physician experiences with and responses to biased patients. JAMA Netw Open. 2020;3(11):e2021769. https://doi.org/10.1001/jamanetworkopen.2020.21769. PMID: 33226429; PMCID: PMC7684448.
24. Alexis DA, Kearney MD, Williams JC, Xu C, Higginbotham EJ, Aysola J. Assessment of perceptions of professionalism among faculty, trainees, staff, and students in a large university-based health system. JAMA Netw Open. 2020;3(11):e2021452. https://doi.org/10.1001/jamanetworkopen.2020.21452. PMID: 33226428; PMCID: PMC7684446.
25. Acholonu RG, Oyeku SO. Addressing microaggressions in the health care workforce-a path toward achieving equity and inclusion. JAMA Netw Open. 2020;3(11):e2021770. https://doi.org/10.1001/jamanetworkopen.2020.21770.

26. Elks ML, Herbert-Carter J, Smith M, Klement B, Knight BB, Anachebe NF. Shifting the curve: fostering academic success in a diverse student body. Acad Med. 2018;93(1):66–70. https://doi.org/10.1097/ACM.0000000000001783. PMID: 28678099; PMCID: PMC5753825.
27. Association of American Medical Colleges. Diversity in medicine: facts and figures 2019. https://www.aamc.org/data-reports/workforce/interactive-data/figure-15-percentage-full-time-us-medical-school-faculty-race/ethnicity-2018. Accessed 12 June 2022.
28. Ramanan RA, Taylor WC, Davis RB, Phillips RS. Mentoring matters. Mentoring and career preparation in internal medicine residency training. J Gen Intern Med. 2006;21(4):340–5. https://doi.org/10.1111/j.1525-1497.2006.00346.x. PMID: 16686809; PMCID: PMC1484727.
29. Bonifacino E, Ufomata EO, Farkas AH, et al. Mentorship of underrepresented physicians and trainees in academic medicine: a systematic review. J Gen Intern Med. 2021;36:1023–34. https://doi.org/10.1007/s11606-020-06478-7.
30. Serchen J, Doherty R, Atiq O, Hilden D, et al. A comprehensive policy framework to understand and address disparities and discrimination in health and health care: a policy paper from the American college of physicians. Ann Intern Med. 2021;174(4):529–32. https://doi.org/10.7326/M20-7219. Epub 2021 Jan 12.
31. Dossett LA, Mulholland MW, Newman EA. Building high-performing teams in academic surgery: the opportunities and challenges of inclusive recruitment strategies. Acad Med. 2019;94(8):1142–5.
32. Lin SY, Francis HW, Minor LB, Eisele DW. Faculty diversity and inclusion program outcomes at an academic otolaryngology department. Laryngoscope. 2016;126(2):352–6. https://doi.org/10.1002/lary.25455. Epub 2015 Jul 7.
33. Deas D, Pisano ED, Mainous AG 3rd, Johnson NG, Singleton MH, Gordon L, Taylor W, Hazen-Martin D, Burnham WS, Reves JG. Improving diversity through strategic planning: a 10-year (2002-2012) experience at the Medical University of South Carolina. Acad Med. 2012;87(11):1548–55. https://doi.org/10.1097/ACM.0b013e31826d63e0.
34. Wingard D, Trejo J, Gudea M, Goodman S, Reznik V. Faculty equity, diversity, culture and climate change in academic medicine: a longitudinal study. J Natl Med Assoc. 2019;111(1):46–53. https://doi.org/10.1016/j.jnma.2018.05.004. Epub 2018 Jun 18.
35. Gutierrez-Wu J, Lawrence C, Jamison S, Wright ST, Steiner MJ, Orr CJ. An evaluation of programs designed to increase representation of diverse faculty at academic medical centers. J Natl Med Assoc. 2022;114(3):278–89. https://doi.org/10.1016/j.jnma.2022.01.012. Epub 2022 Mar 2.
36. Aibana O, Swails JL, Flores RJ, Love L. Bridging the gap: holistic review to increase diversity in graduate medical education. Acad Med. 2019;94(8):1137–41. https://doi.org/10.1097/ACM.0000000000002779.
37. Gonzaga AMR, Appiah-Pippim J, Onumah CM, Yialamas MA. A framework for inclusive graduate medical education recruitment strategies: meeting the ACGME standard for a diverse and inclusive workforce. Acad Med. 2020;95(5):710–6. https://doi.org/10.1097/ACM.0000000000003073.
38. Whitla DK, Orfield G, Silen W, Teperow C, Howard C, Reede J. Educational benefits of diversity in medical school: a survey of students. Acad Med. 2003;78(5):460–6. https://doi.org/10.1097/00001888-200305000-00007.
39. Baugh AD, Vanderbilt AA, Baugh RF. The dynamics of poverty, educational attainment, and the children of the disadvantaged entering medical school. Adv Med Educ Pract. 2019;10:667–76. https://doi.org/10.2147/AMEP.S196840. PMID: 31686941; PMCID: PMC6708885.
40. Perdomo J, Tolliver D, Hsu H, He Y, Nash KA, Donatelli S, Mateo C, Akagbosu C, Alizadeh F, Power-Hays A, Rainer T, Zheng DJ, Kistin CJ, Vinci RJ, Michelson CD. Health equity rounds: an interdisciplinary case conference to address implicit bias and structural racism for faculty and trainees. MedEdPORTAL. 2019;15:10858. https://doi.org/10.15766/mep_2374-8265.10858. PMID: 32166114; PMCID: PMC7050660.

41. Dyrbye L, Herrin J, West CP, Wittlin NM, Dovidio JF, Hardeman R, Burke SE, Phelan S, Onyeador IN, Cunningham B, van Ryn M. Association of racial bias with burnout among resident physicians. JAMA Netw Open. 2019;2(7):e197457. https://doi.org/10.1001/jamanetworkopen.2019.7457. PMID: 31348503; PMCID: PMC6661712.
42. Hall WJ, Chapman MV, Lee KM, Merino YM, Thomas TW, Payne BK, Eng E, Day SH, Coyne-Beasley T. Implicit racial/ethnic bias among health care professionals and its influence on health care outcomes: a systematic review. Am J Public Health. 2015;105(12):e60–76. https://doi.org/10.2105/AJPH.2015.302903. Epub 2015 Oct 15. PMID: 26469668; PMCID: PMC4638275.
43. Hoffman KM, Trawalter S, Axt JR, Oliver MN. Racial bias in pain assessment and treatment recommendations, and false beliefs about biological differences between blacks and whites. Proc Natl Acad Sci U S A. 2016;113(16):4296–301. https://doi.org/10.1073/pnas.1516047113. Epub 2016 Apr 4. PMID: 27044069; PMCID: PMC484348.
44. Terry M. Pushing for more ethnic and racial diversity in clinical trials. Biospace. 2020.
45. Ufomata E, Merriam S, Puri A, Lupton K, LeFrancois D, Jones D, Nemeth A, Snydman LK, Stark R, Spagnoletti C. A policy statement of the society of general internal medicine on tackling racism in medical education: reflections on the past and a call to action for the future. J Gen Intern Med. 2021;36(4):1077–81. https://doi.org/10.1007/s11606-020-06445-2. Epub 2021 Jan 22. PMID: 33483823; PMCID: PMC8042052.
46. Gray DM 2nd, Joseph JJ, Glover AR, Olayiwola JN. How academia should respond to racism. Nat Rev Gastroenterol Hepatol. 2020;17(10):589–90. https://doi.org/10.1038/s41575-020-0349-x.
47. Gimpel N, Kindratt T, Dawson A, Pagels P. Community action research track: community-based participatory research and service-learning experiences for medical students. Perspect Med Educ. 2018;7(2):139–43. https://doi.org/10.1007/s40037-017-0397-2. PMID: 29374389; PMCID: PMC5889376.
48. Smith KL, Meah Y, Reininger B, Farr M, Zeidman J, Thomas DC. Integrating service learning into the curriculum: lessons from the field. Med Teach. 2013;35(5):e1139–48. https://doi.org/10.3109/0142159X.2012.735383. Epub 2013 Jan 15.
49. McNeal MS, Buckner AV. Using mini-grants and service-learning projects to prepare students to serve underserved populations. J Health Care Poor Underserved. 2012;23(2 Suppl):20–6. https://doi.org/10.1353/hpu.2012.0073.
50. Jones K, Blinkhorn LM, Schumann SA, Reddy ST. Promoting sustainable community service in the 4th year of medical school: a longitudinal service-learning elective. Teach Learn Med. 2014;26(3):296–303. https://doi.org/10.1080/10401334.2014.911698.
51. Saha S, Guiton G, Wimmers PF, Wilkerson L. Student body racial and ethnic composition and diversity-related outcomes in US medical schools. JAMA. 2008;300(10):1135–45. https://doi.org/10.1001/jama.300.10.1135.
52. Collins CA, Williams DR. Segregation and mortality: the deadly effects of racism? Sociol Forum. 1999;14:495–523. https://doi.org/10.1023/A:1021403820451.
53. Jackson SA, Anderson RT, Johnson NJ, Sorlie PD. The relation of residential segregation to all-cause mortality: a study in black and white. Am J Public Health. 2000;90(4):615–7. https://doi.org/10.2105/ajph.90.4.615. PMID: 10754978; PMCID: PMC1446199.
54. Popescu I, Duffy E, Mendelsohn J, Escarce JJ. Racial residential segregation, socioeconomic disparities, and the white-black survival gap. PLoS One. 2018;13(2):e0193222. https://doi.org/10.1371/journal.pone.0193222. PMID: 29474451; PMCID: PMC5825109.
55. Torrats-Espinosa G. Using machine learning to estimate the effect of racial segregation on COVID-19 mortality in the United States. Proc Natl Acad Sci U S A. 2021;118(7):e2015577118. https://doi.org/10.1073/pnas.2015577118. PMID: 33531345; PMCID: PMC7896347.
56. Gaskin DJ, Hadley J. Population characteristics of markets of safety-net and non-safety-net hospitals. J Urban Health. 1999;76(3):351–70. https://doi.org/10.1007/BF02345673. PMID: 12607901; PMCID: PMC3456829.

57. Sarrazin MV, Campbell M, Rosenthal GE. Racial differences in hospital use after acute myocardial infarction: does residential segregation play a role? Health Aff (Millwood). 2009;28(2):w368–78. https://doi.org/10.1377/hlthaff.28.2.w368. Epub 2009 Mar 3. PMID: 19258343; PMCID: PMC4182438.
58. Dimick J, Ruhter J, Sarrazin MV, Birkmeyer JD. Black patients more likely than whites to undergo surgery at low-quality hospitals in segregated regions. Health Aff (Millwood). 2013;32(6):1046–53. https://doi.org/10.1377/hlthaff.2011.1365. PMID: 23733978; PMCID: PMC4789147.
59. Zogg CK, Thumma JR, Ryan AM, Dimick JB. Medicar's hospital acquired condition reduction program disproportionately affects minority-serving hospitals: variation by race, socioeconomic status, and disproportionate share hospital payment receipt. Ann Surg. 2020;271(6):985–93. https://doi.org/10.1097/SLA.0000000000003564. PMID: 31469746; PMCID: PMC8106480.
60. Arnett MJ, Thorpe RJ Jr, Gaskin DJ, Bowie JV, LaVeist TA. Race, medical mistrust, and segregation in primary care as usual source of care: findings from the exploring health disparities in integrated communities study. J Urban Health. 2016;93(3):456–67. https://doi.org/10.1007/s11524-016-0054-9. PMID: 27193595; PMCID: PMC4899337.
61. Kaiser Family Foundation. Status of state Medicaid expansion decisions: interactive map. KFF. 2022. https://www.kff.org/medicaid/issue-brief/status-of-state-medicaid-expansion-decisions-interactive-map/.
62. Lukens G, Sharer B. Closing Medicaid coverage gap would help diverse group and narrow racial disparities. Center on Budget and Policy Priorities. 2021. https://www.cbpp.org/research/health/closing-medicaid-coverage-gap-would-help-diverse-group-and-narrow-racial.
63. Walker KO, Calmes D, Hanna N, Baker R. The impact of public hospital closure on medical and residency education: implications and recommendations. J Natl Med Assoc. 2008;100(12):1377–83. https://doi.org/10.1016/s0027-9684(15)31537-6. PMID: 19110905; PMCID: PMC2868965.
64. Williams JP. Code red: the grim state of urban hospitals. US News and World Report. 2019. https://www.usnews.com/news/healthiest-communities/articles/2019-07-10/poor-minorities-bear-the-brunt-as-urban-hospitals-close.
65. Cerdeña JP, Plaisime MV, Tsai J. Race-conscious medicine: a response to critique. Intern Med J. 2021;51(8):1369–70. https://doi.org/10.1111/imj.15460.
66. Louie P, Wilkes R. Representations of race and skin tone in medical textbook imagery. Soc Sci Med. 2018;202:38–42. https://doi.org/10.1016/j.socscimed.2018.02.023. Epub 2018 Feb 23.
67. Martin GC, Kirgis J, Sid E, Sabin JA. Equitable imagery in the preclinical medical school curriculum: findings from one medical school. Acad Med. 2016;91(7):1002–6. https://doi.org/10.1097/ACM.0000000000001105.
68. Bloche MG. Race-based therapeutics. N Engl J Med. 2004;351(20):2035–7. https://doi.org/10.1056/NEJMp048271. Epub 2004 Nov 8.
69. Sankar P, Kahn J. BiDil: ralce medicine or race marketing? Health Aff (Millwood). 2005;(Suppl Web Exclusives):W5-455-63. https://doi.org/10.1377/hlthaff.w5.455.
70. Williams R, Periasamy M. Genetic and environmental factors contributing to visceral adiposity in asian populations. Endocrinol Metab (Seoul). 2020;35(4):681–95. https://doi.org/10.3803/EnM.2020.772. Epub 2020 Dec 23. PMID: 33397033; PMCID: PMC7803598.
71. Alenaini W, Parkinson JRC, McCarthy JP, Goldstone AP, Wilman HR, Banerjee R, Yaghootkar H, Bell JD, Thomas EL. Ethnic differences in body fat deposition and liver fat content in two UK-based cohorts. Obesity (Silver Spring). 2020;28(11):2142–52. https://doi.org/10.1002/oby.22948. Epub 2020 Sep 16.
72. Spence JD, Rayner BL. Hypertension in blacks: individualized therapy based on renin/aldosterone phenotyping. Hypertension. 2018;72(2):263–9. https://doi.org/10.1161/HYPERTENSIONAHA.118.11064. Epub 2018 Jun 25.
73. Helmer A, Slater N, Smithgall S. A review of ACE inhibitors and ARBs in black patients with hypertension. Ann Pharmacother. 2018;52(11):1143–51. https://doi.org/10.1177/1060028018779082. Epub 2018 May 29

74. Olafuyi O, Parekh N, Wright J, Koenig J. Inter-ethnic differences in pharmacokinetics-is there more that unites than divides? Pharmacol Res Perspect. 2021;9(6):e00890. https://doi.org/10.1002/prp2.890. PMID: 34725944; PMCID: PMC8561230.
75. Kuppachi S, Norman SP, Lentine KL, Axelrod DA. Using race to estimate glomerular filtration and its impact in kidney transplantation. Clin Transpl. 2021;35(1):e14136. https://doi.org/10.1111/ctr.14136. Epub 2020 Nov 24.
76. Delgado C, Baweja M, Crews DC, Eneanya ND, Gadegbeku CA, Inker LA, Mendu ML, Miller WG, Moxey-Mims MM, Roberts GV, St Peter WL, Warfield C, Powe NR. A unifying approach for GFR estimation: recommendations of the NKF-ASN task force on reassessing the inclusion of race in diagnosing kidney disease. Am J Kidney Dis. 2022;79(2):268–288.e1. https://doi.org/10.1053/j.ajkd.2021.08.003. Epub 2021 Sep 23.
77. Rossi RM, Requarth E, Warshak CR, Dufendach KR, Hall ES, DeFranco EA. Risk calculator to predict cesarean delivery among women undergoing induction of labor. Obstet Gynecol. 2020;135(3):559–68. https://doi.org/10.1097/AOG.0000000000003696.
78. Vyas DA, Jones DS, Meadows AR, Diouf K, Nour NM, Schantz-Dunn J. Challenging the use of race in the vaginal birth after cesarean section calculator. Womens Health Issues. 2019;29(3):201–4. https://doi.org/10.1016/j.whi.2019.04.007. Epub 2019 May 6.
79. Grobman WA, Sandoval G, Rice MM, Bailit JL, Chauhan SP, Costantine MM, Gyamfi-Bannerman C, Metz TD, Parry S, Rouse DJ, Saade GR, Simhan HN, Thorp JM Jr, ATN T, Longo M, Landon MB, et al. Prediction of vaginal birth after cesarean delivery in term gestations: a calculator without race and ethnicity. Am J Obstet Gynecol. 2021;225(6):664.e1–7. https://doi.org/10.1016/j.ajog.2021.05.021. Epub 2021 May 24. PMID: 34043983; PMCID: PMC8611105.
80. Braun L. Race, ethnicity and lung function: a brief history. Can J Respir Ther. 2015;51(4):99–101. PMID: 26566381; PMCID: PMC4631137.
81. Braun L, Wolfgang M, Dickersin K. Defining race/ethnicity and explaining difference in research studies on lung function. Eur Respir J. 2013;41(6):1362–70. https://doi.org/10.1183/09031936.00091612. Epub 2012 Aug 9.
82. Anderson MA, Malhotra A, Non AL. Could routine race-adjustment of spirometers exacerbate racial disparities in COVID-19 recovery? Lancet Respir Med. 2021;9(2):124–5. https://doi.org/10.1016/S2213-2600(20)30571-3. Epub 2020 Dec 10. PMID: 33308418; PMCID: PMC7867612.
83. Essien UR, He W, Ray A, Chang Y, Abraham JR, Singer DE, Atlas SJ. Disparities in quality of primary care by resident and staff physicians: is there a conflict between training and equity? J Gen Intern Med. 2019;34(7):1184–91. https://doi.org/10.1007/s11606-019-04960-5. Epub 2019 Apr 8. PMID: 30963439; PMCID: PMC6614525.
84. Kelen GD, Catlett CL, Kubit JG, Hsieh YH. Hospital-based shootings in the United States: 2000 to 2011. Ann Emerg Med. 2012;60(6):790–798.e1. https://doi.org/10.1016/j.annemergmed.2012.08.012. Epub 2012 Sep 19.
85. Sotto-Santiago S, Slaven JE, Rohr-Kirchgraber T. (Dis)incentivizing patient satisfaction metrics: the unintended consequences of institutional bias. Health Equity. 2019;3(1):13–8. https://doi.org/10.1089/heq.2018.0065. PMID: 30729230; PMCID: PMC6363594.
86. Takeshita J, Wang S, Loren AW, Mitra N, Shults J, Shin DB, Sawinski DL. Association of Racial/ethnic and gender concordance between patients and physicians with patient experience ratings. JAMA Netw Open. 2020;3(11):e2024583. https://doi.org/10.1001/jamanetworkopen.2020.24583. PMID: 33165609; PMCID: PMC7653497.
87. Sun M, Oliwa T, Peek ME, Tung EL. Negative patient descriptors: documenting racial bias in the electronic health record. Health Aff (Millwood). 2022;41(2):203–11. https://doi.org/10.1377/hlthaff.2021.01423. Epub 2022 Jan 19. PMID: 35044842; PMCID: PMC8973827.
88. Kyle MA, Frakt AB. Patient administrative burden in the US health care system. Health Serv Res. 2021;56(5):755–65. https://doi.org/10.1111/1475-6773.13861. Epub 2021 Sep 8. PMID: 34498259; PMCID: PMC8522562.

89. Office of Management and Budget. Study to identify methods to assess equity: report to the president. Washington, DC: OMB; 2021. https://www.whitehouse.gov/wp-content/uploads/2021/08/OMB-Report-on-E013985-Implementation_508-Compliant-Secure--v1.1.pdf.
90. Ray VE, Herd P, Moynihan, D. (2020). Racialized burdens: applying racialized organization theory to the administrative state. 33(2). https://doi.org/10.31235/osf.io/q3xb8.
91. Cantor JH, McBain RK, Pera MF, Bravata DM, Whaley CM. Who is (and is not) receiving telemedicine care during the COVID-19 pandemic. Am J Prev Med. 2021;61(3):434–8. https://doi.org/10.1016/j.amepre.2021.01.030. Epub 2021 Mar 6. PMID: 33781622; PMCID: PMC7936544.
92. Mitchell M, Kan L. Digital technology and the future of health systems. Health Syst Reform. 2019;5(2):113–20. https://doi.org/10.1080/23288604.2019.1583040. Epub 2019 Mar 25.
93. Obermeyer Z, Powers B, Vogeli C, Mullainathan S. Dissecting racial bias in an algorithm used to manage the health of populations. Science. 2019;366(6464):447–53. https://doi.org/10.1126/science.aax2342.
94. Chien AT, Chin MH, Davis AM, Casalino LP. Pay for performance, public reporting, and racial disparities in health care: how are programs being designed? Med Care Res Rev. 2007;64(5 Suppl):283S–304S. https://doi.org/10.1177/1077558707305426.
95. Markovitz AA, Ryan AM. Pay-for-performance: Disappointing Results or Masked Heterogeneity? Med Care Res Rev. 2017;74(1):3–78. https://doi.org/10.1177/1077558715619282. Epub 2016 Aug 3. PMID: 26743502; PMCID: PMC5858565.
96. Came H, Humphries M. Mopping up institutional racism: activism on a napkin. In: Barter N, Tregidga H, editors. The Journal of Corporate Citizenship: Storytelling: Beyond the Academic Article—Using Fiction, Art and Literary Techniques to Communicate. 1st ed. Oxfordshire: Routledge; 2014. https://doi.org/10.4324/9781351285926.
97. Hassen N, Lofters A, Michael S, Mall A, Pinto AD, Rackal J. Implementing anti-racism interventions in healthcare settings: a scoping review. Int J Environ Res Public Health. 2021;18(6):2993. https://doi.org/10.3390/ijerph18062993. PMID: 33803942; PMCID: PMC8000324.
98. Wyatt R, Laderman M, Botwinick L, Mate K, Whittington J. Achieving health equity: a guide for health care organizations. IHI white paper. Cambridge, Massachusetts: Institute for Healthcare Improvement; 2016. http://www.ihi.org/resources/Pages/IHIWhitePapers/Achieving-Health-Equity.aspx.
99. Ngo VM, Beaverson S, Turkson S, Dow AW. Empowering student antiracist work to overcome inertia in academic health centers. Acad Med. 2021;97:818. https://doi.org/10.1097/ACM.0000000000004557.
100. Smith, DB. Eliminating disparities in treatment and the struggle to end segregation. Commonwealth Fund. 2005. https://www.commonwealthfund.org/publications/fund-reports/2005/aug/eliminating-disparities-treatment-and-struggle-end-segregation.
101. Calderon J, Wise, T. Code of ethics for antiracist white allies. 2014. https://4freedomscoalition.org/wp-content/uploads/2017/04/Cultural-Competence-Code-of-Ethics.pdf.
102. Olaniyan L, Peters C, Darling A, et al. Anti-racist code of conduct. The University of Utah Department of Communication. 2020. https://communication.utah.edu/news/antiracistcode-ofconduct.php.
103. Caverzagie KJ, Cooney TG, Hemmer PA, Berkowitz L. The development of entrustable professional activities for internal medicine residency training: a report from the education redesign Committee of the Alliance for academic internal medicine. Acad Med. 2015;90(4):479–84. https://doi.org/10.1097/ACM.0000000000000564.
104. Alliance for Academic Internal Medicine. Recommendations to Promote Equity in Internal Medicine Clerkship Assessment and Grading. 2020. https://www.im.org/resources/ume-gme-program-resources/resources-clerkship-equity.

Chapter 23
Nurturing a Culture of Diversity and Inclusion in Resident Clinic

Vandana Khungar, Laura Whitman, and Inginia Genao

Introduction

The racial and ethnic makeup of the US population is increasingly diverse, but the same degree of diversity is not reflected in the physician workforce. The American Association of Medical Colleges (AAMC) defines underrepresented in medicine as "those racial and ethnic populations that are underrepresented in the medical profession relative to their numbers in the general population" [1]. In 2020, the USA was 74.3% Caucasian, 18.5% Hispanic/Latino, 13.4% African-American, 5.9% Asian, 1.3% American Indian and Alaskan Native, and 0.2% Native Hawaiian or other Pacific Islander [2]. When focusing on faculty Underrepresented in Medicine (URM) by race and ethnicity in US medical schools, 2018–2019 data reveal that 3.2% of faculty are Hispanic/Latino, 3.6% Black or African-American, 0.2% American Indian or Alaskan Native, and 0.1% Native Hawaiian or Pacific Islander [3]. The pipeline is improving but is not yet where we need it to be, with 6.2% of medical students who are Hispanic/Latino, 7.1% Black or African American, 0.2% American Indian and Alaskan Native, and 0.1% Native Hawaiian or other Pacific Islander [4].

The USA and the world have seen a true and long overdue racial reckoning over the last few years. There is a vast body of literature that focuses on the discrepancy between the burgeoning minority population and underrepresentation of the same groups in medicine and medical education. The clear presence of disparities in care and biases mandate the need for cultural competence, communication skills, and a high degree of professionalism in resident physicians. In a recent welcome development, healthcare organizations and academia are paying growing attention not just

V. Khungar (✉) · L. Whitman · I. Genao
Department of Internal Medicine, Yale School of Medicine, New Haven, CT, USA
e-mail: vandana.khungar@yale.edu; inginia.genao@yale.edu

L. B. Lu et al. (eds.), *Leading an Academic Medical Practice*,
https://doi.org/10.1007/978-3-031-40273-9_23

to recruitment or diversity of the workforce, but also to ensuring equity and inclusion once individuals from diverse backgrounds are recruited. It is arguable that the demographic incongruity between providers and patients is most conspicuous in the clinics staffed by medical residents. Patients who receive primary care in university resident clinics tend to be underrepresented minorities and/or socioeconomically disadvantaged [5]. The distribution of patients and trainees who choose to focus on primary care necessitates proper training and best practices for diversity, equity, and inclusion in the setting of resident clinic. This chapter provides guidance to residency program and resident clinic leadership on methods to foster a culture of diversity and inclusion in resident clinic.

From the now expanding literature on the experiences of minority residents, common themes have emerged. Minority residents from multiple programs nationally noted a barrage of microaggressions and biases, experiencing the "minority tax" or being asked to serve as race or ethnicity ambassadors, and challenges negotiating professional and personal identity while being seen as "other" [6]. Social isolation is another common theme that came out of earlier work on the experiences of minority physicians at all levels [7, 8]. Given these challenges, it is readily apparent that not only recruitment but also retention are critically important. During resident orientation, competing priorities abound, with large amounts of practical knowledge that must be imparted to our new physicians. Devoting a portion of this valuable time to highlight the institution's appreciation for diversity and inclusivity will send a powerful message. Simple introductions by current residents and faculty with a two- to three-sentence summary of their background and interests are a wonderful way to jumpstart networking within a class and to help interns quickly identify potential mentors.

At the Yale New Haven Health System, a Minority Housestaff Organization (MHO) was created. Groups such as this allow for social events during orientation that counteract the sense of being "other" that many URM physicians feel. The MHO underscores the institutional support of diversity. Yale's own MHO can serve as a brief case study. The organization's stated goal is to create a supportive and fecund environment for minorities throughout the Yale New Haven Health System. Additionally, the MHO has said that they wish to promote mentorship, community outreach, and networking/social events. A former co-chair stated, "Our goal is to make it easier for current and future minority residents to find a community and locate the resources and support that are necessary for professional development." The MHO has sent its members to national meetings, organized second-look visits for minority applicants, and sponsored events such as Minority Men in Medicine, a social outing for URM residents with a lively fusion of soul food and rhythm and blues. The MHO has also strategically partnered with medical faculty through the Minority Organization for Retention and Expansion (MORE) and medical students through the Student National Medical Association (SNMA) and Latino Medical Student Association (LMSA). Partnering with similar groups in one's home institution can help to create structure. For those who do not have chapters at their schools, the national groups are wonderful resources.

Residents who are URM bring much-needed skills and experiences to our community. In addition to a heartfelt appreciation for the ethnic diversity of patients and providers, they often feel drawn to provide service to the indigent. They also bolster an environment that is at once welcoming and supportive of minorities [9]. In the authors' experience, active appreciation for the diversity of patients and provision of service to the medically indigent are not typically emphasized enough within most residency training programs. Diversity begets diversity, and the conspicuous presence and promotion of existing minorities as role models and mentors are an important feature to attract and retain other minority physicians. This model has already proven to be quite successful in attracting, recruiting, and retaining women in careers [10]. All centers should aim to proactively recruit minority students rather than passively hoping that they will leap over societal barriers to come to us. In the rest of this chapter, we describe strategies to recruit and retain residents who are underrepresented in medicine.

Outline

- Engagement and beyond: Recruitment and retention efforts to diversify the workforce
- Goal: A climate conducive to appreciation of each other on a cultural and social level
- Definition of community beyond simple demographics
- Cultural competence for all clinic members
- Conclusion

Engagement and Beyond

Recruitment and Retention Efforts to Diversify the Workforce

The success of residency programs depends in part on the recruitment of talented, compassionate physicians, highly qualified leaders, teaching faculty, and residents. Valuing diversity in residency programs offers a host of benefits to all members of the program. On an individual level, school or workplace diversity can result in an increased sense of well-being, decreased levels of stress, and development of genuine respect between colleagues of different backgrounds [11–13]. At the program level, a diversified workforce allows for improved training for all physicians, making them more culturally competent healthcare providers. It also allows for the potential to retain future fellows and faculty from URM groups, thereby increasing the number of physicians to care for patients who may not be used to seeing a doctor of their own ethnic background. Ethnic minority patients are more likely to experience greater satisfaction when they are cared for by a minority physician, improving the interaction and outcome for both patient and physician [14, 15]. In one study where black men were randomized to having a black or non-black physician, the patients agreed to more procedures, particularly invasive ones for preventive services when they had a black doctor. This finding is critically important as many of the diseases that allow for the gap in life expectancy between races are preventable [16]. Consequently, it behooves residency programs to actively promote the recruitment of underrepresented minorities and to sustain an equal amount of men and women in recruitment. In 2019, 36.3% of active physicians in the USA were women [17].

As competition can be intense for programs to recruit from the pool of highly qualified URM students, it is critical that leadership and teaching faculty of residency programs understand how URM and female medical students go about choosing a residency program in internal medicine. Diversity among faculty, residents, patients, and the city are all factors that positively influenced URM candidates' decision to choose a residency program. Additionally, medical students looked for a supportive academic and political environment and a feeling of being desired by the program. Women candidates also valued gender diversity, availability of family-oriented programs, and active discussion regarding potential opportunities for their partners [9]. Recruitment and retention of a diversified workforce, particularly in a resident clinic that cares for an underserved patient population with limited resources, require a solid infrastructure and supportive environment. That environment must also allow faculty members to achieve productive academic careers and to maintain a healthy work-life balance. There are the obvious direct benefits to faculty, but also trainees view the faculty as their role models. If trainees cannot see opportunities for desirable and productive careers, they will be hesitant to remain at the institution in which they train. For example, the Yale internal medicine residency program has several pathways of distinction that residents can participate in, including the Race, Bias, and Advocacy in Medicine (RBAM) pathway, which allows for education, citizenship, and a capstone project. Both the traditional track and primary care track now have associate program directors who are focused solely on DEI issues for each residency program.

One of the most important components of recruitment of URM candidates is creating a pipeline program [18]. Programs can begin as early as elementary school or high school but should have multiple points at which candidates can enter, even later in their studies. Other examples include mentoring programs for college or postbaccalaureate students. One such initiative at Yale, started by one of our URM primary care track residents, Dr. George Agyapong, is titled Service-Learning|Training and Enrichment Programs for Underrepresented Health Professionals (STEP-uHP); more information can be obtained at stepuhp.info. The stated mission of STEP-uHP is that "every aspiring healthcare professional will have social, economic, and academic capital to sustain their career dreams." This program allows undergraduates or post-bac students to work in the hospital as scribes, translators, patient advocates or navigators, or peer mentors, while being paid for these experiences and being assigned to mentors in the department. This program bridges the gap between URM and low-income students and those who have the privilege and opportunity to take unpaid volunteer experiences. It also allows for increased opportunities for students who have not been exposed to medicine earlier in their careers. AAMC data revealed that more than three-quarters of medical students came from families in the top two quintiles of family income [19]. Socioeconomic disadvantage intersects with race and ethnicity. Programs like STEP-uHP aim to avoid URM and low-income students leaving the path upstream.

Another approach the Yale School of Medicine has used is a summer research program for medical students from HBCUs and other schools that have high concentrations of URM students. The students are paired with a mentor, complete a project, and present their findings at a final meeting. This process embeds them in the community, and they are encouraged to apply to our residency programs when the time comes. Their positive experiences are also relayed back to their home institutions.

Support from the highest levels of the institution should be present. In the last few years at our institution, we have created a diversity committee; hired the first deputy dean for diversity and inclusion and first diversity officer, the first medical director of health equity, the first DEI associate chair of medicine, and the first vice chiefs of DEI for each division in the department of medicine; and instituted associate program directors for DEI in the training programs.

Goal: A Climate Conducive to Appreciation of Each Other on a Cultural and Social Level

While residents should create a network of peers and mentors who share characteristics similar to theirs, perhaps in gender or race, and these networks are critical for long-term success and retention, these efforts cannot occur in isolation. At the same time, we do not wish for residents to feel segregated, and all residents should celebrate the ways in which we are similar and different. Intersectionality also becomes an important concept to grasp, as some trainees will be battling multiple challenges related to their identity (for example, a URM resident who also belongs to the LGBTQ+ community). An atmosphere of tolerance, inquiry, and learning should be cultivated. An easy starting point for sharing one's culture is through food as eating is a universal experience. For example, regular potluck meals where people bring their favorite foods are wonderful, low-stress events to connect and learn the basics of another culture. Our primary care clinic holds regular potlucks that are attended by faculty, residents, nurses, and staff. Exposure to a varied group allows for an organic appreciation of one another's cultures, lives, and important roles in healthcare.

Our clinic creates a sense of belonging through multiple activities and structure. Each intern is assigned to a team of three residents, one attending, one nurse, and a medical assistant. The team is the home base for each resident, and it is consistent throughout residency. Clinic groups dictate which patients one care for and the colleagues one works with and often determine who one socializes with. Friendly competitions and social events highlight the team environment. On the first day of clinic orientation, at a welcome ice cream social, interns are given a shirt with their team color; they participate in a clinic scavenger hunt and also receive sign-out on the vulnerable patients for their pod. The games allow for residents to learn about the clinic while team building. It has become the norm for the residents to spontaneously arrange group outings such as dinner, salsa dancing, or indie movie night at the end of each 2-week rotation.

Definition of Community Beyond Simple Demographics

Residents should be acquainted with more than demographic information and textbook-style learning of their patients' communities for a better understanding and sense of belonging with their patients. Introductions that have been successful include neighborhood-guided tours by someone well versed in the community, such as someone who has undertaken a community resident leadership program where they have learned about the mapping of community assets (a focus on community strengths rather than on needs as developed by John Kretzmann and John McKnight) [20]. Trainees can be informed of any community distrust of the healthcare system or home institution and its rationale as well as common health-seeking behaviors and barriers to healthcare as perceived by the community. Home visit programs are another way for trainees to become embedded in the community they serve, in addition to providing much-needed healthcare. Nonprofit organizations are able to conduct community health needs assessments (CHNA) and design strategic plans to address the health needs of a community. Trainees should be introduced to these types of assessments and plans during their training. Many hospitals now have patient and family member advisory councils, and some states even mandate them by law. It is important to ensure adequate representation of all races on these panels. Trainees and faculty can also serve on these committees, which is an excellent opportunity for healthcare providers to hear directly from our patients and their caregivers about important issues that may be affecting their communities. Councils or other similar groups can provide a wonderful collaborative space for community members to inform the institution about opportunities for physicians and the healthcare system to play a constructive role within their community. Projects that have come out of such meetings include community service, social justice organization support, and social functions. In addition, residents should be encouraged to read the local newspaper, listen to community radio, and eat at local restaurants to learn what the community has to offer.

Cultural Competence Training for All Clinic Members

Intern orientation is an exciting, stressful, and promising time. As trainees struggle to retain the information that will allow them to successfully start residency, they often focus on operational and clinical aspects of their first rotation. It is important to emphasize that resident clinic is a longitudinal experience that provides a sense of stability throughout their training. For all residents, we provide a space for them to share their experiences with both implicit and explicit biases. URM, gender minorities, or LGBTQ+ residents often have more of these experiences. A common example is when a resident is mistaken for housecleaning or a multitude of other roles rather than a physician. We recommend structured biweekly or monthly meetings where trainees and faculty openly share experiences of bias that they have experienced or ways in which their patients have been affected by bias. When trainees see that faculty understand their struggles, they do not operate in isolation, and they learn tactics to combat bias and preserve personal well-being.

A large body of literature on cultural competence in healthcare addresses the physician-patient relationship. It is important to ensure that health professionals are culturally competent with a focus on interprofessional relationships. Often, education about one another is the missing ingredient to allow for tolerance. The ability to relate to and understand one another should transcend our degrees, credentials, and academic accomplishments. Cultural introductions can include what truly matters to an individual—personal values, family, and traditions. Social interactions as well as structured activities allow for this sharing. Sharing of stories is an effective way to communicate what is meaningful to an individual, a way to eliminate bias, and a means of introducing conversation that might not otherwise be comfortably broached [21, 22]. Regardless of ethnic or religious background, each of us has a culture, and cultural competence is not solely in the domain of URMs. To some degree, all interactions are intercultural regardless of ethnicity. It is important to define diversity broadly to include race, ethnicity, gender identity, sexual orientation, religion, disability, and even diversity within our country.

Cultural diversity is now at the forefront of multiple domains of life—in family units, at social functions, in the workplace, and in one's online presence. Our patients are diverse, and our workforce is diverse. Training in cultural competence is crucial to create an environment where we acknowledge our differences. The Liaison Committee on Medical Education introduced standards for cultural competence in 2000, and these have been adopted by many medical schools [23]. The AAMC has also developed the Tool for Assessing Cultural Competence Training (TACCT) and a list of resources and guidelines to teach cultural competence [24].

Over the last few years, academic institutions have evolved from small diversity, equity, and inclusion committees to system-wide initiatives and committing to DEI as organization missions. When considering such large-scale goals, leadership is key. One group offered three recommendations for healthcare leaders and their boards: (1) recognize that diversity is necessary but will not, alone, create a just and inclusive culture; (2) be aware that every leader is at risk for blind spots; and (3) appreciate that concepts of leadership and stereotypical traits of leaders among existing leaders may limit efforts for cultural inclusiveness and operational success [25]. We posit that additions to these recommendations should include that leadership needs to articulate a clear message to faculty, trainees, and staff that diversity, equity, and inclusion are now critical to the mission and will be followed in the same way that clinical competence, citizenship, and professionalism are. Stakeholders at all levels need to be visibly engaged in DEI work to all, including department chairs, designated institutional officials, diversity officer, training program directors, clinic directors, faculty, trainees, students, and staff.

Conclusion

The reckoning of the last few years has provided a watershed moment that can be a great impetus for change in academic medicine, for both our trainees and our patients. Given the cultural discordance between faculty, residents, patients, and communities served in resident clinic, it is crucial to create a culture of inclusive diversity that makes everyone feel welcome and promotes a sense of belonging and academic success that is attractive to applicants. It is important to acknowledge the challenges of resident clinic, including poor continuity of care, disenfranchised patient populations, and limited access to resources. Acquainting oneself with the communities one serves allows for alleviation of some of these challenges by instilling compassionate understanding of community needs and a prioritized approach to addressing those needs. Ongoing training in cultural competence can potentially help to decrease misunderstandings and bias. In addition, support from the highest levels of the institution will ensure that all of this is possible. Whether an individual belongs to leadership, faculty, trainees, or staff, we all have room to learn more, to improve our practices to nurture a culture of diversity and inclusion, and to continue to work on this critical topic even when mistakes are made. The current energy and momentum surrounding DEI work must not be lost as we bring new generations of trainees through our clinics.

References

1. aamc.org/what-we-do/equity-diversity-inclusion/underrepresented-in-medicine. Underrepresented in Medicine Definition | AAMC. Accessed 1 May 2022.
2. U.S. Census Bureau Quick Facts. https://www.census.gov/quickfacts/fact/table/US/PST045221. Accessed 01 May 2022.
3. https://www.aamc.org/data-reports/workforce/interactive-data/figure-15-percentage-full-time-us-medical-school-faculty-race/ethnicity-2018. Accessed 01 May 2022.
4. https://www.aamc.org/data-reports/workforce/interactive-data/figure-6-percentage-acceptees-us-medical-schools-race/ethnicity-alone-academic-year-2018-2019. Accessed 01 May 2022.
5. Yancy WS Jr, Macpherson DS, Hanusa BH, et al. Patient satisfaction in resident and attending ambulatory care clinics. J Gen Intern Med. 2001;16(11):755–62. https://doi.org/10.1111/j.1525-1497.2001.91005.x.
6. Osseo-Asare A, Balasuriya L, Huot SJ, Keene D, Berg D, Nunez-Smith M, Genao I, Latimore D, Boatright D. Minority resident Physicians' views on the role of race/ethnicity in their training experiences in the workplace. JAMA Netw Open. 2018;1(5):e182723. https://doi.org/10.1001/jamanetworkopen.2018.2723. PMID: 30646179; PMCID: PMC6324489.
7. Liebschutz JM, Darko GO, Finley EP, Cawse JM, Bharel M, Orlander JD. In the minority: black physicians in residency and their experiences. J Natl Med Assoc. 2006;98(9):1441–8. PMID: 17019911; PMCID: PMC2569716
8. Nunez-Smith M, Pilgrim N, Wynia M, Desai MM, Jones BA, Bright C, Krumholz HM, Bradley EH. Race/ethnicity and workplace discrimination: results of a national survey of physicians. J Gen Intern Med. 2009;24(11):1198–204. https://doi.org/10.1007/s11606-009-1103-9. Epub 2009 Sep 1. PMID: 19727966; PMCID: PMC2771235.

9. Aagaard EM, Julian K, Dedier J, Soloman I, Tillisch J, Pérez-Stable EJ. Factors affecting medical students' selection of an internal medicine residency program. J Natl Med Assoc. 2005;97(9):1264–70. PMID: 16296217; PMCID: PMC2594785.
10. Cook A, Glass C. Diversity begets diversity? The effects of board composition on the appointment and success of women CEOs. Soc Sci Res. 2015;53:137–47. https://doi.org/10.1016/j.ssresearch.2015.05.009. Epub 2015 May 27.
11. Whitla DK, Orfield G, Silen W, Teperow C, Howard C, Reede J. Educational benefits of diversity in medical school: a survey of students. Acad Med. 2003;78(5):460–6. https://doi.org/10.1097/00001888-200305000-00007.
12. Powell C, Yemane L, Brooks M, Johnson C, Alvarez A, Bandstra B, Caceres W, Dierickx Q, Thomas R, Blankenburg R. Outcomes from a novel graduate medical education leadership program in advancing diversity, equity, and inclusion. J Grad Med Educ. 2021;13(6):774–84. https://doi.org/10.4300/JGME-D-21-00235.1. Epub 2021 Dec 14. PMID: 35070089; PMCID: PMC8672828.
13. O'Brien KR, Scheffer M, van Nes EH, van der Lee R. How to break the cycle of low workforce diversity: a model for change. PLoS One. 2015;10(7):e0133208. https://doi.org/10.1371/journal.pone.0133208. PMID: 26217957; PMCID: PMC4517751.
14. Hopkins TJ. Patients are more satisfied with care from doctors of same race. BMJ. 2002;325(7372):1057. PMCID: PMC1124573.
15. Takeshita J, Wang S, Loren AW, Mitra N, Shults J, Shin DB, Sawinski DL. Association of racial/ethnic and gender concordance between patients and physicians with patient experience ratings. JAMA Netw Open. 2020;3(11):e2024583. https://doi.org/10.1001/jamanetworkopen.2020.24583. PMID: 33165609; PMCID: PMC7653497.
16. Alsan M, Garrick O, Graziani GC. Does diversity matter for health? experimental evidence from Oakland, national bureau of economic research. https://www.nber.org/system/files/working_papers/w24787/w24787.pdf. Accessed 5 Jan 2022.
17. https://www.aamc.org/data-reports/workforce/interactive-data/active-physicians-sex-and-specialty-2019. Accessed 1 May 2022.
18. Crews DC, Wilson KL, Sohn J, Kabacoff CM, Poynton SL, Murphy LR, Bolz J, Wolfe A, White PT, Will C, Collins C, Gauda E, Robinson DN. Helping scholars overcome socioeconomic barriers to medical and biomedical careers: creating a pipeline initiative. Teach Learn Med. 2020;32(4):422–33. https://doi.org/10.1080/10401334.2020.1729161. Epub 2020 Feb 25.
19. An Updated Look at the Economic Diversity of U.S. Medical Students. https://www.aamc.org/media/9596/download. Accessed 1 May 2022.
20. Kretzmann JP, McKnight JL. Building communities from the inside out: a path towards finding and mobilizing a community's assets. Chicago: ACTA Publications; 1993.
21. Long A, Jennings J, Bademosi K, Chandran A, Sawyer S, Schumacher C, Greenbaum A, Fields EL. Storytelling to improve healthcare worker understanding, beliefs, and practices related to LGBTQ+ patients: a program evaluation. Eval Program Plann. 2022;90:101979. https://doi.org/10.1016/j.evalprogplan.2021.101979. Epub 2021 Jul 8.
22. Pallai E, Tran K. Narrative health: using story to explore definitions of health and address bias in health care. Perm J. 2019;23:18–052. https://doi.org/10.7812/TPP/18-052. PMID: 30939266; PMCID: PMC6380479.
23. Association of American Medical Colleges. Cultural competence education. https://www.aamc.org/download/54338/data/culturalcomped.pdf. Accessed 1 May 2022.
24. Tool for Assessing Cultural Competence Training (TACCT) Resource Guide. https://www.aamc.org/linkableblob/54328-2/data/tacctresourceguide.pdf-data.pdf. Accessed 1 May 2022.
25. Lee TH, Volpp KG, Cheung VG, Dzau VJ. Diversity and inclusiveness in health care leadership: three key steps. N Engl J Med. 2(3). https://doi.org/10.1056/CAT.21.0166. Accessed 1 May 2022.

Chapter 24
Healthcare Advocacy and Social Justice

Tracey L. Henry, Amber-Nicole Bird, and Sarah Candler

Introduction

In this chapter, we will review the role of Social Justice and Advocacy in academic outpatient primary care practices. For the purposes of our discussion, Social Justice is the equitable distribution of wealth, opportunities, and privileges in a society. Advocacy is the action of speaking up on behalf of a person or specific change in status quo; it can be done informally with colleagues or formally with administrators, lawmakers, or other developers of policy and regulation.

Outline
- Background and definitions
- Social justice
- Advocacy in practice
- Successful initiatives in advocacy and social justice: a review of examples of successful advocacy and social justice efforts
- Conclusion

T. L. Henry (✉)
Emory University School of Medicine, Atlanta, GA, USA
e-mail: tlhenry@emory.edu

A.-N. Bird
University of Pennsylvania, Philadelphia, PA, USA
e-mail: amber-nicole.bird@pennmedicine.upenn.edu

S. Candler
Houston, TX, USA

L. B. Lu et al. (eds.), *Leading an Academic Medical Practice*,
https://doi.org/10.1007/978-3-031-40273-9_24

Background and Definitions

Health care in the United States is in the throes of shifts in payment structures, training requirements, documentation tools, team member roles, federal and state regulations, all while the foundations of medical knowledge and technology continue to grow exponentially. These changes affect physicians at all levels of training and practice, and not always for the better. While engagement in advocacy at the individual patient level has been a cornerstone of the medical profession, an increasing number of training programs and professional societies now recognize the importance of the physician voice in broader discussions of policymaking, regulatory guidance, clinical guidelines, and even development of technology and health system structures. The goal of teaching advocacy and social justice is to ensure equitable opportunities to attain health for all patients as well as equitable learning opportunities for future physicians of all backgrounds and identities. For the purposes of our discussion, social justice is the equitable distribution of wealth, opportunities, and privileges in a society. Health advocacy is "activities related to ensuring access to care, navigating the system, mobilizing resources, addressing health inequities, influencing health policy, and creating system change" [1]. We will use Robert W Johnson Foundation (RWJF) report definition of health equity: "that everyone has a fair and just opportunity to be as healthy as possible. This requires removing obstacles to health such as poverty, discrimination, and their consequences, including powerlessness and lack of access to good jobs with fair pay, quality education and housing, safe environments, and health care" [2]. In contrast, RWJF notes that equality—equal access to resources and efforts—is NOT the same thing because some people require *more* or different resources and efforts to attain equal *opportunities* that would lead to equitable experiences [2]. The same report notes that health disparities (also known as health inequalities) are "plausibly avoidable, systematic health differences adversely affecting economically or socially disadvantaged groups" [2]. Advocacy can be done informally with colleagues or formally with administrators, lawmakers, or other developers of policy and regulation.

There is an increasing recognition of disparities in health outcomes as well as disparities in social drivers of health, which are described in detail in Chap. 21. Here, we will discuss the approach to **addressing those disparities through advocacy in order to achieve a more *just* distribution of resources**. Disparities range from *lack of access to care* due to transportation insecurity, rural geography, or limited access to technology, tools, and services to *inequities in treatment* due to bias, discrimination, and specifically racism in society and medical research. Please see Table 24.1 to review definitions for key terminology for this chapter.

Rather than a hobby or interest of certain physicians, **advocacy is recognized as a mandatory skill that residents are expected to acquire.** In the ACGME Milestones 2.0, where advocacy is often described as an element of "systems-based practice," residents are expected to learn how to navigate the systems ranging from physical clinic spaces to team-based communication therein, but also the payment

Table 24.1 Key definitions

Terminology	
Advocacy	Activities related to ensuring access to care, navigating the system, mobilizing resources, addressing health inequities, influencing health policy, and creating system change
Equity	Fair and just opportunity to be as healthy as possible. This requires removing obstacles to health such as poverty, discrimination, and their consequences, including powerlessness and lack of access to good jobs with fair pay, quality education and housing, safe environments, and healthcare
Equality	Equal access to efforts and resources
Justice	Distribution of wealth, opportunities, and privileges within a society
Health disparities	Systematic health differences adversely affecting economically or socially disadvantaged groups

structures; local, state, and national policies; and even social structures and influences on someone's ability to attain and maintain health.

While advocacy has a longer history of support within clinical education, increasingly social justice is deemed a critical requirement of a well-rounded education. ACGME requires that "Residents must learn to advocate for patients within the health care system" (IV, B, 1, f, (2)). Relatedly, professional organizations like the Society of General Internal Medicine, the *American College of Physicians*, and the American Medical Association dedicate significant resources to members' advocacy to implement their policies. These organizations are increasingly intentional about the impact of unjust distribution of resources and the impact of bias in the medical field.

While not all training programs will have a public health focus, increasingly primary care incorporates tools and metrics based on population health. In this lens, it is imperative that trainees in primary care understand how to recognize disparities and advocate for the just distribution of resources to attain equity in health and healthcare. **In order to address and correct disparities, trainees must be equipped with the skills not only to recognize them, but also to identify the most apt audience for their advocacy.**

In the rest of this chapter, we will define the framework for identifying issues of social justice and provide actionable examples of times, places, and methods to advocate for change.

Case: 68-Year-old woman presents to her primary care physician for diabetes care management and is found to have a hemoglobin A1C of 11.3% up from 8.5% 6 months ago. She is 10 min late and has missed her last two appointments. She shares that she was recently laid off and lost her employer-sponsored health insurance, requiring her to find other coverage after a period of being uninsured. She also lost her transportation and has been unable to afford her insulin. She had been offered a virtual visit and declined due to having minimal data available on her device. Prior to today's visit, the clinic reviewed quality metrics and has set a goal of 85% of all patients with diabetes to have a goal hemoglobin A1C of <7.5%. The primary care physician has 20 min to establish a plan to help this patient reach her goal hemoglobin A1C.

Throughout the chapter, consider the following questions:

1. What *health inequities* does this patient face?
2. What *health disparities* (also known as health inequalities) does she suffer from?
3. How does the system within which the primary care physician works affect this patient adversely, and how could the physician *advocate* for a more *just* system for delivering care?

Social Justice

Social justice, the distribution of wealth, opportunities, and privileges within a society, has history rooted in ethics and law. It consists of four interwoven principles—promoting equal access, removing barriers to participation, protecting individual rights, and promoting equity [3, 4]. More recently, the application of social justice in healthcare has been highlighted in fields like primary care where inequities in access to healthcare, quality of care delivered, and access to finite resources within medicine are routinely encountered [5].

Bioethicists Ruth Faden and Madison Powers developed a social justice theory that states that social injustices arise because of preventable differences in health within a population [6]. In other words, social injustices are seen in what we commonly call health and healthcare inequities and poor health outcomes that arise due to social determinants of health. The social justice theory does not disregard biomedical drivers of poor health, but instead pushes healthcare systems to acknowledge that focusing only on biomedical drivers of health outcomes will never fully address health disparities. This concept is represented in the image below presented in a National Academy of Medicine report on social determinants that emphasized that variation in health outcomes could not be explained by biomedical drivers of health alone and calls for investment in interventions to address the social determinants of health. See Fig. 24.1.

As early as 1999, there have been calls for physicians to engage in social justice as a matter of professional responsibility. A charter put forth by the European Federation of Internal Medicine, the American College of Physicians-American Society of Internal Medicine (ACP-ASIM)—Foundation, and the American Board of Internal Medicine (ABIM) Foundation entitled the "Medical Professionalism Project" argued that the core component of patient care no longer could be defined in the office of the medical professional, but instead existed in the places where "people live their lives, in the home and workplace … the daily choices that determine their health" [7]. To engage in the promotion of health, healthcare workers must focus on social justice, or the fair distribution of healthcare resources, for their communities. Further, the principle of social justice tasks healthcare workers with the active elimination of discrimination within places where care is delivered. The concept of social justice as a professional duty extends into core missions in primary care including the equitable distribution of finite resources, including access to care, and improving the overall quality of care [5, 7].

To understand the role of social justice in the academic primary care practice, it is important to adopt a shared understanding of disparities, equality, and health equity.

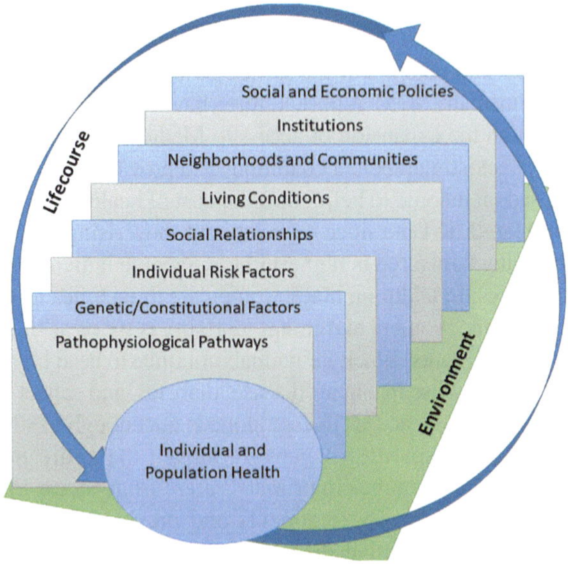

Fig. 24.1 Smedley B. Promoting Health: Intervention Strategies from Social and Behavioral Research. Washington (DC): National Academy Press; 2000

The Healthy People 2020 initiative set forth the goals of eliminating health disparities—health differences linked to social, economic, and/or environmental disadvantage—and achieving health equity—"the attainment of the highest level of health for all people" [8]. Equality aims to provide the same resources to all people to allow them to obtain healthy lives. Equality is founded on the principle of justice but does not account for the fact that all people do not start at the same level of health [9]. Each individual starts at a different level of health, and the resources needed for one individual to attain the highest level of health may be different from another. Equity requires healthcare workers to understand the specific needs of the individual and work to provide the resources they need to obtain healthy lives. It is important to acknowledge that health and healthcare disparities are not only present in populations defined by race or ethnicity. Instead, disparities occur across various dimensions including sexual identity and orientation, disability status, gender, age, socioeconomic status, and citizenship status. Further, disparities can exist within subpopulations including disparities between Asian patients with different primary languages.

In primary care, it is important to understand the impacts of unequal access to care and disparities in quality of care on health outcomes. There is a well-defined inverse relationship between socioeconomic status and disease burden. Individuals with higher socioeconomic status have higher rates of health insurance and longer life expectancy [10]. Individuals with lower socioeconomic status are less likely to be insured, are less likely to utilize primary and preventive care, and experience a higher burden of disease [10]. In 2003, the Institute of Medicine (IOM) report "Unequal Treatment: Confronting Racial and Ethnic Disparities in Healthcare" reviewed existing disparities research that highlighted racial disparities in both access and quality of care [11]. Black and Hispanic patients were found to be offered fewer cardiac procedures, were referred less, waited longer for renal transplant, and had worse diabetes and cancer outcomes. It was also one of the first major publications to highlight the role of bias within populations that had equal access to care. Black and Hispanic patients in the United States had worse health outcomes than white patients of the same age and socioeconomic status.

Since the IOM report, efforts have been made to expand access to healthcare through the expansion of access to Medicaid insurance, disallowing coverage denials for preexisting medical conditions and providing an advanceable, refundable tax credit based on income to help offset the cost of health insurance for low-income individuals and families. Data since its enactment show rising rates of health coverage, but the risk of being uninsured is highest in low-income individuals and black and Hispanic communities. In addition, black women are three times more likely to die from pregnancy than white women, and infant mortality is twice as high in black infants as compared to white infants. Black individuals continue to be at higher risk for poor outcomes from chronic disease like heart disease, diabetes, and cancer than white patients, suggesting that expanding access to care alone is not enough to address health disparities [12].

Health disparities negatively impact the entire medical community. There are often finite resources in primary care—from access to healthcare workers as well as access to necessary treatments and preventative interventions—and an increased burden of preventive disease taxes this system more. A report completed by the W.K. Kellogg Foundation in 2018 estimated that improving the health of the nation by eliminating racial disparities in health would lead to an economic gain of $135 billion per year partially achieved by removing $93 billion in excess costs of care [13]. This type of economic growth would provide an opportunity to shift resources away from the treatment of existing disease toward the assurance that all individuals have access to healthcare and preventive medicine.

It is clear that addressing preventable differences in health outcomes, the social injustices, sits firmly in the responsibility of the primary care clinic. To make this feasible within the already strained academic primary care practice requires a strong investment in population health management and practice improvement. Population health management shifts the focus from the individual patient to the health of the entire primary care population. It creates a systematic approach for ensuring that all members of a primary care population receive the appropriate preventive and chronic care [14]. Through the use of standardized metric review, for example hemoglobin A1C screening in patients with known diabetes mellitus or completed mammography in women of screening age for breast cancer, primary care practices can obtain a holistic view on the quality of care that is being delivered.

Practice improvement involves applying the tools of quality improvement to poor health outcomes within a population [15]. In the academic primary care practice, this involves not only access to timely and accurate metrics for chronic and preventive care but also information on how quality outcomes vary by socioeconomic status, race, ethnicity, or gender. To truly take a social justice lens, academic primary care practices must analyze disparities in the care that is being provided and then work within the healthcare team to increase resources to improve care to those patient populations that are experiencing worse outcomes.

Social Justice Through Population Health: A Case Review

When reviewing colorectal cancer screening outcomes within your practice, you note no overall disparity in screening rates between patient populations defined by race.

However, on closer metric review, you note that your residency practice has a 15% lower rate of colorectal cancer screening and cares for the majority of patients with Medicaid insurance within your practice.

When developing a practice improvement intervention to address disparities in colorectal cancer screening, the just response would be to leverage existing resources to promote increased screening in the resident panel.

Subsequent data review should prioritize not only a review of overall screening rates, but also a review of disparity-based data.

In this case, you should look for rates of screening based on primary insurance, PCP type, and sociodemographic markers. This allows for conscious reflection on the equitable delivery of care within your practice population. Setting standards for review of current disparities in care at the onset of developing your practice improvement interventions will allow the development of obtainable equity metrics alongside more traditional quality metrics.

Advocacy in Practice

A Review of the Levels of Advocacy

Now that we know what advocacy is, our role as clinicians, and how social justice nestles within our sphere of influence, what does advocacy look like in practice? In describing advocacy and our roles, there are multiple ways of categorizing our efforts. In this chapter, we will discuss advocacy using the socioecological model. See Fig. 24.2.

The socioecological model takes into account our role as advocates at all levels within our spheres of influence. It clearly illustrates where we have a role in advocacy as individuals, interpersonally, within our communities and institutions and finally even on the national or legislative levels.

Individual Advocacy

When we speak of individual advocacy, this is the work we do for our patients consistently if not daily depending on your practice demographics. This is where the majority of us will concentrate our efforts and make the most difference for our

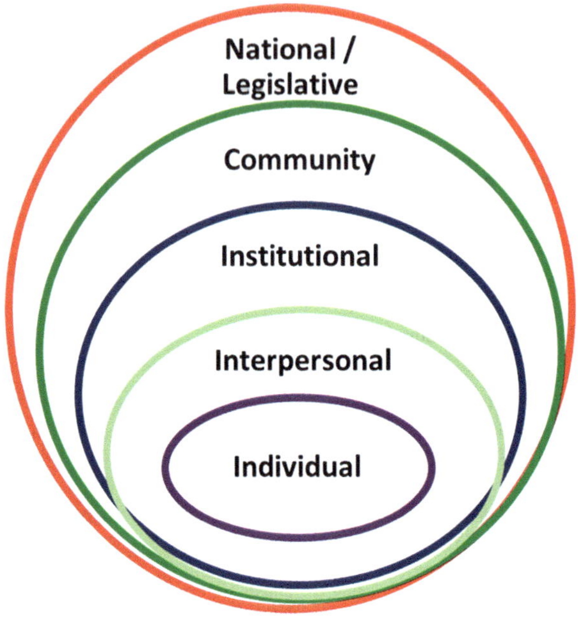

Fig. 24.2 Advocacy categorized via socioecological model adaptation [16]

patients. At the individual level, a clinician or healthcare worker can improve the health and healthcare of our patients, *one* patient at a time. For example, this is where a clinician or healthcare worker can identify your patients' unmet social needs as sometimes unintentionally elucidated by patients but also required by some practices during the social determinants of health screening. However, you can take it a step further. Clinicians can accomplish this goal by physically assisting the patient with their paperwork for free or reduced public transportation, or disability decal when the clinic's social workers are already overbooked, thereby preventing the patient from having to return at a later date, miss further work, juggle to find child care, and pay another co-pay or even another transportation fee that all of which is a strain on the patient's pocket. At the individual level, we can close the loop on prior referrals to social work, connect patients to food banks, and, if English is not their first language, make sure that the summary of the clinic visit and any other medical instructions are written in their language of literacy. If a patient possesses low written literacy, provide instructions in a way that the person can understand and have a chance to adhere to. Other impactful examples include filling out paperwork for patients at a time of the visit and/or mailing the documents to them to save them a trip back to the clinic. The examples are endless. However, what is unique to the individual level of advocacy is that it is all up to us to decide when, what, where, and how we advocate for patients in the clinic, at the bedside, or even beyond as a house call or through mobile integrated care or street outreach. Clinic directors can support their clinicians by providing education on how to be an advocate for your patients, available clinic, and community resources for patients, including working with information technology to incorporate these resources within the EHR and a part of clinic workflow.

Interpersonal Advocacy

The interpersonal level is the next level in our advocacy framework and is the first in the series where our efforts are somewhat dependent on another person. At this level, we have power to speak out against the injustices or biases we see in healthcare interpersonally directly with another person, for example, a professional colleague or even a patient. Efforts at this level center on awareness, knowledge, and empowerment of the individual to seek to mitigate bias or injustice interpersonally. To achieve interpersonal advocacy, scripts or prepared practice language akin to illness scripts are key. As interpersonal advocacy especially in the workplace can be challenging depending on the subject matter such as workplace violence or microaggressions, bias, or racism, you are more likely to speak up in these occurrences if you have prior awareness, practice, or training to address them. See Table 24.2.

Institutional—From an institutional standpoint, this is where our advocacy efforts benefit more than the individual patients that we see in the clinic or the faculty, staff, or other health professional colleagues we encounter interpersonally. At the institutional level, we have the opportunity to, for instance, dismantle systemic racism, as it relates to your institutional practices. Advocacy initiatives at the institutional level can be aimed at benefiting not only patients but also faculty, staff, learners, and other healthcare workers. Examples of these advocacy initiatives include developing equitable hiring and promotion practices, employee professional development programs, and expanding clinical services such as behavioral health and HIV PrEP. At this advocacy level and beyond is also where you need to conduct an analysis of relevant parties. It is imperative to know who is on your side and supports your advocacy initiative, who your opponents are, and whom you should invite to collaborate with you for synergistic efforts. Gaining buy-in and having a strategy for your initiative are essential. In the end, the key is identifying and working toward eliminating institutional practices that perpetuate injustice in healthcare.

Table 24.2 Sample script for responding to racism [17]

When we see or hear racism, call it out:
Seek clarity: "Tell me more about __________."
Offer an alternative perspective: "Have you ever considered __________."
Speak your truth: "I don't see it the way you do. I see it as __________."
Find common ground: "We don't agree on __________ but we can agree on __________."
Give yourself the time and space you need: "Could we revisit the conversation about __________ tomorrow."
Set boundaries. "Please do not say __________ again to me or around me."

Community

At the community level is where academic practices can leverage their existing relationships with community partners and, if nonexistent, begin to develop these partnerships. One example would be bidirectional referrals to address your patient's unmet social needs. As we refer our patients to community resources, food banks, ride share for transportation, and literacy and/or job placement programs, these same programs should also possess the ability to refer patients to establish care in our primary care clinics. Community engagement and advocacy have the distinctive approach of being grass roots in nature, but with the perspective of the individuals, institutions, and community they serve. Real impact at this level of advocacy can be made through cross-sector collaborations with community members, which promote open dialogue, transparency, and trust. By academic centers cultivating community relationships, they are able to identify gaps and develop strategies to address issues in your communities. Academic centers are able to decide based on the gap analysis and the allocation of resources for its center and community. Successful community engagement by academic centers has been initiated using advocacy tools such as town halls broadcasted via social media platforms for topics on COVID-19 vaccine hesitancy [18].

National/Legislative Advocacy

The national or legislative level is what most health professionals think of when they think of advocacy and are often intimidated by the concept of being an advocate. However, as we demonstrated this far, advocacy takes place in many forms on many different levels. At this level, we can advocate for legislative policies at the local city or county governments or even federal government for more resources; better payment policies, for instance, reimbursement for cognitive services; national strategies to address the social determinants; and more research on preventative practices for chronic disease management and investment in the primary care workforce shortage or to expand the number of medical residency slots. Again, at this level, buy-in is required. Further, conducting a relevant party and/or gap analysis of the problem and proposed solutions is needed. It is necessary to determine who is already addressing the identified gap or problem you are attempting to address and consider collaborating for synergistic efforts. Being nonprofit, academic medical centers themselves can advocate or lobby for their organizations. However, ensure that you are aware of the guidelines and/or limits to your lobbying. For example, "a 501(c)(3) organization may engage in some lobbying, but too much lobbying activity risks loss of tax-exempt status" [19]. Many larger practices hire a full/part-time lobbyist or governmental affairs person to advocate on behalf of the organization on a regular basis. The medical director's role is to liaise with the governmental affairs representative via regular meetings to align clinic needs with the clinic/

organization's legislative priorities both on a federal and state/local level. It is important for the medical director to be aware of when your state's legislators are in session.

Successful Initiatives in Advocacy and Social Justice: A Review of Examples of Successful Advocacy and Social Justice Efforts

Implementing a New Clinic Protocol and Workflow

As a new junior faculty member in a hospital-based primary care clinic, Dr. HJ noticed anecdotally that some of her patients, additionally, complained of depressive symptoms and wondered why there was no universal depression screening in their clinic [20]. Dr. HJ approached her medical director and was informed that it was a priority but often not completed in the primary care visit because of time constraints, competing demands, and lack of resources if the depression was positive. Since Dr. HJ's was in a faculty development for new faculty that required a QI project, she decided that implementing universal depression screening in her clinic was the perfect project. Initially met with resistance, Dr. HJ invited key stakeholders such as the medical director to join her team. Initially, no one wanted to work on the depression screening team because even though they saw the value, the perception was that it would be too difficult given the current cultural climate and other competing medical demands such as hypertension and diabetes. Given that health costs nearly double or triple for patients with untreated comorbid depression and the prevalence of depression in our population is nearly 40% and PTSD nearly two-thirds of the population, Dr. HJ was steadfast in her belief that addressing mental health disparities was key to improving the health outcomes and functionality of our patients. In the end, it became one of the three quality initiatives chosen that year. Dr. HJ identified her interested parties, which were many: hospital and clinic leadership; behavioral health department who would manage patients with behavioral health issues beyond the scope of primary care and help us develop appropriate depression screening protocols for our clinic based upon resources; nursing and CMA staff who would be administered the PHQ2 screen and the faculty and residents who will be completing the screening, managing the anxiety and depression in the clinic setting; and residency leadership who worked to deliver the faculty development and residency education about depression screening, brief intervention, and referral when needed.

Dr. HJ sparked the interests of their hospital and clinic leadership and all other stakeholders involved including healthcare providers, medical staff, nurses, mental health specialists, and most importantly our patients and community. Dr. HJ and their team met monthly to advance this initiative. Concretely after implementing the first stage of the depression screening project, our depression screening went from only 20% of patients being screened for depression to over 70% within 6 months and to 95% a few months later. Identifying those patients living and suffering with depression and connecting them to treatment equated to less hospitalizations and improvement in their health outcomes, for instance, in our diabetic patients with comorbid depression. A baseline survey of the clinic providers indicated that providers had many barriers to depression screening, including lack of time, staff, and referral resources. We have addressed many of these issues by providing resources and education to both medical staff and providers. Also, garnering widespread interdisciplinary support and leveraging technology played a substantial role in the ongoing success of this advocacy initiative and have led to its sustainability several years later.

In embarking on advocacy initiatives, especially in academic medical centers, you need top-down buy-in from hospital and/or clinic leadership for approval of system-wide changes like in the depression screening case and you need bottom-up buy-in from the office staff, nursing, physician, faculty, and other healthcare providers for cultural change and sustainability.

Implementing A New Clinic Initiative

Dr. S, a primary care physician in a busy urban academic medical center, was appalled by the number of patients who presented to the clinic with food insecurity. Dr. S wrote a proposal and partnered with a local fruit and vegetable prescription program (FVRx) for his clinic patients suffering from food insecurity. Initial qualitative interviews highlight the many factors that affect food choice and dietary habits, including social and environmental [21]. However, eventually, Dr. S and their team observed the improvement in patient show rates, hemoglobin A1C, and sense of wellness, which led to the clinic investing in a broader food as medicine program that not only supplied fresh fruits and vegetables but also demonstrated how to prepare the food maintaining nutritional value and portion size along with motivational interviewing.

Conclusion

As you can see from the above advocacy examples that took place in the academic medical center setting, they were all successful because the initiatives began with a need, passion, and a sincere desire to improve upon the status quo. Advocacy ultimately requires the ability to identify a problem, perform an analysis of relevant parties (Who are the key players? Which area of need will they address? During which stage are they required?), form strategic partnerships (at each stage of your initiative), and determine which advocacy tool you would use from your tool kit to advance change for your advocacy issue. Finally, create a SMART goal with expected outcomes from your advocacy initiative, describing how you will measure them and when is paramount. Then follow up to review your efforts and to evaluate if your efforts were successful. If not successful, what changes would you make next time? After reviewing your initial needs and your stakeholders', was your ask an overreach? Was the timing right?

In either of the cases, the physician advocate did not have special training, but a commitment to improve the health and wellness of their patients and advance our profession. In general, most advocacy training opportunities are offered through organized medical groups like the Society of General Internal Medicine (SGIM), the American College of Physicians (ACP), or even the American Medical Association (AMA). Given that advocacy training is not yet required for internal medicine training programs although the advocacy skill set itself is an aspirational milestone, we have to be deliberate in offering such training in our medical centers. Intentionally, medical directors can offer monies for CME for training and encourage your clinicians to attend the annual leadership and/or advocacy days offered by SGIM and ACP. These are brief effective learning opportunities to network with colleagues across the country and learn about key advocacy priorities for our patients and profession and mostly importantly how to advocate, culminating in legislative visits with your legislators. Medical directors can even model national advocacy efforts at the local level and invite their legislators to their local clinics for a tour and discussion on the pressing issues for your community and clinic.

References

1. Braveman P, Arkin E, Orleans T, Proctor D, Plough A. What is health equity? And what difference does a definition make? vol. 4. Princeton NJ: Robert Wood Johnson Foundation; 2017. p. 1.
2. Hubinette M, Dobson S, Scott I, Sherbino J. Health advocacy. Med Teach. 2017;39(2):128–35. https://doi.org/10.1080/0142159X.2017.1245853. Epub 2016 Nov 21.
3. Bell LA. Theoretical foundation for social justice education. In: Adams M, Bell LA, Griffin P, editors. Teaching for diversity and social justice. 2nd ed. New York: Routledge; 2007. p. 1–14.
4. ABIM Foundation; ACP-ASIM Foundation. European Federation of Internal Medicine. Medical professionalism in the new millennium: a physician charter. Ann Intern Med. 2002;136(3):243–6. https://doi.org/10.7326/0003-4819-136-3-200202050-00012.
5. Hage SM, Kenny ME. Promoting a social justice approach to prevention: future directions for training, practice, and research. J Prim Prev. 2009;30:75–87. https://doi.org/10.1007/s10935-008-0165-5.
6. Silva D. Powers and Faden's concept of self-determination and what it means to 'Achieve' Well-being in their theory of social justice. Public Health Ethics. 2013;6(1):35–44. https://doi.org/10.1093/phe/pht003.
7. Medical professionalism in the new millennium. A physicians' charter. Lancet. 2002;359(930):520–2. https://doi.org/10.1016/S0140-6736(02)07684-5.
8. Institute of Medicine (US) Committee on leading health indicators for healthy people 2020. Leading health indicators for healthy people 2020: letter report. Washington (DC): National Academies Press; 2011.

9. Braveman PA, Kumanyika S, Fielding J, Laveist T, Borrell LN, Manderscheid R, Troutman A. Health disparities and health equity: the issue is justice. Am J Public Health. 2011;101(Suppl 1):S149–55. https://doi.org/10.2105/AJPH.2010.300062.
10. Singh GK, Daus GP, Allender M, Ramey CT, Martin EK, Perry C, Reyes AAL, Vedamuthu IP. Social determinants of health in the United States: addressing major health inequality trends for the nation, 1935–2016. Int J MCH AIDS. 2017;6(2):139–64. https://doi.org/10.21106/ijma.236.
11. Institute of Medicine (US) Committee on understanding and eliminating racial and ethnic disparities in health care. In: Smedley BD, Stith AY, Nelson AR, editors. Unequal treatment: confronting racial and ethnic disparities in health care. Washington (DC): National Academies Press; 2003.
12. MacDorman MF, Thoma M, Declcerq E, Howell EA. racial and ethnic disparities in maternal mortality in the United States using enhanced vital records, 2016–2017. Am J Public Health. 2021;111:1673–81. https://doi.org/10.2105/AJPH.2021.306375.
13. Turner, Ani. The business case for racial equity: a strategy for growth. WK Kellogg Foundation. 2018; 590(1). https://altarum.org/RacialEquity2018
14. Clarke JL, Bourn S, Skoufalos A, Beck EH, Castillo DJ. An innovative approach to health care delivery for patients with chronic conditions. Popul Health Manag. 2017;20(1):23–30. https://doi.org/10.1089/pop.2016.0076.
15. Practice Improvement. Agency for healthcare research and quality. 2021. https://www.ahrq.gov/practiceimprovement/index.html
16. Bronfenbrenner U. The ecology of human development: Experiments by nature and design. Cambridge: Harvard University Press; 1979.
17. National Museum of African American History and Culture. Talking about race. https://nmaahc.si.edu/learn/talking-about-race. Accessed 22 Jul 2021.
18. Dada D, Djiometio JN, McFadden SM, Demeke J, Vlahov D, Wilton L, Wang M, Nelson LE. Strategies that promote equity in COVID-19 vaccine uptake for black communities: a review. J Urban Health. 2022;99(1):15–27. https://doi.org/10.1007/s11524-021-00594-3.
19. IRS. Lobbying. https://www.irs.gov/charities-non-profits/lobbying. Accessed 8 August 2022.
20. Henry TL, Schmidt S, Lund MB, Haynes T, Ford D, Egwuogu H, Schmitz S, McGregor B, Toomer L, Bussey-Jones J. Improving depression screening in underserved populations in a large urban academic primary care center: a provider-centered analysis and approach. Am J Med Qual. 2020;35(4):315–22. https://doi.org/10.1177/1062860619884639.
21. Cahill E, Schmidt SR, Henry TL, Kumar G, Berney S, Bussey-Jones J, Girard AW. Qualitative research study on addressing barriers to healthy diet among low-income individuals at an urban, safety-net hospital. BMJ Nutr Prev Health. 2020;3(2):383–6. https://doi.org/10.1136/bmjnph-2020-000064.

Part VIII
Population Health, Quality Improvement and Patient Safety

Chapter 25
Population Health Management for Residents

Robert J. Fortuna and Halle G. Sobel

Introduction

Health care expenditures in the United States far exceed any other country in the world, yet the United States lags behind other countries in many quality measures. This has led to the recognition that addressing the health of populations is necessary to improve overall healthcare quality while containing costs. The Institutes for Health Improvement (IHI) has identified improving the health of populations as one of the core elements of the "triple aim" for improving the US health care system [1, 2]. The Accreditation Council for Graduate Medical Education (ACGME) has also established managing the care of patients using population-based data as a core requirement for resident training [3]. To address the triple aim and ACGME requirements, residency training programs must embrace the dual responsibility of training residents in direct patient care and in the care of the broader patient population they serve. Resident physicians must therefore develop the skill set necessary to care for the patient in front of them as well as the larger panel of patients attributed to them, i.e., population health management.

Outline

- Definitions and scope
- Importance of population health management
- Clinical quality measures (CQMs)
- Clinical roles in population health management

R. J. Fortuna (✉) · H. G. Sobel
Internal Medicine, Pediatrics, Community Health, University of Rochester, Rochester, NY, USA

Internal Medicine Residency Program, Division of General Internal Medicine, Larner College of Medicine, University of Vermont Medical Center, Burlington, VT, USA
e-mail: Robert_Fortuna@URMC.Rochester.edu; halle.sobel@uvmhealth.org

L. B. Lu et al. (eds.), *Leading an Academic Medical Practice*,
https://doi.org/10.1007/978-3-031-40273-9_25

- Teaching population health management
- Risk stratification
- Alignment and coordination of population health
- Conclusion

Definitions and Scope

Population health strategies to improve health date back multiple decades, yet there remains a lack of clarity in the various definitions related to population health management [4]. There are many overlapping themes across the definitions of public health, population health, and population medicine [2]. Although public health is a well-established discipline, population health has more recently evolved over the past decade.

Public health, population health, and population medicine all differ in breadth and scope (Fig. 25.1). Public health is a broad discipline encompassing (a) the health of a population in a large geographic region, (b) the many determinants of health (medical, environmental, social), and (c) the regulations of government and community organization to improve the health [5]. Population health and population medicine are less clearly defined. The most commonly accepted definition of population health was defined in 2003 as "the health outcomes of a group of individuals, including the distribution of such outcomes within the

Fig. 25.1 Pyramid of population and public health

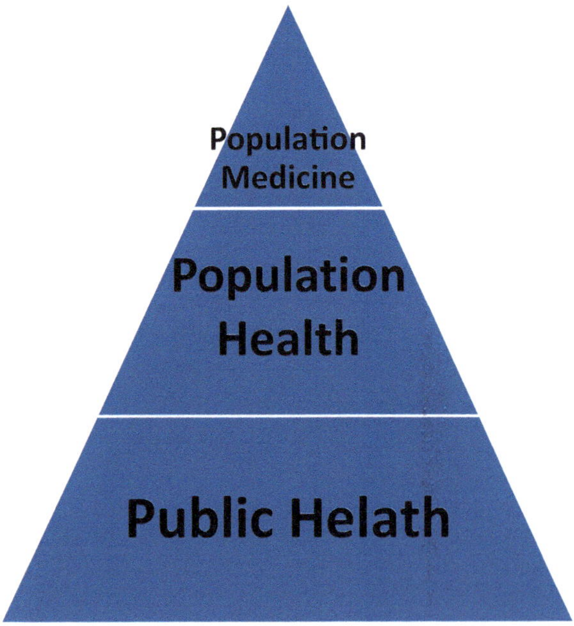

group" [6]. Population health is more narrowly focused than public health and is less tied to governmental agencies, health departments, or broad geographic areas [2, 6, 7].

Population medicine is further focused in clinical scope and how it conceptualizes populations [5, 8, 9]. While population health is slightly broader, population medicine is used to describe "activities limited to clinical populations and a narrower set of health outcome determinants" [9]. Population medicine brings a population view to clinical care and is focused on specific panels of patients [10]. Despite the subtle difference, the terms population health and population medicine are frequently used interchangeably. The terms population health and population health management are most commonly used in resident education and will be used throughout this chapter.

Importance of Population Health Management

Clinical Importance

Population health management has become a vital component of primary care. Resident education has traditionally been focused on direct patient care, or the individual patient the resident is treating [5]. Direct patient care, however, is not mutually exclusive with population health management. Population health management provides the opportunity to improve clinical quality measures across a broad panel of patients. Using clinical dashboards and population health management tools, residents can improve the health of the patient population they serve in a much more effective and efficient manner. Population health complements direct patient care by (a) reinforcing the importance of chronic disease management and preventive care and (b) continuing the relationship with the health care team outside of an appointment.

To optimize the impact, it is important to develop a culture within a practice that prioritizes both individual and population medicine. Fostering this culture may include reviewing dashboard quality data at morning huddles, reviewing overall quality data at resident meetings, and building engagement with population health into semiannual resident assessments.

Financial Importance

In addition to the clinical importance, population health management has significant contractual and financial importance. Academic medical centers are increasingly entering into contracts that incorporate value-based payments, including pay for performance, shared savings, and shared risk contracts [11]. At the same time, the Centers for Medicare & Medicaid Services (CMS) are moving towards more value-based payment structures. Value-based payment structures rely heavily on population health management strategies to improve clinical quality and reduce cost. For instance, pay-for-performance contracts are directly tied to the system's performance on defined clinical quality measures (CQMs), such as the proportion of patients with diabetes who are treated to a goal. Similarly, many shared savings contracts are based on meeting quality metrics in addition to containing cost.

Acknowledging the financial relevance, in broad terms, of population health and value-based payment structures is an important component of resident education.

Clinical Quality Measures (CQMs)

Defining clinical quality goals is an essential step towards establishing a population health management program and measuring the clinical impact. Clinical quality measures are specific definitions of the quality metrics. Over the past several decades, many clinical quality measures have been developed. One of the most widely used sets of measures is the Healthcare Effectiveness Data and Information Set (HEDIS), developed by the National Committee for Quality Assurance (NCQA). In addition to NCQA, the Agency for Healthcare Research and Quality (AHRQ), Centers for Medicare & Medicaid (CMS), and individual states have published their own widely used quality measures (Table 25.1).

All of the quality measures have very tightly defined specifications. These specifications allow for standardization of metrics across the nation but may also limit health systems' flexibility in defining quality. At times, CQMs even lag behind national best-practice standards. Residents must be taught the necessity for standardized definitions of quality but must also understand the need to incorporate individualized clinical judgment.

Table 25.1 Clinical quality measures

Organization	Examples of clinical quality measures (CQMs)
National Committee for Quality Assurance (NCQA)	• Health care Effectiveness Data and Information Set (HEDIS)
Agency for Healthcare Research and Quality (AHRQ)	• Prevention Quality Indicators (PQIs) • Consumer Assessment of Healthcare Providers and Systems (CAHPS)
Centers for Medicare & Medicaid Services (CMS)	• Physician Quality Reporting System (PQRS)
State-based measures	• NYS Quality Assurance Reporting Requirements (QARR) • Massachusetts Health Quality Program (MHQP) • California Cooperative Healthcare Reporting Initiative (CCHRI)

Clinical Roles in Population Health Management

Resident Role

Population health management is quickly becoming an integral component of ambulatory resident practices. The ambulatory clinic is an ideal location to learn and perform these tasks as residents assume responsibility for a panel of patients. Resident panels are typically smaller than faculty panels and thus are a manageable size for residents to develop the skills for population health management.

Population-based approaches include (a) working with patient registries to improve preventive care and chronic disease management, (b) performing outreach between clinical visits to work with patients not meeting goals, (c) engaging with a range of community services, and (d) addressing social determinants of health and disparities [7]. This requires a team-based strategy with all team members working at the top of their training and licensure.

It is important that resident physicians work effectively within an interdisciplinary team to improve the health of their patient panels. This includes remaining aware of the intervisit care and outreach efforts that are delivered to patients. Table 25.2 identifies resident roles in population health management. While residents may not be directly providing that intervisit care, it is important that resident physicians are aware of efforts by team members (care managers, nurses, attendings) to facilitate the necessary care. A structure should be in place to teach residents the principles of leading a multidisciplinary team and provide graduated responsibility. Residents must engage in the process and establish the clinical priorities for population health efforts that are most applicable to their panels. For instance, resident physicians must help determine where to focus efforts and set priorities to maximize the overall health of the population. This requires an in-depth knowledge of the gaps in care and a detailed familiarity with chronic disease and preventive care registries [12].

Table 25.2 Resident role

Resident role in population health management
Establish the clinical priorities
Engage in the process
Remain cognizant of gaps in care
Address gaps in care at visits
Maintain up-to-date disease registries and preventive care registries
Work with multidisciplinary teams to perform outreach to patients

Team-Based Approach

Managing the health of populations between visits is critical and requires a coordinated team approach [12, 13]. While resident physicians must establish the clinical priorities and guide the process, they do not need to assume all of the responsibilities. Managing teams is a critical component of modern medicine and should be a fundamental component of education surrounding population health. These teams commonly include nurses, office support staff, social workers, and care managers, with all team members, ideally, working at the top of their training and licensure [13].

The patient-centered medical home (PCMH) provides a valuable framework to support many elements of population health. This framework includes not only the necessary staffing, but also the operational processes to effectively implement population health initiatives.

Teaching Population Health Management

Population health management curricula are evolving within residency clinics to help to achieve core ACGME resident competencies. Faculty champions are important to help lead and implement the educational curriculum. Curricula should address the importance of population health, elements of the team-based approach, clinical quality measures, and functional tools, such as clinical dashboards, to support population medicine.

The first part of a population health curriculum is to assign resident panels at the beginning of the academic year. Patient panels are commonly transferred from graduating residents to either PGY-1 or PGY-2 residents [14]. Some programs have worked to balance panels based on age, sex, and chronic disease status [15]. Once panels are assigned, residents can learn about the importance of evidence-based medicine and ensure that these standards are applied across populations with chronic diseases, such as diabetes, asthma, COPD, and congestive heart failure. Similarly, preventive care registries provide a mechanism to identify patients eligible for screening and impart an opportunity to teach about recommended preventive measures across populations, such as colorectal cancer screening, breast cancer screening, and immunizations.

Population health curricula should strive for a balance of meaningful clinical team-building, setting population-based goals, and routine reevaluation of progress towards the established goals. Educational space should be reserved for each curricular component of population health. For example, the first year of training may be divided with the first quarter focused on team building, the second quarter focused on chronic disease management (hypertension and diabetes), the third quarter focused on preventive care (cancer screening and immunizations), and the last quarter focused on overall re-evaluation. As residents progress, it is important to develop a more comprehensive approach to monitoring and improving multiple elements of population medicine simultaneously.

Accreditation Council for Graduate Medical Education (ACGME): Competencies and Entrustable Professional Activities (EPAs)

The importance of population health management is increasingly recognized at all levels of education. The updated ACGME core requirements state that residents must "demonstrate the ability to manage the care of patients using population-based data." In addition, the ACGME Milestones 2.0 has faculty assess the residents' ability to utilize EHR data to manage a panel of patients [16, 17]. Residency programs need to establish curricula and develop the ability to capture the work of residents in these required ACGME domains. This may include residents examining opportunities for improvement within their own practice using population-level data and acting on those opportunities.

A comprehensive population health curriculum will provide a structure to reach these competencies [18, 19]. For example, residents may receive a list of all of their patients with diabetes who are not at their hemoglobin A1C goal. They would then receive instruction on standards of care for patients with diabetes and then apply that knowledge to the care of their population of diabetic patients. The residents would work with interdisciplinary teams to identify diabetic patients in their panel not at goal, reach out to uncontrolled patients, and work to improve the care of patients not meeting established clinical goals. As residents progress in their training, they should develop the ability to proficiently manage populations of patients at the level of a practicing physician.

These competencies subsequently lead to Entrustable Professional Activities (EPAs). EPAs integrate competencies, knowledge, skills, and attitudes into discrete work tasks that can be accomplished independently by trainees ready for independent practice [20]. For example, an EPA could focus on improving patient care using quality metrics and dashboards for the ambulatory panel with the collaboration of the care team.

Risk Stratification

Risk assessment is also becoming a crucial element of population health management. Identifying the highest risk patients in a panel is necessary to guide resources and perform outreach. The typical full-time physician has approximately 1800 attributed patients in their panel. Risk assessment tools provide a standardized method for assessing risk across the entire panel.

There are many different risk assessment tools available, some even incorporated into EMRs (Table 25.3). CMS began evaluating different risk stratification instruments in the 1990s to guide clinical payments. In 2004, CMS released Hierarchical Condition Categories (HCCs) [21]. Since that time, HCCs have been revised and are now based on 70 different clinical condition categories obtained from ICD codes

Table 25.3 Risk stratification tools

Risk stratification tool	Description
Hierarchical condition categories (HCCs)	Developed by the Centers for Medicare & Medicaid (CMS). HCC contains 70 condition categories selected from ICD codes
Adjusted clinical groups (ACGs)	Developed at Johns Hopkins University and uses both inpatient and outpatient diagnoses to classify each patient into 93 ACG categories
Chronic comorbidity count (CCC)	CCC is the sum of selected comorbid conditions based on the Agency for Healthcare Research and Quality (AHRQ) clinical classification software
Charlson comorbidity measure	The Charlson model predicts the risk of 1-year mortality based on a range of comorbid illnesses. The model evaluates the presence or absence of 17 health conditions
Impactability scores	Impactability scores extend risk stratification tools to attempt to identify patients amenable to a particular intervention, such as care management

and administrative data. In addition to HCCs, several other risk stratification tools have been developed, most based on clinical conditions and administrative data to predict cost expenditures or resource utilization.

When using risk stratification to guide care management and other population health-based initiatives, it is important to recognize that high risk scores do not necessarily equate to the ability to impact the clinical course. Newer models have begun to incorporate the concept of "impactability." These models strive to identify the combination of high-risk patients and situations that are amenable to intervention.

Alignment and Coordination of Population Health

The importance of population-based strategies crosses many departments at large academic medical centers. Residents will often engage with different elements of population health as they move through different rotations. Inpatient units and subspecialty departments frequently have care managers that engage in elements of population health that will overlap with outpatient efforts. It is important for medical directors leading outpatient population health strategies to align these efforts, as much as possible, across the academic medical center.

Conclusion

As the US health system progresses towards increased accountability throughout medicine, resident physicians must learn to be accountable for the health outcomes of the populations that they serve. Population health management has become an essential component of primary care and residency training. To improve the overall quality of care, residency training programs must embrace the dual responsibility of training residents in direct patient care and population-based management. Programs must also foster the culture that prioritizes population health management and clinical quality initiatives to improve the health of populations of patients.

References

1. Berwick DM, Nolan TW, Whittington J. The triple aim: care, health, and cost. Health Aff (Millwood). 2008;27(3):759–69.
2. Stoto MA. Population health in the Affordable Care Act era. Washington DC: Academy Health; 2013.
3. ACGME. Program requirements for graduate medical education in internal medicine. 2022. IV.B.1.a).(1). (a).(vii).
4. Sharfstein JM. The strange journey of population health. Milbank Q. 2014;92(4):640–3.
5. Gourevitch MN. Population health and the academic medical center: the time is right. Acad Med. 2014;89(4):544–9.
6. Kindig D, Stoddart G. What is population health? Am J Public Health. 2003;93(3):380–3.
7. Kassler WJ, Tomoyasu N, Conway PH. Beyond a traditional payer–CMS's role in improving population health. N Engl J Med. 2015;372(2):109–11.
8. Kindig DA. Understanding population health terminology. Milbank Q. 2007;85(1):139–61.
9. Kindig DA What are we talking about when we talk about population health? 2015.
10. Eggleston EM, Finkelstein JA. Finding the role of health care in population health. JAMA. 2014;311(8):797–8.
11. APM Measurement. Program of alternative payment models. The Health Care Payment Learning & Action Network (LAN). 2021.
12. Rieselbach RE, et al. Ambulatory training for primary care general internists: innovation with the affordable care act in mind. J Grad Med Educ. 2014;6(2):395–8.
13. Hodach R, Chase A, Fortini R, Delaney C, Hodach R. Population health management: a roadmap for provider-based automation in a new era of healthcare. Institute for Health Technology Transformation. 2013.
14. Hern T, et al. Patient care management teams: improving continuity, office efficiency, and teamwork in a residency clinic. J Grad Med Educ. 2009;1(1):67–72.
15. Bennett K, et al. Organized continuity panel reassignment. J Grad Med Educ. 2011;3(3):404–7.
16. Accreditation Council for Graduate Medical Education (ACGME). Internal Medicine Supplemental Guide. 2020. https://www.acgme.org/globalassets/PDFs/Milestones/InternalMedicineSupplementalGuide.pdf?ver=2020-12-02-124831-067&ver=2020-12-02-124831-067A.
17. Accreditation Council for Graduate Medical Education. Milestones accreditation council for graduate medical education. 2022. https://www.acgme.org/what-we-do/accreditation/milestones/overview/.
18. Bodenheimer T, et al. Teaching residents population health management. Washington DC: Association of American Medical Colleges; 2019.
19. Flattery D, Berry L, Subramanian I, Gregory B, Nelson N, Wofsy J. Engaging residents in population-based care through a panel management curriculum. Acad Intern Med Insight. 2016;14(1):7–9.
20. Hauer KE, et al. Identifying entrustable professional activities in internal medicine training. J Grad Med Educ. 2013;5(1):54–9.
21. Pope GC, et al. Evaluation of the CMS-HCC risk adjustment model. Durham NC: Research Triangle Institute (RTI) International Research Triangle Park; 2011.

Chapter 26
Dashboards to Support Academic Practices

Robert J. Fortuna, Gail Berkenblit, and Halle G. Sobel

Introduction

The robust amount of data in the electronic health record is revolutionizing the practice of medicine. These advances provide the necessary data and tools to support population health initiatives with the goal to improve care for patients. The foundation of population health management systems rests upon registries, or databases, of specific clinical conditions. These registries organize the data in a manner that can be presented in dashboards to support clinical and operational activities in faculty and resident practices. Dashboards, in turn, provide a population-based view of the health of the patients based on predefined clinical quality measures (CQMs). Most importantly, dashboards allow the ability to pull gaps in care to support outreach to patients and support quality improvement initiatives. In addition, dashboards offer the opportunity to present the necessary data to support the educational, operational, and financial activities of managing an academic medical practice.

Outline
- Registries
- Patient attribution

R. J. Fortuna (✉)
Internal Medicine, Pediatrics, Community Health, Med-Peds Residency Program, University of Rochester, Rochester, NY, USA
e-mail: Robert_Fortuna@URMC.Rochester.edu

G. Berkenblit
Division of General Internal Medicine, Johns Hopkins University School of Medicine, Baltimore, MD, USA
e-mail: gberken@jhmi.edu

H. G. Sobel
Division of General Internal Medicine, Larner College of Medicine, University of Vermont Medical Center, Burlington, VT, USA
e-mail: Halle.sobel@uvmhealth.org

L. B. Lu et al. (eds.), *Leading an Academic Medical Practice*,
https://doi.org/10.1007/978-3-031-40273-9_26

- Clinical quality measures
- Clinical dashboards
- Operational and administrative dashboards
- Dashboards in resident education
- Conclusion

Registries

The National Institute of Health (NIH) describes a registry as a "collection of information about individuals, usually focused around a specific diagnosis or condition" [1]. At its core, registries provide the foundational data to support the architecture of population health management systems. Disease registries enable teams to identify and manage patients with a particular condition, such as diabetes or hypertension. Similarly, preventive care registries provide the ability to identify the base population of patients eligible for preventive care, such as colorectal cancer screening, breast cancer screening, or immunizations. Registries can also be built based on payor or population demographics.

Overall, registries are simply databases or lists of patients meeting certain criteria, but their underlying coding is often complex. Determining that a patient has a diagnosis of diabetes, for instance, may require the system to examine clinical problem lists, billing claims data, lab data, and medication lists. Institutional informatics teams generally have listings of the parameters of the existing registries available. In addition, most electronic health records (EHRs) also include the capacity to create custom registries.

Patient Attribution

Proper identification of the physician–patient relationship, or primary care physician (PCP) attribution, within registries is essential to the validity of the registries and dashboards. Patient attribution is a foundational component of population health, value-based contracts, and clinical dashboards. Patient attribution, however, is more complex than commonly appreciated, and problems with patient attribution are often at the core of inaccurate reports. Inaccurate patient attribution is especially common in resident practices. One review found that the proportion of patients correctly attributed to their physician ranged from 22% to 45% [2].

Patient attribution can be determined based on several different methodologies [2, 3]. It is important to acknowledge that different attribution methodologies lead to different results.

- *Primary care physician attribution*: Patients are most commonly attributed based on their primary care physician. However, there are multiple ways to determine PCP attribution [2, 3].
  - *Clinician-type attribution*: Most commonly, patients are attributed to resident physicians simply by having the resident listed as the PCP, or equivalent, in the electronic health record.
  - *Visit-type attribution*: Some systems attribute patients to the physician who provided the most, or plurality, of the primary care. This methodology is increasingly used by insurers and should be recognized as a potential cause of variance seen across different reports.
- *Clinical team attribution*: Patients can also be attributed to a physician based on an association with a clinical team. For instance, this is often used to define patient attribution to inpatient teams or assign attribution for quality improvement initiatives.

Independent of the methodology used to determine patient attribution, ongoing maintenance and validation are required to ensure that patient attribution remains current. For instance, patients commonly move or transfer their care to new providers, which may not be captured in the EHR. Out-of-date or inaccurate registries are a common source of inaccurate dashboards. In turn, these inaccurate dashboard reports can be a significant source of frustration for resident physicians, further highlighting the need to maintain accurate attribution. The natural cycle of residency programs necessitates updating the resident PCP on an annual basis after seniors graduate and new interns join the residency program.

Clinical Quality Measures

Clinical quality measures (CQMs) are specific definitions of quality metrics that are generally defined nationally. Typical CQMs include measures related to hypertension control, diabetic control, breast cancer screening, colon cancer screening, medication adherence, and immunizations [4, 5]. Determining which CQMs to focus on is a pivotal step for any population health program. For trainees, programs should optimally focus on metrics that are (i) relevant to the population of the practice, (ii) patient centered, (iii) evidence-based, and (iv) actionable [4]. In addition, healthcare systems will frequently be contractually tied to specific clinical measures as part of their value-based contracts with insurers and the Centers for Medicare & Medicaid Services (CMS). Beyond the contractual obligations, residency programs can determine which specific quality measures are most appropriate for patient care and their educational mission.

Clinical Dashboards

Health-care systems continue to expand their ability to measure and report outcome data with the goal to drive improvements in care [6]. Clinical dashboards provide the user-interface to display data from patient registries in a readable format to support quality initiatives and care delivery. The fundamental purpose of a dashboard is to (i) deliver a broad population-based view of the health of the panel of patients based on defined clinical quality metrics, and (ii) provide the ability to generate reports of gaps in care to support outreach to patients. Figure 26.1 presents an example of a typical clinical dashboard from Epic, a common electronic health record. The dashboard example presents the total patient attribution at the top of the dashboard followed by relevant CQMs. Dashboards generally allow users to toggle between different levels of attribution to visualize performance at a system-level, practice-level, attending-level, or a resident-level.

The most powerful element of dashboards is their ability to generate reports of gaps in care. Clinical care gaps are quality metrics that have yet to be fulfilled at the individual patient level. Gap reports provide an actionable list of patients not reaching clinical goals or patients overdue for preventive care. For instance, a gap report can identify all patients due for colorectal cancer screening or patients not meeting hypertensive care goals. These reports serve as the foundation to guide outreach by the clinical or population health teams.

Dashboards provide a powerful tool to aid residents' understanding of the broader view of the care they are providing. For instance, it is natural for resident physicians to believe that their patients with hypertension are well-controlled based on their experience with the last couple of patients they have treated. However, this may not be reflective of their broader patient panel. The dashboard will provide a population view of the health of their entire panel of patients to guide interventions and care. Dashboards may also be used in efforts to support equity and to reduce disparities in care [7]. This broader context is essential to residents' understanding of populations of patients and system-level care.

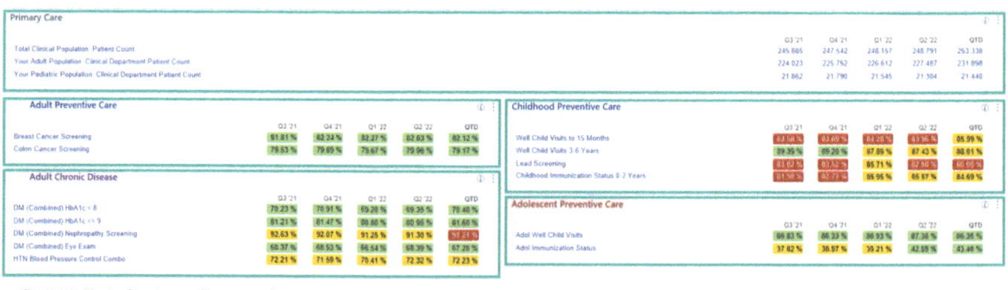

Fig. 26.1 Example of clinical dashboard

Operational and Administrative Dashboards

In addition to presenting clinical quality measures, dashboards can be used to present a myriad of data that may benefit the operational, administrative, and financial processes within the office. These real-time data can support the daily activities of practicing clinicians, front-end support staff, and practice administrators.

Dashboards can provide data on a variety of clinical operational measures, such as number of patients seen per month, number of new patients treated, average wait times for patients at check-in, wait times for the physician, relative value units (RVUs), and summary financial data (Table 26.1). Figure 26.2 presents an example of a clinical operation dashboard. The precise data presented in the operational dashboard can be geared toward the intended user. For medical directors and practices administrators, real-time clinical volume and financial data are critical to managing the practice. For faculty, clinical volume and RVUs may be relevant to compensation. For residents, clinical volume and patient wait times provide valuable information to improve daily performance and monitor Accreditation Council for Graduate Medical Education (ACGME) requirements.

Dashboards can also support medical directors and practice managers in their administrative duties. Administrative dashboards can offer medical directors an overview of scheduling analytics, time lost to no-shows, referrals and referral processing, and financial charges. Figure 26.3 offers an example of an administrative dashboard.

Dashboard data may also benefit front-end clerical staff and schedulers (Fig. 26.4). Front-end staff and office managers can utilize a dashboard to provide visibility to patient wait times, appointment availability, and scheduling trends.

Table 26.1 Example of operational and analytic dashboards

Operational and administrative analytics	
Patient wait times	Practice finances
Physician efficiency measures	Incomplete notes
Office flow	Patient continuity measures
Scheduling analytics	Referral analytics

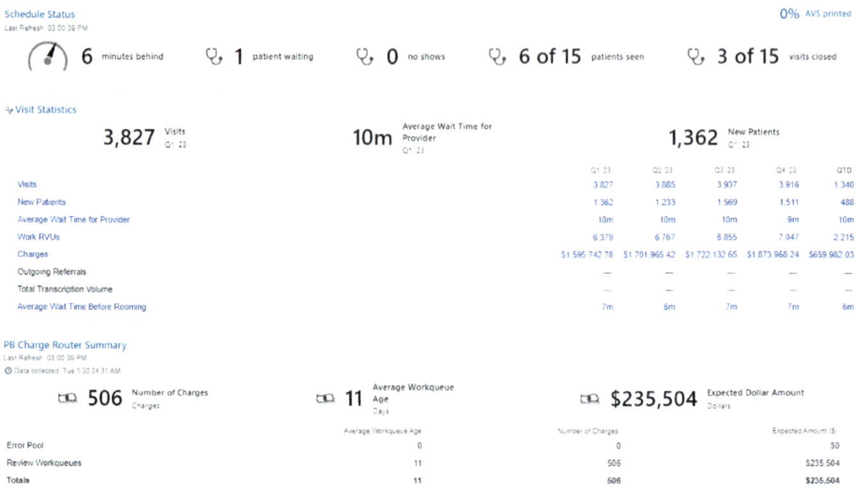

Fig. 26.2 Example of clinical operations dashboard

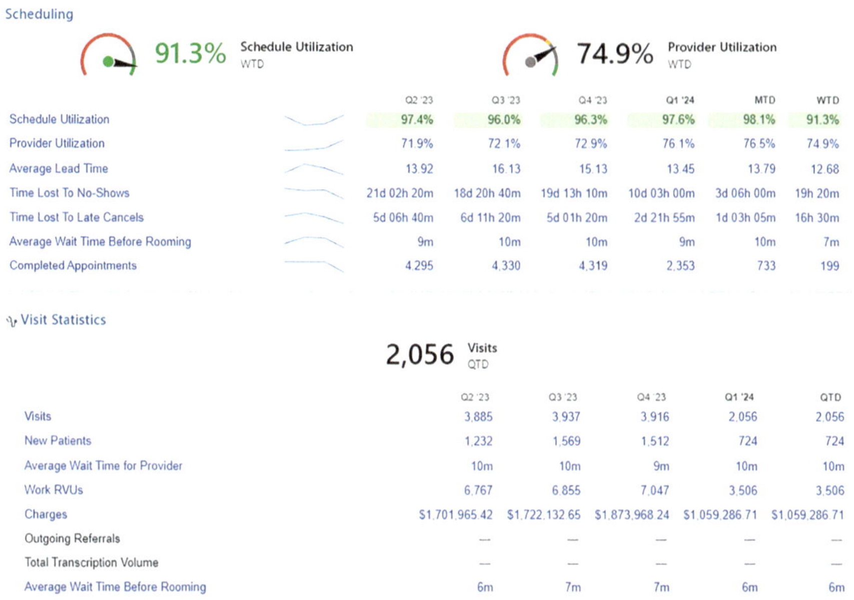

Fig. 26.3 Example of an administrative dashboard

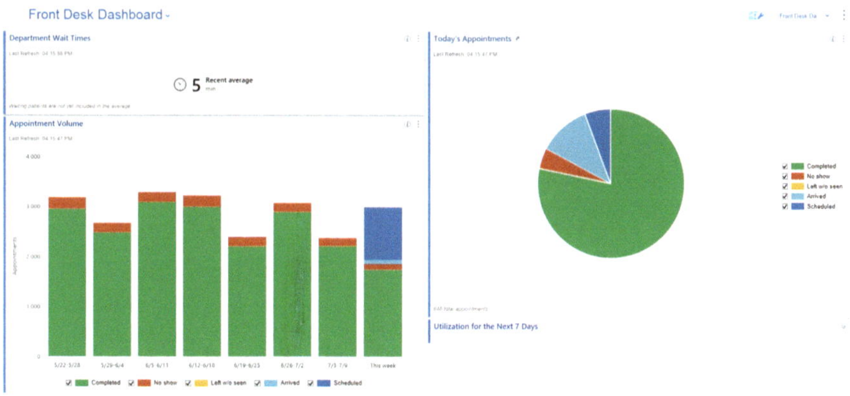

Fig. 26.4 Example of a scheduling dashboard

Dashboards in Resident Education

The ACGME requires that residents receive data on quality measures related to their patient population as one of the core components of patient care [8, 9]. Specifically, the ACGME states "residents need experience using, understanding, and analyzing population health data so that they can develop health care plans to improve health outcomes for their patients" [10, 11]. The use of dashboards and registry data has greatly facilitated resident access to clinical data and augmented teaching curricula aimed at population health. While previous panel management curricula were shown to improve patient outcomes, they often relied on time-consuming chart audits [12]. Current population health curricula combining didactic components with review of dashboard data have been shown to be effective in supporting clinical strategies as well as improving resident attitudes regarding population health management [13, 14].

Dashboards are also a powerful tool to support resident quality improvement (QI) curricula [15]. Curricula that included resident involvement in the selection of metrics, such as adherence to asthma guidelines, have been successful in promoting understanding of dashboard utility and increasing resident engagement in QI. On the other hand, exposure of residents to dashboard metrics without resident input and outside of well-built curricula has not been shown to change performance [16].

Finally, for residents and faculty, education-focused dashboards can support competency-based medical education programs by tracking educational experiences and outcomes [17–19]. For instance, dashboards can display case mix and productivity for residents to ensure adequate exposure to common disorders [18]. Metrics can also be built to capture participation in conferences or online curricula [20]. Faculty evaluations of graduate medical education milestone achievement can be visually displayed, providing a feedback platform for residents and faculty [21]. At a broader level, dashboards that amalgamate data from clinical performance metrics, competency evaluations, and summative experiences, such as in-service examinations, can provide an overall resident assessment (Table 26.2). Linking educational experiences, formative evaluation, and performance data in this way has the potential to identify and address learning gaps and curricular needs [20, 22].

Table 26.2 Example of education dashboards

Educational dashboard components
Clinical case mix
Entrustable professional activities
Completion of board review questions
Completion of rotation evaluations
Faculty feedback to residents

Conclusion

Dashboards serve as a foundational tool for any population health program and can assist in managing the clinical, operational, and educational components of an academic practice. Clinically, dashboards provide a broad summary view of population-level clinical quality data and the ability to identify gaps in care to support patient outreach. Administratively, dashboards can help medical directors and practice managers in monitoring operational and administrative processes, such as patient flow, wait times, and financial performance. Educationally, dashboards can help medical directors and program directors track case mix of resident patients and completion of key educational requirements. Together, these clinical, administrative, and educational dashboards provide a strong foundation of actionable data to manage an academic medical practice.

References

1. NIH Clinical Research Trials and You. 2022. https://www.nih.gov/health-information/nih-clinical-research-trials-you/list-registries.
2. McCoy RG, Bunkers KS, Ramar P, Meier SK, Benetti LL, Nesse RE, et al. Patient attribution: why the method matters. Am J Manag Care. 2018;24(12):596–603.
3. Fiesinger T. Patient attribution: why it matters more than ever. Fam Pract Manag. 2016;23(6):25–30.
4. AAFP Quality measures: AAFP; 2022. https://www.aafp.org/family-physician/practice-and-career/managing-your-practice/quality-measures.html
5. Centers for Medicare & Medicaid Services. Quality measures; 2022. https://www.cms.gov/Medicare/Quality-Initiatives-Patient-Assessment-Instruments/QualityMeasures/index.html
6. Twohig PA, Rivington JR, Gunzler D, Daprano J, Margolius D. Clinician dashboard views and improvement in preventative health outcome measures: a retrospective analysis. BMC Health Serv Res. 2019;19(1):475.
7. Tsuchida RE, Haggins AN, Perry M, Chen CM, Medlin RP, Meurer WJ, et al. Developing an electronic health record-derived health equity dashboard to improve learner access to data and metrics. AEM Educ Train. 2021;5(Suppl 1):S116–s20.
8. ACGME Program Requirements for Graduate Medical Education in Internal Medicine (2022) VI.A.1.b).(2). (a).
9. ACGME Program Requirements for Graduate Medical Education in Internal Medicine (2022) IV.B.1.a).(1). (a).(vii).
10. Accreditation Council for Graduate Medical Education. Milestones; 2022. https://www.acgme.org/what-we-do/accreditation/milestones/overview/
11. ACGME. Internal Medicine Supplemental Guide; 2020. https://www.acgme.org/globalassets/PDFs/Milestones/InternalMedicineSupplementalGuide.pdf?ver=2020-12-02-124831-067&ver=2020-12-02-124831-067A
12. Pickett ME, Azar AS. Rethinking performance audit: chronic illness panel management. J Grad Med Educ. 2020;12(3):353–5.
13. Hadley-Strout EK, Landrey AR, MacLean CD, Sobel HG. Internal medicine resident experiences with a 5-month panel management curriculum. J Grad Med Educ. 2018;10(5):559–65.

14. Hadley Strout EK, Wahlberg EA, Kennedy AG, Sobel HG. A mixed-methods program evaluation of a self-directed panel management curriculum in an internal medicine residency clinic. J Gen Intern Med. 2022;37(9):2246–50.
15. Feld L, Belfer J, Kabra R, Buchan M, Castiglione J, Sayres S, et al. Utility of a Quality Dashboard Established by a Resident Quality Council. Acad Pediatr. 2020;20(7):e50–e1.
16. Kurtzman G, Dine J, Epstein A, Gitelman Y, Leri D, Patel MS, et al. Internal medicine resident engagement with a laboratory utilization dashboard: mixed methods study. J Hosp Med. 2017;12(9):743–6.
17. Carey R, Wilson G, Bandi V, Mondal D, Martin LJ, Woods R, et al. Developing a dashboard to meet the needs of residents in a competency-based training program: a design-based research project. Can Med Educ J. 2020;11(6):e31–45.
18. Epstein JA, Noronha C, Berkenblit G. Smarter screen time: integrating clinical dashboards into graduate medical education. J Grad Med Educ. 2020;12(1):19–24.
19. Friedman KA, Raimo J, Spielmann K, Chaudhry S. Resident dashboards: helping your clinical competency committee visualize trainees' key performance indicators. Med Educ Online. 2016;21:29838.
20. Thoma B, Bandi V, Carey R, Mondal D, Woods R, Martin L, et al. Developing a dashboard to meet competence committee needs: a design-based research project. Can Med Educ J. 2020;11(1):e16–34.
21. Triola MM, Hawkins RE, Skochelak SE. The time is now: using graduates' practice data to drive medical education reform. Acad Med. 2018;93(6):826–8.
22. Harrison R, Tsyrulnik A, Wood DB, Coughlin RF, Della-Giustina D, Goldflam K. An innovative feedback tool leading to improved faculty feedback and positive reception by residents. West J Emerg Med. 2019;21(1):47–51.

Chapter 27
Management of Patients with Complex Needs

Jeremy A. Epstein and Lisa Ochoa-Frongia

Introduction

Academic medical practices serve a valuable role in caring for patients with complex needs and training future internists in the many biopsychosocial components of patient care. Patients with complex needs related to chronic medical conditions, psychosocial factors, and communication barriers frequently require a great deal of resident time and effort. Patient complexity can be defined as "a dynamic state in which the personal, social, and clinical aspects of the patient's experience operate as complicating factors" [1]. This chapter will examine contributors to the challenge of caring for patients with complex needs and propose practical solutions and a framework for the successful management of these patients within resident-inclusive practices.

Outline
- Background
- Defining the patient with complex needs
- Challenges facing the resident primary care physician of patients with complex needs
- Framework for an approach to the complex patient
- Conclusion

J. A. Epstein
Department of Medicine, Divisions of Hospital Medicine and General Internal Medicine, Johns Hopkins University School of Medicine, Baltimore, MD, USA
e-mail: epstein@jhmi.edu

L. Ochoa-Frongia (✉)
Department of Medicine, Division of General Internal Medicine, University of California, San Francisco, San Francisco, CA, USA
e-mail: Lisa.Ochoa-Frongia@ucsf.edu

L. B. Lu et al. (eds.), *Leading an Academic Medical Practice*,
https://doi.org/10.1007/978-3-031-40273-9_27

Background

The experience of serving as a primary care physician (PCP) is not only a formative core clinical experience during residency but is also an Accreditation Council for Graduate Medical Education (ACGME) Common Program Requirement [2]. Based on National Resident Matching Program (NRMP) data from 2021, nearly 9500 residents matched in PGY-1 positions alone [3]. With tens of thousands of resident physicians in categorical or primary care residency programs at any given time, we estimate that three million patients are under the care of resident PCPs at a given time [4]. Even if only 2% of these patients were considered as having complex needs, 60,000 such patients would then be under the care of internal medicine residents.

Resident PCPs face many challenges, particularly early in residency. They are new to the role of physician and PCP while simultaneously trying to get to know their patients and gain clinical and systems knowledge. They are also frequently away from clinic and may have a rotating group of supervisors and team members in the primary care clinic. Resident PCPs may struggle in particular to support and advance the care of primary care patients with complex medical and psychosocial needs compared to more seasoned practitioners. Further, resident PCPs may have patient panels with a higher rate of multiple medical comorbidities and mental health conditions, including substance use disorder and depression compared to staff or faculty physicians [5]. Social determinants of health, including a lack of economic stability, lack of access to quality education or health care, low language or literacy skills, and experiences of racism or violence [6] add to the complexity of patients often seen in resident-inclusive practices. A small number of patients with complex needs may come to dominate the time of a resident PCP unless clear guidance on strategies to address the factors that contribute to their complexity is provided.

Defining the Patient with Complex Needs

What factors define a complex patient? While every PCP can likely quickly compile a mental list of their most complex patients, which factors contribute to this cognitive weight? Patient characteristics, care utilization, number and severity of medical and psychosocial diagnoses, and social determinants of health are broad categories to consider as contributors to complexity [7, 8]. Resident PCPs often have many complex patients empaneled to them. Though there are few studies offering a robust comparison of resident versus faculty physician panel complexity, one recent study found that despite similar levels of medical complexity compared to faculty panels, resident patients had significantly higher levels of psychosocial vulnerability across all measured domains, including health literacy, economic vulnerability, psychiatric illness burden, high-risk behaviors, and patient engagement [9]. Table 27.1 depicts factors increasing patient complexity and how these factors can pose a challenge to the PCP.

Table 27.1 Factors increasing patient complexity and challenges facing resident PCPs in caring for complex patients

Factors increasing complexity	Challenges facing the resident PCP of patients with such factors
Patient demographics	
• Advanced age	• Increased need for advanced care planning • Time and effort to engage with caregivers, family members, and consultants
Care utilization, treatment characteristics	
• Frequent contact with medical system—admissions, ER visits, and primary care visits • High number of prescriptions • Multiple consulting or co-managing specialists	• Need for care coordination, discharge planning, and discharge safety follow-up • Management of polypharmacy • Time and effort to review greater volume of data • Time and effort to manage subspecialist referrals and recommendations
Number and severity of medical conditions	
• High number of conditions • Poor control of condition (high hemoglobin A1c, elevated blood pressure, etc.)	• Increased number of active or severe problems to address during visit • Need for prioritization and prognostication • Increased need for labs or studies • Additional time spent on patient, family education
Psychosocial diagnoses	
• Presence of mental illnesses, particularly poorly controlled or severe mental illnesses • Substance use disorders • Trauma history	• Time and effort to coordinate care with behavioral health team • Increased complexity in communication with patients • Experiences of vicarious trauma
Social determinants of health	
• Lack of safe housing, transportation, and neighborhoods • Racism, discrimination, and violence • Lack of education, job opportunities, and income • Poor access to nutritious foods and physical activity opportunities • Polluted air and water • Lack of language and literacy skills • Lack of insurance or underinsurance	• Feeling of futility of medical interventions when faced with SDOH challenges and barriers • Time and effort spent seeking services • Patient mistrust/fear of the medical system • Increased complexity in communication due to language/literacy barriers • Possible need to advocate for financial assistance if uninsured or underinsured

Challenges Facing the Resident PCP of Patients with Complex Needs

Caring for patients with complex needs requires time and effort to navigate these complex needs and coordinate care with many other members of the health-care system. During a visit when one or more of these factors are present, there may be need for attention to prioritization of the most complex issues, advanced care planning, management of polypharmacy, services referral, care coordination, mitigation of barriers to care, and so on.

The time and effort required for the care of complex patients and the cognitive impact of delivering complex care is substantial. Navigation of these factors represent rich learning and opportunities to build trust and rapport with patients and family members, but residents must have adequate time and support to navigate these challenges. While many clinicians may enjoy the challenge of caring for patients with complex needs and experience satisfaction when patients meet goals or improve, there is often insufficient time or support to care for such patients adequately. Clinic team members, specialists, care managers, and population health teams represent important supports for busy resident PCPs and their patients with complex needs. A key framework to consider in the care of complex patients is that of the patient-centered medical home.

A Framework for the Approach to the Complex Patient

The Patient-Centered Medical Home (PCMH) framework has been recommended as an approach to ensuring the delivery of high-quality primary care for complex patients [10]. Building upon this model, we offer additional recommendations relevant to residency-based practices.

Patient-centered care: The delivery of medical care must be guided by patient goals and wishes, rather than a clinician-driven notion of optimal medical practice. For patients with significant multimorbidity, resident physicians must avoid pursuing treatment or evaluation that, while medically correct, may not be feasible for or desired by the patient. This shift of mindset can be difficult for residents, especially those early on in their training. Traditional teaching in medical school focuses on identifying the ideal diagnostic and treatment pathways for every disease condition. This framework is repeatedly reinforced through standardized testing. This is in contrast to the optimal real-world approach, which may be to establish a strong rapport with a patient and their family, explore their specific care goals and the motivations behind them, and then adjust their care in concordance with those wishes. Preceptors should be mindful of the following signs that may indicate medical care is not appropriately patient-centered:

1. *New initiation of standard of care treatment for a longstanding problem*: While this may indicate that a provider has finally convinced a previously hesitant patient to adopt a key beneficial therapy, it may also suggest that the provider is missing essential information about why this therapy has been withheld historically despite its clear indication.
2. *Reordering tests or referrals that have repeatedly not been completed*: Patients with complex comorbidities may have limited transportation options and require assistance from others to attend appointments. No-shows or cancellations may

reflect underlying transportation barriers or indicate patient disagreement or disengagement with the enacted plan.

3. *Polypharmacy*: Medication regimen complexity is associated with patient nonadherence and frequent hospitalization [11]. The physical process of taking multiple medications a day may be problematic for those with low health literacy or cognitive impairment. For these patients, it can be helpful to switch to a pharmacy that organizes medications into blister or bubble packs by the day and time of administration. The expense associated with polypharmacy also limits patients' access to prescribed treatments [12]. This problem is compounded by the fact that drug pricing is largely unavailable to prescribers at the time of prescribing and patients may be uncomfortable disclosing difficulty affording medications. Preceptors should make use of available resources such as electronic health record (EHR) tools to identify those who are not picking up ordered medications and selecting the cheapest medication options for their patients. In addition to directly contacting a patient's prescription drug plan for price information, other strategies include engaging primary care pharmacists, using prescription price comparison resources (i.e., GoodRx), discount medication lists (i.e., Walmart $4 list), direct to consumer medication suppliers (i.e., Mark Cuban Cost Plus Drug Company), and electronic real-time benefit tools within the EHR (i.e., Surescripts Real-Time Prescription Benefit or RxRevu's SwitftRX).
4. *Patients requesting transfer to different PCP*: Clinic leadership should explore the reason behind these requests by discussing the situation with the patients. To put the patient concerns in appropriate context, it is important to check for patterns. Has the patient repeatedly dismissed previous physicians over similar concerns? Has the physician had several of their patients request transfer to another clinician or raise similar concerns?

Comprehensive care: Resident clinics serving complex patients must be able to connect patients to a variety of health-care resources beyond those of the primary care clinic. Common resources needed include medical subspecialties, imaging, home care services, clinical pharmacists, mental health services, and substance use disorder treatment centers. Community health workers, case managers, and social workers are essential to help address underlying modifiable risk factors responsible for preventable emergency department visits and hospitalizations [13]. Using a team-based care structure helps unburden resident PCPs from having to repeatedly arrange meetings or send messages to facilitate care coordination.

Coordinated care: Having the capability to refer patients to other services is necessary but insufficient for the provision of optimal patient care. Primary care physicians, especially for patients with multimorbidity, need to take an active role in advancing the care of their patients by coordinating and communicating with their different care teams. In the resident clinic setting, care coordination can be particularly challenging. First, given that residents are rotating in and out of outpatient clinical care, it can be difficult to assign to them responsibility for inter-visit care while on other rotations. Second, as trainees, residents may feel uncomfortable directing certain types of messaging to attending-level faculty or staff. Faculty members may similarly have competing obligations and may fail to respond in a timely fashion to messages from trainees. Third, there are immutable barriers to resident-delivered primary care stemming from various billing or regulatory limitations. For example, only nonresident licensed physicians can sign home care orders. In doing so, attendings can supplant resident PCPs as the provider to whom all communication should be sent by the home care team. Several strategies can be employed to enhance the care coordination of complex patients in resident clinics.

1. *Assign an attending to each complex patient*: One mechanism to improve oversight and improve care coordination is to link each complex patient to a particular attending. The designated attending would be someone who knows the patient well from previous health-care contact. They can be copied on all messaging for the patient to help advance their care when the resident PCP is off service. These attendings need to be mindful of the balance of their role. They need to be involved to the extent needed to optimize patient care but not be so involved as to function as the de facto PCP. The patient can be preferentially staffed with this preceptor when they are available, which will also relieve residents from repeatedly retelling complicated past medical histories. The ability to designate other physicians as part of a patient's care team is a common feature of EHRs and can help facilitate the involvement of a longitudinal attending. In some EHRs, this further allows the attending to automatically receive lab results and hospitalization notifications for these patients, serving to keep them up-to-date with their care.
2. *Assign a specific preceptor to each resident*: Residents can be assigned designated longitudinal or primary preceptors who can be a consistent resource and source of guidance for resident patient care. This may be integrated into the existing outpatient structure with attending physicians linked to specific resident outpatient teams or firms. If the associated logistical challenges can be overcome, having the resident's clinic schedule match that of their primary preceptor facilitates continuity not only between the resident and the preceptor but also between the resident's patients and the preceptor.
3. *Shared resident PCP model*: If the complex patient needs to be seen with such frequency that a single resident PCP would not be available, a group of residents or a pair of residents can become the patient's PCP and function as practice partners. This system works particularly well with X + Y resident structures since, at any given time, one of the residents from the PCP's cohort will always be on their ambulatory block and available to see the patient.
4. *Advanced practice provider (APP) integration*: A nurse practitioner or physician assistant can be employed to help manage a cohort of high-risk patients. These advanced practice providers intensely follow a small group of patients and can serve as a second supportive PCP for the resident physician when they are not available. They proactively review charts to ensure that the patient's care plan is proceeding appropriately and take action if needed either by seeing the patient themselves or helping to coordinate care with other clinicians.

5. *Transfer of patients to attending physician:* Some programs will deliberately transfer patients to faculty physicians to avoid the challenges associated with the delivery of complex primary care in the resident clinic setting [14]. Recognizing this may negatively impact resident education, if this approach is going to be considered, it may be best reserved for when the resident PCP is graduating and a new PCP would be needed.

Access to care: Patients with complex medical conditions will need frequent guidance from their medical team. Patients need to be able to easily connect with members of their care team, especially if they are to avoid potentially unnecessary emergency department visits. While some patients may find this most easily accomplished through EHR online health portals, other patients may not have access to or familiarity with internet technology and will rely on traditional phone communication. Both means of communication need to be supported. The ability to schedule future appointments is also a feature of care access. Being able to book an appointment far in advance with a resident PCP can be challenging given logistical constraints and scheduling changes inherent to residency programs. Efforts need to be taken to prioritize clinic scheduling. Strategies to preserve urgent access to resident PCPs include rolling appointments, preserving some appointment slots to open a short time before the appointment date, or holding slots for the resident PCP to use at their discretion.

Appointment length: In addition to rendering appointments available and accessible, perhaps the most meaningful adjustment to improve the care of complex patients is to afford them longer medical appointments. The visit length allotted for a typical follow-up patient will often be insufficient to deliver optimal care in a resident clinic environment. The following two approaches, or both in combination, can facilitate this change. First, selected patient charts can be flagged as preferentially occupying two consecutive slots. Second, specific complex patient appointment slots that are longer in duration can be built into the schedule and reserved for this patient population.

Systems-based approach to quality and safety: For patients with highly complex needs, the number of involved subspecialty physicians and the potential for a shared PCP model makes standardization of documentation important. Providers can use an evidence-supported customized note template with a strong focus on detailed longitudinal management over time [15]. It is helpful for clinic or even health-system leaders to lead the drive toward standardized and succinct documentation. One challenge with using standard progress notes for documentation is that even the most thoughtful and comprehensive notes will become quickly buried—digitally—by other documentation. A complementary strategy can be to use the EHR problem list to document all care, rendering it the most up-to-date representation of a patient's state of health. Incomplete problem lists have been cited to be a widespread problem in primary care practices and a threat to patient safety; problem-based charting can help maintain the problem list while simultaneously providing a common assessment and plan for teams to access [16]. During clinic visits, problems in the list that are addressed and updated would be imported into the standardized templated note to reflect the patient's status at this particular point in time. Digital problem lists that track changes over time can detail historical medical decision-making, further supporting the clinical team.

Conclusion

Caring for patients with complex needs can be a challenging part of the learning and care experience for resident PCPs. These experiences, however, can be satisfying and associated with high-yield learning when coupled with appropriate supports for the resident PCP and their patients with complex needs. Academic medical practices and preceptors can help facilitate the success of resident PCPs and their patients with complex needs alike when they have a clear understanding of the factors contributing to the challenges of caring for such patients, and solutions to these challenges. Applying the framework of the patient-centered medical home to these challenges allows for concrete and specific strategies that may lead to increased patient safety, satisfaction, and resident learning and efficacy.

References

1. Shippee ND, Shah ND, May CR, Mair FS, Montori VM. Cumulative complexity: a functional, patient-centered model of patient complexity can improve research and practice. J Clin Epidemiol. 2012;65(10):1041–51. https://doi.org/10.1016/j.jclinepi.2012.05.005.
2. ACGME Program Requirements for Graduate Medical Education in Internal Medicine. https://www.acgme.org/globalassets/pfassets/programrequirements/140_internalmedicine_2021.pdf. Accessed 25 May 2022.
3. National Resident Matching Program, Results and Data: 2021 Main Residency Match. National Resident Matching Program; 2021.
4. O'Rourke P, Tseng E, Chacko K, Shalaby M, Cioletti A, Wright S. A National Survey of internal medicine primary care residency program directors. J Gen Intern Med. 2019;34(7):1207–12. https://doi.org/10.1007/s11606-019-04984-x.
5. Edwards ST, Kim H, Shull S, Hooker ER, Niederhausen M, Tuepker A. Quality of outpatient care with internal medicine residents vs attending physicians in veterans affairs primary care clinics. JAMA Intern Med. 2019;179(5):711–3. https://doi.org/10.1001/jamainternmed.2018.8624.
6. Healthy People 2030: Social Determinants of Health. https://health.gov/healthypeople/priority-areas/social-determinants-health. Accessed 25 May 2022.
7. Grant RW, Ashburner JM, Hong CS, Hong CC, Chang Y, Barry MJ, et al. Defining patient complexity from the primary care physician's perspective: a cohort study. Ann Intern Med. 2011;155(12):797–804. https://doi.org/10.7326/0003-4819-155-12-201112200-00001.
8. Manning E, Gagnon M. The complex patient: a concept clarification. Nurs Health Sci. 2017;19(1):13–21. https://doi.org/10.1111/nhs.12320.
9. Amat M, Glassman R, Basu N, Doolin J, Flier L, Gonzalez MR, et al. Defining the resident continuity clinic panel along patient outcomes: a health equity opportunity. J Gen Intern Med. 2021;36(9):2615–21. https://doi.org/10.1007/s11606-020-06420-x.

10. Rich E, Debra L, Libersky J, Parchman M. Coordinating care for adults with complex care needs in the patient-centered medical home: challenges and solutions white paper. Rockville, MD: Agency for Healthcare Research and Quality; 2012.
11. Hoel RW, Giddings Connolly RM, Takahashi PY. Polypharmacy management in older patients. Mayo Clin Proc. 2021;96(1):242–56. https://doi.org/10.1016/j.mayocp.2020.06.012.
12. Cong M, Chaisson J, Cantrell D, Mohundro BL, Carby M, Ford M, et al. Association of co-pay elimination with medication adherence and total cost. Am J Manag Care. 2021;27(6):249–54. https://doi.org/10.37765/ajmc.2021.88664.
13. Chang ET, Asch SM, Eng J, Gutierrez F, Denietolis A, Atkins D. What is the return on investment of caring for complex high-need, high-cost patients? J Gen Intern Med. 2021;36(11):3541–4. https://doi.org/10.1007/s11606-021-07110-y.
14. Epstein JA, Wu AW. Delivering complex care: designing for patients and physicians. J Gen Intern Med. 2021;36(3):772–4. https://doi.org/10.1007/s11606-020-06212-3.
15. Epstein JA, Cofrancesco J Jr, Beach MC, Bertram A, Hedian HF, Mixter S, et al. Effect of outpatient note templates on note quality: NOTE (Notation Optimization through Template Engineering) randomized clinical trial. J Gen Intern Med. 2021;36(3):580–4. https://doi.org/10.1007/s11606-020-06188-0.
16. Wright A, McCoy AB, Hickman TT, Hilaire DS, Borbolla D, Bowes WA 3rd, et al. Problem list completeness in electronic health records: a multi-site study and assessment of success factors. Int J Med Inform. 2015;84(10):784–90. https://doi.org/10.1016/j.ijmedinf.2015.06.011.

Chapter 28
Strategies for Optimizing Patient Satisfaction in an Academic Medical Practice

John S. Clark

Introduction

Resident clinic directors face a myriad of challenges today. They must simultaneously deliver high quality medical care to patients, meet resident educational requirements, and perform against increasingly ambitious financial and operational goals. To be successful both in the clinic setting and more broadly in the medical center, resident clinical directors require a broad set of competencies spanning clinical, operational, and educational domains. Indeed, this book and its diverse chapters illustrate the depth and breadth of this required skill set.

One area where clinic directors require foundational knowledge, but which may seem secondary to these other foci, is patient satisfaction. Clinic directors are accountable for the twin responsibilities of improving the satisfaction of patients in the clinic and equipping residents with the skills to interpret and act on patient feedback. Additionally, as the Accreditation Council for Graduate Medical Education (ACGME) mandates 360° resident evaluations and suggests including patient feedback, all clinic directors will benefit from a solid grasp of patient experience measurement and improvement. This chapter seeks to equip clinic directors with a base knowledge of what patient satisfaction is, why it is important, and how to measure and improve it in a resident clinic.

Outline

- History
- What is patient satisfaction
- Patient satisfaction in academic clinics
- Measuring patient satisfaction

J. S. Clark (✉)
UR Medicine Primary Care, University of Rochester Medical Center, Rochester, NY, USA
e-mail: johns_clark@urmc.rochester.edu

L. B. Lu et al. (eds.), *Leading an Academic Medical Practice*,
https://doi.org/10.1007/978-3-031-40273-9_28

- Four key strategies for improving patient satisfaction
- Conclusion

History and Evolution of Patient Satisfaction

Despite its prominence today, patient satisfaction, or more broadly patient experience, is a relatively new concept in health care. Market research using survey research emerged in the 1920s as a method to test advertising effectiveness. Later, George Gallup pioneered the use of scientific methods applied to survey results to assess and predict public opinion, famously predicting the election of Franklin D. Roosevelt in 1936. During the post–Second World War consumer boom of the 1950s, industry looked to market research to better understand their customers' preferences and gauge market opportunity.

By the mid-1980s, during the era of Total Quality Management, customer satisfaction took a firm hold. The leap to patient satisfaction occurred in 1985 when Notre Dame professors Irwin Press, a medical anthropologist, and Rod Ganey, a sociologist and statistician, launched Press Ganey, a health care survey research company [1]. Starting with a few hospitals, the business grew as hospitals saw the potential for tracking their patient satisfaction and comparing it against others.

A few years following Press Ganey's launch, the federal government made its first foray into patient satisfaction. The Centers for Medicare and Medicaid Services (CMS), in partnership with the Agency for Healthcare Research Quality (AHRQ), developed the Hospital Consumer Assessment of Healthcare Providers and Systems (HCAHPS) survey [2]. A year later, CMS and AHRQ launched a survey to measure satisfaction of patients in physician offices, called Clinician and Group Survey, CG-CAHPS. CMS also developed a separate CAHPS survey for measuring and reporting patient experiences with health plans [2]. With the launch of these three standardized surveys, CMS created a novel, powerful measurement apparatus to report on patient experience in America.

In 2001 with the publication of the ground breaking report Crossing the Quality Chasm by the Institute of Medicine, interest in patient experience accelerated [3]. Crossing the Quality Chasm made an urgent argument to improve quality. Providers and health systems, the report argued, must focus on six improvement efforts to address deficiencies and to position health care for success in the twenty-first century. These improvements, the authors wrote, would create a health-care system that is safe, effective, patient-centered, timely, efficient, and equitable [3]. The concept of patient-centeredness was born with this publication, which was described as "providing care that is respectful of and responsive to individual patient preference, needs, and values and ensuring that patient value guide all clinical decisions" [4]. Well-designed patient surveys and other research methods that could capture these dimensions came to be demanded by hospitals, clinics, and health plans.

Looking back, it is clear now that the confluence of patient-centeredness, the federal mandate to collect, report, and compare patient satisfaction coupled with the launch of market research infrastructure created by for-profit research companies, gave rise to the modern-day focus on evaluating patient experience in the United States.

What Is Patient Satisfaction?

Ask any faculty, resident, or health-care administrator what patient satisfaction is, or how to measure it, you will rarely get a consistent response. This lack of consensus reflects that patient satisfaction is somewhat illusive and opaque. This is so because patient satisfaction is largely subjective and depends on the patient perceptions relative to their expectations [5]. This makes the measurement of patient satisfaction through standardizes survey instruments tricky. Ultimately, however, patient satisfaction is interwoven into the fabric of patient-centeredness, which is at the heart of medicine. It is largely about empathy, caring, and communication [4].

So, how can this experience be explored, understood, and improved? Since patient satisfaction is not directly observable, patient satisfaction surveys seek to capture the principal patient experience across several touchpoints of the patient journey [5]. These data are often collected through the CG-CAHPS survey tool and through proprietary surveys developed by companies such as Press Ganey, NRC Health, and others. Today, a vast commercial industry of survey vendors exists to survey patients, tabulate results, and deliver them to their health care clients.

The Importance of Patient Satisfaction

While there are critics of health care's focus on patient satisfaction, there is evidence that patient experience is profoundly important (Fig. 28.1). Patient satisfaction has been found to be associated with clinical quality and risk-adjusted inpatient mortality rates for patients with acute myocardial infarction [6]. Other studies have found that the better the patient experience—even more than adherence to clinical guidelines—the better the outcome [7]. After considering a wide range perceived benefits and shortcoming of patient satisfaction and the available research, Manary and colleagues conclude that both the theory and evidence suggest that patient satisfaction measures are "robust, distinctive indicators of care quality" [7].

Another reason patient experience should be important to physicians is its link to Reduced Malpractice Claims. In a study of the association of inpatient physician satisfaction scores and risk management episodes, Stelfox and colleagues found that when compared to top-rated physicians, mid-tertile physicians experienced a 25% higher rate of malpractice lawsuits [8].

Health system administrators pay close attention to patient satisfaction because not only do regulators believe satisfaction and quality are linked, but payment for hospital and physician services is tied to patient satisfaction performance. In 2012, the Accountable Care Act linked HCAHPS scores with value-based payment. This

Fig. 28.1 Positive associations with patient experience

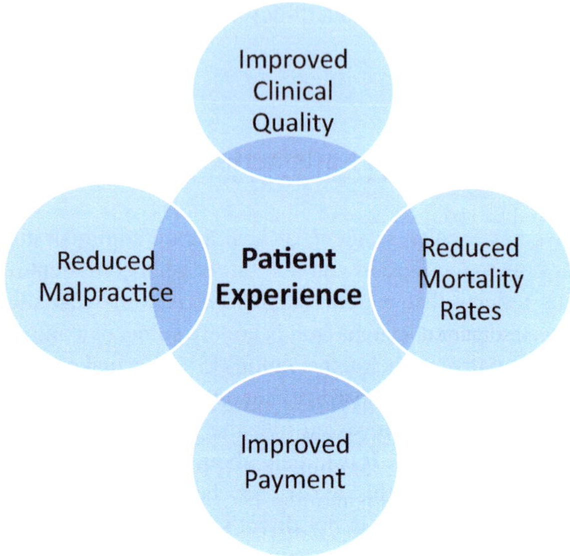

program allows Medicare to withhold 2% of all Medicare payments to fund an incentive pool designed to reward high-quality health care, measured in part by HCAHPS scores. CMS publishes the results of both HCAHPS and CG-CAHPS survey, and this too has spurred health systems to accelerate improvement in scores. Today, most large national health plans integrate satisfaction performance into their value-based contracts for both government-funded health and commercial plans, rewarding doctors and hospitals for top satisfaction performance.

Another reason why administrators care about patient satisfaction scores is that marketing departments can use these data to differentiate a hospital, service line, or physician group from competitors. In fact, several for-profit companies created business units to identify top performing health-care entities and then license an award for use in advertising to support claims of being a top performer. For example, JD Power—best known for its ratings in the auto industry—recognized and certified hospitals as "Distinguished Hospitals" who performed well on their patient survey.

Patient Satisfaction in Academic Clinics

The most important reason that clinic directors must make patient satisfaction a priority is that patient experience is inexorably intertwined with quality, patient outcomes, and patient-centeredness. Quality patient care, the Institute of Medicine argues, is safe, effective, timely, patient-centered, equitable, and designed to improve population health, while reducing per capita costs [3].

ACGME Competencies

In its foundational philosophy, the ACGME underscores the importance of patient-centered care through the core competencies and milestones. The ACGME states, "Residents must be able to provide patient care that is compassionate, appropriate and effective for the treatment of health problems and the promotion of health." One of the six core competencies established by the ACGME, Interpersonal and Communication Skills, requires that residents demonstrate skill at creating a therapeutic relationship with patients, families, and colleagues in the health-care team. The ACGME states, "Residents must demonstrate interpersonal and communication skills that result in the effective exchange of information and collaboration with patients, their families and health professionals. This includes communicating effectively with patient and families across a broad range of socioeconomic and cultural backgrounds" [9].

Residency program directors and the residency's Clinical Competency Committee (CCC) are also required to provide continuous feedback on resident performance against all six core competencies and specialty-specific milestones. ACGME mandates that "... residency program faculty provide frequent feedback throughout the course of each rotation. Further, all programs must provide an objective performance evaluation based on the competencies and the specialty specific milestones. These evaluations must use multiple evaluators, including patients, faculty members, peers, professional staff members and self" [9].

Patient-experience feedback, therefore, has emerged as an important dimension of resident education and development.

Measuring Patient Satisfaction

Patients today have almost unlimited ways of publicly sharing their experience with their doctor through social media channels. Likewise, hospitals and physician practices can choose to collect patient feedback through several means: patient advisory groups, patient focus groups, custom surveys of resident patients, and national surveys of the patient experience.

Challenges Collecting Patient Satisfaction for Resident Physicians

Despite these multiple channels for collecting patient feedback, academic medical centers and resident practices face unique obstacles to collecting patient satisfaction data and performing well. Patients' ease of access to the medical center or clinic—such as the vagaries of public transportation, poor way finding, inconvenient hours of operation—all shape the patient experience before the patient sets foot in the clinic. The model of care, which relies on resident physicians rather than faculty as the primary provider, may impair continuity and the development of longer term doctor–patient relationships. Effective communication with patients due to health literacy, cultural, or language factors may also influence the patient's perception of the quality of provider communication. In addition to these challenges, many academic centers report problems with rates of survey completion. Additionally, it is not given that the hospital's survey vendor will capture data by resident, or if they do, that the vendor will have sufficient sample size by resident to draw reliable conclusions.

Even if patient experience data are available, many residency programs do not make sharing these data a priority. A study conducted by the Council of Residency Directors Emergency Medicine found that less than one-third of emergency medicine residency programs share any patient satisfaction data with residents. Equally concerning, only 27% of these residencies have dedicated curricula on patient experience [10, 11].

Ambulatory CAHPS

The CAHPS platform of surveys is the most widely used standard in measuring consumer experience with health plans, hospitals, and providers. The CAHPS surveys share two goals: to develop standardized surveys that organizations can use to collect comparable information on patient's experience of care; and to generate tools and resources to support the dissemination and use of comparative survey results to inform the public and improve health-care quality.

The CG-CAHPS survey measures patient experience across four domains known as composite measures: access to care, communication between the provider and patients, care coordination, and customer service (Table 28.1) [2].

Table 28.1 Core composite measure in CG-CAHPS

Access to care	Getting timely appointments, care, and information
Communication between patients and providers	How well providers communicate with patients
Care coordination	Providers use of information to coordinate patient care
Customer service	Office staff courtesy and respect

Interpretation of Patient Satisfaction Measures and CG-CAHPS

Health systems will typically receive reports that show data for a current and prior period to allow comparisons. Results will often be reported in a "top box" format, which is the percent of patients who select the "best" response option available. For example, when patients are asked to choose "yes—definitely, yes—somewhat" or "no" in response to a question about whether the provider listened carefully, the top box score represents the percent of patients who select "yes, definitely." Another common report feature is benchmarking, which may compare your clinic's performance to other clinics in your health system, state, or nationally.

While interpreting the results, it is important to be aware of some common limitations of patient satisfaction survey results. Clinic directors should discuss with their survey vendor or quality office:

- Are the data representative of the clinic population? (often these data are not weighted to correct for over- and underrepresented groups)
- Is the sample size adequate to draw reliable conclusions? This is especially important for resident patient panels and when comparing provider performance.
- What potential biases are present due perhaps to online or paper data collection?

Four Key Strategies for Improving Patient Satisfaction

"Where should I begin?" is a question frequently asked by leaders seeking to boost their patient experience scores. This question is not surprising because patient satisfaction reports often identify multiply areas for improvement. Should you focus on sharpening the customer service skills of your receptionists or should your priority be to reduce wait times? Which is more important: improving perceptions of how providers explain things in a way that patients clearly understand or improving performance on after-hour hours phone access? Where, you may wonder, can you achieve the greatest lift in overall patient experience? Table 28.2 identifies four key strategies for improving patient satisfaction.

Focus on Key Drivers of Patient Experience

A powerful strategy to improve performance is to focus on the key drivers of your patients' experience. Begin by identifying those elements of a patient visit that correlate highly with the overall patient satisfaction. This will reveal the relative importance of different domains (such as access to care or physician communication) or

Table 28.2 Key strategies for improving patient satisfaction

Focus on key drivers of patient experience
• Identify the areas that are most important to patients and are in greatest need of improvement
Create a culture focused on patients and the care team
• Culture is at the very heart of the patient experience
• Leaders must cultivate a positive culture that is visible
• Engaged employees are the driving force for delivering a positive patient experience
Improve communication
• Effective patient-centered communication is a fundamental element of patient satisfaction, as well as a core ACGME competency
Deliver training and feedback
• Establish a culture that emphases understanding and sharing patient experience data

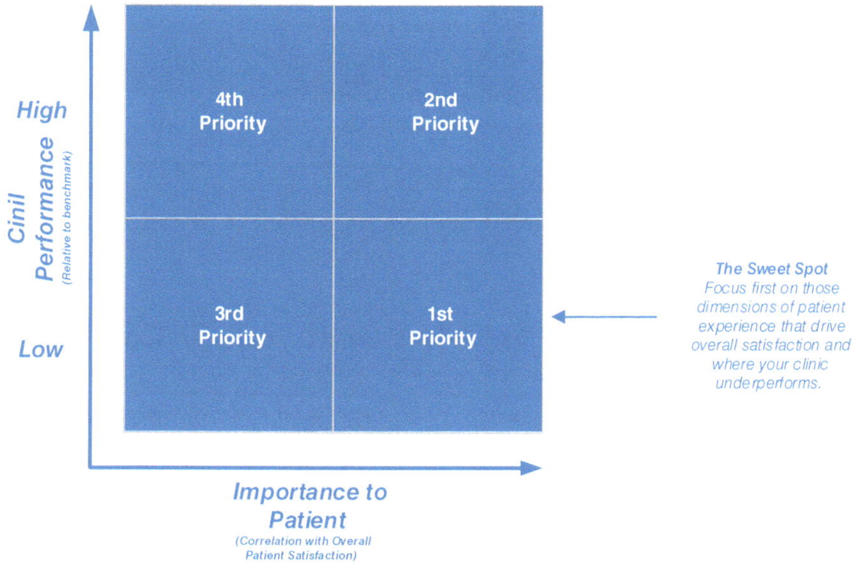

Fig. 28.2 Identify key drivers

individual performance metrics (such as clerk helpfulness or having phone calls returned the same day) to their overall experience with your clinic. Once you have identified those dimensions of the experience that are most correlated with overall satisfaction, you now know what drives their overall experience.

The next step is to identify the "sweet spot" for improvement, which is a key driver where your clinic's performance needs improvement. By plotting different dimensions of patient experience on the map, it helps reveal which dimension(s) of experience, if improved, will have the greatest overall impact (Fig. 28.2). Armed with this information, you can focus with laser precision on those aspects of patient experience that will deliver the greatest impact on your overall performance.

With an improvement goal identified, the next step is to identify the intervention. The good news is that because CG-CAHPS is a standardized tool, there exist multiple strategies for improving most measures on the survey. AHRQ explores many of these strategies. Your survey vendor also likely maintains a portfolio of improvement strategies for each measure. Of course, the medical center's quality office will likely have a deep knowledge of strategies that have delivered results elsewhere in your organization.

Create a Culture Focused on Patients and the Care Team

Foundational to driving performance improvement in patient experience is a clinic culture that focuses on patients and the care team. A culture that is both patient- and team-centered does not happen by accident. In fact, culture is a critical choice of clinic leadership that is at the very heart of patient experience [12]. Expressed another way, culture trumps strategy.

To shape patient experience in a meaningful way, culture requires three essential ingredients. First, it requires that leadership define its mission (why we are here), vision (what we aspire to be), and values (the rules we live by). This needs to broadly appeal to both staff, residents, and faculty. Taken together, these statements should help everyone in the clinic to answer the question of why I am here and connect one's work to a higher purpose [12].

The second important element of culture is a strong and visible desire to know more about the patient experience. Certainly, conducting patient surveys and sharing this information with the residents, faculty, and staff is one vital step. However, there are many other tools that could help reveal a more comprehensive and nuanced picture of how the resident clinic delivers against the goals of patient-centered care. These goals include how well the care team is meeting clinical expectations, but also how well your clinic meets the emotional, mental, spiritual, social, and financial needs of patients. Certainly, the CG-CAHPS survey will fall short of assessing these psychosocial dimensions. Residency directors should consider creating a patient council for the clinic, hosting a focus group with patients or conducting one-on-one interviews with patients. These types of qualitative tools will greatly enhance your ability to view the clinic experience through your patients' lenses.

The third essential ingredient for a patient-focused culture is attentiveness to the engagement of your health-care team. Outside of health care, employee engagement has long been identified as the single most potent driver of patient experience. Many case studies exist on how companies and brands that consumers love—Southwest Airlines, Patagonia, Whole Foods and Harley Davidson—foster employee engagement. Regardless of the industry, engaged employees are the driving force for delivering a positive patient experience.

Any strategy to promote employee engagement begins with an assessment. Your medical center may conduct these studies (often by the same companies who measure patient satisfaction). There are also resources—including a brief, one question assessment tool—that provide easy, intuitive ways to do engagement self-assessments in any business, including a resident clinic [13].

A crucial step in improving staff engagement is to have powerful values, as described above, that link to expected behaviors of the care team. As Greg Lederman—an authority on customer experience and patient engagement—writes, it is not enough to just announce your values and culture, leaders must make if visible [13]. Your hospital or clinics' values or guiding principles are invisible to employees unless your employees know how to act on them. "Companies that make the effort to define the behaviors behind their core values ... create stronger work culture that power a more consistent [and positive] customer experience" [13].

Improve Communication

While all dimensions of the patient experience play a role in shaping a patient's perception of clinic, most often physician communication percolates to the top or near the top of key drivers of patient experience. Improving communication between residents and their patients will pay patient experience dividends and prepare your residents for success.

Patients' most frequent complaints are that physicians do not listen to their concern, care about their problems, or provide enough information about their treatment [14]. It should not be surprising that the quality of physician communication represents the single largest domain in the CG-CAHPS survey. Patients are asked to rate six dimensions of their provider's communication: easy-to-understand explanations, listening carefully, easy-to-understand instructions, knowledge of important medical history, demonstrates respect, and spends enough time with the patient.

Focusing on communication will also pay rewards beyond patient experience improvement. In addition to their alignment with ACGME core competencies, communication skills have a positive impact—treatment adherence and self-management of chronic diseases [15]. Compelling evidence exist that communication improves clinical outcomes in the management of diabetes, hypertension, and cancer. Conversely, poor communication is linked with higher malpractice claims [15].

Deliver Training and Feedback

The use of feedback has long been a vital component of medical student and resident learning. Almost always, achieving high patient satisfaction entails the combination of patient satisfaction training with feedback to the care team. Allenbaugh and colleagues demonstrated that a curriculum comprised of didactics, video, and role-play at the University of Pittsburgh for internal medicine residents and nurses was associated with significant improvements in communication skills across several HCAHPS domains for both doctors and nurses [16].

In another study, conducted with internal medicine residents at the University of California, Los Angeles, researchers demonstrated an improvement in patient satisfaction following implementation of a program that comprised education on improving patient–physician communication skills, frequent individualized patient feedback, and an incentive (movie tickets, popcorn, and a drink) along with recognition [17]. In this study, volunteers—armed with a photograph of the resident—interviewed inpatients using one of two surveys. Survey data were shared weekly with the residency program director as well as the interns and residents. In response to this training and feedback, measurable improvement was made across multiple HCAHPS communication dimensions, including physician courtesy and respect, listening carefully, and explaining in ways the patients could understand. Moreover, there was a significant improvement in the percentage of patients that would definitely recommend the hospital to their friends and family.

The lessons for residency directors are twofold. First, to improve patient experience (and align with ACGME guidelines), one must measure patient experience at the resident and intern level. As some hospital-wide patient satisfaction measurement programs may not provide this level of granularity, the residency program may need to develop its own survey or collect data using the CG-CAHPS. The second lesson is that these programs to support patient satisfaction need not be expensive. They do require, however, a culture in the resident clinic that places an emphasis on understanding and sharing patient experience data.

Conclusion

The demands placed on resident clinic directors today are immense. ACGME sets high expectations for education, training, and evaluation of residents. Lofty financial performance, productivity, and quality goals also place considerable stress on the clinic director. Patient satisfaction, however, must be a priority for resident clinic directors if they seek to have a positive impact on quality, patient-centeredness, and resident education and development.

References

1. Siegriest RB. Patient satisfaction: history, myths, and misperceptions. Am Med Assoc J Ethics. 2013;15(11):982–7.
2. The CAHPS Ambulatory Care Improvement Guide: Practical strategies for improving patient experience. Agency for Healthcare Research and Quality, Rockville, MD. https://www.ahrq.gov/cahps/quality-improvement/improvement-guide/improvement-guide.html.
3. Institute of Medicine Committee on Quality of Health Care in America. Crossing the Quality Chasm: A New Health System for the 21st Century. 2001, National Academies Press (US). Copyright 2001 by the National Academy of Sciences. All rights reserved.: Washington, DC.

4. Boissy A. Getting to patient-centered care in a post-covid-19 digital world: a proposal of novel surveys, methodology, and patient experience maturity assessment. NEJM Catalyst: Innovations in Care Delivery. 2020.
5. Patient Satisfaction Surveys. NEJM Catalyst: Innovations in Care Delivery; 2018.
6. Glickman SW, et al. Patient satisfaction and its relationship with clinical quality and inpatient mortality in acute myocardial infarction. Circ Cardiovasc Qual Outcomes. 2010;3(2):188–95.
7. Manary MP, et al. The patient experience and health outcomes. N Engl J Med. 2013;368(3):201–3.
8. Stelfox HT, et al. The relation of patient satisfaction with complaints against physicians and malpractice lawsuits. Am J Med. 2005;118(10):1126–33.
9. ACGME Internal Medicine Program Requirements; 2020. https://www.acgme.org/globalassets/pfassets/programrequirements/140_internalmedicine_2020.pdf.
10. Walker LE, et al. Progression of emergency medicine resident patient experience scores by level of training. J Patient Exp. 2019;6(3):210–5.
11. London KS, et al. Teaching the emergency department patient experience: needs assessment from the CORD-EM task force. West J Emerg Med. 2017;18(1):56–9.
12. Berrett B, Spiegelman P. The role of organization culture in a positive patient experience: a leadership imperative. The Beryl Institute; 2012. https://www.theberylinstitute.org.
13. Lederman G. Engaged! Outbehave Your Competition to Create Customers for Life. Ashland, OR: Evolve Publishing; 2013.
14. Hickson GB, et al. Obstetricians' prior malpractice experience and patients' satisfaction with care. JAMA. 1994;272(20):1583–7.
15. Levinson W, Lesser CS, Epstein RM. Developing physician communication skills for patient-centered care. Health Aff (Millwood). 2010;29(7):1310–8.
16. Allenbaugh J, et al. A brief communication curriculum improves resident and nurse communication skills and patient satisfaction. J Gen Intern Med. 2019;34(7):1167–73.
17. Banka G, et al. Improving patient satisfaction through physician education, feedback, and incentives. J Hosp Med. 2015;10(8):497–502.

Chapter 29
Quality Improvement Projects and Indicators

Emily Fondahn and Peter McDonnell

Introduction

Recognition of the significant gaps between the actual care patients routinely experience and the ideal standard of care has led to an increased focus on quality of care at all levels of our health-care system. Individual practitioners, clinics, and hospital systems are increasingly using quality improvement (QI) methods to increase the safety and effectiveness of care. Payors are requiring more information on quality metrics and providing incentives for improvement, while accrediting bodies are requiring quality improvement education to be a part of physician training. Academic physicians are in an ideal role to lead quality improvement initiatives due to the unique combination of medical knowledge, direct patient care, and administrative roles they often hold. It is imperative that academic practices model the implementation of quality improvement projects and engage their residents in quality improvement activities so that they are prepared to lead future quality initiatives.

Outline
- Quality improvement background
  - Healthcare quality aims
  - Ambulatory quality metrics and programs

E. Fondahn (✉)
Department of Medicine, University of Missouri, Columbia, MO, USA
e-mail: efhfr@health.missouri.edu

P. McDonnell
Department of Medicine, Washington University School of Medicine, St. Louis, MO, USA
e-mail: pmcdonnell@wustl.edu

L. B. Lu et al. (eds.), *Leading an Academic Medical Practice*,
https://doi.org/10.1007/978-3-031-40273-9_29

- Designing a quality improvement project
  - Model for improvement
  - Root cause analysis
  - Quality measures
  - Setting an aim
  - Involving interested parties
- Engaging residents in quality improvement
  - Models for resident engagement
  - Clinical learning environment review (CLER)
- Conclusion

Quality Improvement Background

In 2001, the Institute of Medicine (IOM) published a groundbreaking report, *Crossing the Quality Chasm*, which stated that the US health-care delivery system does not provide consistent, high-quality medical care to all people [1]. Patients do not always receive the necessary components of care, yet often receive care that is unnecessary. The IOM proposed six aims for health care (Table 29.1).

Since the publishing of *Crossing the Quality Chasm*, improvements have been made within the US health-care system; yet significant gaps still remain. Despite spending more on health care than other countries, the United States continues to have worse health outcomes than international peers [2].

Table 29.1 IOM aims for health care [1]

1. *Safe*: avoiding injuries to patient from the care that is intended to help them. Examples include preventing health-care associated infections or making medication errors.
2. *Effective*: providing services based on scientific knowledge to all who could benefit and refraining from providing services to those not likely to benefit. Examples include screening patients with diabetes for retinopathy or not performing colonoscopy screening on patients with a limited life expectancy.
3. *Patient-centered*: providing care that is respectful of and responsive to individual patient preferences, needs, and values and ensuring that patient values guide all clinical decisions. Examples include discussing benefits and risks of anticoagulation medications for a patient with atrial fibrillation or discussing goals of care for terminally ill patients.
4. *Timely*: reducing waits and sometimes harmful delays for those who receive and those who give care. Examples include reducing the time for patients to establish care with a primary care physician (PCP) or being able to see PCP quickly for urgent conditions.
5. *Efficient*: avoiding waste, including waste of equipment, supplies, ideas/human potential, and energy. Examples of efficient care include having patients go to a PCP rather than the Emergency Room for care of chronic medical conditions or streamlining forms to reduce paperwork.
6. *Equitable*: providing care that does not vary in quality because of personal characteristics such as gender, ethnicity, geographic location, and socioeconomic status. Examples include eliminating racial disparities for cancer screening or reducing variance in care based on geography.

In 2007, the Institute for Healthcare Improvement (IHI) developed the Triple Aim to address quality and cost in health care [3]. The framework was subsequently expanded to include improving the work–life balance of health-care team members with the recognition that widespread issues of burnout can impact patient safety and quality [4]. The Quadruple Aim is composed of four components necessary to optimize a health system performance:

1. Improving the patient experience of care, including quality of care, access, and reliability
2. Improving the health of the population
3. Reducing the per capita cost of health care
4. Improving the work–life of health-care providers

Primary care has been an area of focus within health-care redesign given that it is often the first point of contact for patients in the health-care system. Application of quality improvement principles can allow primary care practices to improve efficiency, optimize clinical outcomes, and reduce costs. To maximize quality efforts, health-care systems need to expand the reach of quality initiatives to include both individuals and populations.

HEDIS Measures

To support quality improvement initiatives, several measures exist to gauge quality at individual and population levels. The Healthcare Effectiveness Data and Information Set (HEDIS) is a set of health-care performance metrics used by the majority of health plans in the United States to measure performance [5]. The HEDIS metrics allow for the comparison of health plans and to benchmark performance on a variety of clinical measures, such as diabetes, hypertension, and cancer screening. The HEDIS data can be used by employers, consultants, and consumers to select the best health plan for their needs. At the clinic level, the data is also a useful starting point for identifying areas for quality improvement opportunities and tracking the success of quality improvement initiatives.

MACRA and MIPS

One of the more definite attempts to shift toward a quality-based health-care system is the Medicare Access and CHIP Reauthorization Act of 2015 (MACRA), which revamped Medicare's reimbursement system for outpatient care. According to the MACRA, providers participating in Medicare must participate in one of two Quality Payment Programs: the Merit-based Incentive Payment System (MIPS) or the Advanced Alternative Payment Model (AAPM) [6]. The MIPS has four categories, including quality, cost, advancing care information, and improvement activities, and requires reporting of quality measures and improvement activities. High-performing providers receive a positive adjustment to their reimbursement, while poor performers will receive a negative adjustment. The AAPMs are programs that, in addition to particular technology and quality requirements, include assuming more financial risk in exchange for a bonus payment.

Designing a Quality Improvement Project

Quality improvement projects can develop in a variety of ways. Sometimes an event causes a problem to become apparent, and other times there is a desire to improve an outcome even if there is not a clear problem with the current process. Regardless of how the project arises, there should be defined steps to investigate an issue, set a goal, make a change, and measure outcomes. Keeping best practices in mind for each of these steps will help avoid common pitfalls and maximize the likelihood of success.

Model for Improvement

The "Model for Improvement" is a framework commonly used for quality improvement projects (Fig. 29.1) [7]. Three framing questions are combined with Plan-Do-Study-Act (PDSA) cycles [8]. The three questions set an aim, identify measures, and choose a change to study. The PDSA cycle is the process of trialing a change by planning it, performing the change, studying the results, and using that information to plan your next action. The goal of PDSA cycles is to be able to relatively quickly test promising changes on a small scale and then refine or combine those changes as needed before implementing them on a broader scale. The Institute of Health has a wealth of resources that adapt this model specifically to the health-care setting [9].

Root Cause Analysis and Identifying Changes

Understanding the current system and potential points of failure is a critical and necessary step at the beginning of any quality improvement project. Studying a problem to determine the underpinning issues is called a root cause analysis. There are many tools that can support root cause analyses, including cause-and-effect diagrams (aka fishbone diagrams) and driver diagrams (Table 29.2). Each tool has advantages and disadvantages and it is usually beneficial to utilize multiple tools for each issue.

After identifying the underlying issues, the next step is to propose changes to help resolve those issues. Multiple methods can be used to assist with change ideas. A literature review to learn how others have approached similar issues can be helpful in generating ideas and reviewing evidence of impact from a change. Brainstorming techniques can assist the group in developing novel ideas. Peers at

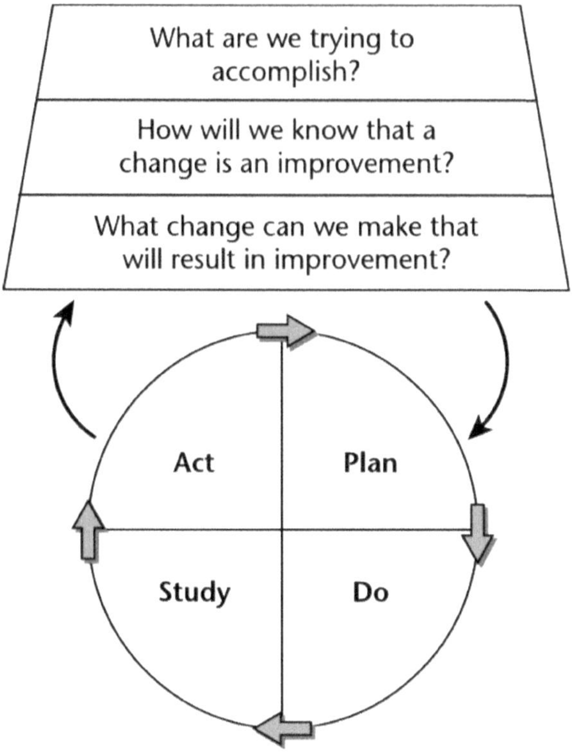

Fig. 29.1 The Model for Improvement. Reprinted with permission from Langley GL, Moen R, Nolan KM, Nolan TW, Norman CL, Provost LP. The Improvement Guide: A Practical Approach to Enhancing Organizational Performance, 2nd ed. San Francisco: Jossey-Bass Publishers; 2009

Table 29.2 Common root cause analysis tools

Tool	Brief description	Comments
5 Whys	Recursively ask "Why?" five times to delve into an issue	Simple and easy, but results are not reproducible and may tunnel in on one aspect of a problem
Cause-and-effect diagram, aka fishbone diagram	Breaks a problem into major categories and graphically sorts causes and sub-causes	Helps identify the causes leading to an effect and their relationship to each other in a structured way
Driver diagram	Identifies the primary "drivers" of an issue, the secondary drivers behind those, and ideas that can affect the drivers	Similar to a cause-and-effect diagram, tends to be a little less structured and more flexible in categories
Flowchart	Maps out all of the steps involved in a process	Helps clarify the current process and identify areas of concern in the process
Failure modes and effect analysis	Systemically reviews a process to identify areas that can fail and the effect of a failure	Can be used proactively to assess for potential problems before they occur. Often valuable before implementing a new process

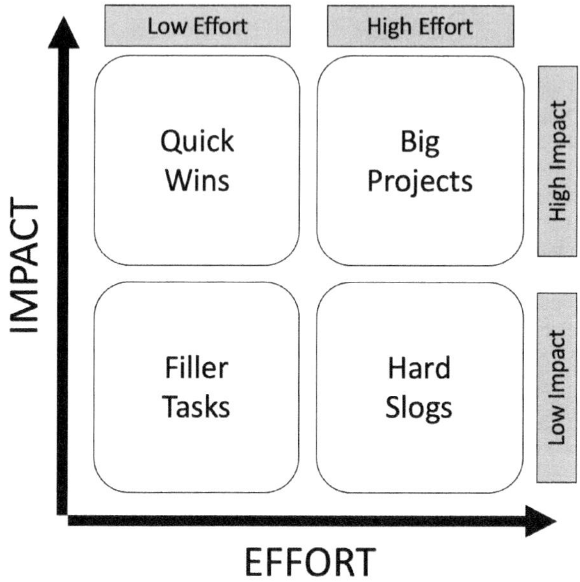

Fig. 29.2 The action priority matrix

other institutions are a useful resource to learn about how they identified and addressed a problem. The team will then need to prioritize change ideas by considering the likely impact of a change versus the effort required to implement the change. Tools like the action priority matrix and the payoff matrix can assist with this classification (Fig. 29.2). The priority matrix can help identify changes that will result in the highest impact with the least effort.

Measurement in Quality Improvement

Measurement is key to knowing if a change has led to an improvement. Health-care measurement generally uses a combination of structural, process, and outcome measures. Table 29.3 describes these types of measures and provides examples of each [10]. Additionally, balancing measures are used to monitor for any unintentional changes caused by the project, usually to ensure that there are not any negative effects of the intervention on the system. Metrics can be obtained through multiple sources, such as claims data, patient surveys, clinician surveys, practice surveys, electronic health record reports, or chart audits. Collecting and analyzing these metrics can create a large administrative burden. When possible, measures that can be automated or easily collected should be used to ease this administrative burden.

Table 29.3 Types of measurements to assess quality

Types	General description	Health-care description	Clinic example
Structural measures	Quantify available resources	Quantify available resources of providers and health-care systems	Number of diabetes educators in a primary care clinic
Process measures	Identify the process steps necessary to achieve the desired outcome	Quantify the diagnostic and therapeutic processes used to care for patients	Number of diabetic patients with a HbA1c checked every 3 months
Outcome measures	Measure the degree to which consumer specifications are met	Quantify the health status of patients	Number of diabetic patients with a HbA1c less than 7
Balancing measures	Quantify if changes to one process worsens other processes	Measure changes in baseline health characteristics aside from the primary outcome	Number of diabetic patients who develop hypoglycemia

Adapted from Institute of Healthcare Improvement, Science of Improvement: Establishing Measures. http://www.ihi.org/resources/Pages/HowtoImprove/ScienceofImprovementEstablishingMeasures.aspx

Developing an Aim

Every project needs an aim or goal. Developing aims can start as little more than a general topic when first considering a project, but they should become specific as the project evolves. Having a clear aim helps keep the team focused on the goal of the project, assists with quantitatively tracking progress, and helps avoid inadvertently backing away from the goal. A commonly used mnemonic for creating strong aims is SMART: Specific, Measurable, Actionable, Realistic, and Timely [11]. For example, a SMART aim would be: "We will increase our rate of screening for colorectal cancer clinic wide by 20% within 12 months."

Involving Interested Parties

Most projects will have multiple interested parties that need to be identified along with the essential project participants. Depending on the size and scope of the project, interested parties may all work in the clinic or include other departments, such as the laboratory or Emergency Department. The team should include someone who is familiar with and can represent each area. This inclusion of all the relevant perspectives will help with project design and generate wider support for the project. Team members can have varying roles from project design to day-to-day implementation to technical expertise, but the responsibility of team members should be clearly defined.

Resident Considerations

Including resident physicians in quality improvement is essential to the success of projects in academic medical practices. Resident physicians are frontline workers who can offer the necessary insight to effectively implement quality improvement initiatives. Including residents, however, can be challenging due to residents' competing clinical responsibilities and complex schedules. To accommodate resident physicians, systems should be established to regularly reorient residents to the project when they rotate through clinic. In addition, the time periods for quality improvement interventions may need to be lengthened. Multiyear projects should plan to accommodate graduating and incoming residents.

Engaging Residents in Quality Improvement

In 2003, the Accreditation Council for Graduate Medical Education (ACGME) added systems-based practice (SBP) and practice-based learning and improvement (PBLI) as part of the six major competencies in medical training [12]. Competency in SBP includes understanding complex systems and the physician's role navigating them for the benefit of patients [13]. For a resident, engagement in SBP could include participating in a clinic QI project, reporting a patient safety event, or adeptly navigating the patient through a complex transition of care. Practice-based learning and improvement encompasses a trainee's ability to reflect on their personal practice, identify opportunities for improvement and create effective plans to improve [14]. Examples of PBLI in residency education include reviewing practice panel-level data for diabetes and making changes in daily practice to improve diabetes metrics. Creating opportunities for residents to engage in QI in clinic can improve patient outcomes as well as be an opportunity to assess residents in these milestones.

Residents, as frontline physicians, are vital members to the clinic's quality improvement team. However, a struggle often exists to successfully engage residents in meaningful quality improvement work. Creating alignment between health system priorities, patient care needs, and resident workflow is critical [15]. The goal is to have resident physicians be part of high-functioning teams that work on projects aligned with clinical site priorities [16]. Table 29.4 depicts models for resident involvement in QI projects [16]. Initiatives that are picked by residents and focus on their patient panel may lead to a small improvement for their patients, but may not be sustainable or generalizable across the clinic. Alternatively, clinics may pick priority areas, then require residents to focus on one of those priorities for their project. Regardless of the project, engaging the clinical leadership and interprofessional team members can lead to stronger interventions that are sustainable over time. Projects that align with the health system and clinical site priorities will likely have the most administrative support, buy-in, data, and resources.

Table 29.4 Models for resident involvement in QI projects

QI project	Description	Involvement of interprofessional care team	Alignment with site priorities	Impact
Individual resident project	Residents choose own QI project with little clinic engagement	Low	Low	Limited: Few sustainable improvements
Small shared projects (resident-directed)	Residents choose QI project and engage clinic staff	High	Low	Moderate: May have some sustained improvements, often small "Just-do-it" projects
Small shared projects (clinic-directed)	Residents choose project from clinic priorities	Variable	High	Limited: May lack engagement from residents since less autonomy to choose project
Clinic-based projects	Residents join interprofessional team	High	High	High: More resources to support project

Challenges to quality improvement work include faculty time, faculty expertise, funding, multiple competing educational and clinical demands, variable participation by a subset of residents, and limitations from the electronic health record for aggregating data and providing performance reports [17]. For residents, barriers to engaging in quality improvement work included challenges with understanding the vision for certain QI initiatives, lack of knowledge for QI methodologies, a sense that resident contributions are not valued, and challenges prioritizing QI work with other tasks [18]. Clear goals set by clinic leadership can help create alignment among residents, faculty, and clinic staff, allowing interprofessional teams to focus on projects that will have the most impact rather than multiple small individual projects by residents that may not be sustainable.

Clinical Learning Environment Review (CLER)

In 2012, the ACGME created the CLER initiative to explore and understand the clinical learning environment in which trainees learn and practice [19]. The CLER initiative aims to improve how clinical sites engage physician trainees in learning to provide safe and high-quality patient care [20]. The CLER program addresses the following six areas:

1. Patient Safety
2. Healthcare Quality
3. Care Transitions

4. Supervision
5. Duty Hours/Fatigue Management and Mitigation
6. Professionalism

The CLER initiative revealed that there is often lack of coordination of Patient Safety and Quality Improvement (PSQI) activities across institutions. For example, resident QI projects may not align with the clinical practice site's overall goals. Additionally, different residency programs within one institution may have different patient safety and quality improvement goals and curricula, hindering the potential to collaborate and standardize. Overall, the CLER initiative highlights the importance of engaging residents in quality improvement and provides leverage for academic medical practices to develop PSQI programs that involve the trainees.

Conclusion

Academic medical practices have the vital role of both providing excellent patient care and training future physicians. A culture of continuous learning and quality improvement creates a rich clinical learning environment that ideally improves patient outcomes and maximizes resident learning. Residents and faculty should collaborate with interprofessional teams and leadership to advance the quality improvement activities within a clinic. At a minimum, practices should provide QI training for residents and faculty, identify key areas of improvement and barriers to success, and develop quality goals that are reviewed regularly [21]. Practices should strive to realize the Quadruple Aim to improve the health of their patients, enhance patient experience, reduce costs, improve team member well-being.

References

1. Institute of Medicine (IOM). Crossing the Quality Chasm: A New Health System for the 21st Century. Washington DC: National Academy Press; 2001.
2. Squires D, Anderson C. U.S. Health Care from a Global Perspective: Spending, Use of Services, Prices and Health in 13 Countries. The Commonwealth Fund, October 2015.
3. Bisognano M, Kenney C. Pursuing the triple aim: seven innovators show the way to better care, better health, and lower costs. San Francisco, CA: Jossey-Bass Publishers; 2012.
4. Bodenheimer T, Sinsky C. From triple to quadruple aim. Ann Fam Med. 2013;12(6):573–6.
5. HEDIS Measure and Technical Resources. https://www.ncqa.org/hedis/. Accessed 1 Feb 2022.
6. Executive Summary: Medicare Program; Merit-Based Incentive Payment System (MIPS) and Alternative Payment Model (APM) Incentive under the Physician Fee Schedule, and Criteria for Physician-Focused Payment Models. Centers for Medicare & Medicaid Services (CMS), HHS, 2016 Contract No.: 42 CFR Parts 414 and 495 [CMS-5517-FC], RIN 0938-AS69.
7. Langley GL, Moen R, Nolan KM, Nolan TW, Norman CL, Provost LP. The improvement guide: a practical approach to enhancing organizational performance. 2nd ed. San Francisco, CA: Jossey-Bass Publishers; 2009.

8. Institute for Healthcare Improvement: Plan-Do-Study-Act (PDSA) Worksheet. http://www.ihi.org/resources/pages/tools/plandostudyactworksheet.aspx. Accessed 1 Feb 2022.
9. Institute for Healthcare Improvement: How to Improve. https://www.ihi.org/resources/Pages/HowtoImprove/default.aspx. Accessed 22 Jul 2022.
10. Donabedian A. Evaluating the quality of medical care. Milbank Q. 2005;83(4):691–729.
11. Doran GT. There's a S.M.A.R.T. way to write management's goals and objectives. Manag Rev. 1981;70(11):35–6.
12. The Internal Medicine Milestone Project. The Accreditation Council for Graduate Medical Education and The American Board of Internal Medicine; 2015.
13. Guralnick S, Fondahn E, Amin A, Bittner EA. Systems-based practice: time to finally adopt the orphan competency. J Grad Med Educ. 2021;13(2 Suppl):96–101.
14. Fondahn E, Burke AE, Padmore JS, Ollendorff AT. Assessing for practice-based learning and improvement: distinguishing evidence-based practice from reflective learning. J Grad Med Educ. 2021;13(2 Suppl):86–90.
15. Clemo R, Parsons AS, Boggan JC, Shieh L, Miller BP. Learning by doing: practical strategies to integrate resident education and quality improvement initiatives. J Grad Med Educ. 2021;13(5):631–4.
16. Thomas Bodenheimer W, Dickinson P, Kong M. Quality improvement models in residency programs. J Grad Med Educ. 2019;11(1):15–7.
17. Mosser G, Frisch KK, Skarda PK, Gertner E. Addressing the challenges in teaching quality improvement. Am J Med. 2009;122(5):487–91.
18. Butler JM, Anderson KA, Supiano MA, Weir CR. "It feels like a lot of extra work": resident attitudes about quality improvement and implications for an effective learning health care system. Acad Med. 2017;92(7):984–90.
19. Wagner R, Patow C, Newton R, Casey BR, Koh NJ, Weiss KB. The overview of the CLER program: CLER National Report of Findings 2016. J Grad Med Educ. 2016;8(2 Suppl):11–3.
20. Weiss KB, Bagian JP, Wagner R. CLER pathways to excellence: expectations for an optimal clinical learning environment (executive summary). J Grad Med Educ. 2014;6(3):610–1.
21. Guinane C, Davis N. Improving quality in outpatient services. Boca Raton, FL: CRC Press; 2011.

Chapter 30
Patient Safety in an Academic Medical Practice

Emily Fondahn, Claire Horton, and Natalie Baumann

Introduction

This chapter provides an overview of causes and types of patient safety errors in resident-based primary care clinics. Types of errors include medication errors, diagnostic errors, communication errors, laboratory and testing errors, administrative errors, and clinical knowledge errors. High-risk situations, such as transitions of care, and the impact of social determinants of health are also discussed. Finally, the chapter reviews the role of risk management and how to engage residents and faculty in improving patient safety.

Outline

- Background
- Common errors in ambulatory care
  - Medication errors
  - Diagnostic errors
  - Communication errors
  - Laboratory and diagnostic test errors
  - Administrative errors
  - Clinical knowledge errors

E. Fondahn (✉)
Washington University in St. Louis, St. Louis, MO, USA

University of Missouri, Columbia, MO, USA
e-mail: efondahn@wustl.edu

C. Horton
San Francisco Health Network, San Francisco, CA, USA
e-mail: claire.horton@sfdph.org

N. Baumann
Washington University in St. Louis, St. Louis, MO, USA
e-mail: nbaumann@wustl.edu

L. B. Lu et al. (eds.), *Leading an Academic Medical Practice*,
https://doi.org/10.1007/978-3-031-40273-9_30

- Transitions of care
- Social determinants of health
- Risk management
- Improving patient safety in an ambulatory practice
  - Building a culture of safety
  - Initiatives to strengthen patient safety
  - Educational opportunities
  - Faculty leadership
- Conclusion

Background

The Agency for Healthcare Research and Quality (AHRQ) defines patient safety as the "prevention of diagnostic errors, medical errors, injury, or other preventable harm to a patient during the process of health care and reduction of risk of unnecessary harm associated with health care" [1]. Patient safety research has largely focused on the inpatient setting with less known about patient safety issues in the clinic. Ambulatory patient safety concerns include harm that occurs to patients in primary care, outpatient specialty care, and the home and community [2].

As many as 4 in 10 patients are estimated to be harmed in the ambulatory setting, and up to 80% of this harm is avoidable [3]. However, the frequency of error reporting in the clinic setting is very low. A review of an ambulatory safety reporting system found that primary care practices only reported 2.1% of the patient safety events out of 2701 events. Nurses were the most common event reporter (29.9% of known event reporter roles) followed by pharmacists (3.9%) and clinicians (3.2%) [2]. Multiple barriers exist for reporting patient safety events in ambulatory care, including lack of knowledge about how and what to report, lack of clarity on who is responsible for reporting, fear of disciplinary action or litigation, and the belief that reporting is time consuming or not be worth the time [4]. A small survey of general practitioners identified several additional barriers to reporting including fear of embarrassment or blame, concern of damage to reputation and loss of patient confidence, and lack of feedback [5]. Some ambulatory practices may not have event reporting systems, and there is no standard taxonomy for classifying incidents in primary care [6]. However, adverse event and near miss reporting systems have been shown to be effective in creating quality improvement activities in primary care [7].

In academic medical practices, residents often act as the primary care physician for a cohort of patients. The resident assumes the responsibility of managing patients and coordinating their care within the health-care system. Residents frequently have other clinical responsibilities, such as night float and the intensive care unit, which can distract from their outpatient clinic responsibilities. Additionally, residents are often caring for complex patients with negative social determinants of health in an understaffed, under-resourced care setting [8]. When coupled with resident inexperience and the unique workflows of a resident-based clinic, these factors may exacerbate the risk for an error to be made in the ambulatory setting.

The Theory of Active and Latent Failures, also known as the "Swiss Cheese Model," is a fundamental concept in patient safety proposed by James Reason. Latent errors, or inherent failures in the system, are represented by the "holes" in the cheese and exist at multiple levels, predisposing the system to error [9]. While a single latent failure is unlikely to cause an error, an alignment of multiple latent failures in the system coupled with an active failure such as human error or cognitive bias leads to harm. The Swiss Cheese Model emphasizes that preventing errors and preserving patient safety requires a focus on addressing failures in systemic processes in addition to human factors. The organizational influences and supervisory, environmental, individual, and team factors that can lead to "holes" in the Swiss cheese are applicable and present in academic medical practices.

Common Errors in Ambulatory Care

The American Medical Association defined the top six errors that occur in the ambulatory setting as medication errors, diagnostic errors, communication errors, laboratory errors, administrative errors, and clinical knowledge errors [10]. In addition, academic medical practices with resident-based clinics have specific patient safety challenges, such as frequent end-of-year patient handoffs, resident scheduling, variable attending supervision and result handling.

Medication Errors

A medication error is defined as a "preventable event that may cause or lead to inappropriate medication use or patient harm while the medication is in the control of the health care professional, patient or consumer" [11]. Medication errors are extremely common in the outpatient setting; an estimated 530,000 Medicare beneficiaries experience a medication-related error yearly [12]. Additionally, up to 25% of inpatient hospitalizations are related to adverse drug events [13]. Medication errors may include several aspects of care, including challenges with medication prescribing, monitoring, reconciliation, and patient adherence.

Given a lack of experience, trainees may make mistakes prescribing, reconciling, and monitoring medications. For interns, each clinic session could represent their first time prescribing a medication that faculty commonly use such as insulin, amoxicillin, or metformin. Residents may not recognize the need for more careful follow-up for medications with a narrow therapeutic range or be aware of medication side effects that need to be relayed to patients.

Despite these barriers, residents are expected to write prescriptions correctly at the start of residency training [14]. Errors can be made while writing a prescription regardless of whether the prescription is hand-written or sent through an electronic health record (EHR). For example, a resident may mean to prescribe guaifenesin, but could mistype into the EHR, leading to guanfacine being prescribed. Additionally, a medication could be written correctly but is not appropriate for the clinical context such as a resident prescribing ondansetron without realizing the patient has a history of a prolonged QTc interval. Pharmacists who receive outpatient prescriptions verify their accuracy and safeguard against errors with prescription writing, although some will undoubtedly be missed.

The increased use of the EHR for documentation, medication management, and communication has benefitted ambulatory patient safety, but there are still opportunities for improvement. Computerized decision support (CDS) tools have shown effectiveness in identifying potentially inappropriate medications [15]. The use of CDS needs to be evaluated comprehensively given the need for workflow changes and the potential for unintended consequences such as alert fatigue, which can limit their overall effectiveness [16]. The EHR also provides opportunities for enhanced medication monitoring for high-risk medications such as anticoagulation and immunosuppression. One study found that being listed on a clinician-specific monitoring bulletin doubled the chances of patients receiving appropriate laboratory monitoring for a number of medications [17].

Medication reconciliation is a systematic and comprehensive review of all the medications a patient is taking to ensure that medications being added, changed, or discontinued are carefully evaluated [18]. A full medication reconciliation can be a difficult and time-consuming task. As a result, many clinicians in primary care clinics do not give this important process the attention it deserves. In video-recorded sessions of ambulatory visits, medication reconciliation took a median of 2.1 min (IQR 1.0–4.2) and comprised a median of 10% (IQR 3–17%) of the visit time; during 47% of this time, the clinician was multitasking in their EHR use. This multitasking creates risk of error in medication entry, prescribing or patient–clinician communication about medication management [19]. Literature has shown that a pharmacist-led medication review reduced the number of medication errors and improved patient outcomes [20]. In one academic resident clinic, nurses were educated by pharmacists on how to complete a medication review during the triage process; they identified multiple medication discrepancies, demonstrating that nursing review may an effective alternative to medication reconciliation by physicians [21].

Medication reconciliation is a critical skill that should be taught to trainees and reinforced across care settings. Medication reconciliation education for internal medicine residents has been effective in reducing medication discrepancies for inpatients [22], and a robust and reliable medication reconciliation process is a key component of a safe discharge. Armor et al. evaluated adult patients attending post-discharge follow-up in an academic family medicine clinic and found that 100% of patients experienced an adverse drug event (ADE) or possible adverse drug event (pADE) and 81% had a medication discrepancy [23]. Educational opportunities to enhance medication reconciliation for residents include didactic sessions, role-play exercises, chart-stimulated recall, and experiential learning.

Finally, medication errors can stem from patient nonadherence such as not taking a medication as prescribed or continuing a medication that was intended to be discontinued. Communication with patients and caregivers regarding medication changes, particularly during a transition of care such as post-hospitalization, is essential to ensure correct medication use at home. Utilizing patient education techniques such as the teach-back method have been shown to increase disease-specific knowledge as well as patient adherence [24].

Diagnostic Errors

A diagnostic error is defined as a delayed, missed, or incorrect diagnosis. A report from the Institute of Medicine reported that 5% of US adults who seek ambulatory care each year experience a diagnostic error [25]. In a resident-based practice, faculty may be particularly vulnerable to committing a diagnostic error as the information received about a patient is filtered by the resident, who may omit pertinent information or frame the case leading to cognitive bias. This can be further exacerbated with the use of the Centers for Medicare & Medicaid Services (CMS) Primary Care Exception billing rule, which allows attending physicians to bill for indirectly supervised outpatient encounters in certain circumstances without personally examining the patient. A study of internal medicine residents found that 100% of residents reported a case of diagnostic error or delay in diagnosis due to cognitive bias [26]. Though these examples occurred during inpatient hospitalizations, diagnostic error can readily occur in the ambulatory setting. The most common cognitive bias, anchoring (making decisions under the influence of a set reference point or "anchor"), was found in 87.8% of cases. This was followed by availability bias (using the information that is most readily available rather than the most representative) in 75.6% of cases. Framing (making decisions based on how information is presented, not based on the facts themselves) was identified in 56.1% of cases and blind obedience (showing undue deference to authority) was identified in 53.7% of cases.

Most studies of diagnostic error focus on physician cognitive bias or systems factors, but patient involvement in the diagnostic process is much less studied. Patients are a unique source of knowledge about their health and should be utilized to mitigate diagnostic error. As a result of the 21st Century Cures Act, most clinical documentation in the EHR, including primary care visit notes, is visible to patients in real-time. A patient survey found that sharing visit notes encourages timely follow-up of test results, which avoids missed or delayed diagnoses, may allow for identification of documentation inaccuracies that contribute to diagnostic error, and strengthens the bidirectional nature of the patient–physician relationship [27].

Communication Errors

Poor communication is frequently cited as a contributing factor to patient safety events. Communication lapses can occur between physicians, other health-care practitioners, clinical support staff, the patient, and many other individuals in the system. In the ambulatory setting, communication lapses can occur at the end of the academic year if a patient is transitioned to a new resident, between inpatient and ambulatory settings, and with specialty consultants.

Physician-to-physician communication is often done through the EHR. Though the transition to the EHR has greatly enhanced patient care, the time ambulatory physicians spend interacting with the EHR has increased [28]. To improve efficiency, many residents and other clinicians utilize the copy-and-paste function, leading to increased errors as inaccurate or outdated information is propagated forward in the medical record. While new technology such as on-demand speech recognition software can improve efficiency and decrease the temptation to copy–paste, a propensity for error still exists as documentation is not reviewed by a certified medical transcriptionist. Zhou et al. found an error rate of 7.4% (7.4 errors per 100 words) in speech recognition generated notes with a reduced error rate of 0.4% following medical transcriptionist review [29]. If on-demand speech recognition software is used by residents, thorough proofreading by the author and supervising attending is key to prevent errors.

Additional physician-to-physician communication occurs via referrals. The majority of primary care physicians report being dissatisfied with the referral process [30]. First, a resident must identify an appropriate clinical question for the referral, determine the urgency of the evaluation, and include supporting documentation. Next, residents must learn the systems-based knowledge needed to send and follow-up on a referral. Though attendings often supervise referral initiation, the discontinuity of resident clinics may still lead to gaps in the referral process, including lack of-follow up with a patient should a referral be processed incorrectly or there be inaction on the consultant's recommendations. Lastly, academic hospital-based clinics often care for a disproportionate number of uninsured or underinsured patients. The lack of insurance is an additional barrier to obtaining timely specialty care. Wait-times may be exaggerated for uninsured patients seeking specialty care, and many specialty services will require cost-prohibitive co-pays. Many clinics have resources for patients to receive financial assistance for co-pays, but this paperwork often takes several weeks to be processed.

Communication errors may also occur between the resident and the attending physician. Many resident clinics operate under the CMS primary care exception rule (PCER), where attending physicians rely on residents to accurately complete the patient evaluation, concisely present information, and communicate the plan to the patient without direct supervision. The PCER can be employed after the resident has completed 6 months of training; however, there are no standardized assessments to determine competency for this progression. Residency clinic leadership should employ evaluations of individual residents based on the Accreditation Council for

Graduate Medical Education (ACGME) milestones and entrustable professional activities to ensure safe practice under the PCER [31].

Even after competency for indirect supervision has been assessed, residents may not present all pertinent information to the attending or appropriately communicate the plan to the patient. Clinic flow may also hinder resident and attending communication. A patient may raise an issue with the resident after a case is presented, and the resident may initiate a plan that is never reviewed with the attending. Residents may receive follow-up information about a patient, such as an abnormal lab value or imaging finding, but not contact the attending to discuss an appropriate treatment plan. With the increase in block schedules, residents may have less continuity with their patients than previously [32]. This loss of continuity may lead to communication errors between the primary resident physicians and other resident team members.

Finally, communication errors can occur between the patient and the resident or attending physician. One study found that over one-third of patients who were prescribed a new medication during an outpatient visit could not recall all details discussed, such as how and when to take the medication and side effects [33]. Thoughtful communication strategies, such as using the teach-back method or sharing recommendations with the patient when a caregiver present, can be helpful to enhance retention. Clear, concise instructions summarizing key visit discussion points, medication changes, and pending orders such as imaging or referrals are also essential.

Laboratory and Diagnostic Test Errors

Primary care physicians order lab tests during an estimated 29–38% of encounters, and these laboratory tests can contribute to 15–54% of errors in primary care [34]. Types of errors include order entry errors, lab collection or transport errors, reporting errors, and errors with patient follow-up. Result management poses a significant challenge in residency clinics. Interpreting and managing test results is a skill that develops over time and can be challenging for trainees [35]. Clinics vary in levels of attending supervision of test results. Some EHRs can send test results to multiple clinicians (e.g., resident and supervising attending physician), while other EHRs can only send test results to the ordering doctor. The rotational nature of a resident's schedule can also pose challenges to viewing and responding to an abnormal test result.

Variability exists within and across practices for how patients are notified of their test results and who is responsible for patient notification [36]. Patient satisfaction has been shown to correlate with physician response time to test results [37]. Streamlining the notification process and providing clear expectations has been shown to effectively increase the rate of laboratory test notification by residents from 16% pre-intervention to 91% post-intervention [38]. Academic practices need to have defined workflows for how to manage test results and follow-up with patients.

Administrative Errors

Administrative errors can be defined as a failure to carry out a planned action or undertaking an incorrect action as part of the systems and processes involved in delivering primary care [39]. The classification of administrative errors can overlap with other types of errors, such as test management or communication. A key concept of administrative errors is to assess the roles and contributions of nonclinical office and administrative staff in patient safety. They create a first impression of the practice for the patient and act as gatekeepers to the clinicians. One study evaluating near-misses in primary care found the most common types of errors were breakdowns in office processes such as filing, chart data entry errors, and problems with appointments or referrals [7]. Events such as the front desk inappropriately routing a patient call, creating a new EHR chart for a patient instead of using the existing chart, or forgetting to schedule a follow-up appointment can lead to adverse events.

Clinical Knowledge Errors

Undergraduate and graduate medical education is often highly inpatient focused. Interns commonly start residency uncomfortable, evaluating and managing common ambulatory topics and feel like they did not receive enough outpatient training in medical school [40]. For example, the average score on an assessment gauging residents' knowledge of ambulatory care for older adults was only 60% [41]. Significant efforts have been enacted to diversify undergraduate ambulatory medical education. A 2016 survey of internal medicine clerkship directors showed that nearly all respondents had dedicated ambulatory experiences that are increasingly interdepartmental. However, significant barriers such as faculty time, physical space, and financial compensation are still present and hinder high-quality teaching in the clinic setting [42].

Concerns about ambulatory education were also noted by the Accreditation Council for Graduate Medical Education (ACGME) as early as 2009 when Internal Medicine program requirements were revised to emphasize the outpatient experience. In 2019, Coyle et al. found that significant clinic redesign initiatives, particularly the movement to X + Y program design, and educational efforts related to transitions of care, substance use, and quality improvement have been successfully developed and implemented. Given the concern for patient safety and quality, there remains opportunity for higher level analysis, including multicenter, randomized controlled trials, to evaluate best practices for ambulatory education [43]. Though there is increasing emphasis on ambulatory education in both undergraduate and graduate medical education, attending physicians should be vigilant for clinical knowledge errors, particularly early in a resident's training.

Transitions of Care

Poor care coordination between the inpatient and ambulatory settings during a transition of care can lead to many high-risk situations, such as lack of scheduled follow-up or inappropriate medication administration, that jeopardize patient safety. Several factors, including ineffective team-based care, inaccurate medication reconciliation, poor communication, and non-standardized handoffs, all contribute to challenges at transitions of care. A large study of heart failure patents in Taiwan found that low care continuity and coordination led to increased 1-year post-discharge mortality and health-care costs [44].

Given that resident clinics tend to care for populations with higher disease burden and increased effects of the social determinants of health when compared with nonacademic practices, resident clinics may struggle to provide optimal post-hospitalization care [45]. Patients followed by a resident primary care clinic were more likely to be readmitted to the hospital and less likely to have follow-up appointments compared to patients followed by a faculty primary care clinic [46]. Programs have initiated quality improvement and educational initiatives to improve accuracy of medication reconciliation, discharge planning for patients, quality of the discharge summary, and communication between inpatient teams and primary care physicians [47–50]. Post-discharge clinics are one option to bridge the patient between the inpatient setting and their primary care physician. These clinics can be housed within a resident primary care clinic and have shown a decrease in time to post-hospital follow-up appointment and readmission rates [51]. Post-hospital visits should include reviewing the discharge summary, coordinating care with consultants or home health, following up on test results, performing drug monitoring, doing a comprehensive medication reconciliation, discussing current symptoms, providing instructions for warning signs and how to seek after-hours care, and ensuring that all appropriate follow-up appointments are made [52]. However, the outpatient clinic physician is dependent on timely and accurate information from the inpatient team. Patients may present to clinic without a completed discharge summary or a discharge summary that lacks important elements from the hospitalization [53]. Given the complexity of post-hospital visits, clinic directors should consider granting extra time for these visits or creating a structured note template.

End-of-year handoffs have received little attention compared to inpatient handoffs and inpatient-to-outpatient transitions of care. Based on an average resident panel size between 50 and 150 patients, an estimated 640,000 to 1.92 million patients per year have a change in their primary care physician when residents graduate from their training program [54]. In internal medicine, family medicine, and pediatrics training programs, patients transition physicians approximately every 3 years—and sometimes more frequently. The incoming residents will not have the same level of expertise as the departing residents, and many programs have no standard way of supervising or requiring end-of-year handoffs. These transitioning patients are at risk of missing visits due to poor follow-up care and scheduling difficulties, resulting in missed test results and delayed medication refills [55, 56]. Pincavage et al. implemented a standardized handoff protocol for high-risk patients at an academic internal medicine primary care clinic including a departure letter to patients, enhanced resident education, improved scheduling coordination, automatic missed visit rescheduling, safety audits, and time for residents to call patients to establish care. This protocol was further enhanced the following year to include a patient-centered transition packet. These interventions significantly decreased the number of acute care visits and patients lost to follow up during the months following the primary care physician transition [57].

Clinics should also have a system to manage laboratory or radiology studies that are completed at the academic year transition. Reports from these tests could be sent to a graduated resident who is no longer in that health-care system, leading to a delay in diagnosis and treatment for a patient. Enhanced handoff protocols that proactively alert incoming residents to pending labs or testing may help reduce delays. If possible, having results sent to the attending physician in addition to the resident could also prevent a missed result during a care transition. Among ambulatory medical practices, 52% reported having a system to record tests ordered while only 32% of practices had systems to detect if patients had missed tests [58]. New residents may not have developed a system to track test results, especially independent of the EHR, and may not fully use all the capabilities of the EHR to track results and follow patients [59].

Social Determinants of Health

Many academic practices care for a patient population significantly impacted by the social determinants of health including high rates of poverty, limited English proficiency, unstable housing, food insecurity, lack of transportation, immigrant and refugee status, low health literacy and numeracy, and high rates of comorbid psychosocial conditions. These social determinants of health negatively affect morbidity and mortality and also contribute to the potential for error in the clinical setting [60, 61]. For example, low-income people with diabetes are more likely to become hypoglycemic from aggressive insulin regimens at months'-end when food budgets are tight [62]. Limited English proficiency contributes to a variety of errors, particularly those focused on health system–patient communication [63].

Due to the impact of the social determinants of health on patients in academic practices, resident and faculty training on social determinants of health, cultural competency, bias reduction, and trauma-informed care are necessary to provide safe, high-quality patient care. A 2019 review by Gard et al. identified significant variation in the development, implementation, and evaluation of social determinant of health curricula created for residents and highlights the need for a systematic approach to this important topic [64]. In addition, many academic practices have embedded social workers to provide additional support and connect patients to community resources.

Risk Management

Risk management in health-care focuses on the detection, assessment, and prevention of risks to safeguard patient safety as well as the institution's assets and community standing [65]. Risk management departments work closely with patient safety leaders to assist with investigations of sentinel events, ensure compliance with regulatory bodies such as the Joint Commission, and utilize tools like the Failure Mode and Effects Analysis to identify all possible failures in a system or design as a way to proactively mitigate risks. Given that risk management practices will vary by institution, residents must be familiar with their institutional practices.

Risk management staff are important partners in cases of patient harm due to medical malpractice. In the event that a malpractice claim is made, risk managers help to coordinate information regarding the case [66]. Early reporting of patient events helps ensure accurate recall of the event, fulfills legal reporting requirements, allows for early patient disclosure and discussion, and offers the opportunity to adjust medical bills. The medical malpractice statute of limitations varies by state; reportable events vary by malpractice insurance carrier but usually include events such as death, paralysis, or loss of limb. Residents should be aware of how to handle record requests from an attorney, lien letters, subpoenas, and summons. In general, legal documents should quickly go to the Risk Management office for review. Documentation in the chart should include information about informed consent, conversations with the patient/family, provisional diagnosis and medical decision-making, and conversations with consultants.

Primary care ranked third of nine specialties for malpractice claims. The most common cause of a claim was a failure to or delay in diagnosis [67]. Often, two or more physicians contributed to the missed diagnosis. The most common missed or delayed diagnoses were cancer (breast most common), infection, fracture, myocardial infarction, embolism, and appendicitis [68]. Missed cancer diagnoses often are errors of high severity. The majority of missed cancer diagnosis errors involved errors in clinical judgment, such as a failure or delay in ordering a diagnostic test or delay in obtaining a consult or referral [69]. The second most common cause of malpractice claims was medication errors. Key reasons cited for medication errors included prescriber's training, drug knowledge and experience, perception of risk, high workload and time pressures, and patient characteristics such as language barriers and complexity of the presentation [67].

Disclosure of adverse events is a key component of the response to a patient safety event. Physicians often have reluctance to disclose adverse events due to a fear of litigation, uncertainty about how/what should be disclosed, doubting the benefits of disclosure, lack of time to disclose errors and feeling a sense of personal failure [70]. However, institutions that have employed early disclosure of errors have shown a reduction in liability payments and legal expenses [71]. Risk management and/or patient safety specialists can help coach physicians on adverse event disclosure and advise if discussion with the insurance carrier is required. In general, the disclosure should be done by the attending physician. Based upon the situation and institution, residents may participate in the disclosure with the attending present. If multiple clinicians are involved, then collaborating on the conversation is useful prior to disclosure. Physicians should not discuss errors made by other health-care practitioners without including those individuals in the conversation, nor should they blame other clinicians. The conversation should be documented in the medical record, including the names of the health-care team and patient's family/friends that were present.

Finally, if a resident or faculty member is involved in a patient safety event, receiving peer support after the event is an important step. After a patient safety event, physicians often have feelings of increased anxiety about future errors, loss of confidence, sleep difficulties, reduced job satisfaction, and concern about harm to their reputation [72]. For residents, self-perceived errors were associated with increased risk of depression and burnout [73]. Physicians often rely on informal support systems, such as discussing an event with a colleague, partner, or supervising physician. Institutions are developing formal peer support programs to prevent or reduce the emotional and psychological distress after a patient safety incident [74]. The importance of recognizing the resident as a "second victim" in a medical error may be even more important in the ambulatory setting. Unlike the wards setting, where the structure supports ongoing daily team-based decision-making, residents in the ambulatory setting may feel isolated in their role as the primary care physician of a patient who has experienced an error. As a clinic director, being aware of patient safety events and the need to support residents and faculty after an event is critical.

Improving Patient Safety in an Ambulatory Practice

Building a Culture of Safety

Safety interventions are most likely to work in a practice culture that is supportive of reporting errors and near-misses without concerns for negative consequences of reporting. AHRQ found that 66% of respondents in medical offices perceived that mistakes were held against them [75]. Overall and domain-specific safety culture scores (teamwork climate, safety climate, working conditions, and perceptions of local management) were positively associated with the practice event reporting rates [76]. This information implies that in these practices with strong patient safety cultures, staff felt more comfortable sharing patient safety events. Having a strong governance model for ambulatory systems can be critically important to establish priorities and create nurse–physician leadership teams [77].

Initiatives to Strengthen Patient Safety

The potential for safety issues in an academic practice and the impact of those errors on both patients and clinicians can seem daunting. In addition to involving risk management in critical issues, it is also important to seek systems-based solutions to reduce the potential for error in an academic clinic. Involving residents in these efforts can be a valuable educational opportunity, as well as a chance to channel anxiety over errors and near-misses into productive change. For example, separating internal medicine resident's inpatient and outpatient duties promoted outpatient safety (34% pre-intervention to 87% post intervention) and led to increase in continuity and total patient visits [78]. While there is no one-size-fits-all approach, some ideas that have been successfully implemented in academic practices include the following:

- A mid-level clinician lab-review to prevent abnormal labs from slipping through the cracks
- Practice partner systems that incorporate lab and diagnostic imaging results review for absent residents
- Structured off-service notes for patients of graduating residents
- Panel review sessions in which a clinic registry tool is used to pull panel-level data for all residents, with structured review techniques residents can follow
- Team-based roles for medical assistants and clerks to help residents outreach to patients between visits when follow-up is needed
- Educational sessions focused on medication reconciliation and medication safety
- Curricula on cognitive errors in medicine to help residents learn to reduce cognitive bias in practice
- Formative feedback initiatives to allow faculty to give residents real-time feedback on their diagnostic skills
- Root cause analysis sessions when errors do occur, in conjunction with faculty and with risk management guidance (These can help residents process and come to terms with errors that have happened, teach them to take a systems-based approach to error prevention, and simultaneously help the practice learn how to become more error-resistant in the future.)

Educational Opportunities

Acknowledging and addressing patient safety issues in residency is important not only for clinical care of patients but it also represents a significant opportunity to educate residents about important patient safety concepts and skills. Educational conferences focused on patient safety can improve residents' comfort level and likelihood to report errors in future practice [46]. These educational opportunities can take many forms, but several programs have had success with the use of ambulatory morbidity and mortality conference (M&M's), root cause analysis sessions, or conferences focused on cognitive error in diagnosis [79]. Patient safety tools such as a fishbone diagram or cause map can help delineate the different factors that contributed to the error. Training on communication skills and disclosure of adverse events are also critical areas in which residents need training to prepare them for their future careers [80]. Ideally, quality improvement and patient safety education are strategically linked to the clinical care and patient outcomes along with having a strong leadership commitment to make improvements [79].

Faculty Leadership

Finally, the importance of faculty leadership in ambulatory patient safety initiatives cannot be overemphasized. Faculty should support and mentor residents in this area, especially when residents are involved in errors and near-misses. While it can be difficult for faculty to openly discuss their own mistakes with residents, doing so sends a powerful message that open discussion of error is not only permissible but also a path toward creation of a greater safety culture.

Conclusion

The ambulatory setting is vulnerable to multiple types of errors, and resident-based primary care clinics present challenges, such as frequent transitions of care and unique workflows, that impact patient safety. Continued research and focus on ambulatory errors will be critical for identifying failure points and building safer systems. Health systems will need to partner with patients to empower them to engage in their care as well as listening to their voice on how we improve our care in ambulatory clinics. Engaging residents and faculty in quality improvement efforts, encouraging robust event reporting, and building a culture of safety with a focus on systems-based solutions are key components to addressing the many opportunities to ensure the delivery of high-quality care.

References

1. Agency for Healthcare Research and Quality; 13 June 2022. https://www.ahrq.gov/topics/patient-safety.html.
2. Sharma AE, Yang J, Del Rosario JB, Hoskote M, Rivadeneira NA, Stakeholder Research Advisory C, et al. What safety events are reported for ambulatory care? Analysis of incident reports from a patient safety organization. Jt Comm J Qual Patient Saf. 2021;47(1):5–14.
3. Auraaen A, Slawomirski L, Klazinga N. The economics of patient safety in primary and ambulatory care: flying blind. Paris: Organisation for Economic Co-operation and Development; 2018.
4. Kaldjian LC, Jones EW, Wu BJ, Forman-Hoffman VL, Levi BH, Rosenthal GE. Reporting medical errors to improve patient safety: a survey of physicians in teaching hospitals. Arch Intern Med. 2008;168(1):40–6.
5. Rea D, Griffiths S. Patient safety in primary care: incident reporting and significant event reviews in British general practice. Health Soc Care Community. 2016;24(4):411–9.
6. Panesar SS, deSilva D, Carson-Stevens A, Cresswell KM, Salvilla SA, Slight SP, et al. How safe is primary care? A systematic review. BMJ Qual Saf. 2015;25:544.
7. Crane S, Sloane PD, Elder N, Cohen L, Laughtenschlaeger N, Walsh K, et al. Reporting and using near-miss events to improve patient safety in diverse primary care practices: a collaborative approach to learning from our mistakes. J Am Board Fam Med. 2015;28(4):452–60.
8. Keirns CC, Bosk CL. Perspective: the unintended consequences of training residents in dysfunctional outpatient settings. Acad Med. 2008;83(5):498–502.
9. Wiegmann DA, Wood LJ, Cohen TN, Shappell SA. Understanding the "Swiss cheese model" and its application to patient safety. J Patient Saf. 2022;18(2):119–23.
10. Lorincz CY, Drazen E, Sokol PE, Neerukonda KV, Metzger J, Toepp MC, Maul L, Classen DC, Wynia MK. Research in ambulatory patient safety 2000–2010: a 10-year review. Chicago, IL: American Medical Association; 2011.
11. National Coordinating Council for Medication Error Reporting and Prevention 2015. 24 March 2016. http://www.nccmerp.org/about-medication-errors.
12. Aspden P, Wolcott J, Bootman JL, Cronenwett LR. Preventing medication errors: committee of identifying and preventing medication errors. Washington, DC: Institute of Medicine; 2006.
13. Samoy LJ, Zed PJ, Wilbur K, Balen RM, Abu-Laban RB, Roberts M. Drug-related hospitalizations in a tertiary care internal medicine service of a Canadian hospital: a prospective study. Pharmacotherapy. 2006;26(11):1578–86.
14. Colleges AoAM. Core Entrustable professional activities for entering residency: faculty and learners' Guide: Association of American Medical Colleges; 2014.
15. Ruhland DJ, Bellone JM, Wilkes E. Implementation and assessment of an ambulatory prescribing guidance tool to improve patient safety in the geriatric population. Consult Pharm. 2017;32(3):169–74.
16. Ranji SR, Rennke S, Wachter RM. Computerised provider order entry combined with clinical decision support systems to improve medication safety: a narrative review. BMJ Qual Saf. 2014;23(9):773–80.
17. Bundy DG, Marsteller JA, Wu AW, Engineer LD, Berenholtz SM, Caughey AH, et al. Electronic health record-based monitoring of primary care patients at risk of medication-related toxicity. Jt Comm J Qual Patient Saf. 2012;38(5):216–23.
18. Medication Reconciliation (MedRec): Institute for Safe Prescribing Practices Canada; 16 Feb 2017. https://www.ismp-canada.org/medrec/.
19. Matta GY, Khoong EC, Lyles CR, Schillinger D, Ratanawongsa N. Finding meaning in medication reconciliation using electronic health records: qualitative analysis in safety net primary and specialty care. JMIR Med Inform. 2018;6(2):e10167.
20. Mekonnen AB, McLachlan AJ, Brien JA. Effectiveness of pharmacist-led medication reconciliation programmes on clinical outcomes at hospital transitions: a systematic review and meta-analysis. BMJ Open. 2016;6(2):e010003.

21. Holt KM, Thompson AN. Implementation of a medication reconciliation process in an internal medicine Clinic at an Academic Medical Center. Pharmacy (Basel). 2018;6(2):26.
22. Arundel C, Logan J, Ayana R, Gannuscio J, Kerns J, Swenson R. Safe medication reconciliation: an intervention to improve Residents' medication reconciliation skills. J Grad Med Educ. 2015;7(3):407–11.
23. Armor BL, Wight AJ, Carter SM. Evaluation of adverse drug events and medication discrepancies in transitions of care between hospital discharge and primary care follow-up. J Pharm Pract. 2016;29(2):132–7.
24. Ha Dinh TT, Bonner A, Clark R, Ramsbotham J, Hines S. The effectiveness of the teach-back method on adherence and self-management in health education for people with chronic disease: a systematic review. JBI Database System Rev Implement Rep. 2016;14(1):210–47.
25. National Academies of Sciences E, and Medicine. Improving diagnosis in health care. Washington DC, National Academies Press; 2015.
26. Ogdie AR, Reilly JB, Pang WG, Keddem S, Barg FK, Von Feldt JM, et al. Seen through their eyes: residents' reflections on the cognitive and contextual components of diagnostic errors in medicine. Acad Med. 2012;87(10):1361–7.
27. Blease CR, Bell SK. Patients as diagnostic collaborators: sharing visit notes to promote accuracy and safety. Diagnosis (Berl). 2019;6(3):213–21.
28. Arndt BG, Beasley JW, Watkinson MD, Temte JL, Tuan WJ, Sinsky CA, et al. Tethered to the EHR: primary care physician workload assessment using EHR event log data and time-motion observations. Ann Fam Med. 2017;15(5):419–26.
29. Zhou L, Blackley SV, Kowalski L, Doan R, Acker WW, Landman AB, et al. Analysis of Errors in dictated clinical documents assisted by speech recognition software and professional transcriptionists. JAMA Netw Open. 2018;1(3):e180530.
30. Gandhi TK, Sittig DF, Franklin M, Sussman AJ, Fairchild DG, Bates DW. Communication breakdown in the outpatient referral process. J Gen Intern Med. 2000;15(9):626–31.
31. Tobin DG, Doolittle BR, Ellman MS, Ruser CB, Brienza RS, Genao I. Modifying the primary care exception rule to require competency-based assessment. Acad Med. 2017;92(3):331–4.
32. Wieland ML, Halvorsen AJ, Chaudhry R, Reed DA, McDonald FS, Thomas KG. An evaluation of internal medicine residency continuity clinic redesign to a 50/50 outpatient-inpatient model. J Gen Intern Med. 2013;28(8):1014–9.
33. Tarn DM, Flocke SA. New prescriptions: how well do patients remember important information? Fam Med. 2011;43(4):254–9.
34. Hickner JM, Fernald DH, Harris DM, Poon EG, Elder NC, Mold JW. Issues and initiatives in the testing process in primary care physician offices. J Comm J Qual Patient Saf. 2005;31(2):81–9.
35. Kwan JL, Cram P. Do not assume that no news is good news: test result management and communication in primary care. BMJ Qual Saf. 2015;24(11):664–6.
36. Litchfield IJ, Bentham LM, Lilford RJ, Greenfield SM. Test result communication in primary care: clinical and office staff perspectives. Fam Pract. 2014;31(5):592–7.
37. Ai A, Desai S, Shellman A, Wright A. Understanding test results follow-up in the ambulatory setting: analysis of multiple perspectives. Jt Comm J Qual Patient Saf. 2018;44(11):674–82.
38. Benton W, Snyder ED, Estrada CA, Bryan TJ. Signed, sealed, delivered: increasing patient notification of test results in an internal medicine resident continuity clinic. South Med J. 2019;112(2):85–8.
39. Administrative Errors. Technical series of safety primary care. Geneva: World Health Organization; 2016.
40. Esch LM, Bird A-N, Oyler JL, Lee WW, Shah SD, Pincavage AT. Preparing for the primary care clinic: an ambulatory boot camp for internal medicine interns. Medical education Online 2015: 20. https://doi.org/10.3402/meo.v20.29702.
41. Kalender-Rich JL, Mahnken JD, Dong L, Paolo AM, Hayley DC, Rigler SK. Development of an ambulatory geriatrics knowledge examination for internal medicine residents. J Grad Med Educ. 2013;5(4):678–80.

42. Shaheen AW, Alexandraki I, Fazio SB, Lo MC, Packer CD, Jasti H, et al. The state of ambulatory undergraduate internal medicine medical education: results of the 2016 clerkship directors in internal medicine annual survey. Am J Med. 2019;132(5):652–7.
43. Coyle A, Helenius I, Cruz CM, Lyons EA, May N, Andrilli J, et al. A decade of teaching and learning in internal medicine ambulatory education: a scoping review. J Grad Med Educ. 2019;11(2):132–42.
44. Chang GM, Chen JY, Kuo WY, Tung YC. Associations of continuity and coordination of care with outcomes and costs after discharge among patients with heart failure: a nationwide population-based study. Int J Cardiol. 2022;353:54–61.
45. Nadkarni M, Reddy S, Bates CK, Fosburgh B, Babbott S, Holmboe E. Ambulatory-based education in internal medicine: current organization and implications for transformation. Results of a National Survey of resident continuity clinic directors. J Gen Intern Med. 2011;26(1):16–20.
46. Doctoroff L, McNally D, Vanka A, Nall R, Mukamal KJ. Inpatient-outpatient transitions for patients with resident primary care physicians: access and readmission. Am J Med. 2014;127(9):886 e15–20.
47. Ramjaun A, Sudarshan M, Patakfalvi L, Tamblyn R, Meguerditchian AN. Educating medical trainees on medication reconciliation: a systematic review. BMC Med Educ. 2015;15:33.
48. Axon RN, Penney FT, Kyle TR, Zapka J, Marsden J, Zhao Y, et al. A hospital discharge summary quality improvement program featuring individual and team-based feedback and academic detailing. Am J Med Sci. 2014;347(6):472–7.
49. Aboumatar H, Allison RD, Feldman L, Woods K, Thomas P, Wiener C. Focus on transitions of care: description and evaluation of an educational intervention for internal medicine residents. Am J Med Qual. 2014;29(6):522–9.
50. Kalanithi L, Coffey CE, Mourad M, Vidyarthi AR, Hollander H, Ranji SR. The effect of a resident-led quality improvement project on improving communication between hospital-based and outpatient physicians. Am J Med Qual. 2013;28(6):472–9.
51. Booth KA, Vinci LM, Oyler JL, Pincavage AT. Using a resident discharge clinic for resident education and patient care: a feasibility study. J Grad Med Educ. 2014;6(3):536–40.
52. Coleman EA. The post-hospital follow-up visit: a physician checklist to reduce readmission. Sacramento, CA: California HealthCare Foundation; 2010.
53. Kripalani S, LeFevre F, Phillips CO, Williams MV, Basaviah P, Baker DW. Deficits in communication and information transfer between hospital-based and primary care physicians: implications for patient safety and continuity of care. JAMA. 2007;297(8):831–41.
54. Young JQ, Wachter RM. Academic year-end transfers of outpatients from outgoing to incoming residents: an unaddressed patient safety issue. JAMA. 2009;302(12):1327–9.
55. Pincavage AT, Ratner S, Prochaska ML, Prochaska M, Oyler J, Davis AM, et al. Outcomes for resident-identified high-risk patients and resident perspectives of year-end continuity clinic handoffs. J Gen Intern Med. 2012;27(11):1438–44.
56. Pincavage AT, Lee WW, Beiting KJ, Arora VM. What do patients think about year-end resident continuity clinic handoffs?: a qualitative study. J Gen Intern Med. 2013;28(8):999–1007.
57. Pincavage AT, Prochaska M, Dahlstrom M, Lee WW, Beiting KJ, Ratner S, et al. Patient safety outcomes after two years of an enhanced internal medicine residency clinic handoff. Am J Med. 2014;127(1):96–9.
58. Poon EG, Gandhi TK, Sequist TD, Murff HJ, Karson AS, Bates DW. "I wish I had seen this test result earlier!": dissatisfaction with test result management systems in primary care. Arch Intern Med. 2004;164(20):2223–8.
59. Cho AH, Namdari NT, Bowlby L, Zipkin DA, Greenblatt L, Causey HE, et al. Multiyear outcomes of a population-oriented care redesign in an internal medicine residency continuity clinic. J Health Care Poor Underserved. 2020;31(2):724–41.
60. Minkler M, Fuller-Thomson E, Guralnik JM. Gradient of disability across the socioeconomic spectrum in the United States. N Engl J Med. 2006;355(7):695–703.
61. McDonough P, Duncan GJ, Williams D, House J. Income dynamics and adult mortality in the United States, 1972 through 1989. Am J Public Health. 1997;87(9):1476–83.

62. Seligman HK, Bolger AF, Guzman D, López A, Bibbins-Domingo K. Exhaustion of food budgets at month's end and hospital admissions for hypoglycemia. Health Aff (Millwood). 2014;33(1):116–23.
63. Divi C, Koss RG, Schmaltz SP, Loeb JM. Language proficiency and adverse events in US hospitals: a pilot study. Int J Qual Health Care. 2007;19(2):60–7.
64. Gard LA, Peterson J, Miller C, Ghosh N, Youmans Q, Didwania A, et al. Social determinants of health training in U.S. primary care residency programs: a scoping review. Acad Med. 2019;94(1):135–43.
65. What is Risk Management in Healthcare? NEJM Catalyst Innovations in Care Delivery. 2018.
66. Kraman SS, Hamm G. Risk management: extreme honesty may be the best policy. Ann Intern Med. 1999;131(12):963–7.
67. Wallace E, Lowry J, Smith SM, Fahey T. The epidemiology of malpractice claims in primary care: a systematic review. BMJ Open. 2013;3(7):e002929.
68. Gandhi TK, Kachalia A, Thomas EJ, Puopolo AL, Yoon C, Brennan TA, et al. Missed and delayed diagnoses in the ambulatory setting: a study of closed malpractice claims. Ann Intern Med. 2006;145(7):488–96.
69. Aaronson EL, Quinn GR, Wong CI, Murray AM, Petty CR, Einbinder J, et al. Missed diagnosis of cancer in primary care: insights from malpractice claims data. J Healthc Risk Manag. 2019;39(2):19–29.
70. Kaldjian LC, Jones EW, Rosenthal GE, Tripp-Reimer T, Hillis SL. An empirically derived taxonomy of factors affecting physicians' willingness to disclose medical errors. J Gen Intern Med. 2006;21(9):942–8.
71. Boothman RC, Blackwell AC, Campbell DA Jr, Commiskey E, Anderson S. A better approach to medical malpractice claims? The University of Michigan experience. J Health Life Sci Law. 2009;2(2):125–59.
72. Waterman AD, Garbutt J, Hazel E, Dunagan WC, Levinson W, Fraser VJ, et al. The emotional impact of medical errors on practicing physicians in the United States and Canada. Jt Comm J Qual Patient Saf. 2007;33(8):467–76.
73. West CP, Huschka MM, Novotny PJ, Sloan JA, Kolars JC, Habermann TM, et al. Association of perceived medical errors with resident distress and empathy: a prospective longitudinal study. JAMA. 2006;296(9):1071–8.
74. van Pelt F. Peer support: healthcare professionals supporting each other after adverse medical events. Qual Saf Health Care. 2008;17(4):249–52.
75. Famolaro T, Hare R, Thornton S, Yount ND, Fan L, Liu H, Sorra J. Surveys on Patient Safety CultureTM (SOPSTM) Medical Office Survey: 2020 User Database Report. Rockville, MD: Agency for Healthcare Research and Quality; 2020. 2020 March 2020. Contract No.: AHRQ Publication No. 20–0034
76. Miller N, Bhowmik S, Ezinwa M, Yang T, Schrock S, Bitzel D, et al. The relationship between safety culture and voluntary event reporting in a large regional ambulatory care group. J Patient Saf. 2019;15(4):e48–51.
77. Kravet SJ, Bailey J, Demski R, Pronovost P. Establishing an ambulatory medicine quality and safety oversight structure: leveraging the fractal model. Acad Med. 2016;91(7):962–6.
78. Bates CK, Yang J, Huang G, Tess AV, Reynolds E, Vanka A, et al. Separating residents' inpatient and outpatient responsibilities: improving patient safety, learning environments, and relationships with continuity patients. Acad Med. 2016;91(1):60–4.
79. Wong BM, Baum KD, Headrick LA, Holmboe ES, Moss F, Ogrinc G, et al. Building the bridge to quality: an urgent call to integrate quality improvement and patient safety education with clinical care. Acad Med. 2020;95(1):59–68.
80. Schiff G, Griswold P, Ellis BR, Puopolo AL, Brede N, Nieva HR, et al. Doing right by our patients when things go wrong in the ambulatory setting. Jt Comm J Qual Patient Saf. 2014;40(2):91–6.

Part IX
Models of Care Delivery

Chapter 31
Hospital Based Clinics

Emily Mullen and Jason Worcester

Introduction

There are multiple venues in which a resident primary care clinic can be housed. One such venue is a hospital-based outpatient clinic. Approximately 90% of internal medicine residency training programs utilize hospital-based clinics and as of 2001, approximately 60% used hospital-based clinics exclusively [1]. A more recent survey of internal medicine program leaders shows a similar trend, with hospital-based clinics accounting for 63% of programs surveyed [2]. Hospital-based clinics can be in a VA hospital, academic hospital, or community teaching hospital. The regulations for practicing in a hospital setting can be complex; however, the rewards can be substantial. It will be important for a medical director in this setting to appreciate the many nuances related this location.

Outline

- General considerations when practicing in the hospital
  - Governance

    Hospital accreditation organizations
    Regulatory concerns

  - Billing for patients

E. Mullen (✉)
Internal Medicine Residency Program, Cone Health, University of North Carolina—Chapel Hill, Greensboro, NC, USA
e-mail: Emily.mullen@conehealth.com

J. Worcester
Boston Accountable Care Organization, Boston Medical Center, Boston University Chobanian & Avedisian School of Medicine, Boston, MA, USA
e-mail: jason.worcester@bmc.org

L. B. Lu et al. (eds.), *Leading an Academic Medical Practice*,
https://doi.org/10.1007/978-3-031-40273-9_31

  - Emergencies
- Educational opportunities
  - Engagement in clinic initiatives
- The patient experience
  - Navigating the system
  - Emergency care
- Conclusion

General Considerations When Practicing in the Hospital

Governance

Hospital-based clinics are required to follow different rules than their community counterparts. The rules will be based on the expectations of the larger health system or hospital and enforced by clinic leadership. In addition, the specific accreditation organization (see below) may have guidelines or regulations that further add to the complexity of running an ambulatory site embedded within the hospital. Therefore, when planning to open a hospital-based clinic, it will be important to coordinate closely with your hospital's leadership to fully understand and stay in compliance with the requirements of their accreditation council.

Hospital Accreditation Organizations

Multiple organizations exist to accredit hospital systems. Accreditation in this instance is defined as a form of external audit against predetermined standards, using a mixture of self-assessment and external surveys [3]. Two of the largest private organizations offering hospital accreditation are the Joint Commission and Der Norske Veritas (DNV). Approximately 75% of hospital systems pay to have an organization accredit their system. The Joint Commission in turn controls more than 80% of this market. If not accredited by a private organization, systems can opt to be reviewed by a state survey agency as part of an agreement with Centers for Medicare & Medicaid Services [4].

Regulatory Concerns

Regardless of accrediting body, there are several regulatory concerns that may differ from those required in community-based ambulatory sites. For example, in the Joint Commission standards, there are hospital-specific regulations concerning the size of the hallways, ability to access emergency care, location and availability of eye wash stations, the presence and composition of code carts, ventilation systems, and many other examples that will differ from free-standing ambulatory site standards. Community-based ambulatory sites likely would not be required to stock a code cart and train staff on emergency response situations in the same way, for example [5]. Though these nuances will often be beyond the scope of a residency program's control, the medical directors of the clinic will need to collaborate with hospital leadership to ensure these standards are followed.

Billing for Patients

There are typically two fees that a patient is charged when visiting a hospital-based clinic, a professional fee, and a facility fee. The professional fee is the charge that the physician or the physician's billing organization levies for the services rendered during the outpatient visit. The evaluation and management code submitted by the physician determines this fee [6]. A new patient is defined as having not being seen by any clinician in the same specialty group within the last 3 years. New visit billing codes can be used if the patient was seen more than 3 years ago. It is common for a patient to be cared for in the hospital by a clinician and later seen by another clinician of the same group in the hospital-based clinic. In this instance, the visit by the clinician in the hospital-based clinic would typically be billed as an established visit, even if the patient had never been to the hospital-based clinic before. That said, readers are encouraged to check with their billing and compliance offices to review how their institution handlesthis and similar circumstances. Like community-based clinics, the use of the primary care exception rule may be permitted if the Centers for Medicare and Medicaid Services criteria are met and should be used selectively to promote resident independence.

The facility fee is charged by the hospital to cover the cost of maintaining the facility and the clinic. The amount of the facility fee can vary from hospital to hospital. A patient or their insurance plan may get two separate bills for each of these fees. It is important for patients to know that care in these facilities is considered as being given "within the hospital" and not in a physician's stand-alone office [7]. This may have billing implications for patients.

Emergencies

Medical emergencies in the hospital-based clinic are infrequent but should be anticipated. Emergency medical equipment should be organized in a central location in the clinic. It should include such items as an automated external defibrillator (AED), oxygen supplies, appropriate personal protective equipment (PPE), and medications (e.g., intramuscular epinephrine, diphenhydramine, naloxone, aspirin, glucose tabs, and sublingual nitroglycerin). As a hospital-based clinic also has to interface with other departments such as pharmacy and central supply, it is imperative that the compliance of stocking and maintaining emergency supplies is assigned and monitored. Emergency protocols should be established by the hospital-based clinic clearly outlining roles and responsibilities of the team members. Unique to hospital-based clinics, the proximity of the clinic to the emergency department and inpatient units allows the possibility of expedited access to a hospital's rapid response or code team. It is important for a hospital-based clinic to establish clear guidelines on the roles and responsibilities of the various teams (i.e., clinic, emergency department, rapid response, hospital security, and/or code team) so that all are aware of how an unstable patient will be managed and transferred to the emergency department.

Clinic staff should be made aware of the location of the emergency equipment and protocols. Team-based simulation of emergency situations is an important step to ensuring medical emergencies proceed as efficient and safe as possible [8]. Please also see section on regulatory concerns.

Educational Opportunities

In a hospital-based clinic, one educational benefit is enhanced access to inpatient didactic activities such as noon conference and morning report. However, a dedicated ambulatory medicine curriculum is still an essential part of outpatient training. Some options noted in the literature include clinic conferences, academic half days, and team-based learning [9–11]. There are many existing programs such as the Yale Office Based Medical Curriculum and some programs create their own didactics [12].

Another educational opportunity for residents is the recruitment of admitted inpatients to the clinic after discharge. Given the location of a hospital-based clinic, patients may be more familiar with the facility and may better understand how to access the resident clinic, thus making it more likely they will transition to or initiate outpatient care after their hospital stay. This can be a very useful addition to a residents' education; following a patient full circle from admission to a hospital follow-up appointment. In fact, multiple studies show that one of the most important factors in resident satisfaction with primary care clinic is continuity of care with patients [13, 14].

Resident satisfaction and interest in outpatient education are often at odds with their inpatient or research responsibilities. Two additional ways to improve resident satisfaction, as reported in the systematic review by Stepczynski et al., are to limit conflict between outpatient and inpatient responsibilities and to provide consistent physician role models [15]. These two factors can be implemented readily in a hospital-based practice. Having the clinic housed in the hospital or close to the hospital allows for day-to-day physical access to the clinic without need for travel. This proximity may allow for closer interaction with the ambulatory interdisciplinary team and may facilitate residents' engagement in clinical workflows. For example, there are many clinical and administrative tasks that still occur outside the electronic medical record (EMR), so residents working in hospital-based clinics may have an easier time completing paperwork and interfacing with other members of the team. If a clinic is located in close proximity and/or in the same building as inpatient medicine responsibilities, this could serve to decrease that conflict and improve satisfaction. It also makes working in the clinic easier and more accessible for core faculty who may have other academic and research pursuits in the hospital system.

It has also been noted in the pediatric literature that community-based clinics tend to have volunteer faculty as opposed to core faculty. These faculty members are often not afforded the same opportunities for professional development and may not have as much experience with teaching residents [16]. These factors could impact the consistency of the education provided at a community-based ambulatory site. Hospital-based ambulatory sites can, of course, face the same problem if many attendings rotate within the clinic, leading to an inconsistent experience of resident education. One way to combat this and add to resident satisfaction is to adopt a "focused faculty model," which promotes a dedicated group of ambulatory faculty to provide most of the supervision and teaching for a group of residents [17].

Engagement in Clinic Initiatives

It is common for residents to feel disengaged from their outpatient clinic experiences, and this is not different for hospital-based clinics. The dominance of inpatient schedules often results in inconsistent clinic schedules, inability to attend team-based clinic meetings, lack of familiarity of other clinic team members, and a sense of lack of ownership of the clinic. Together, these factors may contribute to this perception of not being part of the team. Hospital-based clinics also tend to utilize their facility's centralized services like call centers and consolidated registration centers as opposed to dedicated ambulatory resources. This too may result in a sense of dissociation from clinic team members and may be a barrier to team development.

However, there are several strategies that can help to promote resident engagement in clinic. For example, the use of huddles and team-based meetings can build relationships with other team members and allow residents to refocus on ambulatory care. Huddles can also serve as an opportunity to discuss best practices and improve efficiency [18]. Allowing residents to participate in clinic-based projects can also be effective. For example, population health management, quality improvement initiatives, group medical visits, and interdisciplinary team efforts can successfully integrate residents into clinic operations [19].

The Patient Experience

There are many potential benefits for patients who receive their clinical care in a hospital-based clinic. These benefits can be broadly categorized as technological, financial, geographical, and other. Technological benefits might include access to the hospital's centralized scheduling resources and patient portal that allows patients to easily review the results of lab work and imaging studies as well as to communicate with their health-care team. One systematic review found such access has several benefits for patients including reduced anxiety/reassurance, improvement in the doctor–patient relationships, and increased adherence to medical therapy [20]. Financial advantages might include reduced-cost pharmacy benefits, coordination of care with less travel, and increased access to case managers and social workers. Easy access to an online patient portal can have financial benefits as well, including reduced emergency department utilization and fewer hospital stays [20]. Geographical benefits include, as mentioned above, less travel for the patient, possibly same-day appointments in radiology or with specialists, and also access to the hospital cafeteria for sustenance.

Navigating the System

One important factor of patient experience is ability to accurately navigate the health-care system. This includes the physical navigation to the hospital and within the hospital grounds. A few ways to address this challenge include providing appropriate signage with directions to the clinic, developing specific handheld maps that are patient friendly, and also deploying patient navigators. Ranaghan et al. looked systematically at the role of patient navigator and found mixed results; however, there was a positive effect on patient satisfaction [21]. This could be an interesting area of research for development within the arena of Graduate Medical Education. There are other options for assisting patients within the hospital-based clinic as well; these could include automated appointment reminders and access to a patient portal with reminders and facilitated communication to the health-care team [20].

Emergency Care

Access to Emergency Department

As noted previously, a clinic located in a hospital will also have easier access to hospital-based services such as the emergency department. This feature can improve patient care by allowing patients in need of emergency care to avoid an expensive ambulance fee or the risk of family or self-driving to the hospital. One potential con could be patient confusion regarding when to access each care type. For example, patients may inappropriately utilize emergency room services out of convenience rather than seeking assistance within the primary care setting. Conversely, a very ill patient may present to the clinic inappropriately rather than to the emergency department because of complacency due to their close proximity. This issue can be improved with appropriate patient education.

Conclusion

There are many unique benefits and challenges to starting and maintaining a hospital-based ambulatory site for residency programs. Awareness of and adherence to hospital-specific regulatory requirements is crucial, and the hospital-based clinic must pay special attention to their relationship with the greater hospital community. At the same time, residency programs must prioritize educational objectives and follow the regulations placed on clinical education by the Accreditation Council for Graduate Medical Education (ACGME). A medical director and/or program director will need to focus on these nuances and seek advice from the hospital system to ensure adequate compliance with regulations as well as oversight when starting a hospital-based clinic. Education in a hospital-based clinic is rewarding and can allow for greater faculty flexibility and enhanced patient care. Given what we know about resident satisfaction, working in a hospital-based clinic might allow programs to develop schedules that help further de-accentuate the tension between inpatient and outpatient medicine and thus encourage residents to seek a career in ambulatory primary care.

References

1. Fiebach NH, Wong JG. Taking care of patients in resident clinics: where do we stand. J Gen Intern Med. 2001;16(11):787–9.
2. Babbott S, et al. Ambulatory Office Organization for Internal Medicine Resident Medical Education. Acad Med. 2010;85(12):1880–7.
3. Mumford V, et al. Health services accreditation: what is the evidence that the benefits justify the costs? Int J Qual Health Care. 2013;25(5):606–20.
4. Lam MB, et al. Association between patient outcomes and accreditation in US hospitals: observational study. BMJ. 2018;363:k4011.
5. https://www.jointcommission.org/standards/. Accessed 1 Dec 2021.
6. https://www.cms.gov/Medicare/Medicare-Fee-for-Service-Payment/PhysicianFeeSched. Accessed 24 Jan 2022.
7. Hospital-Based Outpatient Clinics | Atrium Health Wake Forest Baptist (wakehealth.edu). Accessed 1 Dec 2021.
8. Monachino AM, et al. Medical emergencies in the primary care setting: an evidenced based practice approaching using simulation to improve readiness. J Ped Nur. 2019;49:72–8.

9. Wartmann S, et al. Ambulatory-based residency education: improving the congruence of teaching, learning, and patient care. Ann Intern Med. 1992;116(12 Pt 2):1071–5.
10. Batalden M, et al. Beyond a curricular design of convenience: replacing the noon conference with an academic half day in three internal medicine residency programs. Acad Med. 2013;88(5):644–51.
11. Balwan S, et al. Use of team-based learning pedagogy for internal medicine ambulatory resident teaching. J Grad Med Educ. 2015;7(4):643–8.
12. Yale Office Based Medicine Curriculum. https://medicine.yale.edu/intmed/obm/. Accessed 27 Sep 2022.
13. Peccoralo LA, et al. Resident satisfaction with continuity clinic and career choice in general internal medicine. J Gen Intern Med. 2013;28(8):1020–7.
14. Holt SR, et al. Creating a satisfying continuity clinic experience for primary care trainees. Am J Med. 2021;134(4):547–53.
15. Stepczynski J, et al. Factors affection resident satisfaction in continuity clinic—a systematic review. J Gen Intern Med. 2018;33(8):1386–93.
16. Cohen G, et al. Comparing board examination scores between pediatric residents in continuity clinics at different sites. WMJ. 2019;118(1):35–8.
17. Bodenheimer T, et al. Models of faculty involvement in primary care residency teaching clinics. Acad Med. 2020;95(2):190–3.
18. Soones TN, et al. Internal medicine residents' perceptions of team-based care and its educational value in the continuity clinic: a qualitative study. J Gen Int Med. 2015;30:1279–85.
19. Chandran R, et al. Training family medicine residents to build and remodel a patient centered medical home in Rhode Island: a team based approach to PCMH education. R I Med J. 2015;98:35–41.
20. Tapuria A, et al. Impact of patient access to their electronic health record: systematic review. Inform Health Soc Care. 2021;46(2):192–204.
21. Ranaghan C, et al. Effectiveness of a patient navigator on patient satisfaction in adult patients in an ambulatory care setting: a systematic review. JBI Database System Rev Implement Rep. 2016 Aug;14(8):172–218.

Chapter 32
Patient Centered Medical Home

Priya Radhakrishnan

Introduction

The Patient Centered Medical Home (PCMH) is a care delivery model that is team based and aimed at providing coordinated care for patients with complex, chronic medical problems. The PCMH model of care is ideal for residency and faculty practice clinics that typically care for patients who have a high burden of chronic disease and belong to populations that are traditionally underserved. The PCMH delivery model paved the way for Accountable Care Organizations (ACOs), previously called medical neighborhoods. Both models rely on care coordination as a mechanism of improving outcomes. This chapter focuses on providing an overview of the benefits and implementation of the PCMH model of care delivery and will also touch upon the implementation of ACOs within the Academic Internal Medicine clinic structure.

Outline
- PCMH history and evolution
- Accountable care organizations
- PCMH certification/recognition
- Residency clinic director's role
- Maintaining certification
- Engaging patients and patient advisory councils
- Understanding data and value-based payment
- Conclusion

P. Radhakrishnan (✉)
HonorHealth, University of Arizona College of Medicine-Phoenix, Scottsdale, AZ, USA
e-mail: pradhakri@honorhealth.com

L. B. Lu et al. (eds.), *Leading an Academic Medical Practice*,
https://doi.org/10.1007/978-3-031-40273-9_32

PCMH History and Evolution

The Patient Centered Medical Home (PCMH) is a model of care delivery that is designed around the needs of patients and has its foundational elements in care coordination and communication. Originally developed as a method of delivering primary care to patients with complex chronic conditions, it has evolved into one of the building blocks for health care delivery reform and now includes the entire patient population [1]. The term was first coined in 1967 by the American Academy of Pediatrics to describe care models for children with special needs and modified in 1978 by the Hawaiian pediatrician Calvin Sia [2]. The principles were later adopted and ratified by several national primary care organizations including the American Academy of Family Physicians, American Academy of Pediatrics, American College of Physicians, and American Osteopathic Association who together developed the Joint Principles of the Patient Centered Medical Home [3]. The Society of General Internal Medicine took a leadership role in 2009 and convened a series of conferences aimed at evaluating the efficacy of the PCMH movement.

Adapted from the Agency for Healthcare Research and Quality (AHRQ) definition [4], the Patient Centered Primary Care Collaborative (PCPCC) describes the medical home as "an approach to the delivery of primary care that is:

- *Patient Centered*: A partnership among practitioners, patients, and their families ensures that decisions respect patients' wants, needs, and preferences and that patients have the education and support they need to make decisions and participate in their own care.
- *Comprehensive*: A team of care physicians and other providers is wholly accountable for a patient's physical and mental health care needs, including prevention and wellness, acute and chronic care.
- *Coordinated*: Care is organized across all elements of the broader health care system, including specialty care, hospitals, home health care, community services, and supports.
- *Accessible*: Patients can access services with shorter waiting times, 'after-hours' care, 24/7 electronic or telephone access, and strong communication through health information technology (HIT) innovations.
- *Committed to quality and safety*: Clinicians and staff enhance quality improvement to ensure that patients and families make informed decisions about their health."

The early evidence regarding the outcomes of the PCMH model was mixed: it resulted in improved quality but a higher workload for team members [5]. However, as the model matured, the data reporting systems have improved, and there is increasing evidence of the efficacy of the PCMH transformation. Increased adoption of the PCMH domains of function (such as the use of communication tools, an all-payer registry, generation and use of performance reports, tracking of metrics, and 24/7 access) correlated positively with improvements in cost and quality. As with any systematic change, the impact of the PCMH model of care has become more apparent and impactful over time; incremental process improvements have yielded cost savings and broadened implementation of the model [6, 7].

PCMH primary care practices vary in their structure based on geography, size of the practice, patient population, and so on. It is not a "one-size-fits-all" framework. Some of the factors that inform the unique characteristics of a medical home include its location (e.g., urban versus rural setting), composition (e.g., solo/small practice, midsize primary care practice, large multispecialty practice, and academic-affiliated practice), the patient population it serves (e.g., health status and social determinants of health), and whether financial or performance incentives are provided [8].

Regardless of the specifics of the practice, PCMH adoption starts with the practice leadership committing to transformation and a payment structure to support the process. The clinic director is instrumental in driving and sustaining the change needed. As the primary care payment model becomes clearly linked to the demonstration of quality metrics (e.g., implementation of the Merit-based Incentive Payment System, or "MIPS"), academic practices have the unique opportunity to design quality improvement projects with the residents [9–11]. The PCMH model has demonstrated improved health outcomes and reduced inappropriate emergency room visits and readmissions, so quality improvement efforts linked to the PCMH model are likely to be impactful [12].

Accountable Care Organizations

The term ACO was originally coined by researchers and policy experts to describe organizations such as hospitals, medical centers, and clinics that were integrated by way of technology and financial interests, working together toward achieving common clinical goals and outcomes. The ACO model was developed to provide efficient, high value care within a multifaceted physician and provider setting.

It was not until the Patient Protection and Affordable Care Act (also known as the ACA or "Obamacare") was signed into law by President Barack Obama in 2010 that the PCMH model truly gained national attention and the pathways for value-based payment using PCMH principles began at the federal level [13]. The ACA supported increased Medicare and Medicaid reimbursement for enhancing primary care and medical homes. This led to widespread pursuit of PCMH certification among clinics and organizations seeking enhanced reimbursement for the transformation. Subsequently, the Centers of Medicare and Medicaid Innovation (CMMI) launched several demonstration projects such as Comprehensive Primary Care Plus (CPC+) that sought to strengthen primary care through the development of regionally based multi-payer payment reform and care delivery transformation [14].

The ACA provided the beginning of Value-Based Care payment reform and ACOs [15]. This was based on incentivizing medical groups, health systems, and other healthcare providers to coordinate clinically efficient and cost-effective patient care. The physicians, clinics, and healthcare providers become eligible for various benefits (financial and/or other bonuses) when clinical care is delivered effectively with quality outcomes. Hospitals and physicians must meet specific quality benchmarks, which focus on disease prevention, managing patients with chronic diseases, and keeping patients healthy. In order to form an ACO, a formal legal entity with an organizational structure needs to be formed to both receive and distribute shared savings.

Like in the PCMH model, ACOs must develop processes to promote evidence-based medicine, to report on quality data, and to coordinate care and meet the criteria of patient centered care [16]. While ACOs refer to Medicare value-based payment models, several Medicaid and other insurances have similar models. It is essential that academic medical centers align their training missions with high value care [17].

PCMH Certification/Recognition

There are several organizations that have accreditation or recognition programs that clinics can apply to get "official" PCMH status . The National Council on Quality Assurance (NCQA) PCMH recognition program is one of the most widely adopted models for transforming primary care practices into medical homes . Other programs include the Utilization Review Accreditation Commission (URAC), the Joint Commission Primary Care Medical Home Program, and the Accreditation Association for Ambulatory Health Care Medical Home Program. All the certification programs have costs associated with the application and maintenance of the certification [18, 19].

Initial Application

As with any major program that has an impact on the fundamental structure of the clinic, it is important to engage leadership (system/hospital/medical group/health center) to establish stakeholder buy-in. In addition, it is important to have support from the residency program. Although these efforts can be spearheaded by the academic clinic directly, in large health systems it is not unusual for the system leadership to decide to pursue NCQA recognition and bring in the clinic and residency leadership in later to implement the process.

All certification pathways (NCQA or alternative certification) require a feasibility analysis and it is important for the clinic director or manager to assemble a small leadership team who will spearhead the initiative. This team should include representatives from all stakeholder groups (e.g., patients, clinical and administrative staff, nurses, faculty, residents, and HIT personnel). The application process for certification is long and onerous. The group should pick the organization for recognition/certification based on discussions with the health system leadership. Familiarity with the certifying organization (by means of existing centers of excellence, patient safety standards, or preferences from the payer with whom the pilot is considered) should be considered. Champions should be identified early.

The PCMH transformation process must be approached methodically, and a project manager should be assigned. The certifying organizations have clearly organized educational sessions such as conferences, webinars, and checklists, all of which are very helpful. Most electronic health records (EHRs) also have built-in registry functions or population health tools that can aid the process. However, it is important to recognize that considerable work may be needed to improve the quality and attribution of the dataset based on the organizational HIT sophistication.

Taking an inventory of available reports and mapping them to the standards help with organization of the data. This should be followed by development of workflows to manage the transformation.

The team that is involved in the certification or recognition process should meet regularly, with a predetermined agenda using project management techniques to ensure timely completion of the process. Initial certification should take between 3 and 12 months based on the resources available. The PCMH framework includes the six concept areas listed above. The levels of recognition are based on a point system. There are 40 core criteria, and a practice must pass all 40 core criteria. In addition, the practice must demonstrate activities to obtain at least 25 credits of elective criteria across the concept areas that include demonstration of measurement of quality of care and expanded access to care. Patient involvement is a requirement that must begin at the outset of the PCMH recognition process. It is not unusual for clinics to start the process and add patients to the implementation team or develop a Patient Advisory Council (PAC) as an afterthought. In order for the process to be truly patient centric, the planning team must invite patients to join the transformation early on, with clear goals and educational sessions for the patients. Patient representatives can provide the clinic with insight into most of the processes and are typically willing partners for transformation [20]. Additionally, inviting residents and staff to attend the PAC meetings and giving them a formal seat at the table should be encouraged; this promotes collaboration and involvement of the entire team in the transformation process.

Residency Clinic Director's Role

As with any transformative process, the clinic director plays a significant role in championing the project, marketing it to faculty colleagues and residents, and developing small quality improvement projects that involve faculty, residents, and students to help with the certification process.

Engaging the residency program director and faculty is advantageous to both the clinic leadership and the residency program. PCMH transformation fits well into the Clinical Learning Environment Review (CLER) focus areas [21] defined by the Accreditation Council of Graduate Medical Education (ACGME). Involving residents and faculty will also ensure that the residency program is enhanced by the process. For example, many residency clinics care for large populations of patients with significant health care disparities; integrating the PCMH competencies into the population health curriculum within residency training can inspire residents to make changes in their practices and witness real-time transformation. Using a standard process for quality improvement such as the Plan-Do-Study-Act (PDSA) cycle and following the Standards for Quality Improvement Reporting Excellence (SQUIRE) [22] guidelines on reporting quality improvement make this exercise into an academic project worthy of scholarship.

Maintaining Certification

Achieving certification or recognition is the first step in the process of PCMH transformation. To ensure that the process is woven into the fabric of the clinic, the clinic director and leadership should model the patient centered behaviors such as ensuring expanded access to care, timely reporting of test and referral results, accommodating patient preferences, and shared decision-making. For example, it is not unusual for patients to arrive late to clinic and be turned away, and then subsequently coded as a "no-show" in the scheduling system. Depending on clinic policy, this may result in discharge from the clinic. Instead, clinics might consider implementing some form of open access scheduling to accommodate patients who have transportation issues. Having a care coordinator to maintain contact with patients to follow up on referrals and address patient access issues such as transportation etc. ensures that the care is patient centered. Unless clinics pay attention to the continuous process of quality improvement, they may experience lapses. Presenting PCMH reports (based on the reporting criteria) at faculty and resident meetings as a standing agenda item is recommended to improve awareness, transparency, and continuous improvement.

In an academic medical practice, access to care is often limited by conflicting schedules, teaching conferences, and other educational activities. Redesigning the process of health care delivery is essential and can be accomplished by expanding care team to include pharmacists and nurses [23]. Staff and physician training is essential [24]. Special effort must be placed on standardizing Health Insurance Portability and Accountability Act (HIPAA)-compliant communication methods between patients and also between members of the care team; email, text messaging, and telemedicine often improve access to care.

For clinics with many high-risk or vulnerable patients (i.e., significant needs around the social determinants of health, behavioral health problems, pain and addiction, or homelessness), multidisciplinary rounding has been shown to be effective (with the involvement of the entire care team including home visit nurses and social workers when indicated) [25]. Developing multidisciplinary team-based rounding requires a significant preparation of agendas, process for identification or referral of patients, and regular follow-up.

Engaging Patients and Patient Advisory Councils

As previously noted, patients are a valuable and a necessary partner during PCMH transformation. One common error during the process is that when PACs are developed, these advisory councils may not be clear on their roles, nor feel empowered to make recommendations to improve care. While developing a PAC, it is important to spend time defining the makeup of the PAC and to identify the resources needed. The PAC must represent the community of patients. Clinics with high numbers of non-English-speaking patients should make a special attempt to bring interpreters and present materials (agendas and information) in the appropriate language and level of health literacy. It is also important to share data with the PACs to seek their help in the improvement process. In the author's experience, patients can help with setting agendas, improving satisfaction scores by serving as "secret shoppers," and developing pre-visit questionnaires. Academic clinics with empowered PACs are also positioned to apply for Patient Centered Outcomes Research Institute (PCORI) grants. They are also helpful in piloting initiatives around shared decision-making and providing the patient perspective on high-value care.

Understanding Data and Value-based Payment

Increasingly, there is an almost visceral reaction that most physicians display while being given their data. Per Sandy et al., "In today's health care environment where the practice of medicine is increasingly data-driven, it is important for physicians to develop appropriate practice management actions based on the data, and avoid both overreaction and underreaction" [25]. This source further notes that there is a positive association between the NCQA recognition program and achieving *quality* benchmarks, but it may also be negatively associated with achieving *efficiency* benchmarks. The efficiency benchmark tends to be achieved at a later stage of PCMH transformation/ACO implementation. This is likely due to the addition of new workflows early in the transformation process while simultaneously failing to remove redundant or ineffective processes. In order to ensure that efficiency and costs are contained while applying for and subsequently maintaining certification, it is important for the clinic leadership to manage overall processes using strategies such as the Situation, Background, Assessment, and Recommendation (SBAR) model for standardized communication process improvement, and quality improvement strategies (e.g., PDSA or Lean Six Sigma) to reduce the additional burden on staff and faculty [26–28]. The clinic data team involved in developing the reporting framework must initially educate themselves on the quality of data. Despite significant widespread adoption of electronic health records, lack of good quality data is often the norm rather than the exception. Being prepared to evaluate and help "clean the data" is an important step that will determine the success of the transformation. It is important that the faculty members who are responsible for the standards be accountable to the leadership team to ensure that the standards and metrics are met. In the author's experience, increasing numbers of residency clinics have dedicated administrative time built into block clinic rotations to achieve this objective. It is important both for the residents and supervising faculty that there exist clear expectations and a curriculum that defines coordination essential for patient centered care. This is an important venue of engaging the learners (residents as well as the faculty who may not be familiar with the process of data measurement and improvement). Having a robust PCMH/ACO care coordination program can lead to innovative curricula and programs that may, in turn, attract a higher caliber of residents and faculty [29, 30].

Conclusion

While the journey of transformation toward becoming a Patient Centered Medical Home is long and arduous, the impact on improved care, patient satisfaction, and joy of practice is worth the effort. PCMH certification is the first step toward improving the health system, and the clinic director plays an important role in leading the transformation efforts as well as acting as a cheerleader for them. PCMH transformation is vital for academic clinics to ensure that they truly provide high-value care; taking care of patients with complex chronic diseases should be at the forefront of population health initiatives. Clinic directors are in the unique position to help lead the redesign of primary care health care delivery and guide projects to ensure that the transformation efforts support the scholarly activities needed to fulfill ACGME requirements for residents and faculty. The clinic director is instrumental when adopting a PCMH model of care.

References

1. Adamson M. The patient centered medical home: an essential destination on the road to reform. Am Health Drug Benefits. 2011;4(2):122–4.
2. Sia C, Tonniges TF, Osterhus E, Taba S. History of the medical home concept. Pediatrics. 2004;113(5 Suppl):1473–8.
3. American Academy of Family Physicians; American Academy of Pediatrics; American College of Physicians; American Osteopathic Association (March 2007). "Joint principles of the patient centered medical home" (PDF). Retrieved 2009-06-30.
4. Defining the PCMH. US Department of Health and Human Services. https://www.pcmh.ahrq.gov/page/defining-pcmh
5. Reid R, Fishman P, Yu O, Ross T, Tufano J, Soman M, Larson E. Patient centered medical home demonstration: a prospective, quasi-experimental, before and after evaluation. Am J Manag Care. 2009;15(9):e71–87.
6. Paustian M, Alexander J, El Reda D, Wise C, Green L, Fetters M. Partial and incremental PCMH practice transformation: implications for quality and costs. Health Serv Res. 2014;49(1):52–74. Epub 5 July 2013

7. Carlin C, Flottemesch T, Solberg L, Werner AJ. System transformation in patient centered medical home (PCMH): variable impact on chronically ill patients' utilization. J Am Board Fam Med. 2016;29(4):482–95.
8. Tanenbaum JE, Votruba M, Einstadter D, Love TE, Cebul RD. Adoption of health system innovations: evidence of urban-rural disparities from the Ohio primary care marketplace. J Gen Intern Med. 2021;36(6):1584–90. https://doi.org/10.1007/s11606-020-06440-7. Epub 2021 Jan 29. PMID: 33515196; PMCID: PMC8175515
9. Doolittle B, Tobin D, Genao I, Ellman M, Ruser C, Brienza R. Implementing the patient centered medical home in residency education. Educ Health. 2015;28:74–8.
10. The Merit-based Incentive Payment System (MIPS). Centers for Medicare and Medicaid Services. The Medicare Access and Chip Reauthorization Act of 2015. https://www.cms.gov/Medicare/Quality-Initiatives-Patient-Assessment-Instruments/Value-Based-Programs/MACRA-MIPS-and-APMs/Quality-Payment-Program-MIPS-NPRM-Slides.pdf
11. About the Law. US Department of Health and Human Services. https://www.hhs.gov/healthcare/about-the-law/read-the-law/
12. Nielsen M, Langner B, Zema C, Hacker T, Grundy P. Benefits of implementing the PCMH: a review of cost & quality results; 2012
13. Abrams MK, Nuzum R, Zezza MA, Ryan J, Kiszla J, Guterman S. The affordable care act's payment and delivery system reforms: a progress report at five years. Issue Briefs Commonwealth Fund. 2015;12:1–6.
14. Comprehensive Primary Care Plus. Centers for Medicare and Medicaid Services. https://innovation.cms.gov/initiatives/Comprehensive-Primary-Care-Plus
15. Moy HP, Giardino AP, Varacallo M. Accountable care organization. [Updated 2022 Feb 10]. In: StatPearls [Internet]. Treasure Island, FL: StatPearls Publishing; 2022.
16. https://innovation.cms.gov/innovation-models/aco
17. Gupta R, Sehgal N, Arora VM. Aligning delivery system and training missions in academic medical centers to promote high-value care. Acad Med. 2019;94(9):1289–92. https://doi.org/10.1097/ACM.0000000000002573.
18. Gans D. A comparison of the national patient centered medical home accreditation and recognition programs medical group management association. Medical Group Management
19. https://www.ncqa.org/programs/health-care-providers-practices/patient-centered-medical-home-pcmh/process/
20. Sharma AE, Angel L, Bui Q. Patient advisory councils: giving patients a seat at the table. Fam Pract Manag. 2015;22(4):22–2.
21. Accreditation Council for Graduate Medical Education (ACGME). Clinical learning environment review (CLER). http://www.acgme.org/What-We-Do/Initiatives/Clinical-Learning-Environment-Review-CLER
22. Revised Standards for Quality Improvement Reporting Excellence SQUIRE 2.0. http://www.squire-statement.org/index.cfm?fuseaction=Page.ViewPage&PageID=471
23. Strong T. Care team redesign: transforming medical assistant roles in primary care. Healthaffairs.org. 11 Mar 2015. http://healthaffairs.org/blog/2015/03/11/care-team-redesigntransforming-medical-assistant-roles-in-primary-care/
24. Quan X, Joseph A, Keller A, Taylor E. Designing safety-net clinics for innovative care delivery models California Health Care Foundation. March 2011. http://ambulatory.healthdesign.org/sites/default/files/designingclinicsinnovativecaredeliverymodels.pdf
25. Sandy L, Haltson H, Metfessel B, Reese C. Measuring physician quality and efficiency in an era of practice transformation: PCMH as a Case Study. Ann Fam Med. 2015;13(3):264–8.
26. Rizzo E. 10 patient handoff communications tools. Beckers Infection Control and Clinical Quality. 4 Sept 2014. http://www.beckersasc.com/asc-quality-infection-control/10-patienthandoff-communications-tools-2014.html
27. SBAR Toolkit. Institute for Healthcare Improvement. http://www.ihi.org/resources/Pages/Tools/sbartoolkit.aspx

28. Sobek D, Jimmerson C. A3 reports: too for process improvement. https://www.lean.org/Search/Documents/133.pdf
29. Johnson S, Hartigan S, Holt E, Sop D, McHenry C, Lipato T, Elliott T, Ferlis M, Mcmanus C, Smith WR. Using lean six sigma to develop a patient centered medical home for adults with sickle cell disease. Blood. 2019;134(Supplement_1):3408. https://doi.org/10.1182/blood-2019-131117.
30. Shortell SM, Casalino LP. Health care reform requires accountable care systems. JAMA. 2008;300:95–7.

Chapter 33
Federally Qualified Health Centers

Shwetha Iyer, Mary Gover, and Magni Hamso

Introduction

Federally Qualified Health Centers (FQHCs) are part of the nation's medical safety net, with 1400 unique FQHCs serving over 28 million patients annually in underserved, resource-poor areas across the United States [1]. FQHCs are authorized through the Centers for Medicare and Medicaid Services (CMS) and receive enhanced payments (encounter rates) to offset the costs of caring for their largely uninsured and publicly insured patients [2]. Although the missions of FQHCs and internal medicine residency programs largely overlap—providing quality care to underserved populations—few collaborations between FQHCs and internal medicine residency programs exist [3].

It is well known that residents tend to stay within a 100-mile radius of their training site and that those who work at an FQHC during their training are more likely to continue to care for the underserved on graduation [4–10]. Over the last few decades, there have been several attempts to increase the number of postgraduate training programs at FQHCs. These efforts reflect the need to improve the diversity and distribution of the primary care physician workforce and have been led by the Area Health Education Center program, established in 1972 and funded by the

S. Iyer (✉) · M. Gover
Department of Medicine, Albert Einstein College of Medicine/Montefiore Medical Center, Bronx, NY, USA
e-mail: siyer@montefiore.org; mgover@montefiore.org

M. Hamso
Department of Medicine, University of Washington School of Medicine, Boise VA Medical Center, Boise, ID, USA
e-mail: mhamso@uw.edu

L. B. Lu et al. (eds.), *Leading an Academic Medical Practice*,
https://doi.org/10.1007/978-3-031-40273-9_33

Health Resources and Services Administration, and by the Teaching Health Center Graduate Medical Education program, funded under the Patient Protection and Affordable Care Act in 2010 [11–13]. Even so, few residency programs have formal relationships with FQHCs; in fact, per a 2016 analysis of the Accreditation Council for Graduate Medical Education (ACGME) and CMS data, only 4% of family medicine and 5% of internal medicine training sites were at community-based health clinics [3].

There are several barriers to the development and maintenance of affiliations between residency programs and FQHCs that likely contribute to the low number of FQHC-based training sites. However, FQHCs and residency programs share a common commitment to service and providing high quality care to their communities, making collaboration potentially fruitful for both parties. In this chapter, we review the benefits and challenges of FQHC–residency partnerships along with some potential solutions. We also discuss several successful partnerships.

Outline

- Benefits of collaboration
  - Benefits for residency programs
    - Diverse patient population
    - Team-based care
    - Broad clinical experience
    - Social determinants of health
    - High value care
  - Benefits for FQHCs
    - Workforce
    - Finances
    - Quality of care
- Challenges of collaboration
  - Administration and governance
  - Funding
  - Logistics
- Steps toward partnership
- Partnership examples
- Conclusion

Benefits for Residency Programs

Diverse Patient Population

The ACGME requires that residents achieve proficiency in designated competencies prior to graduation, including the ability to demonstrate "respect and responsiveness to diverse patient populations" [14]. Patients served by FQHCs tend to be racially and ethnically diverse, often comprising recent immigrants and refugees in addition to long-established minority communities [1]. This diversity provides residents exposure to different cultures and backgrounds and allows them to practice the skills of cultural humility within their continuity clinics [15]. Even more importantly, by providing primary care training in communities that may have been impacted by structural racism such as police violence and redlining (systematically denying loans to individuals living in poor communities or areas deemed to be of high financial risk), FQHC–residency partnerships provide residency programs the opportunity to explicitly address racism and to train primary care leaders who understand and can work alongside communities to eliminate structural racism [16–18].

Team-Based Care

FQHCs involve residents in team-based primary care. Many FQHCs are leaders in the patient-centered medical home (PCMH) movement, and FQHC–residency partnerships can expose residents to PCMH fundamentals such as team huddles, team-based electronic communication, and physician–staff pairing. In addition, many FQHCs have implemented behavioral health integration. Under the behavioral health integration model, primary care physicians work together with embedded behavioral health counselors and a consulting psychiatrist to diagnose, treat, and monitor patients with common psychiatric conditions such as anxiety and depression. The model includes care coordination, dedicated interdisciplinary meetings, and structured team communication and has been shown to improve patient outcomes and empower physicians to manage behavioral health conditions in primary care [19]. Some FQHCs also employ physician assistants and nurse practitioners who can help manage residents' panels when they are on inpatient rotations or who can refer their more complicated patients to the internal medicine residents for care [12, 15, 20]. The experience in team-based care that residents receive through FQHC–residency partnerships translates into practice: residents trained at PCMH sites are more likely to engage in tasks defined by the National Center for Quality Assurance including providing care between visits, accommodating for language barriers, screening for substance use disorders, and performing medication reconciliation. In addition, they are more likely to advocate for patients and help them connect with community-based resources [21]. FQHC–residency partnerships can thus facilitate primary care training in interdisciplinary teams that will prepare residents for real-world, team-based primary care and help them succeed in caring for psychosocially and medically complex populations in the future.

Broad Clinical Experience

The breadth of patients cared for by FQHCs is tremendous. FQHCs exist in urban and rural underserved areas with patient populations that include young, healthy individuals, the elderly with multiple comorbidities, and people of all ages with conditions that are highly medically complex. Patients in care at FQHCs are more likely to present with serious and chronic conditions compared to patients in care with private practitioners [1]. FQHCs are not only focused on preventative health and routine primary care; many FQHCs are starting to incorporate hepatitis C and HIV treatment into their chronic disease management. In fact, in order to make it easier for people living with HIV/AIDS to obtain quality and culturally appropriate care in their own communities, one component of the National HIV/AIDS Strategy is to expand the number of FQHCs that provide HIV care [22, 23].

FQHC physicians are often on the front lines of screening for and providing mental health care, driven by the tandem forces of the prevalence of mental illness in this population and the paucity of psychologists and psychiatrists in underserved areas [24–26]. These programs are also more likely to have faculty members who prescribe buprenorphine for opioid use disorder and graduates who pursue additional training in addiction medicine [27]. FQHCs thus expose residents to different medical and behavioral health problems, giving them a robust clinical education and preparing them for future practice [28].

Social Determinants of Health

FQHC–residency partnerships prepare residents to address their patients' social determinants of health (SDOH). FQHCs care primarily for individuals living at or near the federal poverty level, with many patients struggling with food insecurity, unstable housing, criminal justice-involvement, and lack of health insurance. When providing primary care at FQHCs, residents must actively consider the impact of SDOH on the well-being of their patients. Although these structural and psychosocial issues can make providing basic primary care more complicated, working with patients whose health is affected by social systems provides real-world experience for residents to develop the skills needed to help their patients navigate community-based resources, social services, and the medical system. In fact, the strongest predictor of resident competence in identifying and addressing SDOH is training in an underserved setting [18, 29].

The ACGME developed the Clinical Learning Environment Review (CLER) program to assess and advance the quality of residents' and fellows' education through accreditation. As part of CLER, residency programs have been tasked with developing specific efforts to reduce disparities and improve community health. FQHC–residency partnerships meet this charge by giving the opportunity for residents to gain competence in working with marginalized communities and by increasing health-care access—through a larger workforce—to communities impacted by SDOH [18]. Furthermore, many FQHCs are closely connected to community organizations such as food banks, shelters, job training programs, and substance use treatment programs. Residencies can collaborate with these community partners who can in turn teach residents about their resources and the biopsychosocial approach to health [1, 15, 24, 25, 30, 31].

High-Value Care

Another benefit of incorporating internal medicine residency programs into FQHCs includes exposing residents to cost-conscious care. FQHCs offer care on a federally set sliding scale for uninsured and underinsured patients, but costs quickly add up, forcing residents to prioritize diagnostic testing and care in partnership with their patients. Similarly, FQHCs have access to a low-cost federal formulary of medications (i.e., the 340b program); however, as patients often struggle to afford multiple medications, residents need to think critically about which medications are truly crucial for that patient's care [2]. The literature is mixed regarding the impact of working in an FQHC on the development of cost-conscious physicians [32, 33]. However, residency programs can increase the culture of high-value care by including explicit training in these areas, increasing access to financial data, and encouraging regular discussions about value [33]. FQHC–residency partnerships can give residents real-world experience with high-value care.

Benefits for FQHCs

Workforce

In addition to internal medicine training programs benefiting from having their ambulatory training at FQHCs, FQHCs can benefit from partnerships with academic medical centers. Many FQHCs struggle with regular turnover in their workforce, often because of lower pay. Turnover has also been blamed on excessive workload and issues regarding autonomy and work control often present in community health center work [18, 34–36]. Partnerships with academic medical centers guarantee a stable workforce through supervising attending physicians and three classes of residents that are replenished each year. Moreover, residents who train at FQHCs often continue to care for underserved patients in the area after graduation [4–8, 18], and FQHCs have the opportunity to recruit and retain them at their clinic. Residency programs retain control over the number of patients residents are scheduled to see each session, protecting them and their supervising attendings from excessive workloads. At the same time, each attending can see more patients through supervision than they can on their own, facilitating the FQHC's goal of increasing patient access and maximizing visit numbers. Additionally, retained physicians are uniquely equipped to contribute to strategic planning of the FQHC by making sure the needs of the community are met based on their training experience [18].

While some aspects of working at an FQHC can be more challenging for practicing physicians, educating students and residents can reduce burnout and connect attendings to the reasons they went into medicine to begin with [18]. This connection to medical education can help retain faculty at these sites.

Finances

Federal rules governing Medicare and Medicaid payments to FQHCs incentivize volume over complexity [2]. FQHCs therefore may emphasize the number of patient encounters more than hospital-based residency clinics and residency programs. However, having residents at an FQHC can facilitate this process. As residents progress through their training and can see more patients per session, they can together see more patients than their supervising physicians could on their own. This allows FQHCs to generate more revenue and offsets the cost of accommodating junior physicians who need more time per encounter [37].

Quality of Care

By partnering with a residency program, an FQHC builds a connection with the affiliated hospital system. This affiliation can create a structured and reliable referral system for the patients of the health center, which previously may not have been available. Physicians can be confident in the quality of their referral system and communication around referrals, and patients benefit by improved access to necessary specialists [38].

Additionally, CLER has required residency programs to formulate patient safety curricula and provide training in quality improvement [39, 40]. This directive has led FQHC–residency partnerships to formally build quality improvement into their work—an endeavor that FQHCs want to engage in but do not often have the time or resources to implement [14, 18, 41].

Challenges

Significant benefits exist in partnerships between residency programs and FQHCs, especially when it comes to learning opportunities for residents and retaining and expanding the primary care physician workforce. At the same time, there are real challenges that can hinder successful, long-term relationships if not appropriately addressed.

Many of these challenges have also been experienced by family medicine residency programs partnering with CMS-certified Rural Health Clinics (RHC), which have a similar goal to FQHCs of increasing access to care in underserved areas. Unlike FQHCs, however, RHCs provide less comprehensive primary care services, must be located in rural shortage areas, and rely heavily on non-physician practitioners by law [42]. New formal partnerships between internal medicine residency programs and RHCs exist; however, family medicine residency programs have long collaborated with RHCs through rural training tracks (RTT) and their lessons learned also inform this section [38].

Administration and Governance

The biggest barriers to a successful FQHC–residency partnership center around governance, administration, and funding. In fact, nearly 30% of program directors cite governance (adhering to the rules and regulations of the supervising body) as a significant barrier to a successful working relationship between FQHCs and residency programs [43]. Residency programs are subject to the rules and requirements of the ACGME and the Resident Review Committee (RRC) that focus on education, while FQHCs are governed by a board of directors that focus on delivering primary care as well as accrediting bodies such as the Joint Commission and federal agencies such as CMS. The different priorities of the bodies governing the residency and the FQHC can make it difficult to meet the goals and needs of the respective organizations [43, 44].

While governance is the most frequently mentioned barrier to successfully maintaining an FQHC–residency partnership, gaps in leadership are highlighted as the most important initial barrier. Hospital administrators or residency program directors may fail to initiate an affiliation with an FQHC due to a lack of knowledge about FQHC–residency program collaborations. They also often have misconceptions about disorganization and poor management at community health clinics and—for those programs that intend to utilize FQHC physicians as resident educators—may be skeptical about the quality of teaching provided by FQHC physicians [30]. Poor communication between the residency program director and the FQHC can exacerbate this potential barrier [43]. Family medicine residency programs with RTTs at RHCs also cite the importance of leadership. In fact, program directors suggest that a strong leader and faculty member who is on site, is passionate about and connected to the local community, and understands the competing demands of both the RHC and the residency is instrumental for not just initiating but also maintaining the partnership [45].

Administrative complexity can also make collaboration difficult. FQHCs must ensure that there are enough support staff to deal with large fluctuations in the number of physicians while remaining flexible with frequently changing resident schedules. The discontinuity of residency clinic scheduling directly challenges the provision of continuity of care provided at the FQHC. Additionally, the frequent cycles of privileging and training of new physicians associated with residency programs can lead to extra administrative burdens not usually dealt with by FQHCs. Ultimately, for a partnership to be successful, there needs to be a balance between the clinic's needs and the residency's needs and an understanding from both programs' leadership about how to address those needs simultaneously [38, 43, 44].

Funding

The issue of funding is another crucial barrier to FQHC–residency partnerships. Underfunding on both sides is common. Each organization needs to protect its own funding streams and often cannot absorb costs that are not directly associated with their primary mission. Each entity may feel as though the other has more resources to help pay for salaries and other costs [30, 43–45]. Moreover, there may be unique costs associated with the affiliation including salaries for additional support staff and for supervising attendings who precept residents. There is significant discrepancy as to the financial implications of training residents, with studies citing anywhere from a cost of $7000–$14,000 per resident per year to a profit of about $1000 per resident over expenses, depending on the availability of volunteer preceptors, FQHC contributions, and the number of patients seen by residents [37].

Actively addressing these potential financial risks and identifying diverse funding streams can be crucial for initiating and maintaining an FQHC–residency partnership [45]. There are creative ways for FQHC–residency partnerships to bring down costs. When the FQHC–residency partnership is affiliated with the residency program's home hospital, inpatient revenue from supervising physicians can contribute to residency training and offset some costs lost to precepting. Additionally, the number of patients seen by residents can be modified as long as the numbers do not exceed RRC standards, allowing attending physicians to care of more patients per hour while precepting than they could seeing patients on their own. Pursuing grant funding and working with state legislatures and Medicaid programs to fund residency slots may also improve the financial viability of FQHC–residency partnerships [37, 45–48]. Ultimately, financial considerations can be complex, and it is essential for the FQHC and residency program to address funding together at the initiation of the partnership.

Logistics

The logistics of practicing at an FQHC can also make it a challenging primary care experience for residents. FQHCs may utilize a different electronic medical record (EMR) system from their affiliated hospitals, and many FQHCs leverage complex multi-hospital referral systems to accommodate their uninsured and underinsured patients [49]. Residents also complain about inefficiencies in the clinic system related to triage, medication refills, paperwork, and wait times for referrals and diagnostic tests [30, 49, 50]. Additionally, although likely mitigated by the move toward X + Y residency scheduling models and team-based care, some residency programs still require residents to follow up on clinic tasks during non-clinic rotations. This work can be especially complex in an FQHC environment both for the reasons described above and because patients at FQHCs often have complex social determinants of health. Ironically, although X + Y residency scheduling models may simplify clinic follow-up work somewhat for residents, the periodic rotation of new residents into the clinic setting can still make logistics difficult for the FQHC. For example, the FQHC staff may struggle to understand and accommodate resident schedules, especially if the residency program is not large enough to maintain a continuous presence at the FQHC.

No-shows present a frequent challenge to FQHCs as well, with rates varying from as low as 5% to as high as 55% [38, 51]. The low-income patients that FQHCs serve frequently have difficulty affording health-care costs even at the FQHC sliding scale price, struggle with transportation and childcare, and have trouble getting time off from work [1]. Patients are also often scheduled months ahead of time, and too much time between scheduling an appointment and the appointment date can affect attendance rates [51, 52]. No-shows reduce physician productivity, increase costs, and ultimately prevent clinics from effectively serving their patients by reducing their functional capacity [52]. FQHCs must consider options in dealing with this high no-show rate, including overbooking and sending out patient reminders, especially as residents with less consistent schedules are added to their workforce. However, despite these challenges, morale among academic FQHC physicians is typically high, reflected in enhanced recruitment and retention, making the partnership a desirable one [44, 49].

Another unique logistical barrier at FQHCs is the need to adapt to the diversity of the patient population and the many languages spoken by patients. In fact, according to recent national surveys, 63% of hospitals and 54% of general internal medicine physicians treat patients with limited English proficiency on a weekly basis, while 84% of FQHCs do so every day [53]. Some potential solutions for this issue include developing operating procedures to support language access, scheduling appointments to take into account the availability of language services, making telephone language lines available in all exam rooms, providing periodic training on communication skills, and developing patient education materials and forms in multiple languages and at a low literacy level [53]. Language services, however, are expensive [54]. While FQHCs often try to hire staff that are at least bilingual with the primary language of their patient population to cut down on the costs of interpreting services, this is not possible within residency training, so the cost of interpretation services may go up when incorporating trainees into an FQHC.

Steps Toward Partnership

As real benefits and challenges exist, it is important to highlight best practices when establishing FQHC–residency partnerships. Structured interviews and focus groups with practice administrators, medical directors, primary care association members, university faculty members, residency program directors, FQHC board members, and government representatives from ten states identified three ways to overcome barriers to successful affiliation: (1) a shared mission of service and education; (2) new funding sources that facilitate the shared mission, account for costs associated with training residents, and protect existing funds; and (3) clear communication regarding governance and administrative responsibilities [44].

First and foremost, there has to be a shared mission regarding service to the community and providing excellent clinical care to the population served by the FQHC. Training residents at the FQHC must be consistent with the goals of the residency program. In addition, an in-depth examination of the financial status of the residency is necessary; if financial barriers are identified, possible solutions need to be generated. These parallel steps must take place at the FQHC once an appropriate FQHC has been identified [30].

The next step should include forming a joint FQHC and residency task force to devise a partnership plan. The members of this task force may include the residency program director, an administrator from the residency and/or sponsoring hospital, an FQHC executive or clinic medical director, an FQHC board of directors representative, and a lawyer for the FQHC. This group will need to outline the financial, service, educational, and legal responsibilities of the residency (and/or sponsoring hospital if appropriate) and the FQHC as the partnership is developed [44].

Introducing residents to the FQHC could begin with block rotations or participation in a community health project and eventually extend into longitudinal training experiences such as continuity clinic. Lastly, a joint strategic planning committee for ongoing monitoring and evaluation of the partnership is recommended [30] (see Fig. 33.1).

Partnership Examples

There are several examples of successful FQHC–residency partnerships described in the literature [31, 34, 55]. These FQHC–residency partnerships have been successful because the FQHC and residency program had a shared mission,

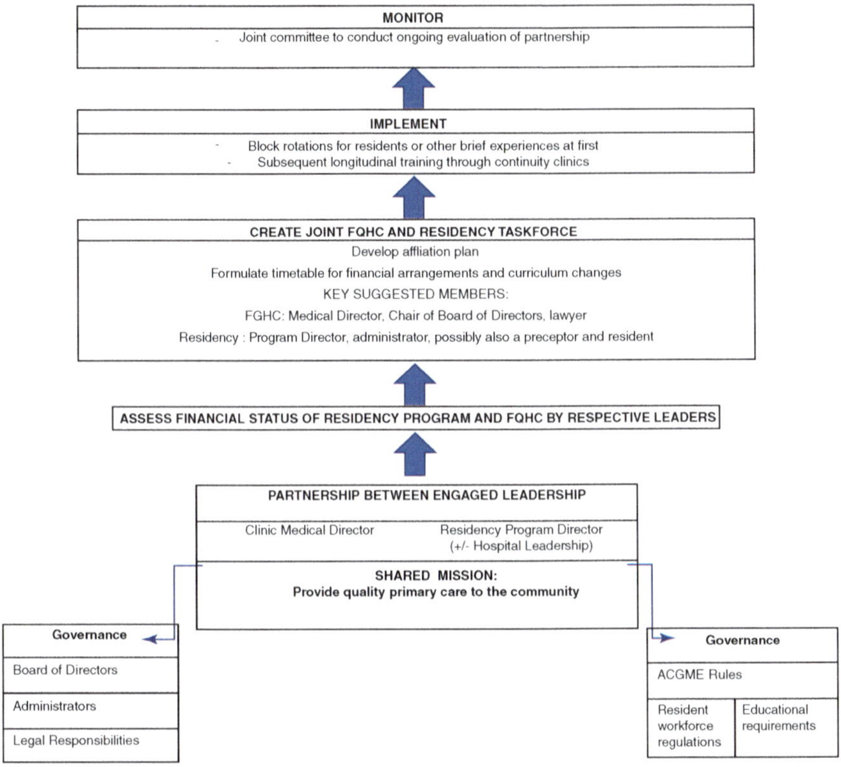

Fig. 33.1 Steps toward FQHC and residency program partnership. Figure developed based on research by Gordan and Hale [30] and Morris and Chen [44]

communicated openly about their governing bodies' priorities, and decided on funding streams from the beginning of their partnerships.

California

The Keck School of Medicine of the University of Southern California successfully merged their struggling residency training clinic with a local hospital and community health center in 2012, in order to forward their shared mission of caring for the underserved and meet the short- and long-term goals of each institution. The residency program needed to increase its residents' numbers of outpatient sessions in order to comply with ACGME training program requirements, the local hospital needed to expand its referral base, and the community health center needed to improve its quality assurance activities and technological/EMR infrastructure. As a result of the collaboration, the residency program was able to recruit an increasingly competitive class of residents and to meet ACGME outpatient encounter requirements. The community health center obtained FQHC status, implemented an EMR, and expanded its patient volume. In turn, the local hospital began receiving more referrals for hospital-based specialty care and diagnostics. Although it took about eighteen months to establish, the collaboration was successful because the institutions had a shared mission, and the leadership at each site was willing to prioritize each partner's goals equally and committed to making the collaboration happen [34].

Connecticut

An internal medicine program at Norwalk Hospital in Connecticut developed a partnership with an FQHC in order to improve their residents' outpatient training and better serve the community. In exchange for moving all of their primary care services and outpatient training to the FQHC, Norwalk Hospital and the residency program helped the FQHC renovate its premises and subsidized the cost of internal medicine staff. The relationship was successful, expanding patient encounters and improving patient satisfaction, as well as reducing clinic staff turnover. Although it took two years to negotiate, the partnership worked because the leadership at both the hospital-based residency program and the FQHC recognized their shared mission of caring for the community and were able to identify mutually beneficial outcomes from the partnership [56].

New York

The Residency Program in Primary Care/Social Internal Medicine (PC/SIM) at Montefiore Medical Center has a successful partnership with an FQHC that demonstrates the multiple benefits a residency program can reap from such a partnership. In this section the authors share their personal knowledge and experience.

Montefiore is a large academic hospital located in the Bronx, NY, with a mission to deliver quality care to the underserved. In the 1980s, it opened the first hospital-based Department of Social Medicine in the country. As part of its mission to expand primary care access in the Bronx, Montefiore partnered with a coalition of FQHCs and school-based health centers, which is now known as the Bronx Community Health Network. The PC/SIM Residency Program specifically collaborated with the Comprehensive Health Care Center (CHCC), one of the FQHCs from this coalition, in the early 1990s. This relationship has been successful because of the hospital, residency, and FQHC's shared mission of providing quality primary care to the Bronx community; a close working relationship between the programs' administrators; and the hospital's willingness to financially back the collaboration. Some highlights of this collaboration include having residency core faculty supervise residents and see their own patients at the same FQHC, as well as established education for residents around caring for specific patient populations seen at the FQHC. The faculty, many of whom are graduates of PC/SIM, have created formal, long-standing partnerships with community-based organizations that work with recent immigrants, justice-involved individuals, persons in supportive housing, and individuals struggling with substance use disorders, giving residents excellent community-oriented training in addressing SDOH and improving care for vulnerable patients.

This FQHC–residency partnership is one in which the FQHC has become an ambulatory site of the hospital system with dual governance from the hospital ambulatory care network and the Bronx Community Healthcare Network. Consequently, while clinical time generates most of their salaries, the core faculty receive additional support from hospital departments to cover teaching and administrative time. The medical director of the FQHC also serves as an associate department chair for the hospital's Department of Medicine and the assistant medical director is the associate program director of the residency program. The close collaboration and even overlap between hospital, residency, and clinic leadership has been crucial for maintaining this long-standing, successful FQHC–residency partnership. The affiliation between Montefiore, CHCC, and PC/SIM highlights the importance of having a shared mission between the organizations and establishing a strong and continued partnership between leadership of all groups. It also illustrates the many training opportunities a long-standing partnership with an FQHC can facilitate.

Conclusion

Although there are challenges to establishing partnerships between FQHCs and residency programs, there are many benefits. Not only can residents receive superb outpatient medical training at FQHCs, but they will also obtain experience caring for a medically and psychosocially diverse patient population, have the opportunity to grapple with SDOH, learn how to work in an interdisciplinary team, and practice cost-conscious care. FQHCs benefit by having a stable workforce and by having the opportunity to recruit well-trained, prepared physicians dedicated to caring for the underserved. In order to create a successful FQHC–residency partnership, it is vital to have a shared mission of service and education, explore reimbursement streams that facilitate the shared mission and account for the costs associated with training residents, understand governance requirements, and clearly delineate administrative tasks and roles for both the residency program and the FQHC.

References

1. National Association of community health centers. America's Health Centers August 2021. https://www.nachc.org/wp-content/uploads/2020/10/2021-Snapshot.pdf. Accessed 23 Feb 2022.

2. Department of Health and Human Services Center for Medicare and Medicaid Services. Medicare Learning Network Booklet: Federally Qualified Health Center. ICN MLN006397. January 2021. https://www.cms.gov/Outreach-and-Education/Medicare-Learning-Network-MLN/MLNProducts/Downloads/fqhcfactsheet.pdf. Accessed 23 Feb 2022.
3. Blanchard J, Petterson S, Bazemore A, Watkins K, Mullan F. Characteristics and distribution of graduate medical education training sites: are we missing opportunities to meet US health workforce needs? Acad Med. 2016;91(10):1416–22.
4. Ferguson WJ, Cashman SB, Savageau JA, Lasser DH. Family medicine residency characteristics associated with practice in a health professions shortage area. Fam Med. 2009;41(6):405–10.
5. Lebel D, Hogg W. Effect of location on family medicine residents' training. Can Fam Physician. 1993;39:1066–9.
6. Morris CG, Johnson B, Kim S, Chen F. Training family physicians in community health centers: a health workforce solution. Fam Med. 2008;40(4):271–6.
7. Phillips RL, Petterson S, Bazemore A. Do residents who train in safety net settings return for practice? Acad Med. 2013;88(12):1934–40.
8. Reese VF, McCann JL, Bazemore AW, Phillips RL. Residency footprints: assessing the impact of training programs on the local physician workforce and communities. Fam Med. 2008;40(5):339–44.
9. Meyers P, Wilkinson E, Petterson S, Patterson DG, Longenecker R, Schmitz D, et al. Rural workforce years: quantifying the rural workforce contribution of family medicine residency graduates. J Grad Med Educ. 2020;12(6):717–26.
10. Parlier AB, Galvin SL, Thach S, Kruidenier D, Fagan EB. The road to rural primary care: a narrative review of factors that help develop, recruit, and retain rural primary care physicians. Acad Med. 2018;93(1):130–40.
11. Bacon TJ, Baden DJ, Coccodrilli LD. The National Area Health Education Center Program and primary care residency training. J Rural Health. 2000;16(3):288–94.
12. Reynolds PP. Commentary: the teaching community health center: an idea whose time has come. Acad Med. 2012;87(12):1648–50.
13. Rich EC. Commentary: teaching health centers and the path to graduate medical education reform. Acad Med. 2012;87(12):1651–3.
14. ACGME. ACGME Program Requirements for Graduate Medical Education in Internal Medicine. 2021. https://www.acgme.org/globalassets/pfassets/programrequirements/140_internalmedicine_2021.pdf. Accessed 19 June 2022.
15. Chen C, Chen F, Mullan F. Teaching health centers: a new paradigm in graduate medical education. Acad Med. 2012;87(12):1752–6.
16. Bailey ZD, Feldman JM, Bassett MT. How structural racism works—racist policies as a root cause of U.S. racial health inequities. New Eng. J Med. 2021;384(8):768–73.
17. Oldfield BJ, Clark BW, Mix MC, Shaw KC, Serwint JR, Desai SV, et al. Two novel urban health primary care residency tracks that focus on community-level structural vulnerabilities. J Gen Intern Med. 2018;33(12):2250–5.
18. Alweis R, Donato A, Terry R, Goodermote C, Qadri F, Mayo R. Benefits of developing graduate medical education programs in community health systems. J Community Hosp Intern Med Perspectives. 2021;11(5):569–75.
19. Archer J, Bower P, Gilbody S, Lovell K, Richards D, Gask L, et al. Collaborative care for depression and anxiety problems. Cochrane Database Syst Rev. 2012;10:Cd006525.
20. Rieselbach RE, Crouse BJ, Frohna JG. Teaching primary care in community health centers: addressing the workforce crisis for the underserved. Ann Intern Med. 2010;152(2):118–22.
21. Block L, LaVine N, Verbsky J, Sagar A, Smith MA, Lane S, et al. Do medical residents perform patient-centered medical home tasks? A mixed-methods study. Med Ed. 2017;22:1352434.
22. The White House. National HIV/AIDS strategy for the United States 2022-2025. The white house Office of National AIDS policy, Washington, DC. 2021. https://hivgov-prod-v3.s3.amazonaws.com/s3fs-public/NHAS-2022-2025.pdf. Accessed 19 June 2022.

23. AIDS Education training center. The AETC Program and the National HIV/AIDS Strategy https://aidsetc.org/about/aetcs-and-nhas. Accessed 19 June 2022.
24. Sharac J, Stolyar L, Corallo B, Tolbert J, Shin P, Rosenbaum S. How community health centers are serving low-income communities during the COVID-19 pandemic amid new and continuing challenges. Kaiser Family Foundation San Francisco, CA 2022.
25. Sharac J, Markus A, Tolbert J, Rosenbaum S. Community health centers in a time of change: results from an annual survey. Kaiser Family Foundation; 2020.
26. Chen C, Chong N, Luo Q, Park J. Community health center residency training: improving staffing, service, and quality. Fam Med. 2021;53(8):689–96.
27. St. Louis J, Worringer E, Barr WB. Residency setting association with resident substance use disorder training: a CERA secondary data analysis. Fam Med. 2020;52(3):198–201.
28. Lardiere M, Jones E, Perez M. NACHC 2010 assessment of behavioral health services in federally qualified health centers. Washington, DC: National Association of Community Health Centers; 2011. http://www.nachc.org/wp-content/uploads/2015/06/BHReport.pdf. Accessed 19 June 2022
29. Gard LA, Cooper AJ, Youmans Q, Didwania A, Persell SD, Jean-Jacques M, et al. Identifying and addressing social determinants of health in outpatient practice: results of a program-wide survey of internal and family medicine residents. BMC Med Ed. 2020;20(1):18.
30. Gordon PR, Hale F. The service-education linkage: implications for family practice residency programs and community and migrant health centers. Fam Med. 1993;25(5):316–21.
31. Strelnick AH, Swiderski D, Fornari A, Gorski V, Korin E, Ozuah P, et al. The residency program in social medicine of Montefiore medical center: 37 years of mission-driven, interdisciplinary training in primary care, population health, and social medicine. Acad Med. 2008;83(4):378–89.
32. Chen C, Petterson S, Phillips R, Bazemore A, Mullan F. Spending patterns in region of residency training and subsequent expenditures for care provided by practicing physicians for Medicare beneficiaries. JAMA. 2014;312(22):2385–93.
33. Gupta R, Steers N, Moriates C, Wali S, Braddock CH, Ong M. High-value care culture among the future physician workforce in internal medicine. Acad Med. 2019;94(9):1347–54.
34. Cousineau MR, Flores H, Cheng S, Gates JD, Douglas JH, Clute GB, et al. Transforming a family medicine center and residency program into a federally qualified health center. Acad Med. 2013;88(5):657–62.
35. Rosenblatt RA, Andrilla CHA, Curtin T, Hart LG. Shortages of medical personnel at community health centers: implications for planned expansion. JAMA. 2006;295(9):1042–9.
36. Cole AM, Doescher M, Phillips WR, Ford P, Stevens NG. Satisfaction of family physicians working in community health centers. J Am Board Fam Med. 2012;25(4):470–6.
37. Jones TF. The cost of outpatient training of residents in a community health center. Fam Med. 1997;29(5):347–52.
38. Lee M, Newton H, Smith T, Crawford M, Kepley H, Regenstein M, et al. The benefits of physician training programs for rural communities: lessons learned from the teaching health center graduate medical education program. JHPCU. 2016;27(4a):83–90.
39. Nasca TJ, Weiss KB, Bagian JP. Improving clinical learning environments for tomorrow's physicians. New Eng J Med. 2014;370(11):991–3.
40. Weiss KB, Bagian JP, Wagner R. CLER pathways to excellence: expectations for an optimal clinical learning environment (executive summary). J Grad Med Educ. 2014;6(3):610–1.
41. Moushey E, Shomo A, Elder N, O'Dea C, Rahner D. Community partnered projects: residents engaging with community health centers to improve care. Fam Med. 2014;46(9):718–23.
42. U.S. Department of Health and Human Services. Health Resources and Services Administration. Comparison of the Rural Health Clinic and Federally Qualified Health Center Programs. June 2006. https://www.hrsa.gov/sites/default/files/ruralhealth/policy/confcall/comparisonguide.pdf. Accessed 24 Feb 2022.
43. Sunshine JE, Morris CG, Keen M, Andrilla CH, Chen FM. Barriers to training family medicine residents in community health centers. Fam Med. 2010;42(4):248–54.

44. Morris CG, Chen FM. Training residents in community health centers: facilitators and barriers. Ann Fam Med. 2009;7(6):488–94.
45. Patterson DG, Schmitz D, Longenecker RL. Family medicine rural training track residencies: risks and resilience. Fam Med. 2019;51(8):649–56.
46. Bruksch-Meck K, Crouse B, Quinn G, McCart L, Traxler K. Graduate medical education initiatives to develop the physician workforce in rural. Wisconsin. 2018;117(5):201–7.
47. Epperly TM. Graduate medical education in Idaho: a ten year strategic plan. Idaho State Board of Education; 2017. https://boardofed.idaho.gov/wp-content/uploads/2018/01/Graduate-Medical-Education-10yr-Plan.pdf. Accessed 20 June 2022.
48. Rittenhouse DR, Ament AS, Grumbach K. Sponsoring institution interests, not national plans, shape physician workforce in the United States. Fam Med. 2020;52(8):551–6.
49. Pincavage AT, Razi RR, Arora VM, Oyler J, Woodruff JN. Resident education in free clinics: an internal medicine continuity clinic experience. J Grad Med Educ. 2013;5(2):327–31.
50. Long T, Chaiyachati K, Bosu O, Sircar S, Richards B, Garg M, et al. Why aren't more primary care residents going into primary care? A qualitative study. J Gen Intern. 2016:1–8.
51. George A, Rubin G. Non-attendance in general practice: a systematic review and its implications for access to primary health care. FPJ. 2003;20(2):178–84.
52. LaGanga LR. Clinic overbooking to improve patient access and increase provider productivity. Decis Sci. 2007;38(2):251–76.
53. Barrett SE, Dyer C, Westpheling K. Language access: understanding the barriers and challenges in primary care settings: perspectives from the field. Association of Clinicians for the Underserved; 2008. https://healthlaw.org/resources/language-access-understanding-the-barriers-and-challenges-in-primary-care-sett/. Accessed 20 June 2022.
54. Ku L, Flores G. Pay now or pay later: providing interpreter services in health care. Health Aff. 2005;24(2):435–44.
55. Fancher TL, Keenan C, Meltvedt C, Stocker T, Harris T, Morfín J, et al. An academic–community partnership to improve care for the underserved. Acad Med. 2011;86(2):252–8.
56. Mazur EM, Cleary JP, Pols KB, Neligan P, Karish DO, Breen T, et al. Collaboration between an internal medicine residency program and a federally qualified health center: Norwalk hospital and the Norwalk community health center. Acad Med. 2001;76(11):1159–64.

Chapter 34
Veterans Affairs Continuity Clinics

Rebekah Kaplowitz and Himabindu Kadiyala

Introduction

Outpatient primary care clinics in the Veterans Affairs (VA) Healthcare System provide a learning environment where medicine residents can train using a multidisciplinary team-based structure. Medicine residents with VA continuity clinics can establish longitudinal relationships with staff and patients, as well as utilize the data analysis resources of the VA to monitor and improve quality of care. This chapter describes the structure of VA continuity clinics within many graduate medical education training models and suggests strategies to ensure educational rigor while providing primary care for male and female military veterans with many physical and mental health challenges.

Outline
- Background
- PACT and academic PACT
- Maintaining continuity for the resident and the patient

R. Kaplowitz (✉)
Lt. Col. Luke Weathers, Jr. VA Medical Center, University of Tennessee Health Science Center, Memphis, TN, USA
e-mail: rkaplowi@uthsc.edu

H. Kadiyala
Primary Care, Baylor College of Medicine, Michael E. DeBakey VA Medical Center, Houston, TX, USA
e-mail: himabindu.kadiyala2@va.gov

L. B. Lu et al. (eds.), *Leading an Academic Medical Practice*,
https://doi.org/10.1007/978-3-031-40273-9_34

- Patient care between clinic sessions
- Patient and resident engagement with the APACT
- Demographic and clinical differences between VA and continuity clinic populations
- Primary care-mental health integration in the educational setting
- Care in resident continuity clinic for women veterans
- General considerations when establishing a resident clinic in the VA
- Maintaining educational quality
- Conclusion

Background

Since 1946, the Department of Veterans Affairs (VA) has partnered with US medical and allied health professional schools in its mission to train generations of health professionals [1]. A key requirement for residency training in internal medicine is the continuity clinic [2], and the VA academic medical center provides opportunities for this outpatient experience. In VA primary care clinics, residents are embedded within an interdisciplinary team of health-care professionals such as nurses, clinical pharmacists, social workers, dietitians, nurse practitioners, and physician assistants to meet the needs of a demographically and clinically unique population of patients. The VA has a distinctive organizational structure as a publicly funded health maintenance organization for a patient population limited to US military veterans and in rare cases their non-veteran spouses [3–5]. Residents who are trained in VA clinics must still obtain adequate case mix for gender, age, and comorbidities in order to receive high-quality medical training as defined by the Accreditation Council for Graduate Medical Education (ACGME). This chapter will explore strategies to leverage the resources of the VA primary care clinics to improve graduate medical education and the quality of patient care, including discussion of different scheduling models for integration of residents within the primary care team [6].

PACT and Academic PACT

The health-care team in academic as well as nonacademic VA primary care settings is aligned according to patient-centered medical home principles called the Patient Aligned Care Team (PACT) [7]. The model has an emphasis on multidisciplinary care, care coordination, nontraditional encounters such as tele-health monitoring and group visits, and patient-centered communication [8–10]. Since the PACT model's national implementation in 2010, there is evidence that it reduces the number of emergency room visits and hospital admissions secondary to ambulatory care sensitive conditions [8, 11].

The PACT model is based on assigning veterans eligible for primary care to a team consisting of an attending physician, registered nurse care manager (RNCM), medical assistant (licensed practical nurse, licensed vocational nurse, or health technician depending on the facility's staffing preferences), and clerk [12]. A fully developed PACT will also have psychologists, pharmacists, social workers, and dieticians who are integrated into the PACT and primary care setting. VA attending physicians are employed by the VA but hold volunteer or paid appointments at affiliated medical schools and residency programs. The VA residency continuity clinic strives to incorporate features of the PACT to assist with communication between the patient and teamlet members [13]. Each VA academic medical center has integrated its residents into the PACT system in its own way, but there is an influential PACT variation that incorporates training environments from several disciplines of internal medicine and allied health care, called the Interprofessional Academic PACT (iAPACT). The iAPACT leverages the clinical expertise of all VA staff with teaching appointments at their health science affiliate to improve trainee education as well as patient care [14–16].

Maintaining Continuity for the Resident and the Patient

Given that longitudinal continuity of patient care is a critical aspect of resident clinics, the PACT system optimizes continuity when assigning patients to teams [17]. Once an unassigned patient has an encounter with a resident, that patient is assigned to the panel of the resident's supervising attending. In this system, the attending becomes the "primary care provider" and the resident is identified as the "associate provider" [18]. Some VA hospitals have groups of associate providers who share responsibility for a panel of patients, while others consolidate responsibility to individual resident-attending dyads. The former program design may be most useful for a rotating block schedule (e.g., X weeks inpatient block alternating with Y weeks in the outpatient setting, or "X + Y") (Table 34.1), while the latter may be most practical when the continuity clinic schedule is one session per week regardless of the clinical rotation. Both the block schedule model and the weekly clinic model can generate continuity of resident–patient care when all staff are mindful of the return scheduling interval. Whether weekly or monthly, resident schedules are made well in advance by residency programs to plan leave and should be referenced by both the resident who is advising the patient on a return visit and the clerk who is scheduling that appointment. The reward of resident–patient continuity builds over the course of the training process as residents have more return visits with patients with whom they have established rapport and a clinical relationship over time.

Residents are expected to have a graduated level of responsibility in patient care as their training progresses to allow for a depth and breadth of clinical experience with the management of medical issues in the ambulatory setting. The patient may interact with the PACT by face-to-face encounter, telephone encounter,

Table 34.1 Example of continuity clinic scheduling model for X + Y. Non-clinic blocks can include ambulatory experience such as quality improvement, specialty outpatient learning, research, and administrative follow-up time

	Monday	Tuesday	Wednesday	Thursday	Friday
Inpatient block for X weeks	No clinic				
Ambulatory AM	VA Women's Clinic	Main VA campus clinic	Ambulatory lectures and asynchronous patient care	VA Women's Clinic	Subspecialty outpatient clinic
Ambulatory PM	Subspecialty outpatient clinic	Main VA campus clinic	Main VA campus clinic	Quality improvement curriculum	Simulator training experience and board review

telemedicine device, or health portal (www.MyHealtheVet.gov). Whether the veteran has VA insurance only, private insurance, Medicare, or Medicaid, in-person and electronic patient contact is coded per Medicare guidelines to track utilization of services [19, 20]. The intent of the PACT and iAPACT is full utilization of all team members in the care process, and Bowen et al. have written eloquently about the modalities needed to maintain continuity for best practices of patient care and medical education [21].

Patient Care Between Clinic Sessions

As previously alluded to, the structure of resident continuity clinic affects the logistics of patient care within the APACT or iAPACT. For example, the VA requirement to notify patients of all laboratory and imaging results in a specified time frame demands that the ordering resident and the veteran's team account for all pending labs [22]. Ordering tests and arranging follow-up is an opportunity to develop a team approach for the patient's care. Planning lab testing for chronic disease management prior to the appointment is an efficient method of having lab information available to discuss at the visit. There is no one-size-fits-all strategy for communicating lab results and clinical information to patients between visits. Patients can be notified of results by phone, letter, or health portal. Residents are expected to follow up on the tests they order, whether at the next clinic session or by arranging appropriate time-sensitive follow up with the help of their PACT. The default recipient of lab results is to the clinician (attending or resident) who ordered the test, so if the resident will not be available to review results (on vacation, night float, ICU), then alternative arrangements utilizing the electronic medical record are available. For example, labs ordered by the resident can be routed back to a coresident, the attending, or the team nurse if the ordering resident will be unavailable to follow up within the mandated period [23]. In the X + Y system, where the resident may be off-site from the VA for weeks, establishing an effective system of communication and hand-off about pending labs to co-residents and other PACT members is critical for patient safety.

Patient and Resident Engagement with the APACT

Patient education is a crucial feature of participation with the APACT or iAPACT to inform the veteran of the array of their clinical resources for care of acute and chronic issues [24–27]. Resident patients may call the team directly or send an encrypted email message through www.MyHealtheVet.gov for clinical concerns or medication refills. The PACT RNCM can triage the clinical concern or place a medication renewal order for the attending's (or covering resident's) signature. If the clinical concern is nonurgent, the team clerk may be alerted to schedule the patient at the next available clinic opening for the resident provider. A complaint that requires a same-day appointment when the resident is not available should be addressed within the PACT structure (e.g., a nurse assessment in conjunction with the attending, or an overbooked appointment into a collaborating resident's clinic).

The PACT experience is designed to maintain as much continuity between patient, Primary Care Provider, Associate Provider, and ancillary team members as possible to provide coordinated multidisciplinary care [26, 27]. All members of the core PACT "teamlet" of Primary Care Provider, RNCM, clinical associate, and clerk are responsible for delivery of evidence-based clinical preventive measures (according to the US Preventive Services Task Force recommendations [28]). When patients are assigned to individual residents as Associate Providers, resident-level quality of care data can be extracted and used to develop quality improvement projects. When patients are assigned to multiple residents (as in the X + Y system), individual residents are encouraged to monitor quality of care for the patients that they see over time, and to take up team-level projects. The attending is ultimately responsible for the clinical care provided by the residents, but the VA system provides numerous resources to assist the whole team.

Demographic and Clinical Differences Between VA and Continuity Clinic Populations

The population that uses VA primary care services is overwhelmingly male and has a high burden of chronic mental and physical illness [29]. Residents assigned to a VA continuity clinic will develop a fund of knowledge regarding medical and mental health risks specific to veterans of different periods of service. For instance, certain health issues are associated with Agent Orange exposure, and others more commonly in the Iraq and Afghanistan conflicts [30, 31]. All women and men should be screened for military sexual trauma (MST) given its prevalence and the availability of patient-centered trauma recovery services [32, 33]. Attendings who have specific expertise caring for veterans with service-related injury can offer invaluable training to residents who may not have had exposure to these conditions and are not aware of the VA's substantial resources to assist in evaluation and management. Regardless of a resident's ultimate career goal, awareness and appropriate management of health sequelae related to military service will be essential, and a strong outpatient experience can be invaluable in that training [34].

Primary Care–Mental Health Integration in the Educational Setting

According to the National Institute of Mental Health, about one in five US adults live with a mental illness. As many mental health illnesses are diagnosed in primary care and patients are reluctant to see mental health specialists, there was an imminent need to integrate primary care and mental health services. In 2007, VA began nationwide implementation of Primary Care–Mental Health Integration (PCMHI) in all VA facilities [35]. The goals of PCMHI involve supporting primary care clinicians in identifying patients with mental health diagnoses, promoting effective treatment of subclinical and moderate mental health conditions, and improving access and quality of care for patients across the spectrum of illness severity. PCMHI is considered population-based mental health clinical care where service delivery is simultaneously colocated, collaborative, and integrated within the primary care clinic. PCMHI colocated behavioral health clinicians are typically psychologists, psychiatrists, clinical social workers, physician assistants, and RN Care Managers. Each member of the PCMHI team utilizes evidence-based protocols to treat common mental health conditions such as depression, anxiety, trauma, alcohol misuse, and other substance use disorders. As PCMHI visits are provided in the primary care clinic, patients are encouraged to consider meeting with a behavioral health clinician as part of their routine primary care visit. The holistic nature and coordinated approach help patients overcome the stigma associated with seeking care for behavioral health disorders conditions and also increases patient engagement and compliance to treatment plans [36]. PCMHI visits are generally brief, usually lasting 20–30 min, and may be limited to 1–6 visits [37]. When extended behavioral health care is needed or patients require specialized services for diagnoses such as bipolar disorder or schizophrenia, a referral is made to specialty mental health care.

VA policy requires annual screening for depression, post-traumatic stress disorder, alcohol use disorder, and suicide risk assessment. Patients who need to see a behavioral health clinician are referred to PCMHI and are usually seen on the same day, except when patients prefer to come back on another day. The same-day access is a key factor of successful PCMHI. One of VA's top priorities is preventing suicide among all veterans. When patients have a positive suicide screen or exhibit suicide warning signs, a warm hand off is given to the mental health clinician to ensure safety and continuity of patient care.

During their continuity clinic experience, residents develop a toolbox of skills for managing behavioral health issues, utilizing all the resources available to PACTs and care coordination with PCMHI team member. The educational benefit from a colocated care model like PCMHI is invaluable. Hemming et al. reported that comanagement in behavioral health integration improved residents' confidence in providing care for patients with behavioral health conditions [38].

Care in Resident Continuity Clinic for Women Veterans

Although women veterans are a distinct minority within the VA system, the percentage of enrollment is increasing steadily [39, 40]. Design of a continuity experience to include the care of women veterans must take into account the veteran's need for a consistent locus of care, such as in a PACT with an attending who is a designated women's health provider [41]. Most VA Medical Centers have a Women Veterans Program Director or Women's Program Medical Director who can assist the residency program in achieving appropriate clinical care along with the educational goals of ambulatory training, thus establishing a clinic structure with gender balance in mind [42–44].

Because the gender balance in the VA setting is still highly skewed toward the care of male patients, an educational structure must be in place to develop an adequate case mix of female and male patients that is more reflective of the general population. The particular construct used will vary depending on the existing framework in each VA location but must be addressed for certification by the Residency Review Committee of the ACGME [2]. Both VA academic and nonacademic medical centers facilitate health-care access for women veterans by identifying clinicians with special training and experience in women's health care, specifically by comprehensive women's health centers and designated women's health providers [41]. Possible mechanisms for obtaining a case mix balanced for gender include integration of residents into VA Comprehensive Women's Health Centers and ensuring that several attendings are designated women's health providers [45, 46]. For example, a resident's regular attending can be a designated women's provider who has a substantial empaneled proportion of women veterans. Similarly, clinic weeks can alternate between the traditional VA clinic with a predominantly male population and a different clinic setting that has most or all female patients, such as a VA Comprehensive Women's Clinic. Literature on the gender-specific and general health needs of women veterans continues to develop [47, 48].

General Considerations When Establishing a Resident Clinic in the VA

Whether the resident continuity clinic is being newly established or has been in practice for a substantial time, the involvement of highly engaged attendings provides both essential supervision for patient care and resident experience in primary care. The number of preceptors recruited should be more than sufficient to staff the number of residents in the clinic at any given time in accordance with the maximum ratio of one preceptor for every four trainees as prescribed by the ACGME. In addition, a contingency plan for faculty absence should be in place to allow for adequate coverage of resident clinic for both planned and emergency absences. Significant advance notice is required for routine cancellation of both faculty and resident clinics. Advance agreement with the residency program regarding who is responsible for submitting and following up on leave requests for vacation and other planned and unplanned resident absences will improve work functioning in the future.

Maintaining Educational Quality

Ultimately, residents with VA clinic are still accountable to the same graduate medical education standards as their peers at other clinic sites. It is expected that residents with continuity clinic at a VA medical center will have the same didactic curriculum as the rest of the training program's residents. Attendings, residents, and residency leadership can routinely review performance measures and consider performance improvement projects or PDSA (Plan-Do-Study-Act) process cycles [49–51]. Attendings and clinical supervisors have access to clinician- and patient-specific data for hypothesis development and testing. VA electronic data also offers a robust source for monitoring quality of care in the residents' clinic patient population.

Conclusion

Given the vast nature of the Veterans Administration and its network of medical centers, outpatient centers, and large and small clinics, no summary can address every educator's personal and professional experience with a VA clinic. However, the technical and systemic challenges that are posed by the VA setting are offset by the tremendous opportunity for offering high-quality care to a population with substantial medical and mental health risk factors. The VA experience can provide in-depth exposure to high-value, cost-effective care that demonstrates an alternative to the fee-for-service model seen by trainees in many other venues. It is not only vertically integrated and team-based at each site but also fully integrated across the United States [52]. The resident continuity experience in VA clinic provides new opportunities to study systems of care and how they affect care delivery.

Disclaimer Opinions expressed herein are the sole opinion of the authors and not of the Department of Veterans Affairs.

References

1. Affiliations VHAOoA. Medical and Dental Education 2021. 19 March 2022. https://www.va.gov/oaa/medical-and-dental.asp.
2. ACGME program requirements for graduate medical education in internal medicine. Chicago, IL: Accreditation Council for Graduate Medical Education; 2022.
3. Gupta R, Davis E, Horton C. Interval examination: building primary care teams in an urban academic teaching clinic. J Gen Intern Med. 2013;28(11):1517–21.
4. Liu C-F, Chapko M, Bryson CL, Burgess JF, Fortney JC, Perkins M, et al. Use of outpatient care in Veterans Health Administration and Medicare among veterans receiving primary care in Community-Based and Hospital Outpatient Clinics. Health Serv Res. 2010;45(5p1):1268–86.
5. Nadkarni M, Reddy S, Bates CK, Fosburgh B, Babbott S, Holmboe E. Ambulatory-based education in internal medicine: current organization and implications for transformation. Results of a National Survey of resident continuity clinic directors. J Gen Intern Med. 2011;26(1):16–20.
6. Galen BT. In support of residency training at an academic veterans hospital. Acad Med. 2012;87(8):993–4.
7. Schectman G, Stark R. Orchestrating large organizational change in primary care: the Veterans' health administration experience implementing a patient-centered medical home. J Gen Intern Med. 2014;29(Suppl 2):S550–1.
8. Bidassie B, Davies ML, Stark R, Boushon B. VA experience in implementing patient-centered medical home using a breakthrough series collaborative. J Gen Intern Med. 2014;29(Suppl 2):S563–71.
9. Farmer MM, Rose DE, Rubenstein LV, Canelo IA, Schectman G, Stark R, et al. Challenges facing primary care practices aiming to implement patient-centered medical homes. J Gen Intern Med. 2014;29(Suppl 2):S555–62.
10. Yoon J, Rose DE, Canelo I, Upadhyay AS, Schectman G, Stark R, et al. Medical home features of VHA primary care clinics and avoidable hospitalizations. J Gen Intern Med. 2013;28(9):1188–94.
11. Chaiyachati KH, Gordon K, Long T, Levin W, Khan A, Meyer E, et al. Continuity in a VA patient-centered medical home reduces emergency department visits. PLoS One. 2014;9(5):e96356.
12. Rodriguez HP, Giannitrapani KF, Stockdale S, Hamilton AB, Yano EM, Rubenstein LV. Teamlet structure and early experiences of medical home implementation for veterans. J Gen Intern Med. 2014;29(Suppl 2):S623–31.
13. Doolittle BR, Tobin D, Genao I, Ellman M, Ruser C, Brienza R. Implementing the patient-centered medical home in residency education. Educ Health (Abingdon). 2015;28(1):74–8.
14. Brienza RS. At a crossroads: the future of primary care education and practice. Acad Med. 2016;91(5):621–3.
15. Brienza RS, Zapatka S, Meyer EM. The case for interprofessional learning and collaborative practice in graduate medical education. Acad Med. 2014;89(11):1438–9.
16. Chang A, Bowen JL, Buranosky RA, Frankel RM, Ghosh N, Rosenblum MJ, et al. Transforming primary care training—patient-centered medical home entrustable professional activities for internal medicine residents. J Gen Intern Med. 2013;28(6):801–9.
17. VHA Handbook 1101.10. Patient Aligned Care Team (PACT) Handbook. Washington, DC: Veterans Health Administration; 2014. p. 72.
18. Primary care management module (PCMM) user manual. In: Affairs DoV, editor. Washington, DC; 2015. p. 197.
19. Coleman DL, Moran E, Serfilippi D, Mulinski P, Rosenthal R, Gordon B, et al. Measuring physicians' productivity in a veterans affairs medical center. Acad Med. 2003;78(7):682–9.
20. Gao J, Moran E, Almenoff PL, Render ML, Campbell J, Jha AK. Variations in efficiency and the relationship to quality of care in the veterans health system. Health Aff (Project Hope). 2011;30(4):655–63.

21. Bowen JL, Hirsh D, Aagaard E, Kaminetzky CP, Smith M, Hardman J, et al. Advancing educational continuity in primary care residencies: an opportunity for patient-centered medical homes. Acad Med. 2014;90:587.
22. VHA Directive 1088. Communicating Test Results to Providers and Patients. Washington, DC: Department of Veteran Affairs; 2015. p. 10.
23. Long T, Uradu A, Castillo R, Brienza R. Addressing outpatient continuity for ambulatory training: a novel tool for longitudinal primary care sign out. Educ Health (Abingdon). 2016;29(1):51–5.
24. Katz DA, McCoy K, Sarrazin MV. Does improved continuity of primary care affect clinician-patient communication in VA? J Gen Intern Med. 2014;29(Suppl 2):S682–8.
25. LaVela SL, Schectman G, Gering J, Locatelli SM, Gawron A, Weaver FM. Understanding health care communication preferences of veteran primary care users. Patient Educ Couns. 2012;88(3):420–6.
26. Rodriguez HP, Marshall RE, Rogers WH, Safran DG. Primary care physician visit continuity: a comparison of patient-reported and administratively derived measures. J Gen Intern Med. 2008;23(9):1499–502.
27. Rodriguez HP, Rogers WH, Marshall RE, Safran DG. The effects of primary care physician visit continuity on patients' experiences with care. J Gen Intern Med. 2007;22(6):787–93.
28. US preventive services task force published recommendations, Rockville, MD: US Preventive Services Task Force; 2022. https://www.uspreventiveservicestaskforce.org/uspstf/recommendation-topics.
29. Amat M, Glassman R, Basu N, Doolin J, Flier L, Gonzalez MR, et al. Defining the resident continuity clinic panel along patient outcomes: a health equity opportunity. J Gen Intern Med. 2021;36(9):2615–21.
30. Military Exposures. Washington, DC: U.S. Department of Veterans Affairs; 2022 [updated April 28, 2022. http://publichealth.va.gov/PUBLICHEALTH/exposures/index.asp.
31. Troyanskaya M, Pastorek NJ, Scheibel RS, Petersen NJ, McCulloch K, Wilde EA, et al. Combat exposure, PTSD symptoms, and cognition following blast-related traumatic brain injury in OEF/OIF/OND service members and veterans. Mil Med. 2015;180(3):285–9.
32. Conard PL, Young C, Hogan L, Armstrong ML. Encountering women veterans with military sexual trauma. Perspect Psychiatr Care. 2014;50(4):280–6.
33. Glaesmer H. Revealing the importance of military sexual trauma and its consequences. J Clin Psychiatry. 2014;75(10):e1188–9.
34. Lee J, Sanders KM, Cox M. Honoring those who have served: how can health professionals provide optimal care for members of the military, veterans, and their families? Acad Med. 2014;89(9):1198–200.
35. Johnson-Lawrence V, Zivin K, Szymanski BR, Pfeiffer PN, McCarthy JF. VA primary care-mental health integration: patient characteristics and receipt of mental health services, 2008-2010. Psychiatr Serv. 2012;63(11):1137–41.
36. Post EP, Metzger M, Dumas P, Lehmann L. Integrating mental health into primary care within the Veterans Health Administration. Fam Syst Health. 2010;28(2):83–90.
37. Dundon M, Dollar K et al. Primary care-mental health integration. Co-located, Collaborative Care: An Operations Manual. 2011. p. 71.
38. Hemming P, Hewitt A, Gallo JJ, Kessler R, Levine RB. Residents' confidence providing primary care with behavioral health integration. Fam Med. 2017;49(5):361–8.
39. Bastian LA, Mattocks KM, Rosen AK, Hamilton AB, Bean-Mayberry B, Sadler AG, et al. Informing policy to deliver comprehensive care for women veterans. Med Care. 2015;53(4 Suppl 1):S1–4.
40. Bastian LA, Trentalange M, Murphy TE, Brandt C, Bean-Mayberry B, Maisel NC, et al. Association between women veterans' experiences with VA outpatient health care and designation as a women's health provider in primary care clinics. Women's Health Issues. 2014;24(6):605–12.

41. VHA directive 1330.01(4). Healthcare Services for Women Veterans. Washington, DC: Veterans Health Administration; 2021. p. 48.
42. Bean-Mayberry B, Yano EM, Bayliss N, Navratil J, Weisman CS, Scholle SH. Federally funded comprehensive women's health centers: leading innovation in women's healthcare delivery. J Women's Health. 2007;16(9):1281–90.
43. Reddy SM, Rose DE, Burgess JF Jr, Charns MP, Yano EM. The role of organizational factors in the provision of comprehensive Women's health in the Veterans Health Administration. Women's Health Issues. 2016;26:648.
44. Yano EM, Bastian LA, Frayne SM, Howell AL, Lipson LR, McGlynn G, et al. Toward a VA Women's Health Research agenda: setting evidence-based priorities to improve the health and health care of women veterans. J Gen Intern Med. 2006;21(Suppl 3):S93–101.
45. Bean-Mayberry B, Yano EM, Washington DL, Goldzweig C, Batuman F, Huang C, et al. Systematic review of women veterans' health: update on successes and gaps. Women's Health Issues. 2011;21(4 Suppl):S84–97.
46. Hsieh E, Nunez-Smith M, Henrich JB. Needs and priorities in women's health training: perspectives from an internal medicine residency program. J Women's Health. 2013;22(8):667–72.
47. Chrystal JG, Dyer KE, Gammage CE, Klap RS, Carney DV, Frayne SM, Yano EM, Hamilton AB. Increasing engagement of women veterans in Health Research. J Gen Intern Med. 2022;37(1):8.
48. Danan ER, Krebs EE, Ensrud K, Koeller E, MacDonald R, Velasquez T, Greer N, Wilt TJ. An evidence map of the women veterans' Health Research literature (2008–2015). J Gen Intern Med. 2017;32(12):18.
49. Tentler A, Feurdean M, Keller S, Kothari N. Integrating a resident-driven longitudinal quality improvement curriculum within an ambulatory block schedule. J Grad Med Educ. 2016;8(3):405–9.
50. Wong BM, Etchells EE, Kuper A, Levinson W, Shojania KG. Teaching quality improvement and patient safety to trainees: a systematic review. Acad Med. 2010;85(9):1425–39.
51. Ogrinc G, Ercolano E, Cohen ES, Harwood B, Baum K, van Aalst R, et al. Educational system factors that engage resident physicians in an integrated quality improvement curriculum at a VA hospital: a realist evaluation. Acad Med. 2014;89(10):1380–5.
52. O'Hanlon C, Huang C, Sloss E, Anhang Price R, Hussey P, Farmer C, et al. Comparing VA and non-VA quality of care: a systematic review. J Gen Intern Med. 2016;32:105.

Part X
Crisis Management, Trauma Informed Care, Burnout and Wellness

Chapter 35
Crisis Management: The Pandemic

Leslie Harris Jr, Juhee C. McDougal, and Louisa Whitesides

Introduction

Pandemics cause major disruptions to clinic structure, program administration, and resident education. Institutions must be flexible to adjust to the rapidly changing and inherently unpredictable circumstances that pandemics bring; there are specific approaches that residency programs can use to adapt. First, it is crucial to follow public health recommendations, identify a pandemic director, and create a structure of remote administration and virtual meetings while maintaining patient and provider safety in the clinic. Second, it is essential to maintain the integrity of residency education, training, and wellness at pre-pandemic levels. Third, programs must be prepared to make accommodations for staffing shortages caused by illness or remote work. Although pandemics create numerous challenges, they may also provide the impetus for innovations that transform the delivery of patient care and residency education.

L. Harris Jr (✉)
University of Alabama at Birmingham Heersink School of Medicine, Birmingham, AL, USA
e-mail: Harrisjr@uab.edu

J. C. McDougal
Boston University Chobanian & Avedisian School of Medicine, Boston, MA, USA
e-mail: jcmcd@bu.edu

L. Whitesides
Internal Medicine, Division of Geriatrics and Palliative Care, George Washington University School of Medicine, Washington, DC, USA
e-mail: lwhitesides@mfa.gwu.edu

L. B. Lu et al. (eds.), *Leading an Academic Medical Practice*,
https://doi.org/10.1007/978-3-031-40273-9_35

Outline

- Clinic structure and administration
  - Public health recommendations
  - Pandemic director
  - Patient and provider safety
  - Managing the pandemic in clinic
  - Clinic staffing and resource challenges
  - Remote administration and virtual meetings
  - Dissemination of information
- Residency education and training
  - Changes to patient care
  - Educational challenges and strategies
  - Resident health
- Conclusion

Clinic Structure and Administration

Public Health Recommendations

Pandemics create an urgent need to follow state public health, Centers for Disease Control and Prevention (CDC), and World Health Organization (WHO) guidelines. To successfully navigate a pandemic, providers, institutions, and individuals must recognize the need for following properly resourced guidelines and recommendations [1].

Due to the sizable impact of pandemic-level threats to the public at large, early involvement of public health officials is an essential part of disease containment. At the state level, public health officials can assist by promulgating pandemic-specific instructions to prevent or mitigate the spread of communicable disease. Importantly, public health departments have access to resources, data, experts, and infrastructure for rapid and accurate dissemination of information. Residency programs should reference the public health department guidance when generating new protocols.

At the national level, the CDC actively communicates the latest guidelines for disease management in the form of frequent press releases, distribution of public health officials, and up-to-date evidence-based recommendations. Government recommendations have the advantage of access to both national and state data to guide the best course of action [2]. Depending on the structure or type of therapy available for the disease (oral/parenteral medications, vaccine) and the need for equipment (respirators, protective equipment, etc.), the State Department may be the local point of contact to access government created or stockpiled supplies [3].

Pandemic Director

Residency programs require successful integration of administrative, clinical, and educational functions. Although each of these components has discrete responsibilities, many components are interdependent and require organized collaboration, especially in a pandemic setting. Proper management of a pandemic requires early recognition of the scope of the problem followed by rapid selection of a leadership committee or a Pandemic Director/Manager. Duties of the pandemic director may include:

- Utilizing official guidelines to create residency-specific protocols
- Coordinating between different residency departments
- Communicating with the Institutional Graduate Medical Education (GME) office to align policies
- Developing contingency plans for personnel shortages
- Overseeing trainee/patient/employee safety
- Establishing clear, simple lines of communication
- Maintaining order during the frenetic phase of pandemic management

An appointed pandemic director with dedicated time will allow for a focused response to salient matters. This will improve organization, situational reaction time, facility preparedness, and allocation of resources. A central individual responsible for pandemic oversight also creates an opportunity to manage programs created for staff safety, stress management, and wellness. The authority and confidence in this director by program leadership can induce trust in employees, directly improving the communication and acceptance of recommended policies. A key function of this leader is to build community, transparency, stability, and positivity in the face of crisis [4, 5].

Patient and Provider Safety

One of the primary tasks of the Pandemic Director is to ensure the safety of patients, staff, and providers. It is of utmost importance that government agency guidelines are followed, including all risk mitigation procedures, such as proper use of protective equipment. Appropriate surveillance testing, early detection, risk assessment, and quarantine and isolation protocols are important for outbreak management. In addition, pathogen-specific evidence-based sanitization/cleaning protocols must be initiated [6–8].

Managing the Pandemic in Clinic

In the midst of a pandemic, clinics must prioritize safety protocols to effectively care for contagious patients (Table 35.1). Clinic visits create many points of contact and thus multiple opportunities for transmission to employees and other patients.

Table 35.1 Examples of clinic safety techniques used in the COVID-19 pandemic

Affected area	Safety technique
In-person clinic visits	• Increase appointment intervals (decreases clinic population density) • Use telemedicine for nonurgent patients • Closure or redesign of waiting room layout • Decrease elevator capacity
Providers	• Appropriate spacing in charting areas • Surveillance testing • Sanitization/cleaning protocols
Other clinical staff	• Shift to remote work where possible • Utilize messaging service/video/phone to limit unnecessary patient contact

Clinics may mitigate these risks in several ways. Depending on the spreading pathogen, offices may implement a screening questionnaire with specific questions regarding current symptoms, travel history (if applicable), and personal contact with positive cases. Those that answer the questions affirmative may be directed to an alternative path for "sick" patients to prevent transmission to other visitors [9].

Staff should plan for the possibility of suspected contagious individuals arriving at the clinic, and it is important that action plans are initiated quickly and followed accordingly. Resident physicians and clinical staff should be briefed on location and proper use of personal protective equipment (PPE) and be notified of a suspected case with ample time to prepare. Protocols should be set in place for rapid testing and results reporting. Finally, patients with suspected disease need to be able to leave the clinic safely with minimal collateral exposures [9].

Next, clinics need to develop workflows that ensure patients are notified of results in a timely manner after testing. One option is creating a specific team dedicated to following up on results. These team members can also serve as educators on the isolation/quarantine guidelines if necessary; these dedicated individuals are better positioned to stay up to date on the latest national recommendations. Clinics also need to be prepared to provide treatments as they become available, or to develop a process to direct patients efficiently to sites of therapy [9].

Finally, clinics must find ways to ensure the health and well-being of their frontline employees while delivering medical care. It may also be helpful to suggest or require surveillance testing of employees if there is asymptomatic spread of disease. If surveillance testing is required, then the infrastructure should be developed to optimize testing (i.e., test locations or on-site testing) and ensure that appropriate protocols are followed [6, 10]. Further, in order to reduce the risk of workforce dissolution if quarantine were required, programs may consider dividing residents into cohorts [11].

Telemedicine

Telemedicine is a safe and effective method to deliver or augment health care provided during a pandemic. In addition to increased convenience and access, remote care allows continued high-quality patient contact while decreasing risk of exposure for patients and providers. The standard of care provided remotely has been shown to equal in-person care delivery across many specialties, making this a highly attractive option during times when health-care crises necessitate physical distancing [12].

Clinic Staffing and Human Resource Challenges

Clinic staffing shortages can present a significant problem in the midst of a pandemic. In the setting of staffing challenges, it is vital that the essential functions of the residency practice are covered. This requires (1) identifying essential roles and functions, (2) taking stock of existing resources and personnel, (3) ensuring vital roles are covered, including possible reassignment of personnel. The communication between the pandemic director and medical director are vital in addressing these issues.

Employee safety and wellness is also a serious human resource concern. Staff who become ill are unavailable to the workforce, and exposures to illness may result in imposed quarantines. Early in a pandemic, entire departments may be impacted before appropriate measures are defined. Mitigation of negative effects can be facilitated by:

- Early recognition of a pending pandemic threat,
- Selection of Pandemic Director,
- Review of current evidence-based management strategies, and
- Appropriate flexing of staff scheduling

Remote Administration

In the midst of a pandemic, it may be necessary for administrative and academic-adjacent sections of the residency program to work remotely. Successful continuation of essential duties while working remotely requires careful planning and preparation. Above all, clear pathways of reliable communication beyond solely email must be established. Modes of communication may include virtual meetings using video platforms, scheduled phone calls, business messaging applications or group chats. This is essential for schedule coordination, as flex type scheduling means a number of staff/faculty/residents will be away from the hub of the program for extended periods.

Virtual Meetings

Virtual platforms are an essential tool in the struggle to continue operations. These meetings share many similarities with in-person meetings, with several important challenges outlined in Table 35.2.

Table 35.2 Virtual meeting challenges and solutions

Challenges	Possible solutions
Decreased audience engagement due to multitasking, which may increase speaker isolation and dissatisfaction	• Set expectations to activate video except in extenuating circumstances • Create intentional interactive opportunities (polls, breakout rooms)
Technical issues—Audio/visual equipment, connection, or network failure	• Designate real-time technical support staff
Background interference (people, pets, ambient noise, etc.)	• Encourage participants to use appropriate environment • Use virtual backgrounds or blurring • Set expectations to mute oneself except when speaking
Virtual fatigue (more meetings than usual, many new protocols/new issues)	• Meeting planner should be mindful of duration/number of meetings and to only invite people essential to the meeting
Distribution of material, especially large files	• Utilize file-sharing cloud platforms

Dissemination of Ever-changing Information

Early in a pandemic, information on novel pathogens is frequently not available, forcing health-care providers, patients, and government entities to act without the benefit of well-established research. In the internet and social media age, misinformation can spread quickly. Distributed information may range from unvalidated and inaccurate to false, which can have a harmful impact on public health. It is important for each clinician not only to stay up to date, but also to help patients understand messages from local, regional, and national public health authorities. Patients often cite their primary care physician as a credible source and authority of health information, and this relationship may facilitate helping patients sift through the voluminous amount of public information.

As new data evolve, public health recommendations will also naturally evolve. It is important that physicians are prepared to acknowledge these new data and help patients understand the changes. Patients actively and passively consume information and misinformation from a variety of sources. These include credible sources like health care providers and health officials as well as those likely to be less accurate—social media and untrained family or friends. Social media does have advantages such as rapid dissemination of information, but it also raises the potential risk that the information is not current, has not been peer reviewed, or is false.

Furthermore, uptake of pandemic-related information may not be uniform. During the COVID-19 pandemic, a study found that participants 55 years and older and those with higher educational background reported a higher average COVD-19 knowledge score. Black/African American and Native American/Alaska Native participants reported a lower average COVID-19 knowledge score than white participants. This underscores the need to reach all communities utilizing different strategies, especially segments of the population with lower uptake [1].

Table 35.3 Categories of pandemic data

Pandemic data	Description
Safety data	Information regarding individual and population safety is rapidly generated during a pandemic. Initial information is likely to be more conservative, with refinement occurring as new data becomes available
Clinical data	As the pandemic progresses, ponderous amounts of clinical information will be generated regarding all aspects of the condition—causative agent/s, possible treatments, and quarantine recommendations. This information may change significantly over time. Clinical leadership in residency programs will play a significant role in creating pandemic-specific educational materials and ensuring sharing of valid protocols
Administrative data	For a variety of reasons, schedules are dramatically affected in a pandemic—ill clinicians, staff, and flex coverage lend to this. Programs must establish a mechanism to quickly share updates and communicate changes to all staff and providers
Organizational data	Pandemics are extraordinarily stressful situations. Leadership of residency programs are responsible for providing frequent accurate updates. Program-wide communications provide an opportunity to share policies, clarify clinical recommendations, address wellness of providers and staff, and express appreciation for performance and resilience during difficult times. Sharing of this type of information needs to be consistent, appropriate, frequent, and accurate

One possible method of organizing the available data is by using categories, for example safety, clinical, administrative, and organizational. Rapid dissemination of information in each of the following categories is essential to an academic medical practice (Table 35.3).

Communication Methods

Email: Programs frequently use email to communicate on a day-to-day basis. Email is especially useful for large, detailed, comprehensive, or specialized organizational messages.

Messaging: Due to the ubiquitous nature of mobile devices, messaging is the most efficient means of rapid communication. Messaging applications, such as WhatsApp, allow for the creation of multiple types of groups in a much more efficient manner than traditional SMS text messaging.

Forum: For town-hall or state-of-the-program type communication, program leadership may elect to speak in open forum or lecture type settings. This method is useful for addressing high level topics, large policy changes, particularly critical news, or important facility changes. As the ability to mobilize and gather staff during a pandemic is compromised, this method of communication has limited application [13].

Residency Education and Training

Through a pandemic, it is critical to maintain the integrity, quality, and mission of residency educational programs. In order to preserve these elements, programs may need to design and manage a new virtual curriculum, create protocols for workforce quarantine and isolation, implement more robust wellness programs, and provide further education on patient care and telemedicine.

Changes to Patient Care in Residency Training

Residents should be involved in the care of patients during a pandemic; however, it is important to balance these learning opportunities with safety. While the focus may shift to the sickest patients in the middle of a pandemic, it is important that all physicians continue chronic disease management and routine health maintenance—both fundamental to our health care system and paramount to resident learning. To maintain accessibility for established patients, clinics must be able to provide a myriad of contact options, including in-person and telehealth visits [14]. While much of chronic care management can be performed through telehealth, some patients need to be seen in person. Residents need to be able to manage their panels, identify patients that are more appropriate for in-person visits, and ensure safety when those patients come to clinic.

Educational Challenges and Strategies

Maintaining resident educational experiences during a pandemic is essential but requires thoughtful planning to address the many challenges. These challenges include absent learners (illness, quarantine, flex schedule coverage, overwhelming numbers of ill patients, sick family members, infrastructure failure, provider fatigue), absent presenters/facilitators, absent administrators/schedulers, lack of materials due to supply line interruption, and loss of conference space.

Resident education requires a broad complement of educational experiences geared toward learners at different levels. Multiple factors determine the optimal education formats used during a pandemic, including presenter preference, type of information, learner proficiency, and availability of technology. Educational experiences can be broadly categorized by type: teacher-centered or learner-centered.

Teacher-centered experiences: In teacher-centered forums, knowledge is shared by an experienced presenter and learning generally happens in a unidirectional manner, such as a traditional didactic lecture. Large lectures and didactic education are typically the least interactive of the experience types, but lend themselves well to virtual education. When virtual educational sessional are held, learners should be encouraged or required to maintain camera activation during live conferences. In addition, participants should be encouraged to actively participate, when appropriate, but should mute devices when not talking. For large groups, an administrator or other individual should be designated to monitor the chat stream.

Learner-centered experiences: In learner-centered experiences, learning happens in multiple directions between all participants, with more experienced members functioning as facilitators. Virtual platforms work well for case-based and didactic presentations but are less effective for hands-on work. One option for virtual hands-on and practical training is distributing equipment to learners prior to the session to use remotely while the speaker demonstrates. Another option is a one-to-one session with a learner and trainer. Individual training during a pandemic is attractive due to the low number of people making contact but will be limited by instructor time available to hold individual sessions [15].

Resident Health

Quarantine and isolation: Resident health is a priority for all programs during a pandemic. Residents who are sick should be provided medical leave without required responsibilities. There may be times, however, when residents must quarantine due to exposure or isolate with asymptomatic illness and should have the opportunity to learn while at home. In these circumstances, programs should develop ways for residents to participate in virtual learning or virtual patient care. Similarly, residency programs should anticipate and plan for resident quarantine and isolation. This planning may include flexibility in residents' schedules to cover for peers and/or non-patient facing electives to reduce exposure risk [16].

Resident wellness: Promoting resident wellness in a time of potential social isolation and fear of morbidity and mortality from occupational exposure is of utmost importance. There are numerous ways to promote resident wellness. Strategies include:

- Regularly scheduled small group discussions held online between program faculty and residents including stress management, mental health, or resident-led well-being topics.
- Frequent reminders of institutional resources for well-being and stress management [16].
- Dedicated, predictable times for decompression. This may include protected times when residents are assured that they will not be pulled for "surge" teams or clinical responsibilities.

Conclusion: Returning to a New Normal

Pandemics require a shift in the ways academic clinics are managed. To navigate the rapid changes, academic centers must analyze clinic structure and administrative duties to best serve their patients and learners. Programs must identify clear leadership, allocate resources appropriately, disseminate properly vetted information in effective ways, and potentially move patient care and learning to virtual platforms. During this transition, patient, learner, and employee safety must remain a priority. Additionally, clinical educators may need to explore new methods of remote learning while maintaining the integrity of the training program and paying specific attention to resident health and well-being.

References

1. Shafiq M, Elharake JA, Malik AA, McFadden SM, Aguolu OG, Omer SB. COVID-19 sources of information, knowledge, and preventive behaviors among the US adult population. J Public Health Manag Pract. 2021;27(3):278–84.
2. Centers for Disease Control and Prevention. Infection Control [Internet]. United States; 2020 [updated 2020 April 29; cited 2021 September 2]. https://www.cdc.gov/InfectionControl
3. Melvin SC, Wiggins C, Burse N, Thompson E, Monger M. Peer reviewed: the role of public health in COVID-19 emergency response efforts from a rural health perspective. Prev Chronic Dis. 2020:17.
4. Mendy A, Stewart ML, VanAkin K. A leader's guide: communicating with teams, stakeholders, and communities during COVID-19. McKinsey & Company; 2020. p. 1–9.
5. Allameh SF, Khajavirad N, Labaf A, Mirzazadeh A, Sadeghniiat-Haghighi K, Mortazavi SJ, Jafarian A. Twelve lessons on hospital leadership during COVID-19 pandemic. Arch Bone Jt Surg. 2020;8(Suppl 1):277.
6. Wee LE, Sim XY, Conceicao EP, Aung MK, Goh JQ, Yeo DW, Gan WH, Chua YY, Wijaya L, Tan TT, Tan BH. Containment of COVID-19 cases among healthcare workers: the role of surveillance, early detection, and outbreak management. Infect Control Hosp Epidemiol. 2020;41(7):765–71.
7. Khanaa R, Cicinella MV. COVID-19 pandemic: lessons learned and future directions. Indian J Ophthal. 2020;68(5):703–10.
8. MacIntyre CR, Wang Q. Physical distancing, face masks, and eye protection for prevention of COVID-19. Lancet. 2020;395(10242):1950–1.
9. Kwon J, Hedges M, Jackson KD, Keimig A, Francis D. Creating a dedicated pandemic ambulatory clinic: lessons learned from COVID-19. Qual Manag Health Care. 2022;31(2):92.
10. Coppeta L, Somma G, Ippoliti L, Ferrari C, D'Alessandro I, Pietroiusti A, Aurilio MT. Contact screening for healthcare workers exposed to patients with COVID-19. Int J Environ Res Public Health. 2020;17(23):9082.
11. Sabharwal S, Ficke JR, LaPorte DM. How we do it: modified residency programming and adoption of remote didactic curriculum during the COVID-19 pandemic. J Surg Educ. 2020;77(5):1033–6.
12. Kichloo A, Albosta M, Dettloff K, Wani F, El-Amir Z, Singh J, Aljadah M, Chakinala RC, Kanugula AK, Solanki S, Chugh S. Telemedicine, the current COVID-19 pandemic and the future: a narrative review and perspectives moving forward in the USA. Fam Med Community Health. 2020;8(3):e000530.
13. Leng JC, Tirumalai AA, Kou A, Brun C, Coffman C, Harrison TK, Howard SK, Shum C, Hammons A, Mariano ER. A tale of two surges: messaging app and public COVID-19 data summarize one anesthesiology practice's pandemic year in review. Can J Anaesth. 2021;68(12):1828–30.
14. Kyle MA, Tipirneni R, Thakore N, Dave S, Ganguli I. Primary care access during the COVID-19 pandemic: a simulated patient study. J Gen Intern Med. 2021;36(12):3766–71.
15. Althwanay A, Ahsan F, Oliveri F, Goud HK, Mehkari Z, Mohammed L, Javed M, Rutkofsky IH. Medical education, pre-and post-pandemic era: a review article. Cureus. 2020;12(10)
16. Abdel-Razig S, Ahmad W, Shkoukani MA, Nusair A, Ramirez A, Siddiqi K, Akmal Y, Al Khusaibi Z, Tuzcu EM. Residency training in the time of COVID-19: a framework for academic medical centers dealing with the pandemic. Perspect Med Educ. 2021;10(2):135–40.

Chapter 36
Managing Patients in Crisis in the Outpatient Medical Setting

Kimberly Parks, Joslyn Fisher, and Elizabeth McCord

Introduction

Health-care professionals face multiple challenges treating patients in crisis in the outpatient setting. Primary care clinicians may not be comfortable assessing and addressing social and mental health crises in clinic. This chapter serves as an overview of mental health and social crises that clinicians are likely to encounter while in clinic and provides strategies on how these may be addressed through preparation, identification, intervention, and post-event debriefing.

Outline

- Background
  - Challenges addressing crises in clinic
  - Crises in clinic presentation, prevalence, and risk factors
  - Epidemiology

K. Parks (✉)
Department of Psychiatry and Behavioral Sciences, Baylor College of Medicine, Houston, TX, USA
e-mail: kimberly.parks@bcm.edu

J. Fisher
Department of Medicine, Baylor College of Medicine, Houston, TX, USA
e-mail: joslyn@bcm.edu

E. McCord
Department of Psychiatry and Behavioral Sciences, Emory University School of Medicine, Atlanta, GA, USA
e-mail: emccor4@emory.edu

L. B. Lu et al. (eds.), *Leading an Academic Medical Practice*,
https://doi.org/10.1007/978-3-031-40273-9_36

- Preparation: before the crisis
  - Establishing a trauma-informed care setting
  - Protocol development and training
  - Training the interdisciplinary team on trauma-informed care practices and responding to crises
- Addressing the crisis
  - Screening and risk assessment
  - Action plan
  - Collaborative team resources
- After the crisis
  - Post-event debriefing
  - Performance improvement
  - Prevention
- Conclusion

Background

Challenges Addressing Crises in Clinic

Within the outpatient setting, health-care professionals face multiple challenges treating patients in crisis including limited time, resources, knowledge, and experience. Primary care physicians may encounter many different psychiatric and social crises during their practice. The aim of this chapter is to provide an overview of crises stemming from mental health and social issues and how these may be addressed in the academic outpatient setting through preparation, identification, intervention, and post-event debriefing.

Crises in Clinic: Presentation, Prevalence, and Risk Factors

Mental health and social crises may require urgent or emergent intervention. This chapter focuses on guidance for the most likely scenarios that may arise in an outpatient setting. Specifically, it is common for clinicians to encounter mental health crises such as suicidal ideation, homicidal ideation, severe post-traumatic stress disorder (PTSD), and acute psychosis. Health-care teams must also be prepared to address patients requiring urgent intervention related to the social issues of interpersonal violence (abuse of child, elderly, disabled, or intimate partner violence) or human trafficking (see Tables 36.1 and 36.2 for definitions).

Table 36.1 Adapted definitions of mental health crises

Suicidal ideation	Suicidal ideation refers to thoughts about attempting suicide. It may or may not come with plans or intent to perform the suicide and die. Plans would include details such as the mechanism someone would use to kill themselves, the timing, and the location. Intent refers to the urge to act on these thoughts and plans [1]
Homicidal ideation	Homicidal ideation refers to thoughts about killing another, which can also coincide with plans or intent. Similar to suicide, homicidal plans may include a time, place, and mechanism to kill another person or multiple other people but will further include either a specific or general target. Homicidal intent would refer to the urge to follow through with these plans
Post-traumatic stress disorder (PTSD)	PTSD is a disorder (defined by DSM-5 Diagnostic Criteria) [2] that develops in some people who have experienced, witnessed, or learned of a shocking, frightening, or dangerous traumatic event. PTSD is characterized by a set of symptoms that most commonly include high levels of anxiety, hypervigilance, re-living/re-experiencing past trauma, nightmares about past traumatic events, and even dissociation [3]
Psychosis	Psychosis refers to psychotic symptoms such as hallucinations, delusions, or disorganized thought processes. These may be part of a larger disorder such as schizophrenia, or may be related to another issue such as substance intoxication or a mood episode [4]

Table 36.2 Social issues that may contribute to crises in the outpatient setting[a]

Child abuse and neglect	Abuse and/or neglect of a child under the age of 18 includes acts by a parent, caregiver, or another person in a custodial role (such as a religious leader, a coach, a teacher) that results in harm, the potential for harm, or threat of harm to a child
Abuse and neglect of elder adults or of persons with disabilities	Elder abuse is an intentional act or failure to act that causes or creates a risk of harm to an older adult. An older adult is someone age 60 or older. The abuse occurs at the hands of a caregiver or a person the elder trusts. Elder abuse may include physical, sexual, emotional, psychological, or financial abuse
Intimate partner violence (IPV)	Intimate partner violence is an act or threat of violence that occurs in a current or former intimate relationship (dating or spouse). It may include physical, sexual, emotional, or psychological abuse as well as stalking
Human trafficking	Human trafficking is an umbrella term for many types of crimes. These can be split into both sex and labor trafficking, but a victim of human trafficking may experience both. Within sex trafficking, someone may be forced to perform sex acts of various types, such as forced participation in escort services, pornography, brothels, and massage businesses. Labor trafficking can include being forced to work in various industries such as agriculture, domestic work, restaurants, cleaning services, or carnivals [5]

[a] Definitions/descriptions adapted from the CDC: https://www.cdc.gov/violenceprevention/index.html

Epidemiology

Suicide is the tenth leading cause of death in the United States [1]. Luoma et al. found that approximately 75% of those who completed suicide had been to an outpatient visit within a year before they died and almost half had seen their primary care clinician within a month of their death [6]. However, studies suggest that most patients do not discuss suicidal ideation with their primary care physician, even when seen within a month of their death [7].

As homicide is 2.5 times less common than suicide in the United States [1], encountering a patient with homicidal ideation in the academic medical clinic will occur much less frequently than suicidal ideation. One review found that the most commonly associated mental illnesses with homicide are schizophrenia, antisocial personality disorder, and substance use disorders [8].

PTSD has a lifetime prevalence of 6.8%, with annual prevalence between 3 and 4% [9]. Prevalence of PTSD within primary care clinic patients varies widely, with studies reporting anywhere from 2 to 39% of the population carrying the diagnosis and the diagnosis often goes unrecognized [10, 11]. These patients may be at increased risk for suicide or homicide.

Psychosis and psychotic disorders such as schizophrenia are less common than mood disorders or PTSD. Studies place lifetime prevalence of psychosis at roughly 1.5% of the population [9]. We also know that a psychotic episode is more common in men than women, with an earlier onset of late teens to early 20s for men [4].

Interpersonal violence is common and can impact health. The prevalence of child abuse in the United States varies greatly with 12.5% of children by 18 years old in one study, and up to 37.4% of all children having a Child Protective Services (CPS) investigation in another [12, 13]. Roughly, a third of women and a fourth of all men experience a form of intimate partner violence during their lives. The highest risk group is the 18–24-year olds, but any age, gender, race, socioeconomic status can experience domestic violence [14]. Elder abuse (including neglect and exploitation) may be experienced by one in ten adults over the age of 70 years [15].

Human trafficking prevalence is also difficult to calculate. It is estimated that 2.5 million people worldwide have been trafficked [16]. It can be difficult to recognize human trafficking victims in outpatient care although many do receive some kind of health-care treatment [17].

Compared to those who have not experienced trauma, survivors of trauma are at increased risk for experiencing anxiety, depression, PTSD, and fearfulness of medical care and health-care systems.

Preparation: Before the Crisis

Establishing a Trauma-Informed Care Setting

As noted above, trauma is a common experience among patients and can adversely impact health. The first step in addressing (and preventing) crises in the ambulatory clinical setting is by establishing trauma-informed care practices. Systems to support trauma-informed care should be universally implemented.

The U.S. Substance Abuse and Mental Health Services Administration's (SAMHSA) trauma-informed approach can guide system-wide practices as well as individual clinical management. A trauma-informed approach can reduce triggers that might precipitate a patient crisis, mitigate barriers to patients' accessing care, and aid health-care team members in responding when crises do arise.

SAMHSA's trauma-informed approach includes four components relevant for health-care teams in the outpatient setting:

1. Realization of trauma's widespread impact on patients, families, and staff
2. Recognition of trauma's signs and symptoms
3. Response—institutional and interpersonal
4. Resist re-traumatization

Ambulatory clinical settings approach assessment of the patient's social history and mental health in a variety of ways. Some clinics request completion of a paper or electronic health questionnaire prior to the visit. Other clinics have developed a protocol where a medical assistant or nurse completes aspects of the patient assessment prior to the clinician's exam. Ultimately, in academic medical practices, the physician or advanced practice professional will be primarily responsible for obtaining the social and mental health history and ideally in a trauma-informed manner. Learners in an academic medical clinic can be reminded that adverse childhood experiences are common, and that this past social history can impact health.

A trauma-informed response incorporates traditional good clinical practices such as maintaining confidentiality, ensuring privacy, and demonstrating compassion and culturally competent care. Any assessment of social history or mental health symptoms should be done in private where others cannot see or hear the patient's response. Confidentiality should be explicitly written on any forms or clinic signage and/or stated by health-care team members.

In addition, patients can be empowered when clinical team members collaborate, embrace shared-decision-making, and ask permission. For example, always ask the patient before bringing an additional person into the room including family member, friend, staff, or trainee. In-person or video interpreters are ideal, when possible, to avoid the uncertainty and anxiety-provoking aspect of not knowing who is interpreting via the telephone.

When a patient discloses mental health symptoms or a history of trauma, provide an attentive and non-judgmental response while avoiding pity or blame. It can be a challenge in the age of electronic health records to maintain consistent eye contact. If the listener is not attentive, there is risk that a patient will feel dismissed and therefore not return for care or feel the need to be louder and more aggressive to be heard.

It is equally important for clinical team members to have an awareness of how they are feeling when caring for a patient in crisis. The ability to calm oneself such as through deep breathing can also help with promoting calmness for the patient.

Providing education about their specific condition, local and online resources, and referrals to trauma-specific care without requiring extensive disclosure of trauma details may help avoid emotionally overwhelming the clinician or the patient. Trauma-informed care also means being aware of factors external to the immediate clinical setting. For example, with federal legislation regulating electronic health records, clinicians should be mindful of what the patient can read in the clinical note and, sometimes more importantly, who else may be able to access the medical record or peer over the patient's shoulder when the patient is reading the medical chart or the printed "After Visit Summary." In select situations, the clinician may choose to block patient access to view the electronic note if there is a concern for harm to the patient.

Procedures, certain aspects of the physical exam, and even the clinical environment itself can be triggering for some patients. Patients may feel a loss of control during procedures. Strict policies (such as cancellation for late arrival) in clinic may present an overwhelming barrier for patients. Clinical leaders should review policies and procedures to address the need for modifications or exceptions in cases of potential crisis. Health-care team members must be mindful that the presence of security officers can be frightening and, in turn, provoke patients. To avoid or minimize re-traumatization, explain your plan, seek permission to proceed and collaborate by offering choices and options.

Case Example Ms. Candid is a 32-year-old woman with no significant past medical history who reports palpitations, weight loss, and anxiety. You plan to examine her thyroid. For some patients, a thyroid exam may prompt a memory of strangulation. One example of an approach, "You have mentioned some symptoms that might be related to your thyroid. In order for me to best help you, I would like to ask for your permission to examine your thyroid gland which is located on your neck. I will be placing my fingers on the front of your neck. If you are uncomfortable with this plan, we can discuss other options. If you feel any discomfort during the exam, please let me know—we can stop any time that you request it."

Protocol Development and Training

While system and individual practices may be optimized to reduce the likelihood that an in-clinic crisis might occur, it is an unpredictable reality that, at some point, a crisis will arise in an academic medical clinic.

To best prepare for crises such as acute interpersonal violence, suicidal ideation, or homicidal ideation (or even an active shooter), clinic protocols should be preemptively established, and routine training should be developed and deployed.

National accreditation/regulatory bodies such as the Joint Commission and Det Norske Veritas (DNV) require health facilities to have emergency management protocols and for the health-care team to know how to access them. If a clinic is part of a larger health system, policies and procedures governing management of certain crises will usually be available. In smaller clinics and for some specific crises, health-care leadership should develop procedures for managing crises. It is important to have protocols readily accessible in written (printed) as well as electronic format. Clinical settings may have an emergency management handbook and/or an emergency management link on the organization's website home page.

Key components for a crisis management protocol include:

- Criteria for initiating crisis management protocol
- Establishing who serves as crisis management team leader
- Designate team members and roles/responsibilities (security, police, mental health crisis team, nurse manager, social work, interpreter, etc.)
- Escalation plan (who calls whom)
- Checklist of "to-do's"
- Incorporate relevant laws (such as reporting)
- Documentation standards (who documents which components of event; accurate concise synopsis)
- Relevant resources—such as local community, online—handouts, phone numbers, etc.
- Plan for debriefing after the event

See Fig. 36.1 for crisis assessment algorithm.

Training the Interdisciplinary Team on Trauma-Informed Care Practices and Responding to Crises

While the Joint Commission requires regular ongoing training for health-care settings for workplace violence, the authors are not aware of specific recommendations for training to manage other crises in outpatient clinical settings. The authors suggest crisis training for health-care team members should occur at least annually—particularly for the nurses, medical assistants, and attending physicians who are present longitudinally since trainees often rotate through different sites in academic medical centers. For all learners, part of clinic orientation should involve raising awareness of available crisis protocols, how to access them, and location of resources.

Training for crisis management can include crisis-specific education (e.g., suicidal ideation or active shooter) or more general crisis intervention techniques. Training options include watching a video, didactic presentation, and simulations. Tabletop exercises where health-care team members meet and review processes for managing example scenarios can be a cost-effective strategy.

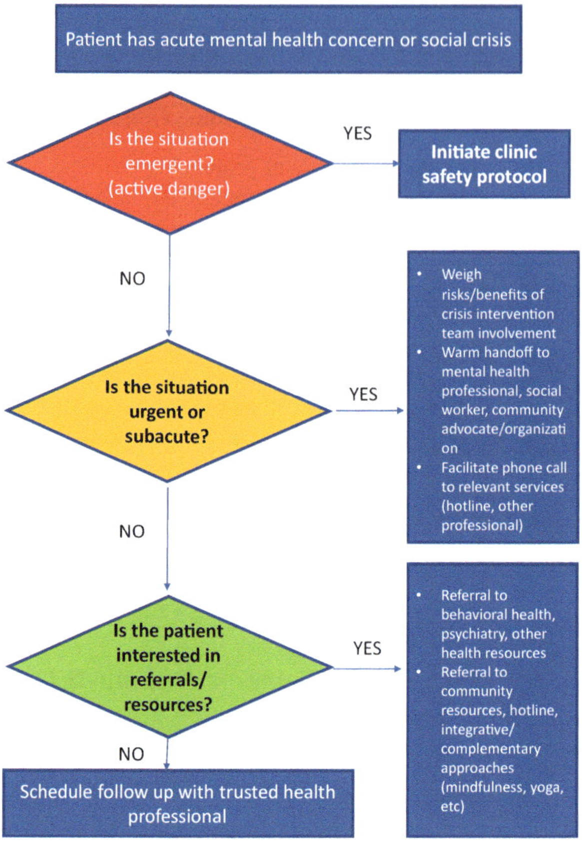

Fig. 36.1 Crisis intervention protocol in clinic

Addressing the Crisis

Screening and Risk Assessment

To identify patients in crisis, we recommend utilizing effective screening tools and conducting a robust clinical interview. The following discussion reviews recommendations for screening for depression and suicidality, homicidal ideation, and interpersonal violence (see Table 36.3 for example tools).

The United States Preventive Services Task Force (USPSTF) recommends screening for depression in adults over age 18 years and should be implemented with adequate systems in place to ensure accurate diagnosis, effective treatment, and appropriate follow-up [18]. However, the USPSTF noted insufficient evidence for routine screening for suicide in the general population, especially if mental health resources are limited or unavailable for at-risk patients [19, 20]. Although the USPSTF acknowledges more research must be done on screening for suicide in the

Table 36.3 Examples of online screening tools

Depression	
PHQ-9 (PHQ-2)	https://www.hrsa.gov/behavioral-health/patient-health-questionnaire-phq-screeners
WHO-5	Regional Office for Europe WHO. Use of Well-Being Measures in Primary Health Care—The DepCare Project. Health for All, Target 12, 1998 https://www.euro.who.int/__data/assets/pdf_file/0016/130750/E60246.pdf
Geriatric depression scale	https://geriatrictoolkit.missouri.edu/cog/GDS_SHORT_FORM.PDF
Intimate partner violence	
https://www.ahrq.gov/ncepcr/tools/healthier-pregnancy/fact-sheets/partner-violence.html (this sheet includes links to several validated tools)	

general population, the authors recommend consistent screening for at-risk individuals seen in the primary care clinic.

There is no universally accepted screening tool to assess a patient for suicidality. However, one of the most common screening tools utilized in the primary care clinic, the Patient Health Questionnaire (PHQ), is a well-validated tool used to screen for depressive symptoms [21]. The questionnaire asks patients to describe how bothered they have been by their symptoms in the last 2 weeks, with response options of "not at all," "several days," "more than half the days," and "nearly every day." The PHQ-2 consists of the first two questions of the PHQ 9-point questionnaire, inquiring about anhedonia and overall depressed state. If the patient screens positive by answering yes to the above questions, this will trigger the health professional to follow-up with the remaining seven items of the PHQ-9 [22]. Some research suggests, that the PHQ-2 may not be adequate alone to identify suicidal ideation [23].

The 15-item Geriatric Depression Scale (GDS) and the 5-item subset of the GDS are additional rating scales used in primary care settings that are sensitive and specific in identifying patients judged to be suicidal via semi-structured clinical interview [24]. While the GDS-15 is historically a screening tool for the elderly, studies support its clinical use in adults aged 18 and older [25].

Although depression is a major risk factor for suicidality, suicidal ideation can be present in nondepressed patients. Clinicians are encouraged to ask about specific thoughts of self-harm, particularly in patients with risk factors such as prior suicide attempt, substance use/dependence, other mental health comorbidities, and social stressors. Merely asking patients about thoughts of death or suicide has not been linked to an increase in suicide attempts [22]. If a patient has shared thoughts of wanting to die, it is the health professional's responsibility to determine whether these thoughts are passive or if they are indicative of active suicidal ideation and intent. If an individual expresses imminent intent to harm themselves or others, the clinician should initiate the appropriate safety protocol.

For patients presenting with acute decompensated psychosis, the mental status exam is a pivotal tool in organizing their presentation, creating a differential, and communicating the patient's condition to peers. It examines the patient's thought content, cognitive ability, and perceptual disturbances (among other things), all of which are important when deciding next steps. It is important to keep in mind that patients may still be a danger to themselves, even without suicidal thoughts.

While more is known about risk factors for suicide, both suicide and homicide share similar risk factors including comorbid mental health diagnoses (such as mood disorders, PTSD, and active psychosis), male gender, prior suicide or homicide attempts, access to weapons, and intoxication or withdrawal from substances. Social stressors such as housing instability, financial stressors, or legal trouble can contribute to either condition as well. Prior experience of interpersonal violence or human trafficking can confer an elevated risk for suicide [26, 27].

Clinicians routinely explore a patient's social history to identify risk factors that can contribute to adverse health outcomes. While it is beyond the scope of this chapter, health professionals should be attentive to signs and symptoms of abuse or neglect in all patients. In addition, the USPSTF recommends screening for intimate partner violence (IPV) in women of reproductive age and offers several evidence-based tools to aid in identification of current or past survivors of IPV [28]. Once clinicians have identified an adult experiencing IPV, a response should include non-judgmental validation and supportive listening. While IPV is common, most patients who disclose IPV exposure will not be in an immediate crisis and thus it would be appropriate to provide resources such as a hotline number or referral to social work. In the situation where someone is in immediate danger (abuser threatening in clinic) or the patient does not feel safe to return home, then the clinical team can contact security and/or facilitate a call to a crisis IPV service for shelter.

Case Continued You realize that Ms. Candid is of reproductive age and you forgot to screen her for intimate partner violence earlier in your exam. You preface your privately conducted screening questions with the comment that intimate partner violence is common, can affect one's health, and you ask all of your patients whether they are experiencing violence. The patient discloses that she is in an increasingly violent relationship and she is actually scared to go home, she fears for her life.

You clarify that her abusive partner is not in the clinic and you facilitate a phone call to a local hotline from an available (empty) exam room. She speaks to the counselor and they plan to provide a taxi to pick the patient up from clinic to bring her to the shelter. You offer and she agrees to allow you to make a follow-up appointment to see you as well as a referral for behavioral health services.

It is important to note that screening tools will never take the place of an effective clinical interview, though they are helpful in identifying level of risk. Each level of risk, whether it be from suicidality, psychosis, or other safety concern, will require a different immediate response and ongoing management plan.

Action Plan

After identifying a patient in crisis, the authors recommend following an action plan that focuses on patient and staff safety. Patients in crisis will fall into one of three categories: subacute, acute/urgent, and emergent (Fig. 36.1). Learners in clinic should discuss all cases of crisis with their faculty preceptor. If it is potentially unsafe to leave the patient alone in the room, the learner can call or page a supervising clinician and/or open the exam room door to call for another nearby health-care team member.

Patients who have been identified as at-risk but not in acute danger can be made aware of and provided with resources and appropriate follow-up. For example: a patient mentions that he had thought about hurting himself last week. However, today he is feeling ok and not actively suicidal. In this case, the clinician can review a safety plan, provide mental health resources, and aid in securing a close mental health appointment. Another example: an elderly patient discloses that she is being neglected on occasion by her caregiver who does not change her soiled clothes within the hour but overall the patient has been doing "ok" and does not feel unsafe. In this case, the clinician can consider contacting a clinic social worker and/or adult protective services, conducting a house call visit if available and arrange for close follow-up with the primary care team (see Table 36.4 for resources).

For patients who disclose they are in distress and in need of more urgent help, it may be appropriate to secure a same-day or next-day mental health appointment with the caveat that the patient may choose to voluntarily go to an emergency room. Another example: if a patient discloses that they are experiencing intimate partner violence and do not feel safe going home, the health-care team can facilitate the patient contacting a shelter or domestic violence hotline.

Once a patient has been identified as having a high-risk emergency, the clinician should notify the care team and follow proper clinic safety protocols. Clinicians should ensure constant observation and monitoring of the patient until a plan is formulated. Having a limited number of staff available to monitor a patient in an exam room can be a significant barrier for the clinic. It may be necessary to recruit

Table 36.4 Crisis resources

Organization/resource	Contact #	Website
Crisis Text Line	Text HOME to 741741	https://www.crisistextline.org/
National Suicide and Crisis Lifeline	988	https://988lifeline.org/
Veterans Crisis Line	988, then PRESS 1 or Text 838255	https://veteranscrisisline.net/
Substance Abuse and Mental Health Services Administration National Helpline	(800) 662-4357 (HELP)	https://www.samhsa.gov/find-help/national-helpline
National Domestic Violence Hotline	(800) 799-7233	https://www.thehotline.org/
National Sexual Assault Hotline	(800) 656-4673	https://www.rainn.org/resources

staff from another area to assist with patient monitoring. For clinics with integrated or onsite behavioral health, the behavioral health specialist may be one of the key responders.

Case Continued Ms. Candid is waiting in an exam room until the taxi to the shelter arrives when she exits the room and starts pacing the hallways, wringing her hands, and states that she cannot go to a shelter, she will never feel safe, and she thinks she would be better off dead. You approach the patient and gently encourage her to return to the exam room. You explore her statement that she would be "better off dead" and learn that she has thought about suicide frequently recently and she plans to take every pill "I can get my hand on so that I can go painlessly out of this world." You are startled but recognize she cannot be left alone in the room. You contact your attending in clinic and activate the clinic's crisis intervention protocol.

Patients in crisis are often experiencing severe psychic distress and anxiety. It is best to match a patient to a professional who can sit with the individual and make them feel "heard." These individuals can add important support for the patient in crisis [29]. Patients in crisis can often act impulsively, especially if there is a perceived threat. It is important to place them in a safe area where there is little to no access to medical equipment that could be used for self-harm (intravenous tubing, scalpels, needles, etc.) [22]. Security personnel can assist with removing the patient's belongings to avoid the risk of overdosing on home medications or accessing a personal weapon. Immediate safety should be prioritized while next steps are being arranged.

For patients presenting with decompensated psychosis, antipsychotic medications or anxiolytics may be given if they are easily accessible in the clinic. In instances where verbal de-escalation is appropriate, the clinician can redirect the situation by demonstrating a willingness to compromise with the patient and validate their concerns. Anger or aggression can manifest as anxiety, guilt, or perceived invalidation; thus, allowing a patient to express their concerns in a nonjudgmental environment may help de-escalate the encounter [30]. Restraints should be used in situations when verbal de-escalation has failed and patients are physically violent (hitting, punching, spitting). The concern of damaging a patient–clinician therapeutic alliance should never interfere with ensuring the patient's or care team's safety in an acute crisis.

In situations where the patient is an imminent risk to self or others, we recommend seeking expert consultation with a mental health professional. Studies show that having access to psychiatric support when managing a patient in crisis reduces clinician anxiety and results in better patient outcomes [31]. Protocols for involuntary psychiatric assessments vary from state to state; thus, it is imperative that clinicians familiarize themselves with local safety protocols for patients needing emergent psychiatric stabilization.

The primary care clinician (or team) should focus on ensuring the safe transportation of the individual to an emergency department if further psychiatric work up is warranted. For nonhospital-based settings, the authors recommend calling emergency services or 911 to safely transport the patient to an emergency department.

Some jurisdictions have a special behavioral health crisis intervention team available to intervene. For others, evaluation and transport might be via an ambulance or regular law enforcement. For patients experiencing an emergent mental health crisis in clinic, the patient's family or friends should not transport the patient. Patients should be transferred using trained personnel following clinic protocols. Law enforcement is usually contacted if the patient has been placed on an involuntary psychiatric hold. Law enforcement can also help ensure the safety of staff and patients during a crisis encounter [32]. If a patient is identified as being in crisis during a telehealth visit, clinicians should contact emergency services to perform a wellness check to assess the need for transfer of the patient to the nearest emergency department.

Collaborative Team Responses

The collaborative care model is an important resource in the primary care clinic that helps engage patients with behavioral health [33]. Collaborative care involves a multidisciplinary approach to treating patients by working with mental health experts, peer support individuals, care managers, nurses, and social workers who are trained in the management of depression and other psychiatric illnesses. Care managers can assist the primary care clinician in monitoring patient outcomes, providing patient education and facilitating communication with patients and their mental health team. Data shows that individuals enrolled in collaborative care have higher rates of remission of major depression as well as decreased suicidality after 24 months of treatment [32]. This data is further supported by the PROSPECT trial, which show that implementing a collaborative care model results in reducing depression rates and suicidal ideations in the primary care clinic [34].

For clinics that do not have access to collaborative, multidisciplinary care, clinicians are encouraged to use local and community psychiatric referrals to manage patients with non-life-threatening mental illness. We recommend close follow-up and frequent visits with the clinical team to assess safety. Patients should be screened for depression and suicide at each follow-up appointment. If a patient was referred to the emergency room for psychiatric stabilization during a previous visit, they should be followed by a mental health specialist for ongoing treatment [32]. We recommend giving patients the National Suicide Prevention Lifeline (1-800-273-TALK or more recently shortened to 988), which is a toll-free crisis line available 24/7. We also encourage outreach from clinical social workers, chaplains, and peer support specialists to help alleviate the burden on the clinician and provide additional support to patients in need.

After the Crisis

Post-event Debriefing

Managing a psychiatric or social crisis in the primary care clinic is not only stressful for the patient and family, but for the health-care professionals as well. Being mindful of one's own well-being when caring for others in distress can aid in reducing clinician burn out and anxiety [29]. Taking a moment to practice deep breathing can be an effective strategy in reducing stress that arises during a crisis. Based on experience and review of online (unpublished) available best practices, the authors encourage clinics to hold a debriefing session to review events that occurred during and after the crisis encounter. This type of forum can help the care team process the challenging and often disturbing nature of the event. Clinic leadership should provide the health-care team members with information on local mental health resources and employee assistance programs offered through their institutions.

Performance Improvement

Clinic leadership should solicit (in both an anonymous and open format) feedback from all team members involved in managing the crisis to improve clinic performance. Team member input can inform specific recommendations on how to improve safety protocols and also highlight what went well during the encounter. The goal of feedback is to improve clinical confidence of the staff as well as troubleshoot issues that may arise in future crisis situations. Standardized evaluation tools can help identify specific areas that require improvement, such as efficient transportation of patients to an emergency department or the absence of appropriate screening techniques [35].

Prevention

Family members and loved ones play a key role in crisis prevention for patients suffering with mental illness and should be engaged on a regular basis as permitted by the patient. The authors recommend counseling the patient and the family/loved ones to foster a safe home environment by removing firearms, medications that can be used in lethal amounts, and other obvious means of self-harm [32]. Families should be encouraged to use the suicide prevention hotline as well as emergency services/911 in the event of a future crisis.

For patients experiencing interpersonal violence or human trafficking, the primary clinical team, the health-care system, as well as local, regional, and national organizations can provide invaluable support. These resources can, in turn, serve to prevent future crises from developing.

Case Continued Ms. Candid returns to clinic. She was hospitalized for a short period to stabilize her mood, after which she was discharged to a women's shelter where she is getting ongoing counseling and support to secure safe long-term housing. You reassure her that her thyroid studies are normal and also assess safety, ensure she has the supportive counseling she wants, and make plans to follow-up with her again for her health maintenance/prevention needs in 3 months.

Conclusion

While crises in the clinic do not happen frequently, health-care team members are encouraged to participate in pre-event preparation, creation of an action plan, and post-event debriefing. Effective teamwork and communication play an integral role in ensuring the safety of patients as well as staff members. With appropriate screening and identification of risk factors, clinicians can feel more empowered to manage a crisis if one should arise.

References

1. National Institute of Mental Health. Suicide. 2022. https://www.nimh.nih.gov/health/statistics/suicide. Accessed 15 Mar 2022.
2. American Psychiatric Association. Desk reference to the diagnostic criteria from DSM-5. Arlington: American Psychiatric Association; 2016.
3. National Institute of Mental Health. Post-Traumatic Stress Disorder. 2022. https://www.nimh.nih.gov/health/topics/post-traumatic-stress-disorder-ptsd. Accessed 15 Mar 2022.
4. National Institute of Mental Health. Schizophrenia. 2022. https://www.nimh.nih.gov/health/topics/schizophrenia. Accessed 16 Mar 2022.
5. Nemeth JM, Rizo CF. Estimating the prevalence of human trafficking: progress made and future directions. Am J Public Health. 2019;109(10):1318–9.
6. Luoma JB, Martin CE, Pearson JL. Contact with mental health and primary care providers before suicide: a review of the evidence. Am J Psychiatry. 2002;159(6):909–16.
7. Isometsa ET, Heikkinen ME, Marttunen MJ, Henriksson MM, Aro HM, Lonnqvist JK. The last appointment before suicide: is suicide intent communicated? Am J Psychiatry. 1995;152(6):919–22.
8. Richard-Devantoy S, Olie JP, Gourevitch R. Risk of homicide and major mental disorders: a critical review. Encéphale. 2009;35(6):521–30.
9. Kessler RC, Berglund P, Demler O, Jin R, Merikangas KR, Walters EE. Lifetime prevalence and age-of-onset distributions of DSM-IV disorders in the National Comorbidity Survey Replication. Arch Gen Psychiatry. 2005;62(6):593–602.
10. Spottswood M, Davydow DS, Huang H. The prevalence of posttraumatic stress disorder in primary care: a systematic review. Harv Rev Psychiatry. 2017;25(4):159–69.

11. Liebschutz J, Saitz R, Brower V, Keane TM, Lloyd-Travaglini C, Averbuch T, et al. PTSD in urban primary care: high prevalence and low physician recognition. J Gen Intern Med. 2007;22(6):719–26.
12. Kim H, Wildeman C, Jonson-Reid M, Drake B. Lifetime prevalence of investigating child maltreatment among US children. Am J Public Health. 2017;107(2):274–80.
13. Wildeman C, Emanuel N, Leventhal JM, Putnam-Hornstein E, Waldfogel J, Lee H. The prevalence of confirmed maltreatment among US children, 2004 to 2011. JAMA Pediatr. 2014;168(8):706–13.
14. Sugg N. Intimate partner violence: prevalence, health consequences, and intervention. Med Clin North Am. 2015;99(3):629–49.
15. Rosay ABP, Mulford CFP. Prevalence estimates and correlates of elder abuse in the United States: the National Intimate Partner and Sexual Violence Survey. J Elder Abuse Negl. 2017;29(1):1–14.
16. Lerche J. A global alliance against forced labour? Unfree labour, neo-liberal globalization and the International Labour Organization. J Agrar Chang. 2007;7(4):425–52.
17. Chisolm-Straker M, Baldwin S, Gaigbe-Togbe B, Ndukwe N, Johnson PN, Richardson LD. Health care and human trafficking: we are seeing the unseen. J Health Care Poor Underserved. 2016;27(3):1220–33.
18. Siu AL, Force USPST, Bibbins-Domingo K, Grossman DC, Baumann LC, Davidson KW, et al. Screening for depression in adults: US Preventive Services Task Force recommendation statement. JAMA. 2016;315(4):380–7.
19. The Joint Commission. Behavioral Health Care and Human Services: 2022 National Patient Safety Goals. 2022. https://www.jointcommission.org/standards/national-patient-safety-goals/behavioral-health-care-national-patient-safety-goals/. Accessed 5 Mar 2022.
20. LeFevre ML, Force USPST. Screening for suicide risk in adolescents, adults, and older adults in primary care: U.S. Preventive Services Task Force recommendation statement. Ann Intern Med. 2014;160(10):719–26.
21. Kroenke K, Spitzer RL, Williams JB. The PHQ-9: validity of a brief depression severity measure. J Gen Intern Med. 2001;16(9):606–13.
22. Raue PJ, Ghesquiere AR, Bruce ML. Suicide risk in primary care: identification and management in older adults. Curr Psychiatry Rep. 2014;16(9):466.
23. Inagaki M, Ohtsuki T, Yonemoto N, Kawashima Y, Saitoh A, Oikawa Y, et al. Validity of the Patient Health Questionnaire (PHQ)-9 and PHQ-2 in general internal medicine primary care at a Japanese rural hospital: a cross-sectional study. Gen Hosp Psychiatry. 2013;35(6):592–7.
24. Heisel MJ, Duberstein PR, Lyness JM, Feldman MD. Screening for suicide ideation among older primary care patients. J Am Board Fam Med. 2010;23(2):260–9.
25. Guerin JM, Copersino ML, Schretlen DJ. Clinical utility of the 15-item geriatric depression scale (GDS-15) for use with young and middle-aged adults. J Affect Disord. 2018;241:59–62.
26. Kiss L, Yun K, Pocock N, Zimmerman C. Exploitation, violence, and suicide risk among child and adolescent survivors of human trafficking in the Greater Mekong Subregion. JAMA Pediatr. 2015;169(9):e152278.
27. Pico-Alfonso MA, Garcia-Linares MI, Celda-Navarro N, Blasco-Ros C, Echeburua E, Martinez M. The impact of physical, psychological, and sexual intimate male partner violence on women's mental health: depressive symptoms, posttraumatic stress disorder, state anxiety, and suicide. J Womens Health (Larchmt). 2006;15(5):599–611.
28. Force USPST, Curry SJ, Krist AH, Owens DK, Barry MJ, Caughey AB, et al. Screening for intimate partner violence, elder abuse, and abuse of vulnerable adults: US Preventive Services Task Force final recommendation statement. JAMA. 2018;320(16):1678–87.
29. Sisler SM, Schapiro NA, Nakaishi M, Steinbuchel P. Suicide assessment and treatment in pediatric primary care settings. J Child Adolesc Psychiatr Nurs. 2020;33(4):187–200.
30. Breen KJ, Greenberg PB. Difficult physician-patient encounters. Intern Med J. 2010;40(10):682–8.

31. Brodsky BS, Spruch-Feiner A, Stanley B. The zero suicide model: applying evidence-based suicide prevention practices to clinical care. Front Psych. 2018;9:33.
32. McDowell AK, Lineberry TW, Bostwick JM. Practical suicide-risk management for the busy primary care physician. Mayo Clin Proc. 2011;86(8):792–800.
33. Blackmore MA, Patel UB, Stein D, Carleton KE, Ricketts SM, Ansari AM, et al. Collaborative care for low-income patients from racial-ethnic minority groups in primary care: engagement and clinical outcomes. Psychiatr Serv. 2022;73(8):842–8.
34. Alexopoulos GS, Reynolds CF 3rd, Bruce ML, Katz IR, Raue PJ, Mulsant BH, et al. Reducing suicidal ideation and depression in older primary care patients: 24-month outcomes of the PROSPECT study. Am J Psychiatry. 2009;166(8):882–90.
35. Barnhill J, Fisher JW, Kimel-Scott K, Weil A. Trauma-informed care: helping the healthcare team thrive. In: Gerber MR, editor. Trauma-informed healthcare approaches: a guide for primary care. Cham: Springer International Publishing; 2019. p. 197–213.

Chapter 37
Addressing Disruptive Patient Encounters: A Trauma-Informed, Equity-Focused Approach

Stacie Schmidt, Elizabeth Norian, and Stan Sonu

Introduction

Understanding the link between psychosocial trauma and poor physical, mental, and social consequences is essential for successfully navigating difficult patient encounters. A growing body of evidence has consistently found that psychosocial adversity has wide ranging and multifaceted effects on health. Toxic stress can embed itself in long-term processes such as behavioral adaptations (e.g., attempts to cope or self-sooth via addiction), chronic low-grade inflammation (a common and shared process in multiple chronic diseases), and a variety of psychiatric disturbances throughout the life course, especially if experienced during the sensitive early years of life.

Trauma-informed care (TIC) employs a preventative, capacity-building approach to improve the quality of clinician–patient communication, foster trust, support patient autonomy, and reduce re-traumatization. TIC provides a series of universal conceptual guardrails that promote patient-centered, humanistic treatment regardless of the patient's personal background. In this chapter, we introduce TIC concepts as a critical perspective for successfully navigating challenging patient encounters. Additionally, a trauma-informed approach includes consideration of how the physical space of the clinic may exacerbate stressful situations.

Finally, there may be circumstances when attempts to integrate TIC and promote a physically safe clinic environment do not prevent or mitigate disruptive behavior.

S. Schmidt (✉) · S. Sonu
Department of Medicine, Emory University School of Medicine, Atlanta, GA, USA
e-mail: srschmi@emory.edu; stan.sonu@emory.edu

E. Norian
Department of Medicine, Harvard Medical School, Boston, MA, USA
e-mail: enorian@bidmc.harvard.edu

L. B. Lu et al. (eds.), *Leading an Academic Medical Practice*,
https://doi.org/10.1007/978-3-031-40273-9_37

In this chapter, we describe a three-tiered approach for making such an assessment, as well as a committee-based approach by which action plans are documented and implemented.

Outline

- Overview of the effects of psychosocial trauma on health and well-being
- Understanding and implementing trauma-informed primary care
  - Components of adverse childhood events and trauma-informed care
  - Six principles of trauma-informed patient care delivery
- Assessing and mitigating factors that contribute to difficult encounters
- Proactive planning for challenging encounters
- Techniques for identifying the agitated patient during a clinic encounter
- Strategies for determining when and how a patient should be discharged from the academic primary care clinic setting
- Conclusion

Overview of the Effects of Psychosocial Trauma on Health and Well-being

Successfully navigating challenging patient encounters *begins* with having a robust understanding of the link between exposure to psychosocial trauma and poor physical, mental, and social outcomes. Mounting evidence spanning at least three decades of research has consistently observed wide-ranging and multifaceted consequences of trauma on health. A framework that translates this understanding to guide clinical encounters is *trauma-informed care* (TIC), which maintains perspectives of empathy and compassion during challenging or emotionally charged encounters with patients [1]. To date, however, knowledge of the link between trauma and health, including TIC, remains low among most graduate medical education programs in the United States [2, 3].

Perhaps the most well-known and seminal work that described the association between negative psychosocial experiences and poor health outcomes is the adverse childhood experiences (ACEs) study, published in the late 1990s [4]. Prior to this work, research on psychological trauma had focused on specific populations, such as combat veterans and survivors of intimate partner violence [5]. The ACE study called attention to the stark reality and multifaceted effect of traumatic experiences to a broader US demography. Individuals who participated in the ACE study were not a group stereotypically viewed as being highly traumatized. Of more than 17,000 adults, 75% were white, with 11% Hispanic, 7% Asian, and 4.5% Black; 75% were college-educated (over 90% graduated high school); and all were insured. Participants were asked about histories of ten categories of adverse experiences encountered within the home before the age of 18. ACE categories included abuse (physical, emotional, and sexual), neglect (physical and emotional), and five types of household stressors (mental health problems and/or substance use disorder in a family member, intimate partner violence, incarceration, and parental separation or divorce). In quantifying the total number of ACEs for each participant, researchers found 64% had ≥1 ACE and 12.5% had ≥4 ACE.

More recent epidemiological work by Merrick et al. (2018), which included over 200,000 participants from a nationally representative sample, found that ACEs were both universal (62% had ≥1, 25% had ≥3) *and* disproportionately common among historically marginalized and neglected groups, such as Black, Hispanic, and multiracial individuals, those with less than a high school education or currently unemployed, and those identifying as lesbian, gay, or bisexual [6]. Additionally, the concept of ACEs itself, which in the original study was limited to adverse events inside the home, has been expanded in recent studies. Wade et al. (2016) surveyed participants from a diverse urban population on conventional ACEs as well as community-level adversities, such as witnessing violence in the community, experiencing discrimination, experiencing bullying, or ever living in foster care [7]. The associations between these expanded ACEs and poor health outcomes were similar to the original ACE study. Thus, over the past 20 years, general understanding of the prevalence and distribution of trauma has evolved. Trauma is no longer understood to be an experience limited to survivors of the most extreme situations or environments (e.g., combat veterans, victims of intimate partner violence or rape) or considered as events only occurring within the home; rather, trauma is both universal across all sociodemographic categories *and also* disproportionately prevalent among historically marginalized and neglected groups; it is a phenomenon of varying scale, occurring at interpersonal, community, and societal levels.

One of the most noteworthy findings from the ACE study was the robust dose-dependent association between the cumulative number of ACEs per individual and the risk of a wide array of undesirable health outcomes. After adjusting for age, sex, race (self-reported), and educational attainment, ACEs were observed to be associated with *health risk behaviors* (tobacco use, heavy alcohol consumption, illicit substance use, high risk sexual activity), *mental health problems* (depression, anxiety, impulse control disorders, history of suicidality, post-traumatic stress disorder), and *chronic disease* (ischemic heart disease, stroke, COPD, diabetes, non-skin cancer, autoimmune disease, and liver disease) [8, 9]. Researchers also observed dose-dependent associations between ACEs and important *social outcomes*, such as job absenteeism, financial problems, and relational challenges [10]. These associations have been observed in both prospective [11, 12] and cross-sectional studies among participants of varying ages, socioeconomic strata, and specific or unique shared experiences (e.g., incarcerated individuals, people living with HIV). Though causality cannot be determined from cross-sectional studies, the exposure variable of ACEs on poor health has been assessed to meet at least seven of nine Bradford-Hill criteria, suggesting the possibility of a causal relationship [13]. Finally, through follow-up assessments over a period of 10 years, ACE researchers observed an alarming disparity in mortality: individuals with ≥6 ACEs lived on average 20 years shorter than those without ACEs [14]. In sum, what is clear from this immense body of research is that psychosocial trauma is inexorably linked with several health and social problems spanning multiple domains of well-being.

The underlying pathophysiologic mechanisms on how psychosocial adversity and trauma promote poor health outcomes has been of increasing interest in recent decades. A convergence of research from neuroscience, medicine, psychology, and child development points to the overwhelmed brain's inability to regulate its stress response system as the key process through which the multitude of physical, mental, behavioral, and social health problems arise. Building on a child's genetic potential, brain development is fundamentally an experience-dependent process [15]. Positive experiences, such as a consistent and stable relationship with a safe, attuned, and nurturing caregiver, powerfully stimulate healthy brain development and formation of synaptic connections [16–18]. In contrast, adverse or traumatic experiences predictably disrupt or derail normal brain development; indeed, the earliest signs of adversity include developmental delays, such as speech/language delay in young children [19, 20]. Because the early childhood years (ages 0–6) are a period of rapid brain growth, these years are particularly vulnerable to the effects of trauma. In the absence of critical protective buffering relationships, ACEs can promote a dysregulated and exaggerated stress response known as toxic stress [21]. Toxic stress disrupts healthy neurodevelopment (altering brain architecture), dysregulates activity of the neuroendocrine and immune systems (often promoting states of chronic, low-grade inflammation), and can promote modifications to the epigenome, altering the expression of genes in the next generation and ultimately highlighting a pattern of intergenerational transmission of trauma. If experienced during the sensitive early years of life, the effects of toxic stress can become embedded into long-term processes, such as behavioral adaptations (e.g., attempts to cope or self-sooth via addiction), chronic low-grade inflammation (a common and shared process in multiple chronic diseases), and a range of psychiatric disturbances throughout the life course.

The psychological and cognitive manifestations of trauma are well described and consistent with the link between trauma, dysregulated activity of the stress response system, and biopsychosocial outputs [22]. In the mid-late twentieth century, post-traumatic stress disorder (PTSD) became a formally recognized condition representing a constellation of signs and symptoms following exposure to an extremely threatening event(s): intrusive reexperiencing of the event (flashbacks, nightmares), avoidant/numbing behaviors, and hypervigilance/hyperarousal [23]. Complex PTSD (cPTSD), a more recently recognized syndrome that was included in the most recent World Health Organization 11th International Classification of Diseases (ICD-11), incudes PTSD items as well as emotional/affect dysregulation, negative self-concept, and challenges in sustaining relationships and intimacy [22]. A recent systematic review including data from over seven million primary care patients estimated the point prevalence of PTSD to be 12.5% [24]; among patients receiving care in urban primary care settings, the prevalence is over 20% [24, 25]. Yet even without formal PTSD diagnosis, the predictable behavioral and cognitive responses due to trauma, coined by the term *post-traumatic stress symptoms* (PTSS), are common among patients in primary care [26, 27]. One study found that despite only 5% of primary care patients having a formal diagnosis of PTSD, over 50% had ≥1 traumatic stress symptom(s) (over 40% of all patients reported avoidance behaviors, 35% reported hypervigilance, and 33% reported detachment/numbing) [26].

Given the relationship between trauma exposure and PTSS, which itself remains vastly underrecognized and thus undertreated in adult primary care settings [26, 28], it follows intuitively that patients with experiences of trauma are more likely to report negative interactions with health providers compared to those without [29]. Compounding this dynamic is the observation that individuals with high trauma exposure are more likely to engage with the health system in counterproductive ways (i.e., overutilization of acute care services, missed appointments, challenges with medication adherence) [30–32]. Lack of awareness of trauma and its effects increases the risk of misunderstanding and miscommunication. For example, a patient with a history of psychosocial trauma and chronic pain managed may express anger or mistrust upon the clinician's suggestion to taper opioids; this behavior is best recharacterized as an adaptive or maladaptive stress response, not as a core personality trait or statement of values on the part of the individual. What underlies the patient's reaction may be deep-seeded fear of uncontrolled pain that then triggers a hypervigilant response, which is an attempt at self-protection, albeit a counterproductive one. The task at hand then is to understand and address underlying fear(s) driving the behavior rather than approaching the issue from a strictly rational or logical point of view. Clinicians who develop the capacity to be receptive and attend to this dynamic can both prevent and mitigate many negative interpersonal interactions with patients. Therefore, it is in this context that the framework of trauma-informed care (TIC) can be a useful resource in challenging ambulatory encounters.

Understanding and Implementing Trauma-Informed Care (TIC)

A trauma-informed care (TIC) framework can enhance the quality of interpersonal communication between clinicians and patients, cultivate trust, support patient autonomy, and mitigate re-traumatization. Centered on the healing potential of relationships and connection, TIC empowers clinicians to maintain a lens of empathy through a rationale grounded in scientific discovery, offering a set of interpersonal guardrails that facilitate patient-centered, humanistic care. Further, the utility of TIC goes well beyond the specific provider–patient dynamic. A trauma-informed perspective can be useful across a wide range of interpersonal relationships, such as with coworkers, supervisors, employees, family members, friends, and more [33].

The Substance Abuse and Mental Health Services Association (SAMHSA) has developed six key principles that are fundamental to a trauma-informed approach to care [34]. These include:

Safety: Safety includes physical, emotional, and cultural forms of safety. Feeling unsafe or vulnerable can promote activation of the stress response system, which can manifest in a wide range of undesired biopsychosocial effects. When a patient feels unsafe, the ability to integrate information shared during the encounter is diminished—in a sense, the patient is in survival mode instead of learning mode. Avoiding re-traumatization is a critical component of implementing TIC; preventing situations that exacerbate stress for a trauma survivor is necessary to move a person through positive and effective medical care. Examples of this include asking permission to examine a patient and approaching care assuming a patient's best intentions [34]. Ensuring a safe environment—whether through thoughtful design of the physical space, emotional safety in which all staff are trauma-informed, or cultural safety through inclusive imagery and shared values and standards in the clinic—is an essential priority in a trauma-informed organization.

Trustworthiness and transparency: Establishing trust is a key component of preventing and mitigating challenging interactions with patients. Individuals with substantial histories of trauma have often experienced broken trust or betrayal by the very people who were supposed to be trustworthy (e.g., primary relationships). This dynamic of fractured trust is not limited to only household members but also includes institutions. For example, the effects of the deeply unethical United States Public Health Service study of Syphilis among Black men in Tuskegee, Alabama, which took place from 1932 to 1972, continue to manifest in mistrust of the US health system and biomedical research to this day [35–37]. Instead of assuming trust is present de novo, clinicians should strive to earn and maintain the trust of patients. This can be better achieved through transparent, consistent, empathetic, and clear communication.

Peer support: Peer support is an effective way to promote the process of recovery, healing, and integration through community building among patients. Individuals with shared or similar experiences of trauma may find deeper understanding, acceptance, compassion, and meaningful connection among each other. Peer support is a powerful mechanism of post-traumatic growth, a process of reintegration after trauma that confers benefits to an individual's perception of self as well as within interpersonal relationships [38]. Opportunities for peer support in a primary care setting may include support groups for substance use disorders, community health workers, and patient advisory boards.

Collaboration and shared responsibility: In contrast to a paternalistic approach to medical decision-making, TIC emphasizes a process of shared decision-making with patients. The dehumanizing force of trauma is that it renders decisions onto survivors in the absence of assent/consent. Patients may experience re-aggravation of traumas in the health-care setting when preferences and values related to care plans are ignored, misunderstood, or overlooked by the clinician. In contrast, creating space for patients to participate in decisions about their care can be an effective way for patients to make positive, health-promoting, and sustainable decisions on their own terms. Further, emphasizing a sense of shared responsibility among clinic staff and medical providers to play an active role in promoting a healing-centered environment is a key component of collaboration. Having a shared understanding of TIC promotes shared responsibility—thus it is imperative that all staff and faculty—such as administrative staff, security, ancillary services—undergo TIC training, not merely care providers.

Empowerment, voice, and choice: Empowering patients, staff, and providers to voice needs and take a primary role in making decisions is an essential way of upholding a person-centered, relationally focused ethos of care. Through an attentive, compassionate, and shared decision-making approach, clinicians can help empower patients toward having agency and autonomy over their health, thereby cultivating resilience and hope that one can overcome future challenges. Encouraging patients to have a primary role in their care lends itself to the development of care plans that are congruent with the patient's values and preferences.

Cultural, historical, and gender issues: Health-care organizations that maintain awareness and engagement with key cultural, historical, and gender issues actively support a trauma-informed culture. Explicit and implicit bias, stereotyping, and willful ignorance about these topics perpetuate dehumanization, fragmentation, and compound the risk of re-traumatization by the health system [39]. Acknowledging and honoring the unique backgrounds, histories, and norms of patients and their communities helps to deepen capacities for empathy and understanding, which can facilitate higher quality communication and care [40]. On a broader level, engagement with relevant social issues can prompt action by the health system to address historical traumas, engage social determinants of health (unmet social needs), and advance health equity.

While by no means a panacea for all types of challenging encounters involving patients, TIC is nonetheless a paradigm-shifting, patient-centered framework that provides universal precautions for healthy interpersonal communication. At its core, TIC is derived from the understanding that psychosocial trauma is common in society, associated with a wide array of undesired physical, mental, and social outcomes, and is a predictable cause of negative cognitive-affective tendencies that promote miscommunication and misunderstanding. For all patient encounters, maintaining a frame of "What's happened to you?" instead of assuming, "What's wrong with you?" [33] can help anchor clinicians to perspectives of compassion and empathy. Asking "What's happened?" nudges the provider to consider what could be occurring behind behavior that is challenging, disruptive, or counterproductive; it holds space for understanding while resisting judgement; it recognizes that traumatic stress reactions are not synonymous with an individual's character or values. Ultimately, when considering effective approaches to navigating challenging patient encounters, integrating a trauma-informed perspective into the philosophy of care and communication is a critical, foundational step that can deepen and strengthen capacities for patience, empathy, and compassion.

Recognizing Health-care Settings at High Risk for Workplace Violence

Patient and Clinician Factors that Contribute to Difficult Encounters

Patients may be perceived as difficult for many reasons, including perceptions by the clinician that they show no improvement in chronic disease outcomes despite repeated visits, feelings that the patient is disinterested in becoming well, the presence of power struggles during visits, or the sense that clinical visits focus on patient concerns that fall outside of their medical care [41]. The estimated prevalence of difficult patients who meet these descriptions is approximately 15% [41].

It is important, however, to note that labels such as difficult, disruptive, or challenging are derived from the perspective of the clinician's feelings, which ascribe pathological attributes and/or character traits to patients. According to the *AMA Journal of Ethics*, focusing on these perspectives tends to represent patients adversely and can negatively affect their experiences receiving medical care [42]. Indeed, the very act of labeling patients may predict certain character traits, feelings, and factors experienced by the clinician during the encounter [42, 43].

Patient factors that contribute to challenging and/or difficult encounters should be viewed though a trauma-informed lens. These patient factors might include: feeling unwell, feeling self-conscious about substance use disorders, feeling anxious or distressed, having unrealistic expectations, feelings of guilt over delayed care for oneself or a loved one, or mistrust in the system due to previous encounters [44]. Recognizing and/or uncovering these issues as they affect patients may prove essential for navigating the visit in productive, affirming, and trust-building ways.

Physician factors that may contribute to difficult encounters include: (1) the clinician's age and experience, with younger age and/or inexperience being associated with more difficult encounters, (2) the perception by the physician that a patient will take up too much of their clinical time, (3) frustrations with managing psychosocial problems and/or substance abuse, (4) defensiveness or anger in response to a patient's behavior, or (5) feelings of fatigue and of being harried [45–47]. Mitigation strategies for these physician factors include reflective learning exercises, and proactively entering/addressing anticipated challenging encounters with courage and compassion, and an understanding that the only control clinicians may have in these scenarios is that of their own emotions, actions, and responses [42, 43].

Achieving Physical Safety in the Academic Primary Care Setting

The most common health-care security challenge involves assault and battery toward medical staff. In health-care settings, 75% of violent incidents are caused by patients hitting, kicking, beating, and/or shoving health-care team members [48]. In fact, health-care workers experience a 20% higher incidence of encountering workplace violence than counterparts in other work settings [49]. It is important to note, however, that workplace violence not only includes physical assault, but also threatening behavior and/or verbal abuse. The aforementioned statistics are likely underestimated, as most reports of workplace violence are only made for physical injuries and not for verbal threats [50]. Many nurses and physicians admit to underreporting due to the presumption that patients with underlying mental health conditions are not to be held responsible for their actions [51]. Indeed, most patients who cause physical injury to health-care workers exhibit "dementia, delirium, substance intoxication, or decompensated mental illness" [48]. That said, a culture of apathy toward verbal abuse or verbal threats "creates an environment conducive to more serious, physical crimes" [48].

The 2018 Joint Commission Sentinel Event Alert states that "each episode of violence or credible threat to health care workers warrants notification to leadership, to internal security, and, as needed, to law enforcement, as well as the creation of an incident report," which can prompt a systematic root-cause analysis and steps that can be taken to prevent a similar incident from occurring in the future. An established timeline for reporting of safety incidents and subsequent root-cause analyses should also be implemented; ideally, workplace safety incidents should be reported within 4 hours and a root-cause analysis completed within 7 days [52]. Such analyses and actionable steps by employers of health systems are imperative for improving health-care worker safety, in accordance with the General Duty Clause, Section 5(a)(1) of the Occupational Safety and Health Act of 1970 [53].

We suggest that, in these situations, a root-cause analysis should be performed. The resulting action plan(s) to mitigate it from occurring again should be shared with the leadership team within the relevant department and/or leadership across the health system. This includes the formation and implementation of a workplace violence mitigation committee that reports to the executive quality or governance board, and/or the formation of "a centralized database that identifies new hazards, trends, and potential strategies for solutions" and is regularly distributed throughout the health system [54]. Health systems that have taken this approach and committed to a multidisciplinary action plan (involving environmental, administrative, and behavioral approaches) to mitigate workplace violence have shown decreases in such work-related injuries approaching 50% [55, 56]. Finally, ensuring appropriate well-being of the person(s) affected by workplace violence is imperative; emotional support should be offered in the form of free and confidential services provided by licensed counselors and/or referral to community resources [52].

Strategies to reduce instances of violence and maintain safety in the health-care setting are outlined in Table 37.1.

Table 37.1 Strategies to maintain safety in the clinic setting

Personal strategies for the clinician	Team-based strategies for health system	Physical environment strategies	Systems-level approaches and solutions
Clinician should be cognizant of the risks that necklaces, dangling earrings, lanyards, ties, and long hair/long ponytails may impart	Communication regarding wait times and use of empathic statements by staff [44]	Consider installing deep surface counters or shatter-proof glass at check-in areas [52] Arrange clinic exam rooms such that clinicians are placed closest to the exit. Avoid clutter	Establish a workplace violence mitigation committee that reports to the executive board
Ensure staff and clinicians have access to emergency exits [48]	Confer with the health system to ensure periodic rotation of security throughout the primary care center, recognizing that the aim in health-care settings is not to provoke anxiety by a forceful security presence	Ensure doors to exam rooms are sliding doors and/or open outwards	Establish "a centralized database that identifies new hazards, trends, and potential strategies for solutions" that is regularly distributed throughout the health system [54]
	Advocate for continuity of scheduling, which allows trusting longitudinal relationships to develop, thereby enabling clinicians to anticipate patient needs and expectations	Consider the installation of a desktop app or call bell that can activate security from each exam room [48] Perform user testing to ensure the app functions as designed, ideally on a biannual basis [52] Train staff to only activate the icon when no other option is available (i.e., inability to exit a room)	Provide follow up, using trauma-informed care and behavioral health supports, for health-care workers who have been affected by workplace violence
	Provide training to clinic staff on de-escalating disruptive behaviors and proactively identifying agitated patients	Ensure entrances to clinic exam areas have automated locks that can require card access for entry. This ensures that unknown persons cannot spontaneously enter areas where physicians are actively delivering care to patients	Improve crowding and wait times through adequate staffing. Establish regular patrols by security and/or behavioral health team members [57]

Table 37.1 (continued)

Personal strategies for the clinician	Team-based strategies for health system	Physical environment strategies	Systems-level approaches and solutions
	All health-care staff should be trained on the early identification of patients who appear agitated during the waiting period, rooming period, and/or triage process If a patient appears agitated but is still amenable to health-care staff recommendations, a staff member should escort them to a room close to an exit and free from an audience as soon as possible [58]	Installing a panic button at check-in desks for clinic staff who register patients; they are the front-line team members most likely to first encounter a disgruntled patient. This button should not be visible to patients	Establish an ongoing safety program involving practice drills for a broad array of workplace violence scenarios, including active shooter situations and issues of patient agitation or verbal abuse [48]
		Be aware of and/or limit environmental factors that can add to patient anxiety Strive for environments with dimmer/natural lighting, limited noise, uncrowded waiting areas, and adequate personal space	Provide crisis prevention institute (CPI) training to clinical staff on an annual basis [52]
		Ensure adequate security and mental health staff presence in the health-care setting	

Proactive Planning for Challenging Encounters Among Patients Who Have Shown Discontent or Agitation at Prior Clinic Visits

Pre-visit planning for an ambulatory clinic visit is a key part of any practice and a valuable tactic for resident learners to develop early in their careers. Pre-visit planning is especially important in preparation for an encounter with a patient who has previously exhibited discontent or agitation.

Pre-visit planning for a potentially challenging patient encounter entails six suggested steps. These include: (1) discussing the case with an attending preceptor prior to the visit, (2) establishing time-specific boundaries, (3) negotiating the agenda, (4) developing a management plan with the attending preceptor, (5) establishing expectations for acceptable behavior and language, and (6) clear and patient-centered documentation that avoids labeling or stereotyping patients [41].

Pre-visit discussion with a precepting faculty member is the first step in preparing for a potentially challenging visit. The resident and attending determine a preliminary agenda that will be reviewed with the patient on the day of the visit; such planning can be particularly effective if sensitive topics are to be discussed. In some situations, role playing may be a helpful tool to review how questions or recommendations may be best articulated, anticipate patient responses, and preemptively discuss strategies should challenging behavior arise.

Establishing time boundaries together with the patient is essential, particularly with patients who present with multiple topics to discuss with limited time available. In isolated cases, it may be helpful to modify a clinician's schedule by increasing the length of the visit. Scheduling the visit either at the beginning or the end of a clinical session can also be effective. Assurance of frequent visits may alleviate a patient's anxiety about not being able to cover all topics in one visit.

During *shared agenda setting*, clinicians elicit patient concerns and develop an agenda in a collaborative manner. The most urgent or acute patient and clinician concerns should be prioritized first. Use of motivational interviewing and maintaining a trauma-informed lens while establishing the agenda can promote a sense of feeling heard for patients, while at the same time keeping space to address urgent clinician concerns. Creating a written list of topics helps to visualize shared expectations for the visit and can support better time management [59].

When caring for challenging patients, it may be helpful for the resident and faculty preceptor to *develop a management plan* in concert. While conducting a clinic visit, if a resident prematurely conveys a plan that ultimately changes after discussion with the attending preceptor, this can erode trust and undercut the patient's confidence in the clinic and providers. Asking residents to discuss the plan with the preceptor does not mean they cannot discuss potential management options with the patient; the request is simply to defer confirming the plan until the case has been discussed with the preceptor. Resident autonomy can still be encouraged as residents articulate preferred plans during sign-out.

Setting expectations for acceptable behavior is an imperative component in proactive planning for a potentially challenging patient visit. Health-care facilities should have institution-wide guidelines that detail a code of conduct for both clinicians and patients. Use of foul language, raised voices, threats, physical harm, and other unacceptable behaviors should be clearly outlined. At times, providing a written summary of this discussion in the form of a note or a behavioral agreement can be helpful for patients and future clinicians.

Documentation using non-judgmental language that avoids stereotyping is extremely important for several reasons. By framing the encounter in this manner, the clinician is able to see the patient as a full person beyond labels and poor behaviors. Second, when other clinicians or clinical staff read notes that include pejorative language, it may influence their own care of the patient. With the advent of open notes, patients routinely read their records and documenting the clinical encounter in a compassionate and unprejudiced manner is essential to a continued positive clinical relationship.

Techniques for De-escalating the Agitated Patient During a Clinic Encounter

It is not always possible to prevent a patient from becoming agitated or upset in a visit. Prior experiences in health care, challenges in daily lives, or a host of other factors can contribute to tension spilling over into unacceptable behavior during a clinical visit. Approaching patients by first managing one's own response to disruptive behaviors and using a trauma-informed care approach to responding can de-escalate a tense situation and ultimately provide a path to move beyond it. Indeed, clinicians react to all patient interactions, both pleasant and challenging. The clinical term for this reaction is countertransference. Countertransference is the complex feeling evoked by a patient and the patient's response to a clinician. Clinicians can be aware or unaware of countertransference. Recognizing our reaction and understanding where it comes from is an important step in managing our reactions to challenging patients [41, 60].

A helpful model to use in managing our own reactions to patients is the CALMER model, first proposed in 2004 as a path to equanimity when managing difficult patient encounters. The CALMER model provides a framework to these encounters that minimizes clinician angst and modulates the clinician's reactions when dealing with a challenging patient. The CALMER model reinforces the demarcation between what clinicians can control (their own feelings and actions) and what they cannot control (patient reaction and experiences outside the clinic). One of the most difficult yet essential trauma-informed practices is to not take a patient's reaction personally. By listening non-judgmentally and then diagnosing, a clinician can focus on what the patient is telling them rather than jumping quickly to a diagnosis and risking early closure or missing essential details of a patient's concern. Agreeing on a health improvement plan should be followed by education and outlining specific, actionable goals [62]. The CALMER model, outlined in Table 37.2, recommends simple, concrete steps to manage our own emotions toward a patient.

Table 37.2 The CALMER approach: six steps to managing difficult clinical encounters [61]

Element	Approach
Catalyst for change	• Identify the patient's progression in the stages of change model • Recommend how the patient can advance to the next stage[a]
Alter thoughts to change feelings	• Identify the negative feelings experienced by the clinician which are elicited by patient behaviors • Clarify how these feelings influence the clinician and the patient during an encounter • Strategize how to reduce negativity and distress
Listen and then make diagnosis	• Remove or minimize barriers to communication • Improve working relationships • Enhance probability of accurate diagnoses
Make an agreement	• Negotiate, agree on, and confirm a plan for health improvement
Education and follow-up	• Set achievable goals and realistic time frames and ensure follow-up
Reach out and discuss feelings	• Ensure a strategy for your own self-care

[a] Stages of change include precontemplation, contemplation, preparation/determination, action, maintenance, and relapse

It is important to remember that body language, vocal tone, and volume also act as significant cues to patients about how clinicians are feeling. The Behavioral Activity Rating Scale (BARS) is one example of a validated tool used to identify physical or verbal overactivity. Such scales can identify patient agitation that is responsive to direction, as compared to overactivity and agitation that continues despite de-escalation attempts. Strategies for de-escalation include:

1. Keeping an open body posture and maintaining a kind and even tone demonstrates respect.
2. Active listening helps manage reactions by letting patient talk without interruption.
3. Asking the patient to explain how they are feeling allows for a deeper understanding of the behavior. Anger and outbursts are usually a secondary emotion, not a primary driver of behavior.
4. Validation and empathy toward a patient's condition or experience aligns us with them as humans who experience suffering. Naming emotions validates how a patient feels and makes them feel understood.

When such attempts fail and continuous agitation persists, prudence in seeking additional support and alerting team members of the situation is paramount.

System-based Strategies for Determining When and How a Patient Should Be Discharged from the Academic Primary Care Clinic Setting

Primary care clinicians and clinic staff often experience challenging patient encounters that leave all parties dissatisfied and distressed. These encounters may involve use of derogatory language and subtle and/or overt threats by patients. Such interactions can take up a significant amount of clinic time and staff energy to resolve, leading to clinician/staff burnout and increased turnover, particularly among nurses and medical assistants who may work hard to protect clinicians from experiencing the brunt of these patient behaviors [52].

When to Discharge a Patient from Clinic and How to Do So with Empathy

We suggest establishing a protocol for determining when a patient should be terminated from a clinic setting and staying consistent to the protocol to prevent actions from being viewed as discriminatory [63]. Barring direct patient threats to staff, clinicians, or other patients, in which case security should be notified, we suggest

AAFP's Managing Difficult Physician–Patient Relationships flowcharts, which follow a three-tiered approach:

- Tier 1 behaviors pose minimal physical risk to staff and might involve a patient missing multiple successive appointments or using inappropriate language in the clinic setting.
- Tier 2 behaviors might involve a continuation of issues identified in tier 1, or any actions that staff perceived as threatening.
- Tier 3 behaviors constitute violent actions or direct threats made toward anyone in the clinic setting [64].

Tier 1 and 2 behaviors should be addressed using the following steps: Form a standing committee to assess and discuss a difficult patient interaction; consider including in the committee the following disciplines: ethics, compliance, psychiatry/psychology, medical clinic leadership and ambulatory chief leadership, patent experience members, and case managers.

1. Encourage resident primary care physicians (PCPs) and clinic staff to proactively push forward cases where they are concerned about a patient's behavior, ideally before the issue escalates to the point where the clinician no longer feels comfortable caring for the patient.
2. Invite the resident PCP, faculty, or clinic staff team members to present their patient's concerns at committee meetings, with the intent to proactively:

   - Develop a strategy to support clinicians and staff in caring for the patient during future visits;
   - Empathically recognize and identify the mental, physical, and emotional issues the patient may be dealing with and bringing to the visit;
   - Strategically think of ways to help the patient by enlisting support from behavioral health, ethics, patient experience, and psychology team members;
   - Identify ethical issues for the patient and/or the clinician/team member in dealing with the situation at hand;
   - Use a standard template note to document the patient's actions, the committee's discussion, and suggested plans for future care delivery. We suggest an iteration of the template shared in Fig. 37.1, which is designed to (i) avoid placing vague or judgmental statements about the patient in the documentation, (ii) consider implicit biases or attitudes by the staff or clinician, and (iii) encourage use of direct and factual statements. Documentation of specific statements and actions made by the patient, as well as specific attempts by the clinician to address and respond to them, should be noted [63]. To avoid personal bias, it may be helpful for the documentation (Fig. 37.1) to be placed by a member of the clinic's leadership team trained in trauma-informed care. Ideally, this should be someone other than the team member experiencing direct action from the patient. Direct quotes are recommended whenever possible, in order to remain true to what was actually said. It is also important to include quotes that not only outline what was said, but also to add comments about any external circumstances leading up to the offensive statement or

It is important as the documenting clinician or staff member to recognize how our own biases and/or the working environment may have impacted the events that transpired. Before moving forward with documenting the event that occurred, please take a moment to note which of the contributing factors listed below played a role in the clinician's and/or staff's attitude and behaviors at the time of the event. While the factors listed below may not need to be documented in the chart, taking pause to consider them should inform how you think about what may have contributed to the event you are planning to document:

- A busy, frazzled waiting room or clinical area, making it hard to focus and remain calm
- Clinicians or staff feeling tired/fatigued
- Clinicians or staff being pulled in many different directions
- Preconceived notions by clinicians and/or staff about the patient, based on the patient's prior actions or based on prior documentation in the chart
- Feeling like the patient has already taken up a lot of our time and energy
- Feeling like the patient is making unreasonable requests of the clinicians and/or clinical staff
- Feeling like no matter what we have done as a healthcare team, the patient is never satisfied
- The clinicians and/or staff were already having a bad day and then this situation occurred
- Other:____________________________________

Please note, patient is <u>of concern</u> for the following actions, dated _______, which occurred in ____________________ department.

Behavioral Concerns

Choose ALL that qualify, as there may be multiple issues at play:

- Used profane language, including name calling and/or racial epitaphs, which responded to verbal de-escalation strategies employed by staff
- Made specific verbal threats of causing bodily harm or injury to healthcare personnel or their families/colleagues
- Attempted physical injury or other inappropriate actions (e.g. spitting) to healthcare personnel or another patient
- Made gestures or comments which felt subjectively threatening to the healthcare team and/or other patients
- Made continued unrealistic and time consuming requests of personnel that have been discussed and/or attempted to be resolved multiple times, to no avail
- Other: ____________________________________

For the above, the direct quotes or exact descriptions of actions that occurred are as follows:

Based on the above actions, we have discussed as a team the appropriate next steps. Our team members included:____
Per the team meeting, the following action steps have been taken [Have a drop down with options to choose from, AND allow multiple options to be chosen]

- Patient should now be scheduled with specified clinicians (e.g. male clinicians only, female clinicians only, etc.) as follows:__________________________
- We have scheduled a meeting with the patient to gain understanding of the situation (e.g. the patient's perspective) and set expectations regarding behaviors/language that are not tolerated. In this meeting, the patient has/will be informed that should these actions reoccur, we will have to consider discharging them from our primary care clinic. This meeting will occur/has occurred on: __________________________
- We have consulted with the following interprofessional team members (e.g. ethics, psychology):__________________________________. Together, we developed the following action plan:_____________________

Fig. 37.1 Sample template note for clinical documentation of a disruptive encounter

- We have made referrals to the following services (these can be internal referrals and/or referrals to community resources):________________________ for the following reasons:_________________________
- We have negotiated a shared agenda with the patient to ensure that specific things occur at future visits. This shared plan involves: ______________________________
- The clinician team has identified one tangible action the clinician can do at future visits to help the patient feel heard and valued regarding their stated concerns:________________________

If behaviors are egregious and/or have persisted despite the above documented action steps, such that the patient must be discharged from the clinical setting, consider documenting the following:

After conferring with our clinic manager and/or the patient experience department, we have determined that the patient can no longer be seen for in-person visits within the Primary Care Center.

- Virtual visits may be considered, if this allows for care to be provided without concern for physical harm to staff or clinicians. Please note, virtual visits may be discontinued if verbal abuse continues during virtual sessions.
- The patient may continue receiving/seeking care within the Emergency Department and certain specialty clinics as outlined: ____________________________________
- Should the patient express a desire to return to the primary care clinical setting in the future, this might be reconsidered after a timeline of____________ with input of the clinic medical director/clinic manager AND demonstrated steps by the patient to resolve the issue of concern (e.g. attendance to virtual visits with demonstrated mutual respect of staff and clinician).

Assuming no further issues after 2-3 years of the incidental behavior, OR if there has been a considerable change in the patient's overall behavior/status (e.g. due to treatment, adherence, etc.), we suggest removing the behavior alert note from view, so as not to perpetuate perceptions of the patient based on remote behaviors that have since been resolved.

Fig. 37.1 (continued)

action, as these circumstances may lend context that better explains why the patient and/or team member may have been stressed or agitated.

- Contact the patient to make them aware of any future action plans and/or expectations moving forward, including a written letter that outlines the plan and that is reviewed/mailed to the patient.
- As themes/systems issues are identified, members of the committee should discuss these themes to their health system's executive and/or ethics committee for further consideration, especially if the question of patient discharge from clinic has arisen.

If discharge is deemed necessary for repeated Tier 1 and 2 behaviors, it is important to consider the AMA Code of Medical Ethics suggesting to "*terminate the patient-physician relationship only when the patient **will not modify** disrespectful, derogatory or prejudiced behavior **that is within the patient's control**, in keeping with ethics guidance*" [65]. In Tier 2 situations, it is also necessary to "*explore the reasons for which a patient behaves in disrespectful, derogatory, or prejudiced ways, insofar as possible*" and to treat and assist in identifying/managing the stressors, coping skills, and emotional issues underlying such behaviors [65].

Tier 3 behaviors threatening the safety of staff or others require immediate actions to de-escalate the situation and/or remove the threat. In many situations, the behavior may warrant immediate consideration for discharge from the primary care clinic. It is important to note that some academic practices are not allowed to discharge patients without the involvement of higher executive leaders, administrators, and compliance team members connected with the health system. Other primary care practices make this decision at the discretion of the local team, which may involve the clinic medical director, practice manager, nurse director, and involved staff. In these scenarios, emergency and behavioral health services should remain available to the patient as applicable and to the degree these services are provided by the health system. The health system might also consider resuming primary care services after a considerable amount of time has elapsed, assuming demonstrable and sustained improvement in behaviors has occurred as observed and documented by the behavioral health team.

When discharge from the clinic is advised, clinicians should work with their leadership to standardize a letter that clearly states (1) the reason for termination, (2) what clinic(s) the discharge is occurring from, (3) what clinical department(s) remain available to the patient, e.g. emergency room, behavioral health clinics, etc., (4) the effective date of discharge, (5) an offer to provide medical records to the new clinician assuming care, and (6) a provision to refill necessary prescriptions for a 30–90-day period post termination until new care is established. Of note, providing care and refills for a reasonable time period is absolutely necessary; in areas where another clinician is not available, there is some legal responsibility to provide care for a longer period of time. If providing care in a safety net setting, consider suggesting nearby health systems available to the patient, taking into consideration their insurance status, financial status, and access to transportation. Legal claims of patient abandonment are becoming more common.

Copies of the letter should be included in the patient's chart for future reference. It is also important to notify insurers if a patient has been discharged from the practice, as some insurers require this [63, 66]. In large health systems, it will be important to establish a standard FYI system within the electronic health record, by which central and local scheduling teams can be easily notified of patients who have been discharged from the practice. Without a standard alert by which scheduling teams are made aware of the discharge decision, patients may try to reenter the system and may inadvertently be rescheduled.

Conclusion

Psychosocial trauma has wide ranging negative impacts on health, and trauma-informed care is one approach that can mitigate its impact in patient encounters. By promoting a safe environment through efforts to enhance trustworthiness, transparency, peer support, collaboration, empowerment, and cultural sensitivity, the clinician can enhance effective communication during otherwise challenging clinical encounters. Even so, conflict and violence in the workplace can occur, so the wise medical director will anticipate and plan for an effective response. When these events require discharging the patient from the clinic, that process should be approached with thoughtful deliberation, in a standardized manner, and with attention to careful documentation

References

1. Harris M, Fallot R. Using trauma theory to design service systems. San Francisco, CA: Jossey Bass; 2001.
2. Tink W, Tink JC, Turin TC, Kelly M. Adverse childhood experiences: survey of resident practice, knowledge, and attitude. Fam Med. 2017;49(1):7–13.
3. Szilagyi M, Kerker BD, Storfer-Isser A, Stein REK, Garner A, O'Connor KG, et al. Factors associated with whether pediatricians inquire about parents' adverse childhood experiences. Acad Pediatr. 2016;16(7):668–75.
4. Felitti VJ, Anda RF, Nordenberg D, Williamson DF, Spitz AM, Edwards V, et al. Relationship of childhood abuse and household dysfunction to many of the leading causes of death in adults. The adverse childhood experiences (ACE) study. Am J Prev Med. 1998;14(4):245–58.
5. Herman JL. Trauma and recovery. New York: Basic Books; 1997.
6. Merrick MT, Ford DC, Ports KA, Guinn AS. Prevalence of adverse childhood experiences from the 2011-2014 behavioral risk factor surveillance system in 23 states. JAMA Pediatr. 2018;172:1038.
7. Wade R Jr, Cronholm PF, Fein JA, Forke CM, Davis MB, Harkins-Schwarz M, et al. Household and community-level adverse childhood experiences and adult health outcomes in a diverse urban population. Child Abuse Negl. 2016;52:135–45.
8. Felitti VJ. Childhood sexual abuse, depression, and family dysfunction in adult obese patients: a case control study. South Med J. 1993;86(7):732–6.
9. Felitti VJ, Anda RF. The relationship of adverse childhood experiences to adult medical disease, psychiatric disorders and sexual behavior: implications for healthcare. In: Lanius RA, Vermetten E, Pain C, editors. The impact of early life trauma on health and disease: the hidden epidemic. 1st ed. Cambridge: Cambridge University Press; 2010.
10. Anda RF, Fleisher VI, Felitti VJ, Edwards VJ, Whitfield CL, Dube SR, et al. Childhood Abuse, household dysfunction, and indicators of impaired adult worker performance. Perm J. 2004;8(1):30–8.
11. Pierce JB, Kershaw KN, Kiefe CI, Jacobs DR, Sidney S, Merkin SS, et al. Association of Childhood Psychosocial Environment with 30-year cardiovascular disease incidence and mortality in middle age. J Am Heart Assoc. 2020;9(9)
12. Flaherty EG, Thompson R, Dubowitz H, Harvey EM, English DJ, Proctor LJ, et al. Adverse childhood experiences and child health in early adolescence. JAMA Pediatr. 2013;167(7):622–9.
13. Anda RF, Felitti VJ, Bremner JD, Walker JD, Whitfield C, Perry BD, et al. The enduring effects of abuse and related adverse experiences in childhood. A convergence of evidence from neurobiology and epidemiology. Eur Arch Psychiatry Clin Neurosci. 2006;256(3):174–86.
14. Brown DW, Anda RF, Tiemeier H, Felitti VJ, Edwards VJ, Croft JB, et al. Adverse childhood experiences and the risk of premature mortality. Am J Prev Med. 2009;37(5):389–96.
15. Perry BD, Pollard RA, Blakley TL, Baker WL, Vigilante D. Childhood trauma, the neurobiology of adaptation, and "use-dependent" development of the brain: how "states" become "traits". Infant Ment Health J. 1995;16(4):271–91.
16. Brown JD, King MA, Wissow LS. The central role of relationships with trauma-informed integrated Care for Children and Youth. Acad Pediatr. 2017;17(7, Supplement):S94–S101.

17. Frosch CA, Schoppe-Sullivan SJ, O'Banion DD. Parenting and child development: a relational health perspective. Am J Lifestyle Med. 2021;15(1):45–59.
18. Sciences NAo. Fostering healthy mental, emotional, and behavioral development in children and youth: a National Agenda. Washington, DC: The National Academies Press; 2019. p. 390.
19. Guinosso SA, Johnson SB, Riley AW. Multiple adverse experiences and child cognitive development. Pediatr Res. 2016;79(1–2):220–6.
20. Jackson DB, Testa A, Vaughn MG. Adverse childhood experiences and school readiness among preschool-aged children. J Pediatr. 2020;230:191.
21. Bucci M, Marques SS, Oh D, Harris NB. Toxic stress in children and adolescents. Adv Pediatr. 2016;63(1):403–28.
22. Ford JD. Progress and limitations in the treatment of complex PTSD and developmental trauma disorder. Curr Treat Opt Psychiatry. 2021;8(1):1–17.
23. Brewin CR, Cloitre M, Hyland P, Shevlin M, Maercker A, Bryant RA, et al. A review of current evidence regarding the ICD-11 proposals for diagnosing PTSD and complex PTSD. Clin Psychol Rev. 2017;58:1–15.
24. Spottswood M, Davydow DS, Huang H. The prevalence of posttraumatic stress disorder in primary care: a systematic review. Harv Rev Psychiatry. 2017;25(4):159–69.
25. Liebschutz J, Saitz R, Brower V, Keane TM, Lloyd-Travaglini C, Averbuch T, et al. PTSD in urban primary care: high prevalence and low physician recognition. J Gen Intern Med. 2007;22(6):719.
26. Coon KA, Miller-Cribbs J, Wen F, Jelley M, Sutton G. Detecting and addressing trauma-related sequelae in primary care. Prim Care Companion CNS Disord. 2021;23(3):20m02781.
27. Berfield JB, Goncharenko S, Forkus SR, Contractor AA, Weiss NH. The differential relation of trauma types with negative and positive emotion dysregulation. Anxiety Stress Coping. 2021;35:1–15.
28. Joneydi R, Lack KA, Olsho LEW, Corry NH, Spera C. Addressing posttraumatic stress disorder in primary care: primary care physicians' knowledge, confidence and screening practices related to PTSD among military populations. Med Care. 2021;59(6):557–64.
29. Green BL, Kaltman SI, Chung JY, Holt MP, Jackson S, Dozier M. Attachment and health care relationships in low-income women with trauma histories: a qualitative study. J Trauma Dissociation. 2012;13(2):190–208.
30. Hargreaves MK, Mouton CP, Liu J, Zhou YE, Blot WJ. Adverse childhood experiences and health care utilization in a low-income population. J Health Care Poor Underserved. 2019;30(2):749–67.
31. Alcalá HE, Valdez-Dadia A, Von Ehrenstein OS. Adverse childhood experiences and access and utilization of health care. J Public Health. 2018;40(4):684–92.
32. Korhonen MJ, Halonen JI, Brookhart MA, Kawachi I, Pentti J, Karlsson H, et al. Childhood adversity as a predictor of non-adherence to statin therapy in adulthood. PLoS One. 2015;10(5):e0127638.
33. Sweeney A, Filson B, Kennedy A, Collinson L, Gillard S. A paradigm shift: relationships in trauma-informed mental health services. BJPsych Advances. 2018;24(5):319–33.
34. Substance Abuse and Mental Health Services Administration. SAMHSA's concept of trauma and guidance for a trauma-informed approach. HHS publication no. (SMA) 14-4884. Rockville, MD: Substance Abuse and Mental Health Services Administration; 2014.
35. Corbie-Smith G, Thomas SB, Williams MV, Moody-Ayers S. Attitudes and beliefs of African Americans toward participation in medical research. J Gen Intern Med. 1999;14(9):537–46.
36. Shavers VL, Lynch CF, Burmeister LF. Knowledge of the Tuskegee study and its impact on the willingness to participate in medical research studies. J Natl Med Assoc. 2000;92(12):563–72.
37. Darcell PS, Katherine JM, Pamela J, Jonathan H, Emeobong M, Dorothy E. More than Tuskegee: understanding mistrust about research participation. J Health Care Poor Underserved. 2010;21(3):879–97.
38. Tedeschi RG, Calhoun LG. The posttraumatic growth inventory: measuring the positive legacy of trauma. J Trauma Stress. 1996;9(3):455–71.

39. Byrd WM, Clayton LA. Race, medicine, and health care in the United States: a historical survey. J Natl Med Assoc. 2001;93(3 Suppl):11S–34S.
40. Lorié Á, Reinero DA, Phillips M, Zhang L, Riess H. Culture and nonverbal expressions of empathy in clinical settings: a systematic review. Patient Educ Couns. 2017;100(3):411–24.
41. Haas LJ, Leiser JP, Magill MK, Sanyer ON. Management of the difficult patient. Am Fam Physician. 2005;72(10):2063–8.
42. Aluri J. Interrogating assumptions about "difficult" patients and situations. AMA J Ethics. 2017;19(4):319–22.
43. Dudzinski DM, Timberlake D. Difficult patient encounters. University of Washington Medicine, Department of Bioethics and Humanities. https://depts.washington.edu/bhdept/ethics-medicine/bioethics-topics/detail/60. Accessed 16 May 2022.
44. Medical Defence Union. https://themdu.com/guidance-and-advice/guides/guide-to-dealing-with-challenging-patients
45. Davis MA. A perspective on cultivating clinical empathy. Complement Ther Clin Pract. 2009;15(2):76–9.
46. Hull SK, Broquet K. How to manage different patient encounters. Ram Pract Manag. 2007;14(6):30–4.
47. Krebs EE, Garrett JM, Konrad TR. The difficult doctor? Characteristics of physicians who report frustration with patients: an analysis of survey data. BMC Health Serv Res. 2006;6(1):128. https://doi.org/10.1186/1472-6963-6-128.
48. The Joint Commission. Sentinel event alert: physical and verbal violence against health care workers. 2018;59, April 17, 2018. Revised June 18, 2021. https://www.jointcommission.org/-/media/tjc/documents/resources/patient-safety-topics/sentinel-event/sea-59-workplace-violence-final2.pdf. Accessed 16 May 2022.
49. Harrell E. Workplace violence. 1993-2009. Washington, DC: Department of Justice, Bureau of Justice Statistics, National Crime Victimization Survey; 2011.
50. Kowalenko T, Gates D, Gillespie GL, Succop P, Mentzel TK. Prospective study of violence against ED workers. Am J Emerg Med. 2013;31(1):197–205.
51. Privitera M, Weisman R, Cerulli C, Tu X, Groman A. Violence toward mental health staff and safety in the work environment. Occup Med (Lond). 2005;55(6):480–6.
52. Emory Emergency Medicine Safety Task Force: A toolkit for workplace violence prevention in the emergency department.
53. U.S. Department of Labor. Occupational Health and Safety administration. Workplace Violence. Enforcement. Washington, DC: OSHA, no date
54. The Joint Commission. Improving patient and worker Safety: opportunities for synergy, collaboration and innovation. Oakbrook Terrace, IL: The Joint Commission. 2012. https://www.jointcommission.org/-/media/tjc/documents/resources/patient-safety-topics/patient-safety/tjc-improvingpatientandworkersafety-monograph.pdf. Accessed 16 May 2022.
55. Beard D, Conley M. Operation safe workplace: a multidisciplinary approach to workplace violence. Philadelphia, PA: Aria-Jefferson Health; 2017.
56. Arnetz JE, Hamblin L, Russell J, Upfal MJ, Luborsky M, Janisse J, Essenmacher L. Preventing patient-to-worker violence in hospitals: outcome of a randomized controlled intervention. J Occup Environ Med. 2017;59(1):18–27.
57. Occupational Safety and Health Administration. Guidelines for preventing workplace violence for healthcare and social service workers (OSHA, 3148-04R). Washington, DC: OSHA; 2015.
58. Kelley EC. Reducing violence in the emergency department: a rapid response team approach. J Emerg Nurse. 2014;40:60–4.
59. Hardavella G, Aamil-Gaagnat A, Frille A, Saad N, Niculescu A, Powell P. Top tips to Deal with challenging situations: doctor-patient interactions. Breathe. 2017;13(2):129–35.
60. Adams J, Murray R. The general approach to the difficult patient. Emerg Med Clin North Am. 1998;16(4):689–700, v
61. Lorenzetti RC, Jacques CHM, Donovan C, Cottrell S, Buck J. Managing difficult encounters, understanding physician patient and situational factors. Am Fam Physician. 2013;87(6):419–25.

62. Pomm HA, Shahady E, Pomm RM. The CALMER approach: teaching learners six steps to serenity when dealing with difficult patients. Fam Med. 2014;36(7):467–9.
63. Salz T. Carefully discharge difficult patients. Medical Economics. July 2012. https://www.medicaleconomics.com/view/carefully-discharge-difficult-patients. Accessed 16 May 2022, 89, 38.
64. AAFP's Managing Difficult Physician-Patient Relationships Flowchart, Developed by Deanna R. Willis, MD, MBA. Copyright © 2005 American Academy of Family Physicians. Related article: https://www.aafp.org/fpm/2005/0900/p34.html.
65. American Medical Association Code of Medical Ethics Opinion 1.2.2. Discrimination and Disruptive Behavior by Patients. https://www.ama-assn.org/delivering-care/ethics/discrimination-and-disruptive-behavior-patients. Accessed 16 May 2022.
66. Adams RK, Roberts LW. Discharging problem patients the right way. Physicians Practice; 4 May 2016. https://www.physicianspractice.com/view/discharging-problem-patients-right-way. Accessed 16 May 2022.

Chapter 38
Burnout and Steps Toward Wellness

Amy Sheer, Nischal Narendra, and Sharon Aroda

Introduction

Wellness and resilience are central to health care as physician burnout rises. Numerous publications have identified this "epidemic" of burnout [1]. Burnout was first published in medical literature in 1974, and since then, it has been identified in many professions. The Accreditation Council for Graduate Medical Education (ACGME) has partnered with the Association of American Medical Colleges (AAMC) and the National Academy of Medicine (NAM) to create the Action Collaborative on Clinician Well-Being and Resilience. This network of more than 60 organizations is committed to reversing trends in clinician burnout [2].

This chapter will define wellness and burnout and review the negative impact of burnout on healthcare professionals, specifically physicians, and physicians-in-training. Tools to assess burnout, well-being, and resilience will be discussed. These methods will be reviewed for efficiency and accessibility. The Liaison Committee for Medical Education (LCME) and the ACGME require all medical and residency programs to establish a framework to support trainee and faculty well-being. We will review individual and organizational initiatives and interventions to reduce burnout among physicians at all stages.

Outline
- Defining the problem of burnout
- Tools to assess physician burnout, wellness, and resiliency

A. Sheer (✉) · S. Aroda
University of Florida, Gainesville, FL, USA
e-mail: asheer@ufl.edu; sharon.aroda@medicine.ufl.edu

N. Narendra
Cone Health, Greensboro, NC, USA
e-mail: nischal.narendra@conehealth.com

L. B. Lu et al. (eds.), *Leading an Academic Medical Practice*,
https://doi.org/10.1007/978-3-031-40273-9_38

- Mandatory requirements for internal medicine resident milestones
  - Liaison Committee for Medical Education (LCME)
  - Accreditation Council for Graduate Medical Education (ACGME)
- Interventions to reduce physician burnout and improve wellness
- Individual-focused, organizational, and systems approaches
- Trainee interventions
- Conclusion

Burnout and Steps Toward Wellness: The Scope of the Problem

The World Health Organization (WHO) defined wellness as a "state of complete physical, mental and social well-being and not merely the absence of disease or infirmity" [3]. Wellness and burnout are two separate entities, and the absence of wellness does not imply the presence of burnout.

Burnout is a state of emotional fatigue or frustration secondary to increased stress from a mismatch of resources to the needs of patients [4]. Burnout is thought to consist of three main components: emotional exhaustion (individual stress response), depersonalization or cynicism (negative reaction to the job as well as others), and inefficacy (decreased sense of personal accomplishment) [4].

In a 2012 survey of more than 7000 physicians, over 45% reported at least one symptom of burnout, with the highest rates noted in front-line physicians (emergency medicine, family medicine, general internal medicine) and only 49% reported satisfaction with their work–life balance [5]. Multiple studies show increased levels of distress among residents, including high levels of burnout [6] and depression during internship [7] and residency [8]. The numbers have quickly worsened during the COVID-19 pandemic with over half of health-care workers surveyed reporting burnout [9].

Burnout in physicians has been associated with increased rates of alcohol abuse or dependence [10]. It also correlates with higher rates of suicidal ideation among medical students [11] and residents [12]. Burnout affects many patient-centered outcomes [13] and has been associated with decreased patient satisfaction and decreased quality of care, [14, 15] including higher rates of medical errors [16]. There is also an economic impact attributable to burnout as it leads to decreased clinical productivity, increased turnover [17], and cost to health-care systems [18].

During the COVID-19 pandemic, the term "moral injury" first described in military personnel, came into the context of front-line healthcare workers [19, 20].

The term "burnout" can suggest that the issue lies with the individual and, therefore, it is the individual's responsibility to find solutions. However, the term does not acknowledge the systemic issues that give rise to these symptoms. Moral injury acknowledges physicians' competing responsibilities in treating patients, such as the insurers, hospitals, healthcare systems, and their own financial incentives [21].

Resilience has been described as the qualities that enable an individual to adapt or thrive in adversity [22]. In a recent study, resilience was inversely related to burnout, and physicians were noted to have higher resiliency scores than the general population. However, even among the most resilient physicians, there was a substantially high burnout rate [23]. Interventions focused on individual measures to improve resilience have shown to be largely unsuccessful, with only a 10% reduction in overall burnout [24]. The introduction of wellness curricula in residency programs also proved ineffective, [25, 26] with only wellness group meetings showing some benefit [26]. As we move forward, it has been proposed that we focus on models that address individual, organizational, and systemic resilience [1].

Requirements of Well-being in Physician Training: LCME and ACGME Guidelines

Recognizing the growing degree of trainee burnout, the LCME and ACGME issued requirements for all medical and residency programs to establish policies and programs supporting optimal trainee and faculty member well-being [27, 28]. The regulations specify ongoing assessments of learner burnout, easy access to mental health counseling, and duty-hour restrictions. Yet, the LCME and ACGME do not specify guidelines, nor do best practices exist in the literature on trainee or faculty burnout prevention and resiliency building.

There has been a call to action among the medical communities, including the American Medical Association Resident/Fellow Section and NAM, to improve physician wellness and resiliency. In 2014, the ACGME Council of Review Committee Residents made recommendations for a national academic policy on wellness to address several goals: (1) increasing awareness of the risk of depression during training and destigmatizing it; (2) building systems to identify and treat depression in trainees confidently; (3) establishing a more formal system of peer and faculty mentoring; (4) fostering efforts to learn more about trainee burnout and wellness [28]. The ACGME Common Program Requirements highlight the importance of building a positive culture of well-being through respect, accountability, support, and self-care, which is paramount to professionalism. This will provide trainees with the skills needed to thrive throughout their careers [29].

Tools to Assess Physician Burnout, Well-being, and Resiliency

For institutions to address physician and trainee burnout, they must first understand how to assess it. Only then can institutional stakeholders evaluate the efficacy of wellness interventions by using appropriate tools.

Tools to Assess Burnout

Maslach Burnout Inventory (MBI)

This self-assessment questionnaire is the most widely used tool in assessing burnout [30]. The MBI has three distinct subsections: emotional exhaustion, depersonalization, and a sense of personal accomplishment. It uses population norms as a benchmark to help compare scores. The most widely used version is the MBI-Human Services Survey (MBI-HSS). This tool has demonstrated high reliability and validity in the measuring burnout [31] and has been used in multiple studies with residents [32, 33]. There is no standard definition of exactly what score signifies the start of burnout. However, people are considered to have at least one symptom of burnout if they have high scores on the emotional exhaustion or depersonalization scales of the MBI-HSS. Higher scores on either of these scales correlate with clinical burnout [34]. Disadvantages to the MBI are that it is expensive to administer, does not consider nonprofessional factors that may be contributors, and the absence of burnout does not necessarily indicate the presence of well-being.

Copenhagen Burnout Inventory (CBI)

The CBI is reliable and valid [35] and has been studied in resident physicians [36]. The CBI has three distinct subsections: personal burnout, work-related burnout, and client-related burnout. The personal burnout section determines how tired or exhausted a person is on the physically and emotionally. The work-related burnout section determines what degree of physical and emotional fatigue is perceived to be attributable to their work. Comparing personal and work-related burnout scores can help identify to what extent nonwork factors are contributing to their exhaustion. The CBI is free to use and easy to access.

Other tools like the Oldenburg Burnout Inventory and the Stanford Professional Fulfillment Index have also been used widely across the healthcare profession. The Oldenburg Burnout Inventory is free to use and the Stanford Professional Fulfillment Index is free to nonprofit organizations for research and operational assessment [37].

The current tools represent an aggregate assessment of burnout that can be based on several external factors in addition to work-related burnout. This makes it difficult to assess the efficacy and need for continued investment of specific interventions that address burnout [38]. It is important to find intermediate outcomes that can help assess specific interventions introduced in an institution. Examples could be surrogate outcomes such as a sense of physician community, decreased physician turnover, and perception of appreciation.

Tools to Assess Well-being

Wellness is not merely the absence of burnout. The exact definition of wellness is ambiguous, but it can be conceptualized as a reservoir that, when replenished, can lead to better resilience and mental health and, when depleted, can manifest as burnout or depression. Wellness has many components, including work–life balance, resilience, mood, and mindfulness. Well-being is a state of mind, and a sense of well-being creates more wellness habits. Some of the tools used to assess wellness and well-being are discussed next.

Physician Well-being Index (PWBI)

The Mayo Clinic School of Medicine developed this and has both validated resident and medical student versions [39]. The PBWI is a seven-item survey that examines six dimensions of psychological distress and well-being, including meaning in work, severe fatigue, quality of life, the likelihood of burnout, work–life integration, and suicidal ideation. It is quick to complete and provides immediate resources to participants as well as comprehensive reports to wellness leaders.

Resident Wellness Scale

This is a 10-item scale covering six dimensions of well-being: meaningful work, personal growth, life security, institutional support, and social support. It can help measure individual resident well-being, evaluate the impact of specific burnout interventions, and track changes in resident wellness over time. It is free for institutions to use through Wayne State University's website.

There has been a recent shift to focus on wellness instead of burnout [40]. Wellness models can help individual physicians and academic programs develop wellness goals, but there are drawbacks. Various dimensions in a wellness model may conflict with each other and can change based on individual circumstances [1]. Residents struggle to balance different aspects of their lives and recognize that they may be investing in professional development at the expense of other aspects of their personal and family life [41]. They may not be able to focus on the physical, spiritual, and intellectual aspects of wellness. Overemphasis on a particular dimension of wellness, like physical activity, may worsen burnout given these constraints.

Micro-stresses arising from daily challenges while practicing can be especially stressful for residents and medical students and may contribute to more psychological distress. Wellness models do not provide ways to reflect on these daily stressors or help one's ability to deal with adversity.

Tools to Assess Resilience

Given the inherent issues with wellness models, a focus is now on improving resilience. Resilience acknowledges the presence of adversity and the conflict between different wellness dimensions. Data suggesting that low levels of resilience are related to higher levels of burnout and depression [42].

Connor-Davidson Resilience Scale (CD-RISC)

This tool is a 25-item scale with each item rated on a five-point scale (0–4). It was thought to have three potential purposes: (1) to study the biological aspects of resilience, (2) to assess the efficacy of interventions to improve resilience, and (3) to use as a screening tool for high-risk, high-stress occupations [22]. There are also modified 10-item and 2-item scales. All versions of the scale have demonstrated validity and reliability and have been used in various populations [43]. The tool was shown to have a possible "ceiling effect," making it unreliable to measure higher levels of resilience [44]. This can limit its utility when assessing professions known for higher levels of resilience.

Individual and Organizational Initiatives

Many interventions have been aimed at the individual to strengthen resilience and teach coping strategies such as positive psychology techniques; unfortunately, these have demonstrated only marginal benefit [45, 46]. Individual training typically includes group didactics on behavioral techniques such as adaptive coping skills, communication skills, mindfulness and stress reduction, psychotherapy, narrative medicine, and group support. Individual-focused initiatives show mixed results, likely due to difficulty in measuring benefits, and changing demands throughout the academic year. Mandatory training on these topics should be avoided, as it can fuel resentment and disengagement and lead to further distress [37]. Importantly, individual-focused initiatives and training do not address the problem of preventable burnout caused by organizational and systems issues.

Organizational-focused approaches have demonstrated more benefit than individual-focused interventions and generally focus on physician empowerment through practice improvements in clinician workload, clinical workflow, and healthcare team communication [47]. Examples include physician-driven committees to launch initiatives, and simple changes such as increasing patient visit time or adjusting physician clinical hours to meet their needs better. Interventions that combined several approaches, such as improving healthcare team communication, cultivating a sense of teamwork and job autonomy, have successfully reduced burnout [48]. The ability of organizations to carry out any specific intervention is likely to be limited by concerns regarding implementation and the incorrect assumption that initiatives to improve physician wellness conflict with other organizational objectives [49].

Burnout is a problem of the entire healthcare system and requires an organizationally embedded approach [37, 49]. Much of the literature focuses on individual versus organizational interventions, with little data on system approaches. In its charter on Physician Well-being [50] and its Oath to Self-Care and Well-Being [51], the Collaborative for Healing and Renewal in Medicine calls for close partnerships between the individual clinician and the academic or community organization to create the culture of well-being. Combating physician burnout is a multifold process that involves mitigating organizational drivers of burnout and building individual and organizational resiliency.

In the Healthy Work Place Study, Linzer et al. [52] explored organizational interventions aimed at different work conditions to see which had the greatest impact on clinician stress and symptoms of burnout. In a cluster-randomized controlled trial in 34 primary care clinics, interventions were grouped into three categories: improved communication, changes in workflow, and quality improvement. While the specific interventions and implementation of the interventions varied by the clinic, workflow interventions (such as changing call schedules and reassigning clinic staff) and targeted quality improvement projects (such as automatic prescription renewal, establishing mechanisms to improve quality metrics) showed the most benefit in reduction of emotional exhaustion scores [52]. Interventions to improve communication among clinicians and staff resulted in improvements in clinician satisfaction. Addressing the work–system factors that contribute to burnout, such as in this intervention, can lead to meaningful improvements in burnout and dissatisfaction.

The Listen-Act-Develop model implemented at the Mayo Clinic is an example of an organizational-sponsored systems improvement initiative [49]. The intention of this model is to identify drivers of burnout, foster healthy physician–organizational relationships, and alleviate burnout by improving system processes, facilitating teamwork, encouraging physician engagement, and supporting the development of physician leadership. This approach mitigates burnout by meeting the psychological needs of people. The steps in this intervention are: (1) acknowledge and assess the problem of burnout while listening to physician concerns; (2) identify physician leaders and champions, empower physicians to implement solutions; (3) develop physician leaders in the context of improvement work; and (4) commit to a continuous cycle of performance improvement. This approach uses the power of leadership, engagement, and professional relationships to improve systems and promote individual and organizational health. Having effective physician leadership alone is a protective factor against burnout [53].

Initiatives that foster interprofessional relationships, work–life balance, engagement, and build trust among team members have shown positive results. A 90-min group session utilizing the Stress Management and Resiliency Training (SMART) program with two follow-up phone interviews significantly improved in perceived stress, anxiety, quality of life, and mindfulness in radiology faculty after 12 weeks [54]. Similarly, internal medicine faculty who underwent the SMART program improved resiliency, perceived stress, anxiety, and overall quality of life after eight weeks [55].

Weill Cornell Medicine has implemented a Well-Being Taskforce to work with department leaders and creating focus groups to address burnout in their institution. Response was monitored with utilization of the Well-Being Index developed by Mayo Clinic, and Weill Cornell has seen an improvement in the overall mean distress score among physicians from 1.84 in June 2019 (above the national mean of 1.57) to 1.08 in late 2019, 1.19 in 2020, and 1.22 as of June 2020 [56]. This example provides a method that could be implemented in more programs as the next step toward wellness and resilience for physicians and trainees.

Poor communication and strained interprofessional teams contribute to physician burnout. The CREW (Civility, Respect, and Engagement at Work) intervention developed by the Veterans Health Administration works to improve social interactions between team members. Participants meet in their groups regularly with a trained facilitator to set goals and discuss shared experiences and ways to work better together. Outcomes in CREW research have shown higher overall satisfaction, increased job satisfaction, reduced sick leave usage, fewer complaints, and better patient care outcomes [57–59]. The Schwartz Center Rounds are another example of an intervention meant to enhance communication and relationships among all members of a multidisciplinary healthcare team and create a supportive learning environment [60]. The rounds are 1-h, case-based, interactive discussions held monthly or biweekly. While there has been no research linking the rounds with a reduction in burnout, there is evidence that they improve teamwork, enhance communication and provider support [60], and improve psychological well-being [61].

Trainee Burnout and Wellness Interventions

In the health profession, trainees work in an amalgam of both nonclinical and clinical settings. Within these different learning environments are complex social interactions and organizational cultures that shape the training experience and professional development. It is here that high degrees of stress and burnout are cultivated [62]. Around 45–56% of medical students [33] and 45–60% of residents [63] report symptoms of burnout. Residents and students often care for the most vulnerable populations with healthcare disparities. Such challenges create a sense of powerlessness and burnout for physicians in training [64]. Several techniques to improve the learner's learning environment, such as schedule flexibility, pass–fail curriculum, and formal mentor–mentee programs, have shown positive outcomes in trainee well-being [41]. The ACGME has included wellness in the Common Program Requirement for residency and fellowship programs. The Action Collaborative on Clinician Well-Being and Resilience is an example program chaired by the ACGME, AAMC, NAM, and more organizations to create a national framework for all programs to share ideas and promote wellness.

Wellness curricula have been widely incorporated across medical school and residency programs [65]. These programs are aimed to encourage self-care, teach coping skills, and increase mindfulness-based stress reduction to learners to promote well-being. In a 2016 survey of select medical schools, over half had a well-being curriculum that offered a variety of emotional/spiritual, physical, financial, and social well-being activities [66]. The implementation and assessment of the curricula varied widely across programs. Several programs have published novel curricula incorporating both didactic and nondidactic components, but little is known about the efficacy of these programs. Williamson et al. published a 12-month multifaceted curriculum for emergency medicine residents based on six common dimensions of wellness, using interactive didactic sessions and extracurricular activities, such as group yoga, group service project, and wellness champions [67]. Another study involving internal medicine residents compared resident-driven and formal resiliency curricula and found no improvement in resident burnout [26]. Several other studies using facilitated small group discussions and wellness and stress management courses have failed to show benefits [68, 69]. Studies on the efficacy of implemented curricula have significant limitations, such as small sample size, lack of control, volunteer bias, and varying levels of participation [14].

While evidence on effective well-being and resiliency curricula is sparse; there are data showing that personal practices and institution-sponsored programs can have benefits. One such technique is mindfulness, which can be taught through various methods, including Mindfulness-Based Stress Reduction (MBSR) and an Embodied Health program of yoga and meditation with a neuroscience didactic component. Multiple studies utilizing these techniques in medical schools have shown favorable results including decreases in perceived stress, and improvements in mindfulness, self-regulation, self-compassion, and empathy [70–72]. Relaxation techniques, including autogenic training, have also been studied in trainee population and found favorable results, including burnout reduction [73, 74].

The bridge between narrative medicine, appreciative inquiry, and resiliency is an emerging pedagogy in medical education [75]. Narrative medicine is a powerful tool for learners to share their clinical work experiences while cultivating listening, empathizing, and reflecting skills. Data supports narrative medicine, specifically Balint groups activities focusing on patient-centered management and strong patient–doctor relationships for reducing burnout, anxiety, and work-related exhaustion. However, most improvements in learners' stress and empathy occurred during the intervention and were not sustained after the intervention ended [76]. Other studies focusing on curriculum topics, including humanism [77] and health advocacy [78, 79] have shown positive results on trainee well-being.

Conclusion

This chapter was written during a time of significant adversity, the rise of a global COVID-19 pandemic when physicians, physicians-in-training, and students are expending long hours toward providing health care. Front-line workers, in particular, are experiencing burnout, leading to a new term of moral injury.

Nationwide, academic institutions are recognizing moral injury in addition to burnout and wellness and opening communication with their physicians and trainees to shape the wellness of the individual and program overall. Vanguard institutions have transitioned to Well-Being 2.0, a shift from awareness to action [80]. By creating an action plan, these organizations first seek out system factors, practice environment, and human factors that negatively impact physicians clinically and emotionally. A collaborative group of administrators and physicians then deliberate on solutions and follow through on implementation and response. This initiative focuses on remembering that physicians are human rather than hero.

The interventions to achieve and maintain resilience must be applied methodically and systemically to allow physicians and trainees to thrive during challenging times. Thus far, organizational-focused approaches have proven effective with a focus on physician/trainee empowerment as a driver of clinical systemic change. The awareness has provided insight into burnout and wellness, and now action should be taken toward physician/trainee self-care for work–life integration.

Next Steps

As noted, the increasing rates of burnout will lead more programs to implement interventions. A suggested method is first to choose a tool to measure the presence of burnout in your program. Once you measure the scope of the problem, identify the systemic, organizational, and individual factors contributing to burnout. Create an action plan to implement changes, include the leadership and physicians/trainees in the planning step, and assess the impact of change on wellness and resilience. Once, a successful approach/action plan is identified, programs can further incorporate a systematic process to evaluate burnout and wellness.

References

1. Vercio C, et al. Shifting focus from burnout and wellness toward individual and organizational resilience. Teach Learn Med. 2021;33(5):568–76.
2. National Academy of Medicine. Action Collaborative on Clinician Well-Being and Resilience 2017 [cited 2020 May 27]; https://nam.edu/initiatives/clinician-resilience-and-well-being/.
3. World Health O. Constitution of the world health organization. 1995.
4. Freudenberger HJ. Staff burn-out. J Soc Issues. 1974;30(1):159–65.
5. Shanafelt TD, et al. Burnout and satisfaction with work-life balance among US physicians relative to the general US population. Arch Intern Med. 2012;172(18):1377–85.
6. West CP, Shanafelt TD, Kolars JC. Quality of life, burnout, educational debt, and medical knowledge among internal medicine residents. JAMA. 2011;306(9):952–60.

7. Sen S, et al. A prospective cohort study investigating factors associated with depression during medical internship. Arch Gen Psychiatry. 2010;67(6):557–65.
8. Mata DA, et al. Prevalence of depression and depressive symptoms among resident physicians: a systematic review and meta-analysis. JAMA. 2015;314(22):2373–83.
9. Ghahramani S, et al. A systematic review and meta-analysis of burnout among healthcare workers during COVID-19. Front Psych. 2021;12:12.
10. Oreskovich MR, et al. Prevalence of alcohol use disorders among American surgeons. Arch Surg. 2012;147(2):168–74.
11. Dyrbye LN, et al. Burnout and suicidal ideation among US medical students. Ann Intern Med. 2008;149(5):334–41.
12. Van der Heijden F, et al. Suicidal thoughts among medical residents with burnout. Arch Suicide Res. 2008;12(4):344–6.
13. Halbesleben JRB, Rathert C. Linking physician burnout and patient outcomes: exploring the dyadic relationship between physicians and patients. Health Care Manag Rev. 2008;33(1):29–39.
14. Tawfik DS, et al. Physician burnout, well-being, and work unit safety grades in relationship to reported medical errors. Mayo Clinic Proc. 2018;93(11):1571–80. Elsevier
15. Shanafelt TD, et al. Burnout and self-reported patient care in an internal medicine residency program. Ann Intern Med. 2002;136(5):358–67.
16. Shanafelt TD, et al. Burnout and medical errors among American surgeons. Ann Surg. 2010;251(6):995–1000.
17. Shanafelt TD, et al. Longitudinal study evaluating the association between physician burnout and changes in professional work effort. Mayo Clinic Proc. 91(4):422–31. Elsevier
18. Hamidi MS, et al. Estimating institutional physician turnover attributable to self-reported burnout and associated financial burden: a case study. BMC Health Serv Res. 2018;18(1):1–8.
19. Williamson V, Murphy D, Greenberg N. COVID-19 and experiences of moral injury in front-line key workers. Oxford: Oxford University Press; 2020. p. 317–9.
20. Shale S. Moral injury and the COVID-19 pandemic: reframing what it is, who it affects and how care leaders can manage it. BMJ Leader. 2020:leader-2020.
21. Dean W, Simon Talbot AD. Reframing clinician distress: moral injury not burnout. Fed Pract. 2019;36(9):400.
22. Connor KM, Davidson JRT. Development of a new resilience scale: the Connor-Davidson Resilience Scale (CD-RISC). Depress Anxiety. 2003;18(2):76–82.
23. West CP, et al. Resilience and burnout among physicians and the general US working population. JAMA Netw Open. 2020;3(7):–e209385.
24. West CP, et al. Interventions to prevent and reduce physician burnout: a systematic review and meta-analysis. Lancet. 2016;388(10057):2272–81.
25. Williamson K, et al. The implementation of a national multifaceted emergency medicine resident wellness curriculum is not associated with changes in burnout. AEM Educ Train. 2020;4(2):103–10.
26. Sheer AJ, et al. Improving burnout and well-being among medicine residents: impact of a grassroots intervention compared to a formal program curriculum. J Educ Health Promot. 2021:10.
27. Accreditation Council for Graduate Medical, E., Summary of changes to ACGME common program requirements Section VI. 2018.
28. Daskivich TJ, et al. Promotion of wellness and mental health awareness among physicians in training: perspective of a national, multispecialty panel of residents and fellows. J Grad Med Educ. 2015;7(1):143–7.
29. Goldman ML, et al. An intervention framework for institutions to meet new ACGME common program requirements for physician well-being. Acad Psychiatry. 2018;42(4):542–7.
30. Schaufeli WB, Leiter MP, Maslach C. Burnout: 35 years of research and practice. Career Dev Int. 2009;14:204.

31. Maslach C, Jackson SE, Leiter MP. Maslach burnout inventory. Lanham: Scarecrow Education; 1997.
32. Kimo Takayesu J, et al. Factors associated with burnout during emergency medicine residency. Acad Emerg Med. 2014;21(9):1031–5.
33. Dyrbye LN, et al. Burnout among US medical students, residents, and early career physicians relative to the general US population. Acad Med. 2014;89(3):443–51.
34. Schaufeli WB, et al. On the clinical validity of the Maslach burnout inventory and the burnout measure. Psychol Health. 2001;16(5):565–82.
35. Ruiz EM, Gómez-Quintero HB, Lluis SM. Validation of the Copenhagen burnout inventory to assess professional burnout in Spain. Rev Esp Salud Publica. 2013;87(2):165–79.
36. Kassam A, et al. Predictors of well-being in resident physicians: a descriptive and psychometric study. J Grad Med Educ. 2015;7(1):70–4.
37. National Academies of Sciences, Engineering, and Medicine. Taking action against clinician burnout: a systems approach to professional well-being. 2019.
38. Rotenstein LS, Sinsky C, Cassel CK. How to measure progress in addressing physician well-being: beyond burnout. JAMA. 2021;326(21):2129–30.
39. Dyrbye LN, et al. Development and preliminary psychometric properties of a well-being index for medical students. BMC Med Educ. 2010;10(1):1–9.
40. Eckleberry-Hunt J, et al. Changing the conversation from burnout to wellness. Physician well-being in residency training programs. J Grad Med Educ. 2015;2009:1.
41. Ratanawongsa N, Wright SM, Carrese JA. Well-being in residency: a time for temporary imbalance? Med Educ. 2007;41(3):273–80.
42. Simpkin AL, et al. Stress from uncertainty and resilience among depressed and burned out residents: a cross-sectional study. Acad Pediatr. 2018;18(6):698–704.
43. Burns RA, Anstey KJ. The Connor–Davidson Resilience Scale (CD-RISC): Testing the invariance of a uni-dimensional resilience measure that is independent of positive and negative affect. Personal Individ Differ. 2010;48(5):527–31.
44. González VBA, et al. An in-depth psychometric analysis of the Connor-Davidson Resilience Scale: calibration with Rasch-Andrich model. Health Qual Life Outcomes. 2015;13(1):1–12.
45. West CP, et al. Intervention to promote physician well-being, job satisfaction, and professionalism: a randomized clinical trial. JAMA Intern Med. 2014;174(4):527–33.
46. Shanafelt TD. Enhancing meaning in work: a prescription for preventing physician burnout and promoting patient-centered care. JAMA. 2009;302(12):1338–40.
47. Zaidi Z, Rosenberg EI, Beyth RJ. Contemporary challenges in medical education: from theory to practice. Gainesville, FL: University Press of Florida; 2019.
48. Panagioti M, et al. Controlled interventions to reduce burnout in physicians: a systematic review and meta-analysis. JAMA Intern Med. 2017;177(2):195–205.
49. Swensen S, Kabcenell A, Shanafelt T. Physician-organization collaboration reduces physician burnout and promotes engagement: the Mayo Clinic experience. J Healthc Manag. 2016;61(2):105–27.
50. Thomas LR, Ripp JA, West CP. Charter on physician well-being. JAMA. 2018;319(15):1541–2.
51. Panda M, O'Brien KE, Lo MC. Oath to self-care and well-being. Am J Med. 2020;133(2):249–5.
52. Linzer M, et al. A cluster randomized trial of interventions to improve work conditions and clinician burnout in primary care: results from the Healthy Work Place (HWP) study. J Gen Intern Med. 2015;30(8):1105–11.
53. Shanafelt TD, et al. Impact of organizational leadership on physician burnout and satisfaction. Mayo Clinic Proc. 2015;90(4):432–40. Elsevier
54. Sood A, et al. Stress Management and Resiliency Training (SMART) program among Department of Radiology faculty: a pilot randomized clinical trial. Explore. 2014;10(6):358–63.
55. Sood A, et al. Stress management and resilience training among Department of Medicine faculty: a pilot randomized clinical trial. J Gen Intern Med. 2011;26(8):858–61.
56. Kjaer K, et al. A grassroots approach to protecting physicians against burnout and building an engaging practice environment. NEJM Catal Innov Care Deliv. 2021;2(12)

57. Leiter MP, et al. Getting better and staying better: assessing civility, incivility, distress, and job attitudes one year after a civility intervention. J Occup Health Psychol. 2012;17(4):425.
58. Osatuke K, et al. Civility, Respect and Engagement at the Workplace (CREW): a national organization development program at the Department of Veterans Affairs. J Manag Polic Pract. 2013;1(2):25–34.
59. Osatuke K, et al. Civility, Respect, and Engagement in the Workplace (CREW) in the USA Veterans Affairs: Predictors of successful outcomes.
60. Lown BA, Manning CF. The Schwartz center rounds: evaluation of an interdisciplinary approach to enhancing patient-centered communication, teamwork, and provider support. Acad Med. 2010;85(6):1073–81.
61. Maben J, Taylor C. Schwartz center rounds: an intervention to enhance staff well-being and promote organisational change. In Connecting healthcare worker well-being, patient safety and organisational change. Springer; 2020. p. 281–98.
62. Rotenstein LS, et al. Prevalence of depression, depressive symptoms, and suicidal ideation among medical students: a systematic review and meta-analysis. JAMA. 2016;316(21):2214–36.
63. Dyrbye L, Shanafelt T. A narrative review on burnout experienced by medical students and residents. Med Educ. 2016;50(1):132–49.
64. West CP, et al. Association of resident fatigue and distress with perceived medical errors. JAMA. 2009;302(12):1294–300.
65. Gardiner P, et al. The incorporation of stress management programming into family medicine residencies-results of a national survey of residency directors: a CERA study. 2015.
66. Dyrbye LN, et al. Medical school strategies to address student well-being: a national survey. Acad Med. 2019;94(6):861–8.
67. Williamson K, et al. Development of an emergency medicine wellness curriculum. AEM Educ Train. 2018;2(1):20–5.
68. Ripp JA, Fallar R, Korenstein D. A randomized controlled trial to decrease job burnout in first-year internal medicine residents using a facilitated discussion group intervention. J Grad Med Educ. 2016;8(2):256–9.
69. Slavin SJ, Chibnall JT. Finding the why, changing the how: improving the mental health of medical students, residents, and physicians. Acad Med. 2016;91(9):1194–6.
70. Kraemer KM, et al. Mind–body skills training to improve distress tolerance in medical students: a pilot study. Teach Learn Med. 2016;28(2):219–28.
71. Rosenzweig S, et al. Mindfulness-based stress reduction lowers psychological distress in medical students. Teach Learn Med. 2003;15(2):88–92.
72. Bond AR, et al. Embodied health: the effects of a mind–body course for medical students. Med Educ Online. 2013;18(1):20699.
73. Wild K, et al. Strategies against burnout and anxiety in medical education–implementation and evaluation of a new course on relaxation techniques (Relacs) for medical students. PLoS One. 2014;9(12):e114967.
74. Shinde V, et al. A study on the effect of relaxation techniques and Shavasana on stress and pulse rates of medical students. J Exerc Sci Physiother. 2015;11(2):123–8.
75. Krasner MS, et al. Association of an educational program in mindful communication with burnout, empathy, and attitudes among primary care physicians. JAMA. 2009;302(12):1284–93.
76. Zwack J, Schweitzer J. If every fifth physician is affected by burnout, what about the other four? Resilience strategies of experienced physicians. Acad Med. 2013;88(3):382–9.
77. Dotters-Katz SK, et al. Developing a pilot curriculum to foster humanism among graduate medical trainees. J Educ Health Promot. 2018;7:7.
78. Coutinho AJ, Dakis KE. Incorporating advocacy training to decrease burnout. Acad Med. 2017;92(7):905.
79. Long T, et al. Expanding health policy and advocacy education for graduate trainees. J Grad Med Educ. 2014;6(3):547–50.
80. Shanafelt TD. Physician well-being 2.0: where are we and where are we going? Mayo Clin Proc. 2021;96(10):2682–93. Elsevier

Index

L. B. Lu et al. (eds.), *Leading an Academic Medical Practice*,
https://doi.org/10.1007/978-3-031-40273-9

B

C

GPSR Compliance

The European Union's (EU) General Product Safety Regulation (GPSR) is a set of rules that requires consumer products to be safe and our obligations to ensure this.

If you have any concerns about our products, you can contact us on ProductSafety@springernature.com

In case Publisher is established outside the EU, the EU authorized representative is:

Springer Nature Customer Service Center GmbH
Europaplatz 3
69115 Heidelberg, Germany

Batch number: 10732632

Printed by Printforce, the Netherlands